Advances in Experimental Medicine and Biology

Volume 867

More information about this series at http://www.springer.com/series/5584

Roberto Scatena
Editor

Advances in Cancer Biomarkers

From biochemistry to clinic for a critical revision

Springer

Editor
Roberto Scatena
Institute of Biochemistry and Clinical Biochemistry
School of Medicine, Catholic University
Rome, Italy

ISSN 0065-2598 ISSN 2214-8019 (electronic)
Advances in Experimental Medicine and Biology
ISBN 978-94-017-7214-3 ISBN 978-94-017-7215-0 (eBook)
DOI 10.1007/978-94-017-7215-0

Library of Congress Control Number: 2015951661

Springer Dordrecht Heidelberg New York London

Printed on acid-free paper

Springer Science+Business Media B.V. Dordrecht is part of Springer Science+Business Media (www.springer.com)

Advances in Cancer Biomarkers: a Preface

Advances in cancer biomarkers – from biochemistry to clinic for a critical revision – would represent a fast and easy contribution to rationalize the use of current and future tumor markers.

In fact, the clinician too often has expectations in terms of diagnosis, prognosis, and monitoring of therapy that the present tumor markers cannot fulfill.

These limits do not only hamper a correct therapeutic approach to the cancer patient but they have a high direct and indirect economic cost.

A lot of national and international guidelines have been published to educate physicians to rationalize the use of these important laboratory parameters, but results appear anyway disappointing.

These limited results also affect the clinical applications of the new cancer biomarkers that too often show a stimulating experimental background not followed by so positive clinical applications.

This tangled situation seems to also depend on a mere clinical approach to the old and new tumor markers while the biochemistry, physiology, and pathophysiology of the molecule, acting as tumor marker, is too often neglected. This inadequate knowledge of the molecular basis of a particular molecule/tumor marker may hamper a careful evaluation of the diagnostic/prognostic potential of these biomarkers.

The aim of this book is to illustrate not only the clinical biochemistry and clinical oncology of some important biomarkers but also to stress their physiological and pathophysiological roles. The knoweledge of these roles may represent a fundamental step to really know tumor markers, ameliorating, in such a way, their use with undeniable clinical and economic advantages.

Importantly, at present there are a plethora of old and new tumor markers, and for our purpose we have considered just some that for their biochemical, laboratory, and clinical peculiarities may better represent the tangled status of these fundamental biomarkers of laboratory medicine.

Rome, Italy Roberto Scatena

Contents

Part I Generality

1 **Cancer Biomarkers: A Status Quo** 3
Roberto Scatena

2 **Cancer Biomarkers Discovery and Validation: State of the Art, Problems and Future Perspectives** 9
Alvaro Mordente, Elisabetta Meucci, Giuseppe Ettore Martorana, and Andrea Silvestrini

3 **Use of Biomarkers in Screening for Cancer** 27
Michael J. Duffy

4 **The Role of Metabolomics in the Study of Cancer Biomarkers and in the Development of Diagnostic Tools** 41
Jean-Pierre Trezzi, Nikos Vlassis, and Karsten Hiller

5 **The Role of Epigenomics in the Study of Cancer Biomarkers and in the Development of Diagnostic Tools** 59
Mukesh Verma

6 **Efficient, Adaptive Clinical Validation of Predictive Biomarkers in Cancer Therapeutic Development** 81
Robert A. Beckman and Cong Chen

Part II Tumor Markers – A Critical Revision: Enzymes

7 **Prostate Specific Antigen as a Tumor Marker in Prostate Cancer: Biochemical and Clinical Aspects** 93
J.W. Salman, I.G. Schoots, S.V. Carlsson, G. Jenster, and M.J. Roobol

8 **The Actual Role of LDH as Tumor Marker, Biochemical and Clinical Aspects** 115
Vladimir Jurisic, Sandra Radenkovic, and Gordana Konjevic

9 **Neuron-Specific Enolase as a Biomarker: Biochemical and Clinical Aspects** 125
Maria Antonietta Isgrò, Patrizia Bottoni, and Roberto Scatena

10 **Components of the Plasminogen-Plasmin System as Biologic Markers for Cancer** 145
Brandon J. McMahon and Hau C. Kwaan

Part III Tumor Markers – A Critical Revision: Hormones

11 **The Role of Human Chorionic Gonadotropin as Tumor Marker: Biochemical and Clinical Aspects** 159
Lorenza Sisinni and Matteo Landriscina

Part IV Tumor Markers – A Critical Revision: Oncofetal Proteins

12 **Biomarkers for Hepatocellular Carcinoma (HCC): An Update** 179
Dave Li and Shinji Satomura

Part V Tumor Markers – A Critical Revision: Cytokeratins

13 **Mucins and Cytokeratins as Serum Tumor Markers in Breast Cancer** 197
Andrea Nicolini, Paola Ferrari, and Giuseppe Rossi

Part VI Tumor Markers – A Critical Revision: Carbohydrate Markers

14 **The Role of CA 125 as Tumor Marker: Biochemical and Clinical Aspects** 229
Patrizia Bottoni and Roberto Scatena

Part VII Tumor Markers – A Critical Revision: Blood Group Antigens

15 **CA 19-9: Biochemical and Clinical Aspects** 247
Salvatore Scarà, Patrizia Bottoni, and Roberto Scatena

Part VIII Tumor Markers – A Critical Revision: Genetic Markers

16 **Non Coding RNA Molecules as Potential Biomarkers in Breast Cancer** 263
Kim De Leeneer and Kathleen Claes

17 **Urinary Prostate Cancer Antigen 3 as a Tumour Marker: Biochemical and Clinical Aspects** 277
Marianne Schmid, Jens Hansen, and Felix K.-H. Chun

Part IX Tumor Markers – A Critical Revision: Various Protein Markers

18 Biomarker in Cisplatin-Based Chemotherapy for Urinary Bladder Cancer 293
Thorsten H. Ecke

19 A Critical Approach to Clinical Biochemistry of Chromogranin A 317
Patrizia Bottoni, Teresa De Michele, and Roberto Scatena

Part X Receptors as Biomarkers

20 The Actual Role of Receptors as Cancer Markers, Biochemical and Clinical Aspects: Receptors in Breast Cancer 327
Matthew Brennan and Bora Lim

Part XI Perspectives

21 The Role of CTCs as Tumor Biomarkers 341
Evi S. Lianidou, Athina Markou, and Areti Strati

Index 369

Part I

Generality

Cancer Biomarkers: A Status Quo

1

Roberto Scatena

Abstract

At present, there are a growing number of biomolecules under investigation to understand their potential role as cancer biomarker for diagnostic, prognostic and therapeutic purposes. Intriguingly, the state of art on cancer biomarkers research shows interesting and promising results together to clamorous failures. Also from a clinical point of view, there are contradictory results on routine clinical use of the present cancer biomarkers. Some patients may be simply monitored in their course by a periodic blood sample, but sometimes this monitoring show dramatic limits. A lot of patients show serious and extensive relapses without significant change in serum concentrations of biomarkers tested. Often the physician who should utilize these biomarkers does not entirely know their limits and the total potential applications as well and sometimes this knowledge is influenced by economical and marketing strategies. This limited and "polluted" knowledge may have dramatic consequences for patient. A critical approach towards old and new cancer biomarkers should foster a deepened and useful understanding of the diagnostic and prognostic index of these fundamental parameters of laboratory medicine and in the same time can facilitate the research of new and more sensitive-specific signals of the cancer cell proliferation

Keywords

Biomarkers • Biomarkers failures • Biomarker research • Cancer cell plasticity • Cancer cell metabolism • Cancer stem cell • Circulating tumor cell • Clinical validation • Clinical and laboratory data integration • Diagnostic purposes • Prognostic purposes • Therapeutic purposes

R. Scatena (✉)
Institute of Biochemistry and Clinical Biochemistry,
School of Medicine, Catholic University,
Largo Gemelli 8, 00168 Rome, Italy
e-mail: r.scatena@rm.unicatt.it

R. Scatena (ed.), *Advances in Cancer Biomarkers*, Advances in Experimental Medicine and Biology 867, DOI 10.1007/978-94-017-7215-0_1

Despite the adoption of increasingly sophisticated multidisciplinary treatment protocols (i.e., biological drugs) cancer mortality has not been significantly reduced for the past 50 years. This dramatically contrasts with the significant reduction in mortality obtained on cardiovascular and infectious diseases. Recently, in his review [1] Jim Watson asserted that "…although the mortality from haematopoietic cells has been steadily falling, the more important statistic may be that so many epithelial cancers and all mesenchymal cancers remain largely incurable".

This statement does not only indicate the limits of current pathophysiological approaches and consequently of anticancer therapeutic protocols but, even if indirectly, it stresses the serious situation about the difficulty of laboratory medicine to really permit precocious and sensitive diagnostic and prognostic procedures in cancer.

A lot of studies have clearly shown that early diagnosis of cancer can lead to superior long-term survival and ameliorate the percent of radical treatment. Thus the need of cancer biomarkers with high sensitivity and specificity is more and more important.

To obtain an early cancer detection, an effective treatment, and consequently a decreased mortality, it become imperative to have valid biomarkers or at least make the most by the current tumor markers.

It is not by chance that the main topic of the actual real translational biomedical research is the discover of valid cancer biomarkers.

But what are the peculiar characteristics of a valid cancer biomarker? A lot of definitions are been already given, all are right but some seem more representative of the actual tangled status of tumor markers.

In fact, an ideal tumor marker should be: (i) easily, quickly measured, not too much expensive; (ii) it must be drawn from readily available sources, such as blood or urine; (iii) it should have a high sensitivity and an high specificity; (iv) its levels should vary rapidly in response to treatment; (v) its basal level should permit a risk stratification and prognostic evaluation; (vi) most importantly, its monitoring should be linked to pathophysiology of cancer, above all in term of evolution.

Regrettably, none of the present markers meets all the illustrated characteristics. Thereby, it should be better, to change their definition, according with Gion [2] suggestions, from tumor marker to tumor associated markers, in a attempt to stress the methodological, pathophysiological and clinical limits of actual markers.

But are these real clinical limits? or more simply the criticism may partially originate by an overvaluation due both to marketing strategies of the diagnostic industry and to too much optimistic experimental and clinical researchers, and above all to the strong expectation for biomarkers really clinically useful for such a dramatic disease?

Considering the ethic, clinical and economic consequences of an inappropriate use of cancer associated markers, similarly to others laboratory parameters, it must be fundamental a continuous critical approach on their evolving pathophysiological aspects and clinical peculiarities. All that could permit not only to realize an appropriate use of the actual tumor associate markers but also a better understanding of biomedical peculiarities of new markers.

Importantly, until now, as cancer associated markers, research is mainly searching for any cell products including proteins (enzymes, serum proteins, metabolites, receptors, carcinoembryonic proteins, and oncoproteins) and more recently DNA, RNA (also microRNA) and whole cells (circulating tumor cells – CTCs), encoded/contained by suppressor/promoter genes which could have a significant pathogenetic role in transformation/dedifferentiation, proliferation, and metastasis of tumor cells and that can be observed in tissues and/or biological fluids.

Theoretically, serum testing should be the ideal methods because of the noninvasive nature, more accurate quantification, and lack of interobserver difference. Moreover, also the progressive improved sensitivities of the assays made serologic tests far superior to other clinical examinations based on physical methods.

Until now, the levels of serum tumor markers are often related to tumor proliferation, tumor dedifferentiation, proteolytic activities in the tumor cell, and abnormal secretion and/or release from necrotic tumor cells. But it could be interesting also to consider the secretion products of microenvironment. Consequently, to learn how to identify, select, and utilize tumor markers for the diagnosis, monitoring of and the management of cancer patients, it is always more important to have a careful knowledge about the physiological and pathological role of each individual marker, in such a way to partially counterbalance their low specificity and/or sensibility.

At present, another aspect that must be always stressed is a right integration of the biomarker level with the clinical picture and the other diagnostic and prognostic parameters. In fact, paradoxically, the progress of technology related to laboratory medicine, are causing an amazing improvement of the assays sensitivity. However this is often associated to a significant reduction of specificity. This interesting new trend of the laboratory medicine in general could imply a revisitation of this discipline above all in terms of interpretation of diagnostic testing that must be carefully integrated with the overall clinical picture. By a qualified data integration, the introduction of high sensitivity diagnostic tests may be considered a real progress because of the possibility to very early advise the physician about the beginning of a "generic" alteration in an organism.

It is important to stress that a valid integration among laboratory and clinical data could be fruitfully realized if some methodological bias are significantly reduced. Specifically, it is fundamental at present and even more with HS-assays, to resolve some problems related to standardization of the processes related to development and reporting of old and new tumor associated markers. In fact, the actual developmental process for tumor markers and the regulatory oversight are not so rigid as with drug development and often result too much influenced by marketing strategies of industry and/or researcher. Yet, several methods are available to measure specific tumor marker, generally there is a good but not perfect concordance between assays; moreover each method has distinct analytic performance impairing a really accurate head-to-head comparison. Moreover, differences in sample collection, handling or storage (i.e. free PSA), and profiling techniques among laboratories may significantly modify the proteome pattern of a single sample, thereby it is imperative to follow a rigid standardization issues to limit biological variation, preanalytical and analytical variability.

At last but not least, there is a great expectation among physicians, clinical and basic researchers, and patients, to rapidly utilize emerging potential tumor markers into clinical care, and that could impairs a rigorous evaluation of the analytic and clinical validity of new associated tumor markers.

At present, two main experimental approaches are used to find out new valid tumor markers with acceptable level of specificity and sensitivity, i.e. genomic and proteomic. These approaches could also theoretically overcome a major problem in the discover of valid cancer biomarkers, that is the very low concentrations of markers obtained from tissues with small, early-stage cancer lesions.

However, results until now did not meet expectations. In fact, meanwhile a lot of new potential tumor markers have been experimentally identified by proteomic and genomic approaches only few come to clinical phase and even less were marketed. None of them, moreover, show a real specificity and sensitivity better than more classic tumor markers.

Erroneous results, due to both chance and bias, were also published, inducing scientific community to promote more rigid protocol approaches for researches conducted in several "-omics" fields to assess molecular markers for diagnosis and prognosis of cancer. In fact, in 2002–2003, studies reported that a blood test, based on pattern recognition proteomics mass spectroscopy analysis of serum, was nearly 100 % sensitive and specific to detect ovarian cancer [3, 4]. The introduction of a commercial screening test was later delayed because results were not reproducible and reliable. Also in genomic area there are nucleic acid-based tests that haven't met inflated expectations originated from experimental results (see Sect. 7.5.1) [5].

To this end, and just as example, it could be useful and explanatory to report the Guidelines for The Use of MALDI-TOF Mass Spectrometry Profiling to Diagnose Cancer edited by National Academy of Clinical Biochemistry realized [6]. These guidelines recommends, that:

- all technologies that directly impact patient health should not be adopted as a diagnostic test for cancer in clinical practice, until extensive validation studies are performed.
- investigators should perform validation experiments based on good laboratory/clinical practice and should provide data in a transparent form.
- appropriate independent validation sets should be employed using inflammatory and benign controls along with high numbers of unaffected controls, since specificity will be an important determining factor of success in the clinic, especially for screening indications.

At last, it is interesting to report that Academy concludes that despite difficulties in extending experimental data in clinical results for genomics and proteomics, at present there is a better understanding of potential sources of bias and instrument variances, as well as the requirements for implementing good laboratory practices such that validation and clinical use for new biomarkers could be quickly obtained.

It is clear that such recommendations could be easily extrapolated to other methodological approaches adopted to discover new tumor biomarkers.

Moreover, the value of this particular approaches and the importance to reduce bias in this research's field is indirectly confirmed by the foundation of the National Cancer Institute's (NCI) Clinical Proteomic Tumor Analysis Consortium (CPTAC) which represents a network of Proteome Characterization Centers, which coordinate and conduct research and data sharing activities to comprehensively examine genomically characterized cancer biospecimens. Importantly, CPTAC data with accompanying assays and protocols are freely available. This multidisciplinary (proteomics, genomics, bioinformatics, experimental design, statistics, cancer biology and oncology) and integrated consortium identifies proteins that result from changes in cancer genomes translating these results in validated clinical applications [7].

The next research on Cancer biomarkers should have the main aim to find out signal molecules which render cancer care increasingly dependent on tumor markers to diagnose, anticipate prognosis, and select optimal therapy. Any circulating biomolecule, cell products exosomes and/or whole tumor cells (the so-called circulating tumor cells) can be used as tumor markers if they are associated with events related to some clinical relevant aspect of cancer pathophysiology.

It is evident that such markers should be indentified and monitored at very low concentrations and that justifies the difficulties related to this research. A particular attention should be due to the albumin molecule as a circulating molecular mop, grabbing and concentrating (more than 100-fold) low-molecular-weight proteins present in blood at very low concentrations. This "microproteome" could better represent the minimal variations related to the beginning of an anaplastic process evolution.

Importantly, from a research point of view, some new tumor markers could be derived from current topics related to molecular biology of cancer, like:

(a) Cancer stem cells/circulating tumor cells. This new paradigm of oncogenesis is progressively changing some fundamental aspects of pathophysiology of cancer. The evidence of a subpopulation of cells with pathogenically relevant role is re-addressing a series of translational and clinical researches on the functional phenotype of these peculiar cancer cells (stemness markers profile, altered signal transduction pathways, ROS metabolism, EMT) which seem to be characterized by a relatively low proliferation index, by an intriguing chemoresistence and to the tendency to give rise recidivism and metastasis.

(b) Genetic markers. Circulating nucleic acids (circulating cell-free DNA circulating, extra-cellular miRNAs and/or exosomes) do represent interesting potential new tumor markers with a biochemical profile that seems to better adhere to the characteristics of an ideal cancer biomarkers. However, such an optimistic expectation must be validated by a right comparison with biological variability and a more accurate knowledge of their pathophysiological role in different diseases other than cancer.

(c) Cancer cell plasticity. Strictly related to the other previous aspects is the peculiarity of cancer cells to finely adapt to particular microenvironment by a Darwinian selective pressure and/or by a particular functional plasticity which anyway seems to be related to typical cancer cell genetic instability. The debated molecular mechanisms at the basis of this instability could represent an useful targets with diagnostic, prognostic and therapeutic implications (i.e., quali-quantitative variations in cells *DNA repair* machinery).

(d) Cancer cell metabolism. At present, this aspect is subjected to a deep revision of the so-called Warburg effect which is clearly an intriguing epiphenomenon of a more complex metabolic adaption of cancer cell metabolism in which not only glycolysis but also the Krebs cycle, beta oxidation, and anabolic metabolism in general are readdressed to respond to the new primary function of this cell (i.e., uncontrolled proliferation) by providing not only energy but also building blocks for the synthesis of nucleotides and amino and fatty acids. This important metabolic shift is not simply related to cell proliferation but imply some important additional characteristics. Specifically, cancer induced mitochondrial metabolic seems to stress a more specific role for some related enzymes as: aconitase, isocitrate dehydrogenase, PKM2, and so on that should be better investigated from a diagnostic point of view. In fact, by carefully clarifying the peculiar metabolic aspects of cancer cell it could be possible to highlight subtle variation of enzymatic proteome in serum that could precociously indicate an abnormal cell growth related to a neoplastic cell proliferation.

In conclusion, the identification of new and valid tumor markers is one of the main topics of cancer research. However, it is a really hard target because of methodological, pathophysiological and clinical difficulties that too often are neglected. We are witnessing to a continual discover of "biomarkers" not only for cancer but for a lot of diseases that, however, do not obtain a clinical validation and, on the other side, it is evident a clear misuse of the present tumor markers with clinical and, above all, economical negative effects.

To clash this misuse, it should be fundamental to know not only the clinical aspects related to a specific biomarkers but also to have a careful understanding of their biochemical, physiological and pathophysiological role. At last but not last, this knowledge should be continuously updated with respect to revisions of related clinical biochemistry aspects and advances of medicine.

References

1. Watson J (2013) Oxidants, antioxidants and the current incurability of metastatic cancers. Open Biol 3:120144. doi:10.1098/rsob.120144
2. Gion M, Fabricio AS (2011) New frontiers in tumor marker studies: from biobanking to collaboration in translational research. Int J Biol Markers 26:73–74
3. Petricoin EF, Ardekani AM, Hitt BA, Levine PJ, Fusaro VA, Steinberg SM, Mills GB, Simone C, Fishman DA, Kohn EC, Liotta LA (2002) Use of proteomic patterns in serum to identify ovarian cancer. Lancet 359:572–577
4. Zhu W, Wang X, Ma Y, Rao M, Glimm J, Kovach JS (2003) Detection of cancer-specific markers amid massive mass spectral data. Proc Natl Acad Sci U S A 100:14666–14671
5. Amaro A, Esposito AI, Gallina A, Nees M, Angelini G, Albini A, Pfeffer U (2014) Validation of proposed prostate cancer biomarkers with gene expression data: along road to travel. Cancer Metastasis Rev 33:657–671

6. Sturgeon CM, Hoffman BR, Chan DW, Ch'ng SL, Hammond E, Hayes DF, Liotta LA, Petricoin EF, Schmitt M, Semmes OJ, Söletormos G, van der Merwe E, Diamandis EP (2008) National Academy of Clinical Biochemistry. National Academy of Clinical Biochemistry Laboratory Medicine Practice Guidelines for use of tumor markers in clinical practice: quality requirements. Clin Chem 54:e1–e10
7. Ellis MJ, Gillette M, Carr SA, Paulovich AG, Smith RD, Rodland KK, Townsend RR, Kinsinger C, Mesri M, Rodriguez H, Liebler DC (2013) Clinical Proteomic Tumor Analysis Consortium (CPTAC). Connecting genomic alterations to cancer biology with proteomics: the NCI Clinical Proteomic Tumor Analysis Consortium. Cancer Discov 3:1108–1112

Cancer Biomarkers Discovery and Validation: State of the Art, Problems and Future Perspectives

2

Alvaro Mordente, Elisabetta Meucci, Giuseppe Ettore Martorana, and Andrea Silvestrini

Abstract

Cancer is one of the major public health problems worldwide representing the leading cause of morbidity and mortality in industrialized countries. To reduce cancer morbidity and mortality as well as to facilitate the evolution from the traditional "one size fits all" strategy to a new "personalized" cancer therapy (i.e., the right drug to the right patient at the right time, using the right dose and schedule), there is an urgent need of reliable, robust, accurate and validated cancer biomarker tests.

Unfortunately, despite the impressive advances in tumor biology research as well as in high-powerful "omics" technologies, the translation of candidate cancer biomarkers from bench to bedside is lengthy and challenging and only a few tumor marker tests have been adopted successfully into routine clinical care of oncologic patients.

This chapter provides an updated background on biomarkers research in oncology, including biomarkers clinical uses, and discusses the problems of discovery pipeline, biomarkers failures and future perspectives.

Keywords

Biomarkers • Biomarkers failures • Cancer • Cancer biomarker: discovery and validation • Cancer control studies • Cancer therapy • Clinical assay development • Clinical uses • Discovery • Pharmacodynamic markers • Preclinical exploratory studies • Predictive markers • Prognostic markers • Prospective screening studies • Retrospective longitudinal repository studies • Risk assessment • Validation

A. Mordente (✉) • E. Meucci • G.E. Martorana
A. Silvestrini
Istituto di Biochimica e Biochimica Clinica,
Università Cattolica del S. Cuore,
Largo F. Vito 1, 00168 Roma, Italy
e-mail: alvaro.mordente@rm.unicatt.it

R. Scatena (ed.), *Advances in Cancer Biomarkers*, Advances in Experimental Medicine and Biology 867, DOI 10.1007/978-94-017-7215-0_2

2.1 Background

"The term *cancer* defines over one hundred different diseases that can arise from virtually any tissue or organ in the body and, while sharing common properties of local invasion and distant spread, may have different causative factors, molecular composition, natural history of disease, methods for diagnosis and methods by which they are treated" [1].

Cancer is a major public health problem worldwide, representing the leading cause of morbidity and mortality in industrialized nations, where the lifetime risk of developing cancer is approximately 40 % (about 43 % for males and 38 % for females) [2].

According to GLOBOCAN 2012 [3], the International Agency for Research on Cancer's online database, the global burden of cancer increased to 14.1 million new cancer cases and 8.2 million cancer-related deaths worldwide in 2012 compared with 12.4 million and 7.6 million in 2008, respectively [4]. Furthermore, GLOBOCAN 2012 predicts that there will be 19.3 million new cancer cases per year by 2025, due to growth and ageing of the global population, environmental exposures, cancer-associated lifestyles (e.g., diet, obesity, smoking and sedentary life) and late diagnosis with low survival rates. More than half of all cancers (56.8 %) and cancer deaths (64.9 %) in 2012 occurred in less developed regions of the world, and these proportions will increase further by 2025.

More than 30 % of cancer deaths could be prevented by modifying or avoiding key risk factors (behavioural and dietary), including high body mass index, low fruit and vegetable intake, lack of physical activity, tobacco and alcohol use.

To reduce cancer morbidity and mortality thereby alleviating both the economic and social costs caused by cancer, there is an urgent need to develop novel tumor biomarker tests which are sensitive and specific enough for early diagnosis, for staging and monitoring disease progression and for predicting and monitoring therapeutic response, paving the way to a "personalized" cancer treatment [5].

Unfortunately, despite the impressive advances in knowledge of tumor biology as well as in "omics" and "lab-on-a-chip" technologies, the translation of candidate cancer biomarkers from bench to bedside is long and challenging and only a few tumor marker tests have been adopted successfully into routine clinical care of oncologic patients.

Here, we review the state of the art on biomarkers research in oncology and discuss the reasons that impede the translation of findings from tumor markers research to standard clinical practice and also the ways in which this is being addressed.

In particular, this review aims to focus on the following questions: what is a cancer biomarker, and which are the potential clinical uses for a tumor biomarker test and the strategies for discovering and validating novel cancer biomarkers; finally, what are the reasons why many cancer biomarkers do not perform well in clinical practice.

2.2 Cancer Biomarkers: Definition, Types and Potential Clinical Uses

2.2.1 Definition of Cancer Biomarker

The Biomarkers Definitions Working Group of the National Institutes of Health defines a biomarker as a cellular, biochemical, and/or molecular (including genetic and epigenetic) characteristic that can be objectively measured and evaluated as an indicator of normal biological processes, pathogenic processes, or pharmacologic responses to a therapeutic intervention [6].

A cancer biomarker, in particular, is a "biological molecule produced either by the tumor cell or by human tissues in response to cancer that is objectively measured and evaluated as an indicator of cancerous processes within the body" [7].

Alternatively, a tumor marker may be defined as a "molecule that indicates the presence of cancer or provide information about the likely future behaviour of a cancer (i.e., likelihood of progression or response to therapy" [8].

Table 2.1 Human specimens for cancer biomarker discovery

Human specimen	Cancer type
Blood (Serum or Plasma)	Broad spectrum
Cerebrospinal fluid	Brain
Nipple aspirate fluid	Breast
Breast cyst fluid	Breast
Ductal lavage	Breast
Cervicovaginal fluid	Cervical and endometrial
Stool	Colorectal
Pleural effusion	Lung
Bronchoalveolar lavage	Lung
Saliva	Oral
Ascites fluid	Ovarian
Pancreatic juice	Pancreatic
Seminal plasma	Prostate and testicular
Urine	Urological

Scientists commonly use the terms "biomarker", "marker", "molecular diagnostic" and "signature molecule", interchangeably.

Biochemically, cancer biomarkers can be DNA (germline or somatic), RNA, proteins, peptides, hormones, metabolites, and even biological processes such as apoptosis, angiogenesis or proliferation.

Cancer biomarkers can be detected in the circulation (whole blood, serum or plasma) or in secretions (stools, urine, sputum or nipple discharge) or in others human biological fluids (Table 2.1) [9] and thus easily assessed non-invasively and serially, or can be tissue-derived and require either biopsy or surgical resection [10, 11].

An ideal tumor biomarker should be [8, 9]:

(a) produced only by the tumor cells;
(b) correlated with tumor burden and endowed with a sufficient lead time (i.e. the time between asymptomatic cancer still localized to the organ of origin and clinical diagnosis; for example, aggressive cancers have shorter lead times than indolent cancers);
(c) present in measurable quantities (or in concentrations significantly higher than normal) in the blood (or other human biological fluids) of cancer patients at early or preclinical stages (preferably in one cancer type only);
(d) undetectable (or present at a very low levels) in the blood (or other biological fluids) of healthy individuals or with benign disease;
(e) easy to measure even in small amounts and with little preparation, by means of a reliable test, cost-effective and associated to high analytical sensitivity (the percentage of individuals with cancer who test positive for the biomarker) and to specificity (the percentage of individuals without cancer who test negative for the biomarker). An ideal biomarker test would have 100 % sensitivity and specificity (i.e. everyone with cancer would have a positive test, while everyone without cancer would present a negative test).

To date, the U.S. Food and Drug Administration (FDA) have just approved 19 protein cancer biomarkers, only 11 of which are detectable in the blood (Table 2.2).

Although these biomarkers are routinely in clinical practice, nevertheless they are far from ideal, for, as the saying goes, "the ideal tumor marker does not actually exist" [8].

2.2.2 Types of Cancer Biomarkers

Based on their clinical use, three major types of cancer biomarkers are currently distinguished: (1) prognostic, (2) predictive, and (3) pharmacodynamic markers [1, 12–15]. Notably, an individual biomarker may serve more than one purpose and thus can fall into more than one of the above categories [16].

2.2.2.1 Prognostic Markers

Prognostic markers are factors that predict "disease outcome in the absence of systemic therapy or portend an outcome different from that of patients without the marker, despite empiric (not targeted to the marker) systemic therapy" [13, 17].

Practically, prognostic markers predict "the natural course of an individual cancer, distinguishing *good outcome* tumours from *poor outcome* tumours, and they guide the decision of whom to treat and/or how aggressively to

Table 2.2 List of FDA-approved protein cancer biomarkers

Biomarker	Specimen	Clinical use	Cancer type	Methodology
α-fetoprotein (**AFP**)	Serum	Staging	Nonseminomatous testicular	Immunoassay
Human chorionic gonadotropin-β (β-**hGC**)	Serum	Staging	Testicular	Immunoassay
Carbohydrate antigen 19–9 (**CA 19–9**)	Serum	Monitoring	Pancreatic	Immunoassay
Carbohydrate antigen 125 (**CA 125**)	Serum	Monitoring	Ovarian	Immunoassay
Carbohydrate antigen 15.3 (**CA 15.3**)	Serum	Monitoring	Breast	Immunoassay
Carbohydrate antigen 27.29 (**CA 27.29**)	Serum	Monitoring	Breast	Immunoassay
Carcinoembryonic antigen (**CEA**)	Serum	Monitoring	Colorectal	Immunoassay
Fibrin/fibrinogen degradation products (**FDP**)	Serum	Monitoring	Bladder	Immunoassay
Human epidermidis protein 4 (**HE4**)	Serum	Monitoring	Ovarian	Immunoassay
Prostate specific antigen (**PSA**)	Serum	Screening and monitoring	Prostate	Immunoassay
Thyroglobulin (**TG**)	Serum	Monitoring	Thyroid	Immunoassay
Epidermal growth factor receptor (**EGFR**)	Tissue	Prediction	Colorectal	Immunohistochemistry
v-kit Hardy-Zuckerman 4 feline sarcoma viral oncogene homolog (**KIT**)	Tissue	Prediction	Gastrointestinal	Immunohistochemistry
Estrogen receptor (**ER**)	Tissue	Prognosis and prediction	Breast	Immunohistochemistry
Progesterone receptor (**PR**)	Tissue	Prognosis and prediction	Breast	Immunohistochemistry
v-erb-b2 erythroblastic leukemia viral oncogene homolog 2 (**HER2-neu**)	Tissue	Prognosis and prediction	Breast	Immunohistochemistry
Nuclear matrix protein 22 (**NMP-22**)	Urine	Screening and monitoring	Bladder	Immunoassay
Bladder tumor antigen (**BTA**)	Urine	Monitoring	Bladder	Immunoassay
High molecular CEA and mucin	Urine	Monitoring	Bladder	Immunofluorescence

treat" [14]. Prognostic markers are therefore particularly important at the time of initial diagnosis of malignancy and in cancers that vary widely in patients' outcome (e.g. prostate and breast cancer) [13, 18].

However, as emphasized by Duffy and Crown [18], "no prognostic marker can accurately predict outcome for an individual patient; it provides a probability estimate of outcome for a heterogeneous population of patients".

Importantly, prognostic markers may be crucial to reduce overtreatment of patients with indolent malignancy and so minimizing the side effects of adjuvant systemic therapies, and to avoid under-treatment of patients with aggressive and life-threatening malignancy for which would be recommended to receive the most appropriate local and systemic therapy [18].

In the last years, hundreds of prognostic biomarkers have been proposed, but few have progressed to clinical use (see Sect. 2.4). Some of the best-validated and/or clinically used prognostic markers as well as other markers proposed but not used routinely in clinical oncology have been recently critically reviewed by Duffy and Crown [18].

2.2.2.2 Predictive Markers

Predictive markers are molecules that "provide upfront information as to whether or not a patient is likely to benefit from a specific therapy" [19]. Predictive biomarkers assess the likelihood that the tumor will respond to the drug, and thereby allow a level of personalization to be introduced into the treatment regimen [1]. There are a small number of predictive biomarkers that have found clinical utility [20], and others are gaining clinical acceptance as objective measurements that inform on the clinical response to the drug (i.e., only patients expressing the marker will respond to the specific treatment or will respond to a greater degree than those without the marker) [1, 17]. Predictive markers, by prospectively differentiating populations of "responder" from "non-responder" patients, can guide the choice of anticancer therapy [17] thereby saving patients from unnecessary side effects [18]. At the same time, predictive markers might result in considerable cost savings (especially for the new biological therapies), as anticancer drugs would be used only in patients likely to derive benefit. Predictive markers, especially the very few ones that are in clinical use or close to entering clinical use, have been critically reviewed by Duffy et al. [19] and La Thangue and Kerr [1]. Again, putative predictive genomic biomarkers for cancer targeted therapies have been recently reviewed by Simon and Roychowdhury [15].

2.2.2.3 Pharmacodynamic Markers

Pharmacodynamic markers provide information on the effects of the drug on the body (i.e., drug targets and mechanisms of action), including both early effects on its molecular target (i.e. whether a drug engages and inhibits a target, and the degree and timing of the inhibition) and also later effects on downstream events [21–23]. On the other hand, pharmacokinetics evaluates the effect of the body on the drug: that is, the process by which a drug is absorbed, distributed, metabolized and eliminated by the body.

Consequently, endpoints of pharmacodynamic markers include assessments of protein phosphorylation markers, measures of cellular proliferation/apoptosis, cell-cycle regulation biomarkers, and epigenetic changes [21, 24]. In oncology, pharmacodynamic biomarkers are utilized in optimizing doses of chemotherapeutic drugs below their cytotoxicity level and in understanding response/resistance mechanisms [21, 22].

2.2.3 Potential Clinical Uses of Cancer Biomarkers

The different types of cancer biomarkers that can be used in multiple clinical settings depend on the disease stage (and hence on patient status). Biomarkers, indeed, can be accounted for before cancer diagnosis (in risk assessment and screening for premalignant lesions or early invasive disease), at diagnosis (in staging, grading, and selection of initial therapy) and after diagnosis (in monitoring therapy, selecting additional therapy and detecting recurrence) (Fig. 2.1).

"Consequently, the spectrum of cancer patient status can range from unaffected individuals who are concerned about whether they should adopt preventive or screening strategies, to patients with early-stage disease for whom considerations of appropriate primary (surgery and radiation) and adjuvant systemic therapies (chemotherapy, hormone therapy, biological therapy or various combinations of these therapies) are critical, to those who are free of disease but are concerned about recurrence, and finally to patients with established metastatic disease" [11].

Remarkably, some biomarkers are only used in a specific setting, whereas other ones can serve in more than one mode [10].

In this regard, tumor biomarkers might be useful for: (1) risk assessment, (2) screening for early cancer detection, (3) diagnosis, (4) prognosis, (5) selection and monitoring of anticancer therapy [10, 11, 25].

2.2.3.1 Risk Assessment

"Risk assessment is the search for factors that provide the earliest evidence of the impending cancer in persons not yet diagnosed with the disease" [26].

Cancer, traditionally viewed as a series of genetic diseases, is now recognized to involve epigenetic modifications along with genetic mutations [27]. Moreover, genetic and epigenetic alterations are not separate events in cancerogenesis, but the "*crosstalk*" between these two mechanisms ultimately promotes genomic instability and abnormal gene expression contributing to the various phases of neoplastic development

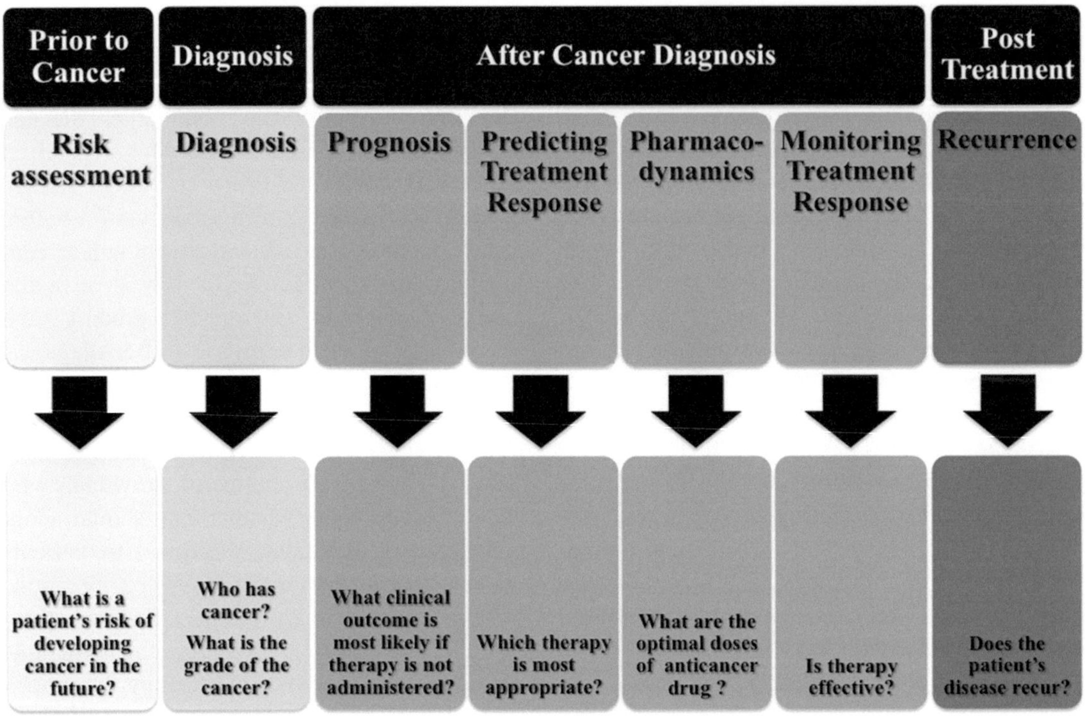

Fig. 2.1 Potential fields of application of a cancer biomarker test

including initiation, promotion, invasion, metastases and chemotherapy resistance [28]. Consequently, genetic (e.g. point mutations, translocations and copy number variations) and, more important, epigenetic materials modifications (e.g. DNA methylation, histone post-translational alterations, chromatin remodeling, and small, noncoding microRNAs expression) may represent an early and promising analytical tool for biomarker discovery, with broad potential applications in risk assessment, screening for early cancer detection, prognosis, and prediction of response to therapy [29].

In particular, because epigenetic modifications may constitute a signature of specific exposure to certain risk factors, they have the potential to serve as highly specific biomarkers for risk assessment [29].

Genetic and epigenetic biomarkers and their clinical implications in risk assessment and early cancer diagnosis are diffusely discussed in recent pivotal reviews [27, 30–33].

2.2.3.2 Screening for Early Cancer Detection

Many cancer types, if diagnosed and treated early, can be cured or, at least, transformed to a chronic disease. Therefore, early cancer detection in asymptomatic patients still remains a priority of cancer research with a high potential of improving both patients' survival and quality of life [34].

A useful screening test for early detection of cancer must exhibit most, if not all, the characteristics previously described for an ideal tumor marker. "First of all, a screening test should be able to detect malignancy at an early and asymptomatic stage thereby resulting in decreased morbidity or increased survival rates" [35]. In addition, the test must be inexpensive and safe enough to be applied to mass populations. Moreover, a screening test should have a very high sensitivity and an exceptional specificity, to avoid too many false positives in populations with a low cancer prevalence.

Unfortunately, besides some notable exceptions (e.g. human choriogonadotropin for germ cell tumors and gestational trophoblastic disease and α-fetoprotein for hepatocellular and testicular carcinoma), none of the biomarker tests currently used in clinical oncology is suitable for population screening or early diagnosis of cancer, that still remains the biggest clinical challenge of all [34, 36, 37].

A list of selected promising molecular markers for early detection of cancer is reported in [38].

2.2.3.3 Diagnosis

Contrary to screening, a diagnostic test would be prescribed to an individual who has already manifested symptoms of cancer. Currently, however, there is no biomarker test recommended in clinical practice guidelines for cancer diagnosis, but many of the well-known markers are widely used as aids in diagnosis and/or sub-classification of a particular malignancy state [8, 35].

2.2.3.4 Prognosis

For prognostic markers see Sect. 2.2.2.1.

2.2.3.5 Selection and Monitoring of Cancer Therapy

For predictive and pharmacodynamic markers see Sects. 2.2.2.2 and 2.2.2.3, respectively.

2.3 Cancer Biomarker: Discovery and Validation

The process of discovering and developing molecular cancer biomarkers "is a work in progress and is evolving" [39], representing an "integral component of contemporary cancer research" [35].

In 2001, the National Cancer Institute's Early Detection Research Network (EDRN), to promote efficiency and scientific rigor in biomarkers research, introduced guidelines "to guide the process of biomarker development" consisting of five "phases that are generally ordered according to the strength of evidence that each phase provides in favour of the biomarker, from weakest to strongest and the results of earlier phases are generally necessary to design later phases" [40].

These guidelines propose specific aims, subject selection, outcome measures, and evaluation of results for each of the five phases of a biomarker discovery pipeline in the context of progress being made in the field and relevant published studies [40–42]. The phase structure of biomarker development pipeline includes: Phase 1 (Preclinical exploratory studies), Phase 2 (Clinical assay development), Phase 3 (Retrospective longitudinal studies), Phase 4 (Prospective screening studies), and Phase 5 (Cancer control studies).

The phases are not rigorously distinct from each other and to proceed from one phase to another a candidate biomarker needs to overcome pre-analytical, analytical and post-analytical challenges at different levels. Only biomarkers that will reach the last step successfully will be implemented in the clinic [9, 35, 43, 44].

A major implication of this framework is that the time required from the initial discovery to clinical adoption of a biomarker is lengthy, generally a decade or more [25].

2.3.1 Phase 1: Preclinical Exploratory Studies

The beginning of the discovery phase in the biomarker development pipeline involves preclinical semi-quantitative studies to identify one or more promising biological molecules ("candidate biomarkers") that, exhibiting discriminating potential between cancer patients and healthy subjects, might be useful to develop clinical tests for early detecting and monitoring cancer or for managing cancer therapy.

The discovery process of new putative tumor markers can involve two major complementary approaches: (a) "knowledge-based" or "hypothesis-driven" or "targeted" method; (b) "unbiased" or "discovery-based" or "untargeted" method [7, 45, 46]. The "hypothesis-driven" approach identifies candidate biomarkers by a deductive method that relies on ever-increasing knowledge of the molecular mechanisms underlying cancer biology and therefore only a specified set of molecules supposed to be involved in cancerogenesis is measured ("targeted" method). In contrast, the "discovery-based" approach identify candidate biomarkers by an inductive method that, exploiting the extraordinary potentiality of new high-throughput-omics technologies (capable of identifying multiple rather than just a single marker by performing parallel rather than serial analyses), select molecular species on the basis of their differential expression between normal (controls) and diseased (cases) states, without an *a priori* target identification ("untargeted" method) [7, 45, 46].

Although high-throughput-omics technologies are frequently used for biomarkers discovery, hypothesis-driven method is now endorsed as the preferred one [7, 35, 47, 48] as the key advantage of this approach is that "defining an intended use for the tumor marker at the early stages of the discovery process allows better control of the variables (other than the cancer itself) that may influence measured levels of the marker during the discovery process" [7].

Regardless of which method is selected, a rigorous and accurate study design is essential to reach the required results. The major topics to be defined when discovery studies are planned include: (a) the number of samples to analyse; (b) inclusion/exclusion criteria for the samples; (c) collection and handling requirements; (d) limitations of the analytical methodology(ies); (e) appropriate statistical analysis of the acquired data; and (f) validation of the findings in independent datasets and by independent investigators. Moreover, complete and transparent reporting of results is also necessary so that other investigators can assess the "soundness of the study" [7, 49].

"Judging by the numerous publications reporting novel candidate biomarkers, the discovery phase seems to be productive" [35], however the majority of cancer biomarkers do not progress beyond this phase. The main reasons for this failure include modest differences in the concentration of the biomarker in cases compared with controls and large variability in the levels of the biomarker in healthy subjects [50].

For an in-depth discussion of these and other issues of the discovery phase of biomarker-development pipeline, the reader is referred to several excellent published reviews [7, 35, 37, 44, 49] and to the references therein.

2.3.2 Phase 2: Clinical Assay Development

Once a promising cancer biomarker is identified, the next crucial step is to develop and validate a robust, accurate and reliable test (at this regard, "it is essential to distinguish a cancer biomarker from a cancer biomarker test, that is a specific assay that measures the marker reliably" [51]) to measure the analyte of interest both in the clinical trials of the biomarker-development pipeline and, more important, in an eventual routine laboratory practice [40].

"Assay development and validation is an iterative process that occurs at every step in the pipeline and may not end even after an assay is marketed" [35]. To progress to clinical practice, a candidate biomarker test, like any other medical technology or intervention, must undergo a rigorous evaluation that involves the assessment of its: (a) analytical validity, (b) clinical validity, and (c) clinical utility (Fig. 2.2). The terms "analytical validity", "clinical validity" and "clinical utility" have been coined in 2009 by the Evaluation of Genomic Applications in Practice and Prevention Working Group in the development and implementation of a rigorous process able to support the translation of scientific evidence on genomic testing into clinical practice [52].

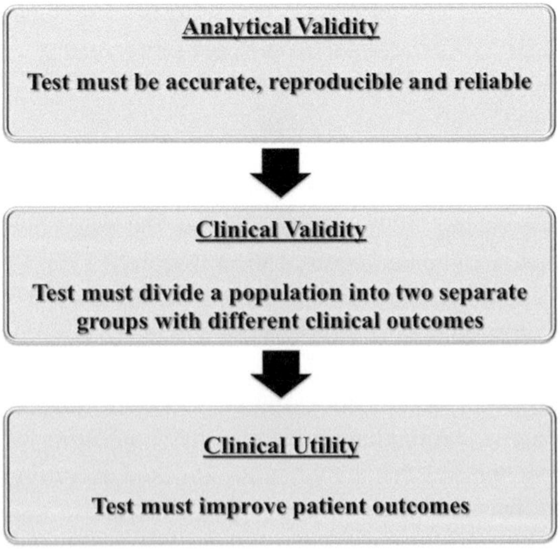

Fig. 2.2 Validation process of a candidate cancer biomarker test

Analytical validity is defined as the "test's ability to accurately and reliably measure the analyte of interest in the clinical laboratory, and in specimens representative of the population of interest" [10, 52–54].

In other words, analytical validation means establishing that the "test measures what it claims to measure, and does so accurately with adequate sensitivity and specificity" [15]. "Analytical validity refers not just to the hardware platform used for measuring test but to the entire process of treating a sample including sample preparation, performing the assay and the computational pipeline for assembling the sequence readouts and calling variants" namely the three different phases of assay development: pre-analytical, analytical, and post-analytical phase [15, 55].

In order to develop an analytically robust biomarker assay, at least the following parameters should be assessed: accuracy, trueness, precision, reproducibility, robustness, linearity, reportable range, reference range, interfering substances, analytical sensitivity and specificity, and limit of detection [7, 10, 56, 57]. Lastly, a useful biomarker test should be easily performed by routine clinical laboratories.

About the analytical platform used for measuring test, since most of the cancer biomarkers have a plasma or serum concentration in the range of picogram to nanogram per milliliter, immunoassays, such as enzyme-linked immunosorbent assay (ELISA) or radioimmunoassay (RIA), remain the method of choice for protein quantification in clinical samples [35, 58–60]. Immunological techniques, indeed, still offer a higher level of sensitivity (two to three orders of magnitude), reproducibility and dynamic range than the more sophisticated nonimmuno-based technologies (e.g. mass spectrometry assay) [58]. At the state of art, mass spectrometry technique, due to their high assay complexity, high cost, and expertise requirements is not yet transferable into routine use in clinical laboratories [35, 60]. It is noteworthy that the majority of FDA-approved protein assays utilize immunoassay (see Table 2.2), and not a single mass spectrometry-based protein assay has been approved for clinical use yet [59, 61].

"Robust analytical performance is an essential but insufficient prerequisite for the successful clinical deployment of a novel tumor marker test" [7], therefore, once verified the analytical (or "technical") validity, the biomarker assay must be tested for evaluating its clinical (or "biological") validity.

Clinical validity is defined as the "test's ability to consistently and accurately identify or predict the intermediate or final clinical outcomes of interest". Practically, clinical validity implies that the cancer biomarker test separates a population into two or more distinct groups with different biological characteristics or clinical outcomes. Clinical validity encompasses clinical sensitivity and specificity (integrating analytic validity), receiver operating characteristic (ROC) curves analysis, as well as positive predictive value (PPV) (i.e. the chance that a person with a positive test has cancer), and negative predictive value (NPV) (i.e. the chance that a person with a negative test does not have cancer) [7, 52, 54, 57]. Clinical validity studies may be conducted retrospectively or prospectively on samples collected from clinical trials, tissue banks or other sources.

Finally, before a cancer biomarker test is introduced into standard clinical management, it must also demonstrate to have what is commonly called "clinical utility". Clinical utility is defined as "the test's ability to significantly improve measurable clinical outcomes, and its usefulness and added value to patient management decision making compared with current management without testing" [52].

Therefore, "whereas analytic and clinical validity transform data into knowledge, demonstration of clinical utility is the critical last step that allows for application of a tumor biomarker test in patient care" [62].

The end point for establishing clinical utility is generally survival or progression-free survival, whereas the end point used for establishing clinical validity is often tumor or clinical response [15]. Key features for evaluations of the clinical utility of diagnostic testing are summarized in [63].

Ideally, the clinical utility of tumor biomarker test is best assessed through prospective randomized controlled trials, as these studies are the least prone to bias. However, such trials are not always feasible because they are often costly, require very large sample sizes, and have ethical challenges [63, 64]. Clinical utility may be alternatively determined either from prospective–retrospective studies using archived specimens from previously conducted prospective clinical trials [64] or, if adequate archived specimens are not available, from prospectively direct clinical trials [17, 65, 66].

At this regard, an experts committee convened by the Institute of Medicine (IOM) of the United States to define the best practices for translation of omics-based tests from the research laboratory into clinical trials, and ultimately to clinical care, has recently proposed a roadmap for development of putative new omics-based tests from initial concept to ultimate clinical utility [67]. Although specifically ideated for omics-based tests, the roadmap is still applicable to any diagnostic test, and in particular to tumor biomarker tests. The roadmap involves two stages: (1) discovery and test validation, and (2) evaluation for clinical utility and use. The first stage can be divided into two separate but linked phases: (a) discovery of a tumor biomarker test of potential biological or clinical interest, and (b) analytical development of a tumor biomarker test with biological/clinical validity.

In the second stage, an analytically-validated tumor biomarker test is further evaluated for clinical utility, either in a prospective-retrospective study using archived specimens or in a prospective clinical trials where the test either is used to direct patient management or is prospectively determined to be the primary objective of the trial [68].

Notably, the potential pathways suggested by the IOM to generate high levels of evidence necessary to demonstrate clinical utility of the biomarker test follow quite closely the recommendations of Simon et al. [64].

Most biomarkers do not progress beyond this phase primarily because the validation study shows that the biomarker test does not have sufficient sensitivity or specificity to be clinically useful (see Sect. 2.4).

2.3.3 Phase 3: Retrospective Longitudinal Repository Studies

With a good clinical assay in hand, a retrospective analysis using stored samples can be employed to determine if the biomarker can truly detect the outcome of interest and define the cut-point for a biomarker with many values [40, 43].

The phase 3 of the biomarker development pipeline is aimed at evaluating the capability of the biomarker test to detect preclinical disease on samples collected and stored longitudinally from research cohorts. Accordingly, the biomarker level is measured in specimens collected from cancer case subjects prior to their clinical diagnosis and compared to that measured from specimens collected from age-matched healthy subjects (i.e., subjects who have not developed cancer). Furthermore, the retrospective longitudinal studies can be useful to compare multiple markers of interest with a view to select those that are most promising and to develop algorithms for combinations of biomarkers. Criteria for ‘positive’ screening defined in this phase are used in the subsequent phase 4.

In contrast to the discovery phase, retrospective longitudinal studies require large numbers of samples to ensure a rigorous statistical analysis, as well as samples that reflect the biological variability of the targeted population.

The retrospective longitudinal studies of phase 3 are not able to establish the stage or nature of the cancer at the time that it can be detected.

2.3.4 Phase 4: Prospective Screening Studies

The phase 4 intends to determine whether a biomarker test can detect a cancer at an early stage of development [40]. In particular, the primary aim of this phase is to determine the “operating characteristics of the biomarker based screening test in a relevant population” by calculating the detection rate or PPV (i.e. the proportion of screened subjects who test positive and have the disease), and the false-referral rate (i.e. the proportion of screened subjects who test positive but do not have the disease).

In other words, in phase 4 "the biomarker is tested to determine if it can do what it is hypothesized to do" [43].

In the prospective studies of phase 4, asymptomatic subjects are screened using the biomarker test, and those with a positive result are followed up to determine if they have cancer and, if so, its stage.

Notably, in contrast to studies in phases 1, 2, and 3, which are conducted on retrospective analysis of stored specimens, studies in phase 4 involve screening people and lead to diagnosis and treatment [40].

2.3.5 Phase 5: Cancer Control Studies

The final phase of the biomarkers development pipeline evaluates how the biomarker test performs in the population [43]. Large-scale population studies are designed to determine whether screening test reduces the burden (in morbidity and mortality) of cancer on the population [40].

2.4 Cancer Biomarkers Failures

Despite the impressive volume of research that has been addressed to identify cancer biomarkers and the increasing number of putative tumor markers reported in literature (and some of them in very prominent journals), "very few, if any, new circulating cancer biomarkers have entered the clinic in the last 30 years" [69].

Paraphrasing the title of a Buchen's article, it seems right to ask: why is it so hard to find a test to predict cancer? [36] Furthermore, why do most cancer biomarkers fail to reach the clinic?

"The problem of identifying novel cancer biomarkers cannot be attributed to the lack of pathophysiological knowledge, powerful techniques, or investment of funds, but it may reside in difficulties that are associated with biomarker discovery, which have apparently been persistently underestimated" [69, 70].

Although "the high failure rates in the cancer biomarker field are no different from those of therapeutics", "therapeutics leading to relatively small improvements in patient survival (weeks to months) are likely to be marketed, diagnostics with relatively small improvements in patient diagnosis or prognosis will likely fall by the wayside. Hence, similar advances in therapeutics and diagnostics can be hailed as *successes* in the former and *failures* in the latter" [69].

Recently, the reasons responsible for cancer biomarker failure to reach the clinic have been widely discussed and classified into distinct categories [69, 71]. The classification is aimed to "help in understanding what goes wrong in each case and offer some lessons on how we could try to avoid similar problems in the future" [71].

According to Diamandis [69], tumor biomarkers failures can be classified into three distinct categories: (a) fraudulent reports, (b) discovery of biomarkers with weak clinical performance, and (c) false discovery or artifactual biomarkers.

The first category involves fraudulent publications that, in spite of the huge attention that they usually receive by scientific community and press, are extremely rare and responsible for a negligible percentage of biomarker failures [72, 73].

The second and largest category of failing biomarkers includes those biomarkers that have been discovered and validated by using robust and reliable techniques (*true discovery biomarkers*), but that never reach the clinic because of poor clinical performance (i.e. low specificity, low sensitivity, low prognostic/predictive value, and information not necessary for clinical decision-making) [35, 69].

Further details regarding this type of failing biomarkers have been discussed elsewhere [35, 58].

The third category includes cancer biomarkers that at first look highly promising (or even "revolutionary") but later on show several shortcomings, either at the discovery or validation phase (pre-analytical, analytical, post-analytical and statistic/bioinformatic artifacts), which invalidate the original performance claims (*false discovery* or *artifactual biomarkers*). Therefore, these cancer biomarkers do not reach the clinic because "the original performance claims cannot be independently reproduced in subsequent validation studies" [69].

Examples of such artifactual biomarkers have been summarized elsewhere [74–76].

Ioannidis [71] has recently proposed a classification of tumor biomarker failures, slightly different from that of Diamandis [69], that recognizes four different types: (A) clinical reversal, (B) validation failure, (C) nonoptimized clinical translation, and (D) promotion despite nonpromising evidence.

Type *A* failure (or clinical reversal) occurs when a "widely used biomarker that has already been implemented in clinical practice is shown to be largely useless or even harmful and therefore needs to be abandoned" [71]. The problem is to eliminate this obsolete test that regularly continues to be used, more frequently for non-scientific reasons, for example because of conflicts of interest of specialist practitioners.

Type *B* failure (or validation failure) occurs when a "biomarker shows great promise in one or more early studies, the claims are later found to be wrong or exaggerated, and the biomarker is eventually never implemented into clinical practice" [71]. Type *B* failure of Ioannidis's classification may be considered analogous to the third category of failing biomarkers (false discovery biomarkers) described by Diamandis [69].

Type *C* failure (or nonoptimized clinical translation) occurs when a "biomarker shows some genuine promise in one or a few early studies but this result is not followed up systematically toward clinical implementation" [71]. Type *C* failure of Ioannidis's classification may be considered analogous to the second category of failing biomarkers (true discovery biomarkers) described by Diamandis [69].

Type *D* failure (or promotion despite nonpromising evidence) occurs when a "biomarker shows no or little promise, but nevertheless is enthusiastically promoted for widespread clinical or population use" [71].

Reasons for biomarker failures and some solutions to overcome these challenges have been discussed in a seminal review [35].

2.5 Concluding Remarks and Future Perspectives

The traditional approach to treat cancer is commonly defined "trial and error" or "one size fits all". This therapeutic approach is largely empirical, costly, and frequently ineffective thus resulting in an inappropriate treatment or, worse, in drug-related toxicity [13]. As a result, "some patients with aggressive malignancy may be undertreated, and some with indolent disease may be overtreated" [13].

In the last years, cancer therapy is evolving from the traditional "one size fits all" to a new "personalized" or "individualized" approach based on the molecular characterization of the tumor and on the concept that cancer is a highly heterogeneous disease (both within a tumour and between a primary tumour and metastases) [77, 78] and consequently "each individual solid tumor and hematologic malignancy in each person is unique in cause, rate of progression and responsiveness to therapy" [79–82]. Therefore, the ultimate goal of personalized cancer therapy is to deliver "the right drug to the right patient at the right time, using the right dose and schedule" [83].

To accomplish this ambitious outcome, personalized oncology needs reliable, robust, accurate and validated cancer biomarker tests [13] in order to:

(a) differentiate patients with indolent malignancy from those with aggressive forms (prognostic markers);
(b) predict response or resistance to specific therapies so that the right patients receive the right drugs (predictive markers);
(c) identify patients who are likely to develop severe toxic side effects from specific treatments (pharmacodynamic markers).

Unfortunately, the cancer biomarkers field, just in the case of protein tumor markers, appears to be currently stagnant [36, 58] and most of the newly discovered cancer biomarkers have been either abandoned or not clinically validated because they failed to satisfy the analytical criteria necessary for clinical implementation [58, 84].

Nevertheless, recent advances in genomic technologies (i.e. next-generation sequencing) as well as in diagnostic platform for the detection of circulating tumor cells (CTCs) have allowed to identify and characterize new circulating cancer biomarkers, which are collectively defined by the scientific community with the term of "liquid biopsy" [85, 86]. *Stricto sensu*, the expression "liquid biopsy" should be restricted to CTCs by analogy with the standard definition of "tissue biopsy" [87]. However, the term "liquid biopsy" is used to identify different circulating cancer biomarkers such as CTCs but also cell-free tumor DNA (ctDNA) and microRNA (miRNA) [85, 86, 88, 89].

In this view, the detection of CTCs, ctDNA and/or miRNA could serve as a true "liquid biopsy" for cancer patients, and results much less invasive compared to surgical or endoscopic biopsy permitting also repeated samplings so tracking the current status of tumor characteristics.

"Liquid biopsy" analysis might be potentially useful at different stages of the diagnostic/therapeutic course of cancer patients, namely for: (a) early diagnosis, (b) monitoring tumor dynamics, (c) identification of genetic determinants for targeted therapy and resistance mechanisms (predictive marker), (d) evaluation of early treatment response, (e) stratification and real-time surveillance of therapies, and (f) estimation of the risk for metastatic relapse or metastatic progression (prognostic marker) [81, 89–91].

The first report on the presence of CTCs in the peripheral blood of a cancer patient was attributed to Ashworth [92]. Since then, CTCs have received enormous attention, representing one of the most active areas of translational cancer research, with more than 15,850 publications listed in PubMed in December 2014. CTCs, moreover, are used as biomarkers in more than 280 clinical trials registered at ClinicalTrials.gov.

"CTCs are rare cells that are shed from primary and metastatic tumour deposits into the peripheral circulation, and represent a means of performing noninvasive tumour sampling" [93], thus providing the opportunity to monitor serial changes in tumour biology [94].

Generally, CTCs occur at very low concentrations in the peripheral blood of cancer patients (one CTC in a background of approximately 10 million leukocytes and 5 billion erythrocytes in 1 ml of blood) [93, 95], therefore the accurate detection of CTCs with sufficient sensitivity and specificity is a major technical challenge. Up to date, the only FDA cleared technology for enumeration of CTCs in whole blood is the CellSearch® system (Veridex, Raritan, NJ) [81, 96].

The main clinical evidence for CTCs detection in various types of cancer (e.g., breast, prostate, lung, and colon cancer) is discussed in several reviews [91, 96–98]. Although CTCs are already used in numerous clinical trials as potential cancer biomarker, their clinical utility in oncology is still under investigation [88, 99].

In parallel to the progress in CTCs research, significant advancement has also been made with circulating cell-free DNA (cfDNA), whose clinical utility has been investigated in many disciplines of medicine. Circulating cell-free DNA exists at steady-state levels and increases, sometimes dramatically, with cellular injury or necrosis [100]. Like normal cells, tumor cells also release DNA fragments (ctDNA) into the circulation and significant differences in the amounts of plasma ctDNA are detected in cancer patients as compared to subjects with benign disease or healthy individuals [89]. Notably, ctDNA, which represents a very small fraction (<1.0 % and possibly as little as 0.01 %) of total cfDNA [100, 101], differs from normal cfDNA by the presence of mutations (commonly single base-pair substitutions) and may be therefore used to reconstruct tumor genomes [89, 102, 103]. The techniques for ctDNA analysis as well as the potential role of ctDNA as a diagnostic, prognostic and predictive cancer biomarker have been extensively reviewed by Ignatiadis and Dawson [104] and by Heitzer et al. [89]. Although the analysis of ctDNA constitutes a promising area of investigation, ctDNA is not yet routinely measured in clinical practice may be because is considered "not yet ready for a starring role in the clinic" [101].

Another cancer biomarker that is gaining popularity and might be used as a "liquid biopsy" is microRNA (miRNA) [105–108]. MicroRNAs are fragments of single-stranded (18–25 nucleotides long) non-coding RNAs that regulate a variety of genes (more than 50 % of all protein-coding genes) by targeting mRNA transcripts and thereby controlling various cell functions such as apoptosis, proliferation and differentiation [105, 109]. Additionally, miRNAs have emerged as critical factors in cancer pathogenesis and progression by modulating many pathological aspects related to tumor initiation, growth, metastasis, and drug resistance.

"Expression patterns of miRNAs are unique to individual tissues and differ between cancer and normal tissues. Some miRNAs are overexpressed or downregulated exclusively or preferentially in certain cancer types" [109]. The high specificity together with the remarkable stability in a wide variety of human biological fluids, including blood, make circulating miRNAs attractive biomarkers in early cancer diagnosis, prognosis and response to therapy [105–107]. The potential roles of circulating miRNAs in various cancer types are summarized in several recent reviews [105, 109, 110]. These initial promising findings notwithstanding, the role of circulating miRNAs is still under investigation and further research is warranted to ascertain the potentiality of these interesting non-coding RNA molecules [108].

Difficult as it may seem, the proposal of "liquid biopsy" looks scientifically sound. The outlook from the bedside will of course remain the same, that is the need to determine when the neoplastic process has effectively started, where is localized, what type of malignancy (aggressive or indolent) is being developed and what therapeutic approach is best for that particular patient.

In conclusion, many important information for early diagnosis, prognosis and treatment of cancer are "*written in one's blood*" whose script is still not fully decoded and made available for an application to a valid biomarker test by present knowledge and technology.

References

1. La Thangue NB, Kerr DJ (2011) Predictive biomarkers: a paradigm shift towards personalized cancer medicine. Nat Rev Clin Oncol 8(10):587–596. doi:10.1038/nrclinonc.2011.121
2. National Cancer Institute (2014) Lifetime risk tables. Available on line: http://seer.cancer.gov/csr/1975_2011/results_merged/topic_lifetime_risk.pdf. Accessed 31 Dec 2014
3. GLOBOCAN (2012) Available online: http://globocan.iarc.fr/Pages/fact_sheets_cancer.aspx. Accessed 31 Dec 2014
4. Ferlay J, Soerjomataram I, Dikshit R, Eser S, Mathers C, Rebelo M, Parkin DM, Forman D, Bray F (2015) Cancer incidence and mortality worldwide: sources, methods and major patterns in GLOBOCAN 2012. Int J Cancer 136(5):E359–E386. doi:10.1002/ijc.29210
5. Makawita S, Diamandis EP (2010) The bottleneck in the cancer biomarker pipeline and protein quantification through mass spectrometry-based approaches: current strategies for candidate verification. Clin Chem 56(2):212–222. doi:10.1373/clinchem.2009.127019
6. Biomarkers Definitions Working Group (2001) Biomarkers and surrogate endpoints: preferred definitions and conceptual framework. Clin Pharmacol Ther 69(3):89–95. doi:10.1067/mcp.2001.113989
7. Fuzery AK, Levin J, Chan MM, Chan DW (2013) Translation of proteomic biomarkers into FDA approved cancer diagnostics: issues and challenges. Clin Proteomics 10(1):13. doi:10.1186/1559-0275-10-13
8. Duffy MJ (2013) Tumor markers in clinical practice: a review focusing on common solid cancers. Med Princ Pract 22(1):4–11. doi:10.1159/000338393
9. Kulasingam V, Diamandis EP (2008) Strategies for discovering novel cancer biomarkers through utilization of emerging technologies. Nat Clin Pract Oncol 5(10):588–599. doi:10.1038/ncponc1187
10. Henry NL, Hayes DF (2012) Cancer biomarkers. Mol Oncol 6(2):140–146. doi:10.1016/j.molonc.2012.01.010
11. Paoletti C, Hayes DF (2014) Molecular testing in breast cancer. Annu Rev Med 65:95–110. doi:10.1146/annurev-med-070912-143853
12. Buyse M, Michiels S, Sargent DJ, Grothey A, Matheson A, de Gramont A (2011) Integrating biomarkers in clinical trials. Expert Rev Mol Diagn 11(2):171–182. doi:10.1586/erm.10.120
13. Duffy MJ, Crown J (2008) A personalized approach to cancer treatment: how biomarkers can help. Clin Chem 54(11):1770–1779. doi:10.1373/clinchem.2008.110056
14. Sawyers CL (2008) The cancer biomarker problem. Nature 452(7187):548–552. doi:10.1038/nature06913
15. Simon R, Roychowdhury S (2013) Implementing personalized cancer genomics in clinical trials. Nat Rev Drug Discov 12(5):358–369. doi:10.1038/nrd3979
16. Febbo PG, Ladanyi M, Aldape KD, De Marzo AM, Hammond ME, Hayes DF, Iafrate AJ, Kelley RK, Marcucci G, Ogino S, Pao W, Sgroi DC, Birkeland ML (2011) NCCN Task Force report: evaluating the clinical utility of tumor markers in oncology. J Natl Compr Canc Netw 9(Suppl 5):S1–32, quiz S33

17. Sargent DJ, Conley BA, Allegra C, Collette L (2005) Clinical trial designs for predictive marker validation in cancer treatment trials. J Clin Oncol 23(9):2020–2027. doi:10.1200/JCO.2005.01.112
18. Duffy MJ, Crown J (2014) Precision treatment for cancer: role of prognostic and predictive markers. Crit Rev Clin Lab Sci 51(1):30–45. doi:10.3109/10408363.2013.865700
19. Duffy MJ, O'Donovan N, Crown J (2011) Use of molecular markers for predicting therapy response in cancer patients. Cancer Treat Rev 37(2):151–159. doi:10.1016/j.ctrv.2010.07.004
20. August J (2010) Market watch: emerging companion diagnostics for cancer drugs. Nat Rev Drug Discov 9(5):351. doi:10.1038/nrd3173
21. Gainor JF, Longo DL, Chabner BA (2014) Pharmacodynamic biomarkers: falling short of the mark? Clin Cancer Res 20(10):2587–2594. doi:10.1158/1078-0432.CCR-13-3132
22. Guchelaar HJ, Gelderblom H, van der Straaten T, Schellens JH, Swen JJ (2014) Pharmacogenetics in the cancer clinic: from candidate gene studies to next-generation sequencing. Clin Pharmacol Ther 95(4):383–385. doi:10.1038/clpt.2014.13
23. Sarker D, Workman P (2007) Pharmacodynamic biomarkers for molecular cancer therapeutics. Adv Cancer Res 96:213–268. doi:10.1016/S0065-230X(06)96008-4
24. Shapiro GI, Rodon J, Bedell C, Kwak EL, Baselga J, Brana I, Pandya SS, Scheffold C, Laird AD, Nguyen LT, Xu Y, Egile C, Edelman G (2014) Phase I safety, pharmacokinetic, and pharmacodynamic study of SAR245408 (XL147), an oral pan-class I PI3K inhibitor, in patients with advanced solid tumors. Clin Cancer Res 20(1):233–245. doi:10.1158/1078-0432.CCR-13-1777
25. Prensner JR, Rubin MA, Wei JT, Chinnaiyan AM (2012) Beyond PSA: the next generation of prostate cancer biomarkers. Sci Transl Med 4(127):127rv123. doi:10.1126/scitranslmed.3003180
26. Negm RS, Verma M, Srivastava S (2002) The promise of biomarkers in cancer screening and detection. Trends Mol Med 8(6):288–293
27. Kanwal R, Gupta S (2012) Epigenetic modifications in cancer. Clin Genet 81(4):303–311. doi:10.1111/j.1399-0004.2011.01809.x
28. You JS, Jones PA (2012) Cancer genetics and epigenetics: two sides of the same coin? Cancer Cell 22(1):9–20. doi:10.1016/j.ccr.2012.06.008
29. Nogueira da Costa A, Herceg Z (2012) Detection of cancer-specific epigenomic changes in biofluids: powerful tools in biomarker discovery and application. Mol Oncol 6(6):704–715. doi:10.1016/j.molonc.2012.07.005
30. Barrow TM, Michels KB (2014) Epigenetic epidemiology of cancer. Biochem Biophys Res Commun 455(1–2):70–83. doi:10.1016/j.bbrc.2014.08.002
31. Coppede F, Lopomo A, Spisni R, Migliore L (2014) Genetic and epigenetic biomarkers for diagnosis, prognosis and treatment of colorectal cancer. World J Gastroenterol 20(4):943–956. doi:10.3748/wjg.v20.i4.943
32. Sandoval J, Peiro-Chova L, Pallardo FV, Garcia-Gimenez JL (2013) Epigenetic biomarkers in laboratory diagnostics: emerging approaches and opportunities. Expert Rev Mol Diagn 13(5):457–471. doi:10.1586/erm.13.37
33. Toiyama Y, Okugawa Y, Goel A (2014) DNA methylation and microRNA biomarkers for noninvasive detection of gastric and colorectal cancer. Biochem Biophys Res Commun. doi:10.1016/j.bbrc.2014.08.001
34. Konforte D, Diamandis EP (2013) Is early detection of cancer with circulating biomarkers feasible? Clin Chem 59(1):35–37. doi:10.1373/clinchem.2012.184903
35. Pavlou MP, Diamandis EP, Blasutig IM (2013) The long journey of cancer biomarkers from the bench to the clinic. Clin Chem 59(1):147–157. doi:10.1373/clinchem.2012.184614
36. Buchen L (2011) Cancer: missing the mark. Nature 471(7339):428–432. doi:10.1038/471428a
37. Diamandis EP (2010) Cancer biomarkers: can we turn recent failures into success? J Natl Cancer Inst 102(19):1462–1467. doi:10.1093/jnci/djq306
38. Dunn BK, Wagner PD, Anderson D, Greenwald P (2010) Molecular markers for early detection. Semin Oncol 37(3):224–242. doi:10.1053/j.seminoncol.2010.05.007
39. Ransohoff DF (2008) The process to discover and develop biomarkers for cancer: a work in progress. J Natl Cancer Inst 100(20):1419–1420. doi:10.1093/jnci/djn339
40. Pepe MS, Etzioni R, Feng Z, Potter JD, Thompson ML, Thornquist M, Winget M, Yasui Y (2001) Phases of biomarker development for early detection of cancer. J Natl Cancer Inst 93(14):1054–1061
41. Ransohoff DF (2007) How to improve reliability and efficiency of research about molecular markers: roles of phases, guidelines, and study design. J Clin Epidemiol 60(12):1205–1219. doi:10.1016/j.jclinepi.2007.04.020
42. Witkowska HE, Hall SC, Fisher SJ (2012) Breaking the bottleneck in the protein biomarker pipeline. Clin Chem 58(2):321–323. doi:10.1373/clinchem.2011.175034
43. Heckman-Stoddard BM (2012) Oncology biomarkers: discovery, validation, and clinical use. Semin Oncol Nurs 28(2):93–98. doi:10.1016/j.soncn.2012.03.003
44. Rifai N, Gillette MA, Carr SA (2006) Protein biomarker discovery and validation: the long and uncertain path to clinical utility. Nat Biotechnol 24(8):971–983. doi:10.1038/nbt1235
45. Frangogiannis NG (2012) Biomarkers: hopes and challenges in the path from discovery to clinical practice. Transl Res 159(4):197–204. doi:10.1016/j.trsl.2012.01.023
46. Schwamborn K (2012) Imaging mass spectrometry in biomarker discovery and validation. J Proteomics 75(16):4990–4998. doi:10.1016/j.jprot.2012.06.015
47. Schiess R, Wollscheid B, Aebersold R (2009) Targeted proteomic strategy for clinical biomarker discovery. Mol Oncol 3(1):33–44. doi:10.1016/j.molonc.2008.12.001

48. Zhang Z, Chan DW (2010) The road from discovery to clinical diagnostics: lessons learned from the first FDA-cleared in vitro diagnostic multivariate index assay of proteomic biomarkers. Cancer Epidemiol Biomarkers Prev 19(12):2995–2999. doi:10.1158/1055-9965.EPI-10-0580
49. McShane LM, Hayes DF (2012) Publication of tumor marker research results: the necessity for complete and transparent reporting. J Clin Oncol 30(34):4223–4232. doi:10.1200/JCO.2012.42.6858
50. Wagner PD, Srivastava S (2012) New paradigms in translational science research in cancer biomarkers. Transl Res 159(4):343–353. doi:10.1016/j.trsl.2012.01.015
51. Hayes DF (2013) OMICS-based personalized oncology: if it is worth doing, it is worth doing well! BMC Med 11:221. doi:10.1186/1741-7015-11-221
52. Teutsch SM, Bradley LA, Palomaki GE, Haddow JE, Piper M, Calonge N, Dotson WD, Douglas MP, Berg AO (2009) The Evaluation of Genomic Applications in Practice and Prevention (EGAPP) initiative: methods of the EGAPP Working Group. Genet Med 11(1):3–14. doi:10.1097/GIM.0b013e318184137c
53. Hayes DF (2013) From genome to bedside: are we lost in translation? Breast 22(Suppl 2):S22–S26. doi:10.1016/j.breast.2013.07.004
54. Linnet K, Bossuyt PM, Moons KG, Reitsma JB (2012) Quantifying the accuracy of a diagnostic test or marker. Clin Chem 58(9):1292–1301. doi:10.1373/clinchem.2012.182543
55. de Gramont A, Watson S, Ellis LM, Rodon J, Tabernero J, Hamilton SR (2014) Pragmatic issues in biomarker evaluation for targeted therapies in cancer. Nat Rev Clin Oncol. doi:10.1038/nrclinonc.2014.202
56. Behrens T, Bonberg N, Casjens S, Pesch B, Bruning T (2014) A practical guide to epidemiological practice and standards in the identification and validation of diagnostic markers using a bladder cancer example. Biochim Biophys Acta 1844(1 Pt A):145–155. doi:10.1016/j.bbapap.2013.07.018
57. Jennings L, Van Deerlin VM, Gulley ML (2009) Recommended principles and practices for validating clinical molecular pathology tests. Arch Pathol Lab Med 133(5):743–755. doi:10.1043/1543-2165-133.5.743
58. Diamandis EP (2014) Present and future of cancer biomarkers. Clin Chem Lab Med 52(6):791–794. doi:10.1515/cclm-2014-0317
59. Drabovich AP, Martinez-Morillo E, Diamandis EP (2014) Toward an integrated pipeline for protein biomarker development. Biochim Biophys Acta. doi:10.1016/j.bbapap.2014.09.006
60. Sahab ZJ, Semaan SM, Sang QX (2007) Methodology and applications of disease biomarker identification in human serum. Biomark Insights 2:21–43
61. Li J, Kelm KB, Tezak Z (2011) Regulatory perspective on translating proteomic biomarkers to clinical diagnostics. J Proteomics 74(12):2682–2690. doi:10.1016/j.jprot.2011.07.028
62. Yu PP, Hoffman MA, Hayes DF (2014) Biomarkers and oncology: the path forward to a learning health system. Arch Pathol Lab Med. doi:10.5858/arpa.2014-0080-ED
63. Bossuyt PM, Reitsma JB, Linnet K, Moons KG (2012) Beyond diagnostic accuracy: the clinical utility of diagnostic tests. Clin Chem 58(12):1636–1643. doi:10.1373/clinchem.2012.182576
64. Simon RM, Paik S, Hayes DF (2009) Use of archived specimens in evaluation of prognostic and predictive biomarkers. J Natl Cancer Inst 101(21):1446–1452. doi:10.1093/jnci/djp335
65. Freidlin B, McShane LM, Polley MY, Korn EL (2012) Randomized phase II trial designs with biomarkers. J Clin Oncol 30(26):3304–3309. doi:10.1200/JCO.2012.43.3946
66. Pepe MS, Feng Z, Janes H, Bossuyt PM, Potter JD (2008) Pivotal evaluation of the accuracy of a biomarker used for classification or prediction: standards for study design. J Natl Cancer Inst 100(20):1432–1438. doi:10.1093/jnci/djn326
67. IOM (2012) Evolution of translational omics: lessons learned and the path forward. Available on line: http://www.nap.edu/openbook.php?record_id=13297. Accessed 31 Dec 2014.
68. Hayes DF, Allen J, Compton C, Gustavsen G, Leonard DG, McCormack R, Newcomer L, Pothier K, Ransohoff D, Schilsky RL, Sigal E, Taube SE, Tunis SR (2013) Breaking a vicious cycle. Sci Transl Med 5(196):196cm196. doi:10.1126/scitranslmed.3005950
69. Diamandis EP (2012) The failure of protein cancer biomarkers to reach the clinic: why, and what can be done to address the problem? BMC Med 10:87. doi:10.1186/1741-7015-10-87
70. Kern SE (2012) Why your new cancer biomarker may never work: recurrent patterns and remarkable diversity in biomarker failures. Cancer Res 72(23):6097–6101. doi:10.1158/0008-5472.CAN-12-3232
71. Ioannidis JP (2013) Biomarker failures. Clin Chem 59(1):202–204. doi:10.1373/clinchem.2012.185801
72. Baggerly KA, Coombes KR (2011) What information should be required to support clinical "omics" publications? Clin Chem 57(5):688–690. doi:10.1373/clinchem.2010.158618
73. Samuel Reich E (2011) Cancer trial errors revealed. Nature 469(7329):139–140. doi:10.1038/469139a
74. Diamandis EP (2003) Point: proteomic patterns in biological fluids: do they represent the future of cancer diagnostics? Clin Chem 49(8):1272–1275
75. Diamandis EP (2004) Analysis of serum proteomic patterns for early cancer diagnosis: drawing attention to potential problems. J Natl Cancer Inst 96(5):353–356
76. Diamandis EP (2007) POINT: EPCA-2: a promising new serum biomarker for prostatic carcinoma? Clin Biochem 40(18):1437–1439. doi:10.1016/j.clinbiochem.2007.09.003

77. Meacham CE, Morrison SJ (2013) Tumour heterogeneity and cancer cell plasticity. Nature 501(7467):328–337. doi:10.1038/nature12624
78. Yap TA, Gerlinger M, Futreal PA, Pusztai L, Swanton C (2012) Intratumor heterogeneity: seeing the wood for the trees. Sci Transl Med 4(127):127ps110. doi:10.1126/scitranslmed.3003854
79. Ginsburg GS, McCarthy JJ (2001) Personalized medicine: revolutionizing drug discovery and patient care. Trends Biotechnol 19(12):491–496
80. Kalia M (2013) Personalized oncology: recent advances and future challenges. Metabolism 62(Suppl 1):S11–S14. doi:10.1016/j.metabol.2012.08.016
81. Rolfo C, Castiglia M, Hong D, Alessandro R, Mertens I, Baggerman G, Zwaenepoel K, Gil-Bazo I, Passiglia F, Carreca AP, Taverna S, Vento R, Peeters M, Russo A, Pauwels P (2014) Liquid biopsies in lung cancer: the new ambrosia of researchers. Biochim Biophys Acta 1846(2):539–546. doi:10.1016/j.bbcan.2014.10.001
82. Ross JS (2011) Cancer biomarkers, companion diagnostics and personalized oncology. Biomark Med 5(3):277–279. doi:10.2217/bmm.11.29
83. Schilsky RL, Doroshow JH, Leblanc M, Conley BA (2012) Development and use of integral assays in clinical trials. Clin Cancer Res 18(6):1540–1546. doi:10.1158/1078-0432.CCR-11-2202
84. Diamandis EP (2014) Towards identification of true cancer biomarkers. BMC Med 12(1):156. doi:10.1186/s12916-014-0156-8
85. Alix-Panabieres C, Pantel K (2013) Circulating tumor cells: liquid biopsy of cancer. Clin Chem 59(1):110–118. doi:10.1373/clinchem.2012.194258
86. Pantel K, Alix-Panabieres C (2013) Real-time liquid biopsy in cancer patients: fact or fiction? Cancer Res 73(21):6384–6388. doi:10.1158/0008-5472.CAN-13-2030
87. Ilie M, Hofman V, Long E, Bordone O, Selva E, Washetine K, Marquette CH, Hofman P (2014) Current challenges for detection of circulating tumor cells and cell-free circulating nucleic acids, and their characterization in non-small cell lung carcinoma patients. What is the best blood substrate for personalized medicine? Ann Transl Med 2(11):107. doi:10.3978/j.issn.2305-5839.2014.08.11
88. Alix-Panabieres C, Pantel K (2014) Challenges in circulating tumour cell research. Nat Rev Cancer 14(9):623–631. doi:10.1038/nrc3820
89. Heitzer E, Ulz P, Geigl JB (2014) Circulating tumor DNA as a liquid biopsy for cancer. Clin Chem. doi:10.1373/clinchem.2014.222679
90. Diaz LA Jr, Bardelli A (2014) Liquid biopsies: genotyping circulating tumor DNA. J Clin Oncol 32(6):579–586. doi:10.1200/JCO.2012.45.2011
91. Toss A, Mu Z, Fernandez S, Cristofanilli M (2014) CTC enumeration and characterization: moving toward personalized medicine. Ann Transl Med 2(11):108. doi:10.3978/j.issn.2305-5839.2014.09.06
92. Ashworth TR (1869) A case of cancer in which cells similar to those in the tumors were seen in the blood after death. Aust Med J 14:146–149
93. Miyamoto DT, Sequist LV, Lee RJ (2014) Circulating tumour cells-monitoring treatment response in prostate cancer. Nat Rev Clin Oncol 11(7):401–412. doi:10.1038/nrclinonc.2014.82
94. Heitzer E, Auer M, Gasch C, Pichler M, Ulz P, Hoffmann EM, Lax S, Waldispuehl-Geigl J, Mauermann O, Lackner C, Hofler G, Eisner F, Sill H, Samonigg H, Pantel K, Riethdorf S, Bauernhofer T, Geigl JB, Speicher MR (2013) Complex tumor genomes inferred from single circulating tumor cells by array-CGH and next-generation sequencing. Cancer Res 73(10):2965–2975. doi:10.1158/0008-5472.CAN-12-4140
95. Paterlini-Brechot P, Benali NL (2007) Circulating tumor cells (CTC) detection: clinical impact and future directions. Cancer Lett 253(2):180–204. doi:10.1016/j.canlet.2006.12.014
96. Joosse SA, Gorges TM, Pantel K (2014) Biology, detection, and clinical implications of circulating tumor cells. EMBO Mol Med. doi:10.15252/emmm.201303698
97. Cristofanilli M (2006) Circulating tumor cells, disease progression, and survival in metastatic breast cancer. Semin Oncol 33(3 Suppl 9):S9–S14. doi:10.1053/j.seminoncol.2006.03.016
98. Truini A, Alama A, Dal Bello MG, Coco S, Vanni I, Rijavec E, Genova C, Barletta G, Biello F, Grossi F (2014) Clinical applications of circulating tumor cells in lung cancer patients by cell search system. Front Oncol 4:242. doi:10.3389/fonc.2014.00242
99. Krebs MG, Metcalf RL, Carter L, Brady G, Blackhall FH, Dive C (2014) Molecular analysis of circulating tumour cells-biology and biomarkers. Nat Rev Clin Oncol 11(3):129–144. doi:10.1038/nrclinonc.2013.253
100. Diehl F, Schmidt K, Choti MA, Romans K, Goodman S, Li M, Thornton K, Agrawal N, Sokoll L, Szabo SA, Kinzler KW, Vogelstein B, Diaz LA Jr (2008) Circulating mutant DNA to assess tumor dynamics. Nat Med 14(9):985–990. doi:10.1038/nm.1789
101. Yong E (2014) Cancer biomarkers: written in blood. Nature 511(7511):524–526. doi:10.1038/511524a
102. Bettegowda C, Sausen M, Leary RJ, Kinde I, Wang Y, Agrawal N, Bartlett BR, Wang H, Luber B, Alani RM, Antonarakis ES, Azad NS, Bardelli A, Brem H, Cameron JL, Lee CC, Fecher LA, Gallia GL, Gibbs P, Le D, Giuntoli RL, Goggins M, Hogarty MD, Holdhoff M, Hong SM, Jiao Y, Juhl HH, Kim JJ, Siravegna G, Laheru DA, Lauricella C, Lim M, Lipson EJ, Marie SK, Netto GJ, Oliner KS, Olivi A, Olsson L, Riggins GJ, Sartore-Bianchi A, Schmidt K, Shih IM, Oba-Shinjo SM, Siena S, Theodorescu D, Tie J, Harkins TT, Veronese S, Wang TL, Weingart JD, Wolfgang CL, Wood LD, Xing D, Hruban RH, Wu J, Allen PJ, Schmidt CM, Choti MA, Velculescu

VE, Kinzler KW, Vogelstein B, Papadopoulos N, Diaz LA Jr (2014) Detection of circulating tumor DNA in early- and late-stage human malignancies. Sci Trans Med 6(224):224ra224. doi:10.1126/scitranslmed.3007094
103. Heitzer E, Auer M, Ulz P, Geigl JB, Speicher MR (2013) Circulating tumor cells and DNA as liquid biopsies. Genome Med 5(8):73. doi:10.1186/gm477
104. Ignatiadis M, Dawson SJ (2014) Circulating tumor cells and circulating tumor DNA for precision medicine: dream or reality? Ann Oncol 25(12):2304–2313. doi:10.1093/annonc/mdu480
105. Cheng G (2014) Circulating miRNAs: roles in cancer diagnosis, prognosis and therapy. Adv Drug Deliv Rev. doi:10.1016/j.addr.2014.09.001
106. Hayes J, Peruzzi PP, Lawler S (2014) MicroRNAs in cancer: biomarkers, functions and therapy. Trends Mol Med 20(8):460–469. doi:10.1016/j.molmed.2014.06.005
107. Shen J, Stass SA, Jiang F (2013) MicroRNAs as potential biomarkers in human solid tumors. Cancer Lett 329(2):125–136. doi:10.1016/j.canlet.2012.11.001
108. Witwer KW (2014) Circulating microRNA biomarker studies: pitfalls and potential solutions. Clin Chem. doi:10.1373/clinchem.2014.221341
109. Schwarzenbach H, Nishida N, Calin GA, Pantel K (2014) Clinical relevance of circulating cell-free microRNAs in cancer. Nat Rev Clin Oncol 11(3):145–156. doi:10.1038/nrclinonc.2014.5
110. Wang J, Zhang KY, Liu SM, Sen S (2014) Tumor-associated circulating microRNAs as biomarkers of cancer. Molecules 19(2):1912–1938. doi:10.3390/molecules19021912

Use of Biomarkers in Screening for Cancer

3

Michael J. Duffy

Abstract

Screening for premalignant lesions or early invasive disease has the potential to reduce mortality from cancer. Because of their ease of measurement, several biomarkers have been evaluated or are currently undergoing evaluation as screening tests for early malignancy. These include the use of AFP in screening for hepatocellular cancer in high-risk subjects, CA 125 in combination with transvaginal ultrasound (TVU) in screening for epithelial ovarian cancer, PSA in screening for prostate cancer, faecal occult blood testing (FOBT) in screening for colorectal cancer (CRC) and vanillymandelic acid and homovanillic acid in screening for neuroblastoma in newborn infants, Of these biomarkers, only the use of FOBT in screening for CRC has unequivocally been shown to reduce mortality from cancer. Although 2 large randomized prospective trials have evaluated PSA as a screening test for prostate cancer, it is still unclear whether the benefits outweigh the harms in this setting. Although biomarkers have many attractive features as cancer screening tests, lack of sensitivity and specificity, when combined with the low prevalence of specific cancer types in asymptomatic subjects, limit their application for the early detection of malignancy.

Keywords

AFP • Asymptomatic subjects • CA 125 • Cancer • Colorectal cancer • Criteria for disease screening • Early malignancy • FOBT • Gestational trophoblastic neoplasia • Hepatocellular cancer • Ovarian cancer •

M.J. Duffy (✉)
Clinical Research Centre, St Vincent's University Hospital, Elm Park, Dublin 4, Ireland

UCD School of Medicine and Medical Science, Conway Institute of Biomolecular and Biomedical Research, University College Dublin, Dublin 4, Ireland
e-mail: Michael.J.Duffy@ucd.ie

R. Scatena (ed.), *Advances in Cancer Biomarkers*, Advances in Experimental Medicine and Biology 867, DOI 10.1007/978-94-017-7215-0_3

Premalignant lesions • Prostate cancer • PSA • Screening • Screening advantages • Screening for cancer • Screening limitation • Screening tests • Tumor biomarkers

Screening has been defined as the systematic application of a test to identify subjects at sufficient risk of a specific disorder to benefit from further investigation or direct preventive action, among persons who have not sought medical attention on account of symptoms of that disorder [1]. To be of value, screening must detect disease earlier and result in an efficacious treatment and the earlier use of efficacious treatment must lead to a better outcome compared to treatment available at the onset of symptoms [2]. Screening for a disease differs from diagnosis in that the aim is to detect disease or a predisease state when subjects are asymptomatic. Diagnosis, on the other hand, involves investigating individuals with symptoms that may or may not be due to cancer.

3.1 Criteria for Disease Screening

Over 40 years ago, the World Health Organization (WHO) published a list of criteria that should be fulfilled prior to the introduction of a screening programme for a specific disease [3]. These criteria are:

- The condition should be an important health problem.
- There should be a treatment for the condition.
- Facilities for diagnosis and treatment should be available.
- There should be a latent stage of the disease.
- There should be a test or examination for the condition.
- The test should be acceptable to the population.
- The natural history of the disease should be adequately understood.
- There should be an agreed policy on whom to treat.
- The total cost of finding a case should be economically balanced in relation to medical expenditure as a whole.

Although these criteria were published several decades ago, they are still highly relevant and should be borne in mind before a new disease screening programme is introduced. A new criterion however, might be added, i.e., the balance of benefits of the screening programme should outweigh the harm. This is important as screening is performed on well or healthy individuals. In this situation, it is therefore important to minimize risk, while attempting to enhance benefit, as much as possible.

3.2 Advantages and Limitation of Screening

Screening and the early detection of disease has intuitive appeal as a process for reducing morbidity and mortality from disease. Indeed, it is widely believed that the early detection of disease followed by treatment results in a better outcome. While this is undoubtedly true in many situations, screening may not always result in improved outcome. There are two main prerequisites in order for screening to reduce death rates from malignancy [4]. Firstly, the process must bring forward the date of diagnosis of cancer that are destined to result in death. Secondly, early treatment of these cancers must confer an advantage relative to treatment at clinical presentation.

Screening for cancer is widely promoted, especially in the lay media. Most of this promotion focuses on the potential benefits of the practice, with little references to its limitations or its potential for harm. Indeed, most of the currently available screening tests have limitations that are not widely known by the individuals undergoing the process.

One of these limitations relates to the lack of sensitivity and specificity of the available screening tests [5]. For example, all screening tests yield false positive results, increasing anxiety and stress as well as the possibility of unnecessary investigations and treatment. In addition, no screening test displays 100 % sensitivity, leading to a false sense of security that the subject is free of the disease being screened for. Another disadvantage of screening is that it may lead to overdetection of disease that may never present clinically or cause major morbidity or mortality [5]. Finally, the performance of some screening tests may cause side effects in subjects undergoing the test. An example of this is the possibility of bleeding or perforation in subjects undergoing screening for colorectal cancer with colonoscopy [6]. Ideally, therefore, before any test is used in population screening, it should be shown in a large prospective randomized trial to reduce mortality and results in overall more benefit than harm.

Because of these limitations, most expert panels currently recommend that prior to undergoing screening, at least for cancer, that the individual be told about the potential benefits and risks associated with the process as well as the possible diagnostic test and treatment that may result from a positive screening test.

Before concluding this section, it is important to stress that although screening may result in harm in some individuals, it can reduce mortality from cancer. Indeed, it is widely believed that although screening may result in harm in some individual, its practice together with the availability of better treatments are the main reasons for the declines in specific cancers observed in a number of Western countries in recent years. A good example of a successful screening test is the use of cytology (PAP test) in screening for cervical cancer. This screening is estimated to have reduced the incidence of cervical malignancy by at least 60 % and death from cervical cancer by 20–60 % [7].

3.3 Established Screening Tests

Currently, only a small number of screening tests have been shown to reduce mortality from cancer. These include mammography in screening for breast cancer (especially in women >50 years of age), the Papanicalaou (PAP) test in screening for cervical cancer, both faecal occult blood testing (FOBT) and flexible sigmoidoscopy in screening for colorectal cancer (CRC) and low-dose computed tomography (CT) in screening high-risk subjects for lung cancer (for review, see refs [8, 9]). The use of mammography to reduce mortality from breast cancer, FOBT to decrease death from CRC and low dose CT to reduce mortality have all been validated in large randomized trials. Although the PAP test has not undergone validation in a prospective trial, large population-based studies have clearly concluded that it reduces mortality from cervical cancer.

3.4 Biomarkers in Screening for Cancer

Biomarkers have several theoretical advantages as cancer screening tests. These include:

- Biomarkers can be measured in biological fluids such as blood and urine that can be obtained with minimal inconvenience to subjects undergoing screening. This in turn should lead to high compliance rates with the screening.
- For many biomarkers, automated assays are available, allowing the processing of large numbers of samples in a relatively short period of time.
- Tests for biomarkers provide quantitative results with objective endpoints.
- Assays for biomarkers are relatively cheap.

In practice however, lack of sensitivity for early invasive disease or premalignant lesions and lack of specificity for malignancy, limit the use of most existing biomarkers in screening asymptomatic subjects for early malignancy [10, 11]. This lack of sensitivity and specificity when combined with the low prevalence of specific cancer types in the general population preclude the use of most biomarkers in screening asymptomatic populations for cancer. This is especially true with single determinations of markers or if

Table 3.1 Biomarker investigated in cancer screening

Cancer	Biomarker	Reduction in mortality
Prostate	PSA	[a]Data conflicting
Ovarian	CA 125	Unknown
[b]Hepatocellular	AFP	Yes, in a single study
Colorectal	FOBT	Yes
Neuroblastoma	[c]VMA, HVMA	No
[d]Gastric	Pepsinogen	Unknown
Gestational trophoblastic disease	HCG	Yes

[a]Results from trials provide conflicting data
[b]High risk patients investigated
[c]Vanillymandelic acid and homovanillic acid
[d]Only used in parts of Asia, where the prevalence of gastric cancer is high

markers are used alone, i.e., without backup testing (e.g., transvaginal ultrasound as a follow-up test in screening for ovarian cancer).

Although these limitations have been known for several years, a number of biomarkers have undergone evaluation as potential cancer screening tests (Table 3.1). The aim of this chapter is to critically review the role of the most widely investigated biomarkers in screening for early cancer.

3.5 AFP in Screening for Hepatocellular Cancer

Although relatively rare in the West, hepatocellular cancer (HCC) is the 3rd most frequent cause of cancer-related deaths world-wide [12]. HCC is particularly prevalent in South-east Asia and sub-Saharan Africa. Overall, almost 80 % of the newly diagnosed cases of HCC diagnosed each year occur in Asia [13]. These wide variations in incidence of HCC are mostly due to variations in risk factors, especially exposure to hepatitis B virus (HBV) or hepatitis C virus (HCV). HBV is responsible for most cases of HCC in China and Africa, whereas HCV accounts for most of the hepatitis-related cases in the Western world [12, 13]. As well as infection with HBV or HCV, other conditions that increase the risk of HCC include alcoholic cirrhosis, primary biliary cirrhosis, obesity and genetic haemochromatosis [14].

Since a group of subjects at high risk of developing HCC can be identified, i.e., patients with cirrhosis and carriers of hepatitis B or hepatitis C, screening using regular surveillance may be performed with the aim of detecting the possible development of early HCC. Two tests are widely used to screen high-risk subjects for HCC, i.e., measurement of serum AFP and performance of liver ultrasound [14].

As mentioned above, the definitive procedure for validating a screening procedure is a large randomized prospective trial. Two such trials using AFP and/or liver ultrasound to screen for HCC in high-risk subjects have been carried out in China. In the one of these trials, almost 19,000 subjects aged 35–55 years of age with hepatitis B infection or chronic hepatitis were offered bi-annual AFP measurement and ultrasound or subjected to the usual standard of care [15, 16]. Using a cut-off value of 20 μg/L, the sensitivity of AFP for HCC was 69 % and the specificity was 95 %. The positive predictive value (PPV) however, was only 3.3 %. Combining ultrasound with AFP increased sensitivity to 92 % but decreased specificity to 92.5 %. Outcome analysis showed that screening reduced mortality from HCC by 37 % [15, 16].

In the second randomised trial, screening with AFP resulted in the earlier diagnosis of HCC but this did not lead to an overall reduction in mortality [17]. A major limitation of this trial was that a high proportion of subjects with screen-detected cancers did not undergo follow-up with surgical resection.

As well as these large randomized trials, several smaller studies have investigated screening for early HCC [18]. Thus, following a systematic review of the literature, Singal et al. [18] identified 13 such studies. Meta-analysis of these 13 studies gave a sensitivity and specificity of 94 % for ultrasound. However, this sensitivity decreased to 63 % in patients with early stage HCC. Addition of AFP to ultrasound only marginally increased sensitivity, i.e., to 69 % ($p=0.65$).

In contrast to this meta-analysis of clinical trial data, a large real world study, i.e., carried out in a clinical setting, rather than as part of clinical trial, concluded that a combination of ultrasound and AFP was the most effective strategy to detect HCC at an early stage [19]. In this clinical study carried out in patients with cirrhosis, AFP had a sensitivity and specificity of 66 % and 91 %, respectively. The corresponding values for ultrasound were 44 % and 92 %. Combining AFP and ultrasound increased sensitivity to 90 % but reduced specificity to 83 %.

Although high-level evidence is lacking, especially in the Western world, several guidelines published by expert panels recommend that high-risk subjects should undergo surveillance and be screened for HCC [20–24]. However, the guidelines differ in the specific tests that they recommend. According to the National Academy of Clinical Biochemistry NACB (USA) [20], AFP should be measured and abdominal ultrasound performed at 6-monthly intervals in subjects at high risk of HCC, especially in those with hepatitis B and hepatitis C-related liver cirrhosis. AFP concentrations that are >20 μg/L and increasing should prompt further investigation, even if ultrasound is negative [20]. Similarly, the National Comprehensive Cancer Network (NCCN) recommends both regular AFP and ultrasound determination in screening high risk subjects for HCC [21]. According to this organization, additional imaging with CT or MRI is necessary if AFP levels are increasing.

In contrast to the NACB and NCCN, the American Association for the Study of Liver Disease (AASLD) state that AFP should not be used in the surveillance of high-risk groups for HCC unless ultrasound is not available [22]. According to the AASLD, AFP lacks the necessary sensitivity as a screening test for early HCC [22, 23]. Similarly, joint guidelines published by the European Association for the Study of Liver (EASL) and the European Organization for Research and Treatment of Cancer (EORTC) are opposed to the use of AFP in surveillance for HCC, claiming that the small increase in sensitivity with AFP measurement does not counterbalance the increased rate of false-positive results [23].

3.6 Use of PSA in Screening for Prostate Cancer

Prostate cancer is the most commonly diagnosed cancer in men, world-wide [25]. In recent, decades the prevalence of this malignancy has greatly increased, mainly due to an aging population and an increased use of PSA screening. Screening asymptomatic men for prostate cancer however is controversial. Some of the reasons for this controversy are as follows [26]:

- Screening may lead to overdiagnosis and consequently overtreatment of indolent disease.
- The optimum treatment for early prostate cancer is unclear, i.e., whether it should be radical prostatectomy, radiotherapy or merely active surveillance.
- PSA alone is a non-ideal screening test for early prostate cancer, lacking sensitivity and specificity.
- Consistent data from randomised prospective trials showing that screening decreases mortality from prostate cancer or does more good than harm is lacking.

In an attempt to address the effectiveness of PSA screening in decreasing mortality from prostate cancer, two large prospective randomized controlled trials have been carried out, i.e., the European Randomized Study of Prostate Cancer (ERSPC) [27] and the Prostate, Lung, Colon and Ovary trial (PLCO) [28]. The ERSPC trial was performed in 7 different European countries while the PLCO trial was based at 10 different sites in the US. Both these trials started in the middle 1990s and by 2002, over 200,000 men had been randomised [29].

Preliminary results from both the ERSPC and PLCO studies were first published in 2009. In the PLCO trial, 76,693 men were randomized to either annual screening or standard care [28]. After 7–10 years of follow-up, the incidence of prostate cancer per 10,000 person-years was 116 (2,820 cancers) in the screened group and 95 (2,322 cancers) in the control group (rate ratio, 1.22; 95 % CI, 1.16–1.29). The incidence of death per 10,000 person-years was 2.0 (50 deaths) in the screened group and 1.7 (44 deaths) in the control group (rate ratio, 1.13; 95 % CI, 0.75–1.70). Thus, after 7–10 years of follow-up, similar rates of death were found in the screened and control groups.

This trial had several limitations [30, 31]. One of these was that approximately 50 % of men in the control group underwent PSA testing during the study. This trial might thus be regarded as a comparison between annual and ad hoc screening. A further limitation was that almost 50 % of the men participating in the study had undergone PSA testing before the trial had commenced. This pre-trial testing was likely to have reduced the number of aggressive cancers in both arms. A further limitation of this trial was that the biopsy rate was only approximately 40 % in men who gave a positive screening test.

In the ERSPC study, 162,243 men, 55–69 years of age, were randomly assigned to PSA screening at an average of once every 4 years or to a control group not subjected to screening [27]. During a median follow-up of 9 years, the cumulative incidence of prostate cancer was 8.2 % in the screened group and 4.8 % in the control group. The rate ratio for death from prostate cancer in the screened group, as compared with the control group, was 0.80 (95 % CI, 0.65–0.98; adjusted $p = 0.04$), i.e., screening reduced death rates by 20 %.

Although PSA-based screening reduced the rate of death from prostate cancer by 20 %, the authors calculated that 1410 men would have to be screened and 48 cases of prostate cancer would have to undergo treatment to prevent one death from prostate cancer. These high rates however, are likely to decrease with further patient follow-up. Updated analysis of the PLCO and ERSPC studies published in 2012 gave essentially similar findings [32, 33], to that in the original analyses.

Because of the uncertainty of whether PSA screening does more good than harm, published guidelines differ as to whether men should undergo screening for prostate cancer [8, 34–37]. Thus, according to the American Cancer Society (ACS) [8], men should "make an informed decision with their doctor about whether to be tested". The ACS also state "that men should not be tested without learning about what we know and don't know about the risks and possible benefits of testing and treatment. If men decide to be tested, they should have the PSA blood test with or without a rectal exam". On the other hand the US Preventive Services Task Force (USPSTF) recommends against PSA-based screening for prostate cancer [34]. According to USPSTF, the benefits of PSA-based screening do not outweigh the harms.

3.7 Use of CA 125 in Screening for Ovarian Cancer

Although epithelial ovarian cancer is relatively rare, it is the 4th most common cause of tumor-related death in women and the most lethal gynaecological malignancy [38]. Unlike the situation in many cancers such as prostate and breast cancer, most (approximately 70 %) cases of ovarian cancer are diagnosed at an advanced stage and thus have poor outcome. Because of this large difference in outcome, it has been argued that early detection by screening should lead to a better prognosis. The main screening tests undergoing investigations for ovarian cancer are CA 125 and transvaginal ultrasound (TVU) [39, 40].

Due to the low prevalence of ovarian cancer in asymptomatic women, it is widely accepted that a screening strategy for ovarian cancer should have a PPV of at least 10 % to be clinically useful [41, 42]. With a PPV of 10 %, 10 women would be required to have surgery for every case of ovarian cancer detected. In order to achieve a PPV >10 %, a highly stringent screening strategy is required, i.e., it should possess a sensitivity of >75 % for early disease and a specificity of >99.6 % [41, 42].

Although widely used in monitoring treatment in patients with diagnosed ovarian cancer, inadequate sensitivity for stage 1 disease and lack of specificity for cancer of the ovary, preclude the use of CA 125 alone, in screening healthy women for ovarian cancer [40–42]. In order to enhance the clinical utility of CA 125 as a screening test for ovarian cancer, a variety of strategies have been attempted, including the assay of biomarkers complementary to CA 125 in addition to CA 125, sequential assays of CA 125 and a combination of CA 125 with TVU (i.e., multi-modal screening) [40–42].

It is the latter approach that has been used most frequently used in the ovarian cancer screening studies reported to date (for review, see refs. [43–49]). In multi-modal screening, CA 125 is assayed initially and TVU only performed if elevated marker concentrations are found. The advantage of this approach is that only a minority of women need to undergo TVU which reduces costs and the need for a clinical examination.

Two large randomized trials have or are currently evaluating the role of CA 125 and TVU in screening for early ovarian cancer in asymptomatic women. One of the trials known as the Prostate, Lung, Colorectal and Ovarian (PLCO) Cancer Screening Trial has been ongoing in the US for over a decade [50, 51]. This trial randomized 78,216 asymptomatic women, aged 55–74 years, to either annual screening or standard care. Women assigned to screening were offered annual CA 125 measurements for 6 years and TVU for 4 years. CA 125 levels >35 kU/L were regarded as positive.

Despite this relatively intensive screening, similar rates of mortality were found in the screened and control groups after a median follow-up of 12.4 years [51]. In addition to having no significant impact on mortality, screening was also associated with a relatively high number of false-positive findings, i.e., 3285 [51]. Due to these false-finding, 1080 (33 %) women were subjected to surgery, of whom, 163 suffered at least one serious complication (15 %).

The second large randomized trial evaluating CA 125 and TVU in screening for ovarian cancer is currently taking place in the UK, i.e., the UK Collaborative Trial of Ovarian Cancer Screening (UKCTOCS) trial [52]. In this trial, approximately 200,000 asymptomatic postmenopausal women, aged 50–74 years were randomized to annual TVU, annual CA 125 assay and a control group. All CA 125 assays were measured in the same center, using the same method.

Rather than relying on an absolute cut-off value for CA 125 concentrations as in the PLCO study, this trial is using a risk of ovarian cancer (ROC) algorithm. The algorithm includes the age of subject, rate of change in CA 125 level and absolute level of CA 125 [45, 47]. The inclusion of the rate of change in CA 125 concentration in the algorithm was based on the prior observation that while women with ovarian malignancy generally have rising marker concentrations, women with benign diseases are likely to have constant or declining values [47]. The algorithm calculates the slope (change in marker levels over time) and intercept (initial value) of the best-fit line between sequential CA 125 values. The greater the slope or intercept, the higher was the risk of ovarian cancer. The ROC algorithm was found in a preliminary analysis to be superior to that of a fixed cut-off concentration of CA 125 in early detection of ovarian cancer in postmenopausal women [45].

Early results from the UK trial have been published [52]. Of the 58 cancer detected through screening, 28 (48 %) were found to be either stage I or II. Overall sensitivity, specificity and PPV for primary and tubal malignancies were 89.4 %, 99.8 % and 35.1 %, respectively, when CA 125 and ultrasound were used in screening. Specificity and PPV but not sensitivity was significantly greater when the combined versus the when multimodal screening was used [52]. Due to inadequate follow-up, results on mortality were not presented but are expected in 2015/2016.

Thus, at present, it is unclear whether screening asymptomatic women with CA 125 measurement and TVU improves outcome in patients with ovarian cancer. Based on our current state of knowledge, it is therefore not surprising that Expert Groups in Europe and the US recommend against using CA 125, either alone or in combination with TVU, in population screening for ovarian cancer [36, 53–55].

Although screening postmenopausal women with CA 125 and TVU has not yet been shown to enhance survival in average-risk women, use of these tests in women at high risk of ovarian cancer might be beneficial, as the prevalence of disease is substantially higher in these women. Thus, in a recent study, Rosenthal et al. [56] screened 3563 women with a ≥10 % life-time risk of developing ovarian or fallopian tube cancer, using annual CA 125 determination and TVU. CA 125 was measured at separate sites using the locally available method.

Using CA 125 cut-off values of 35 and 30 IU/ml for premenopausal and postmenopausal women, respectively, sensitivity for the detection of ovarian or fallopian tube cancer at 1 year after last annual screen was 81.3 % if occult cancers were classified as false negatives and 87.5 %, if classified as true positives. Positive and negative predictive values were 25.5 and 99 %, respectively. Of the 13 incident cancer detected, 4 were either stages 1 or 2, while 9 were stage 3. A follow-up phase 2 trial to above is currently in progress. In this new trial, screening is performed every 4 months and CA 125 is being measured in a single laboratory. This single laboratory measurement should reduce inter-laboratory variation. Furthermore, in this follow-up trial, serial CA 125 levels are being interpreted with the ROC algorithm mentioned above.

3.8 Use of Faecal Occult Blood Tests in Screening for Colorectal Cancer

Colorectal cancer (CRC) is the third most common cancer, worldwide with an estimated one million new cases and a half million deaths each year [57]. CRC possess several characteristic that make it a suitable disease for population-based screening.

- Firstly, as mentioned above, it is a common serious condition and thus a major public health problem.
- Secondly, outcome is closely related to the disease stage at diagnosis. Thus, 5-year survival is approximately 90 % if the disease is detected while still localized, but only approximately 70 % when metastasis to lymph nodes are present and only about 10 % when distant metastasis are present [57].
- Thirdly, most CRCs are derived from precursor lesions known as adenomas, some of which may progress slowly to malignancy via an advanced adenoma state. Removal of these advanced adenomas reduces the risk of developing CRC.
- Fourthly, many of the molecular alterations involved in the progression of adenomas to carcinomas are now known [58]. Indeed, the specific DNA alterations responsible for this transition are potential markers for CRC screening.

Although several types of screening tests are available for CRC such as colonoscopy, flexible sigmoidoscopy and faecal marker testing (Table 3.2) [59–61], this article will focus exclusively on faecal-based markers. It should be stated that compared to endoscopic techniques (e.g., colonoscopy or sigmoidoscopy), measurement of faecal markers is relatively simple, low cost, non-invasive and can be carried out in the individual's own home. These tests are thus suitable for large population-based screening. A positive faecal occult blood test (FOBT) however, must be followed-up with a colonoscopy. A further disadvantage of FOBT is that it must be performed on a regular basis such as annually or biannually.

FOBT may be measured, either by the guaiac test which detects the pseudo peroxidase activity of haem/haemoglobin or with a faecal immunochemical test (FIT) which detects the globin antigen in haemoglobin [60, 62–64]. Of these two methods, the older guaiac test has been the more widely evaluated, especially in large randomized controlled trials. Indeed, to date, FITs have not undergone evaluation in a large prospective trial.

A systematic review of the literature identified 11 articles containing results from 4 prospective randomized controlled trials that evaluated the

Table 3.2 Screening tests for colorectal cancer and advanced colorectal adenomas. FOBT, faecal occult blood test

Colonoscopy
Flexible sigmoidoscopy
Computed tomographic colonography
Guaiac-based FOBT (gFOBTs)
Immunochemical FOBT (FITs)
Stool panel of DNA markers

guaiac FOBT in population-based screening studies for CRC [65]. Overall, the combined trials involved >300,000 subjects, with follow-up ranging from 8 to 18 years. Cumulative results from the four randomized studies showed that the subjects allocated to screening had a 16 % reduction in the relative risk of CRC mortality. Many individual invited however, did not participate in the screening programme. Following statistical adjustment of for non-attendances, the overall predicted relative mortality reduction was 25 % for the screened group. The authors concluded that FOBT screening had the potential to reduce approximately 1 in 6 deaths from CRC. Although deaths from CRC were reduced in this meta-analysis, overall mortality was not decreased.

Although screening with the guaiac test has clearly been shown to reduce mortality from CRC, this test is currently being replaced with FITs. Some of the advantages of the FIT tests compared to guaiac tests include [60–64]:

- FITs have better analytical sensitivity and specificity for human haemoglobin than guaiac-based test.
- Some FITs can be automated, thus increasing throughput and reproducibility.
- Some FITs can be quantitated, enabling adjustment of sensitivity, specificity and positivity rates to meet local requirements.
- Unlike the guaiac tests which may be affected by certain dietary components (e.g., red meat, vitamin C) and some medications (e.g., aspirin), FITs are free from interference by these factors.

FITs however, are more expensive to perform than guaiac-based tests. Furthermore, as mentioned above, FITs have not to-date been shown to reduce mortality from CRC in randomized clinical trials. However, since their accuracy in detecting CRC and advanced adenomas, is at least as good, if not better than guaiac-based tests [60–64], such validation should not be necessary. It is likely that FITs will replace guaiac-based tests in screening for CRC, in the future.

Based on the available evidence, it is not surprising that most, if not all expert panels, recommend that subjects 50 years or older should undergo screening for CRC [36, 59, 66–69]. Since the optimum screening test/strategy is still unclear, some organizations are not prescriptive as to the specific screening procedure to be used. A joint statement from the American Cancer Society, the US Multi-Society Task Force and the American College of Radiology [59] thus, stated that "clinicians should make patients aware of the full range of screening options but at a minimum, they should be prepared to offer patients a choice between a screening test that is effective at both early cancer detection and cancer prevention (e.g., colonoscopy) and a screening test that primarily is effective at early cancer detection (e.g., FOBT)". It was the strong opinion of these three organizations that colon cancer prevention should be the main goal of cancer screening. The EGTM panel, on the other hand, recommend FOBT using a FIT in screening for CRC [69].

3.9 Use of hCG in Screening for Gestational Trophoblastic Neoplasia

Women who develop hydatidiform molar pregnancies have an increased risk of developing gestational trophoblastic neoplasia (GTN) such as an invasive mole or choriocarcinoma. Data from the UK suggests that malignancy can occur in approximately 1 % of women who have had a partial mole and in about 15 % of those with a complete hydatidiform mole. Because of this increased risk, such women undergo regular surveillance with hCG measurements [70, 71]. According to the International Federation of Gynecology and Obstetrics (FIGO) committee on gynaecological oncology [72], early onset of malignancy can be detected when:

- The plateau of hCG lasts for four measurements over a period of 3 weeks or longer; that is, days 1, 7, 14, 21.
- If there is a rise of hCG of three weekly consecutive measurements or longer, over at least a period of 2 weeks or more; days 1, 7, 14.

- If hCG level remains elevated for 6 months or more.
- If there is a histologic diagnosis of choriocarcinoma.

The measurement of serial levels of hCG and the early initiation of chemotherapy when these levels suggest early malignancy, has greatly reduced deaths from GTN in recent decades. Indeed, death from GTD is now extremely rare. In contrast, prior to the use of this strict monitoring with hCG, mortality from GTD was relatively common.

3.10 Conclusion

Although intuitively appealing, the success of biomarkers in screening for early cancer has been disappointing. Indeed, the discovery and validation of biomarkers for this purpose presents a major challenge. Despite efforts by the Early Detection Research Network (EDRN) [73], few new promising cancer screening biomarkers have emerged in recent years. Furthermore, new technologies such as gene expression microarray and proteomics have so far been slow in providing useful leads. The "holy grail" of a simple blood test for the early detection of cancer therefore remains.

Indeed, the question needs to be addressed whether the measurement of a single biomarker in serum can provide a reliable test for the early detection of cancer. Small or surgically resectable cancers are likely to release relatively low concentrations of biomarkers into blood. This, coupled with the large dilution in blood following release, presents a major challenge in devising assays to detect biomarker levels above background. Rather than using blood as the source of biomarker, an alternative might be to use proximal fluids, i.e., fluids that are released from adjacent tumors. In this context, it should be pointed out that preliminary results suggest that the measurement of methylated genes in sputum is a promising new test for the early detection of lung cancer [74]. Similarly, the measurement faecal molecular marker is a promising new approach for the early diagnosis of CRC [75].

Acknowledgements Funding is acknowledged in part from Science Foundation Ireland, Strategic Research Cluster Award (08/SRC/B1410) to Molecular Therapeutics for Cancer Ireland (MTCI)/ National Cancer Research Centre of Ireland (NCRCI) and in part from the BREAST-PREDICT Collaborative Cancer Research Centre programme (CCRC113GAL), of the Irish Cancer Society.

References

1. Wald NJ (1994) Guidance on terminology. J Med Screen 1:76
2. Brawley OW, Kramer BS (2005) Cancer screening in theory and in practice. J Clin Oncol 23:293–300
3. Wilson JMG, Jungner G (1968) Principles and practice of screening for disease. WHO Chronicle Geneva: World Health Organization 22(11):473. Public Health Papers, #34
4. Bleyer A, Welch G (2012) Effects of three decades of screening mammography on breast cancer incidence. N Engl J Med 367:1998–2005
5. Miller AB (2010) Conundrums in screening for cancer. Int J Cancer 126:1039–1046
6. Lieberman DA (2009) Clinical practice. Screening for colorectal cancer. N Engl J Med 361:1179–1187
7. Moyer VA (2012) US preventive services task force. Screening for cervical cancer: US preventive services task force recommendation statement. Ann Int Med 156:880–891
8. Smith RA, Cokkinides V, Brawley OW (2012) Cancer screening in the United States, 2012: a review of current American Cancer Society guidelines and current issues in cancer screening. CA Cancer J Clin 63:88–105
9. Bretthauer M, Kalager M (2013) Principles, effectiveness and caveats in screening for cancer. Br J Surg 100:55–65
10. Duffy MJ (2001) Clinical uses of tumor markers: a critical review. Crit Rev Clin Lab Sci 38:225–262
11. Roulston JE (1990) Limitations of tumor markers in screening. Br J Surg 77:961–962
12. Maluccio M, Covey A (2012) Recent progress in understanding, diagnosing, and treating hepatocellular carcinoma. CA Cancer J Clin 62:394–399
13. Song P, Tang W, Tamura S, Hasegawa K, Sugawara Y, Dong J, Kokudo N (2010) The management of hepatocellular carcinoma in Asia: a guideline combining quantitative and qualitative evaluation. Biosci Trends 4:283–287
14. Parikh S, Hyman D (2007) Hepatocellular cancer: a guide for the internist. Am J Med 120:194–202
15. Zhang B, Yang B (1999) Combined alpha fetoprotein testing and ultrasonography as screening tests for primary liver cancer. J Med Screen 6:108–110
16. Zhang B-H, Yang B-H, Tang ZY (2004) Randomized controlled trial of screening for hepatocellular carcinoma. J Cancer Clin Oncol 130:417–422
17. Chen J-G, Parkin DM, Chen Q-G, Lu J-H, Shen Q-J, Zhang B-C et al (2003) Screening for liver cancer:

results of a randomised controlled trial in Qidong, China. J Med Screen 10:204–209
18. Singal A, Volk ML, Waljee A, Salgia R, Higgins P, Rogers MA, Marrero JA (2009) Meta-analysis: surveillance with ultrasound for early-stage hepatocellular carcinoma in patients with cirrhosis. Aliment Pharmacol Ther 30:37–47
19. Singal AG, Conjeevaram HS, Volk ML, Fu S, Fontana RJ, Askari F, Su GL, Lok AS, Marrero JA (2012) Effectiveness of hepatocellular carcinoma surveillance in patients with cirrhosis. Cancer Epidemiol Biomarkers Prev 21:793–799
20. Sturgeon C, Duffy MJ, Hoffman BR, Lamerz R, Fritsche H, Gaarestrom K et al (2010) National Academy of Clinical Biochemistry Laboratory Medicine Practice Guidelines for use of tumor markers in liver, bladder, cervical and gastric cancers. Clin Chem 56:e1–e48
21. National Comprehensive Cancer Network (NCCN) (2012) Clinical practice guidelines in Oncology, Hepatobiliary cancers version 2. http://www.nccn.org/. Accessed 18 Apr 2013
22. Bruix J, Sherman M (2005) Management of hepatocellular carcinoma. Hepatology 42:1208–1236
23. Bruix J, Sherman M, American Association for the Study of Liver Diseases (2011) Management of hepatocellular carcinoma: an update. Hepatology 53:1020–1022
24. Verslype C, Rosmorduc O, Rougier P, ESMO Guidelines Working Group (2012) Hepatocellular carcinoma: ESMO-ESDO clinical practice guidelines for diagnosis, treatment and follow-up. Ann Oncol 23(Suppl 7):vii41–vii48
25. Jemal A, Bray F, Center MM, Ferlay J, Ward E, Forman D (2011) Global cancer statistics. CA Cancer J Clin 61:69–90
26. Duffy MJ (2011) Prostate-specific antigen: does the current evidence support its use in prostate cancer screening? Ann Clin Biochem 48:310–316
27. Schröder FH, Hugosson J, Roobol MJ, Tammela TL, Ciatto S, Nelen V et al (2009) Screening and prostate-cancer mortality in a randomized European study. N Engl J Med 26(360):1320–1328
28. Andriole GL, Crawford ED, Grubb RL 3rd, Buys SS, Chia D, Church TR et al (2009) Mortality results from a randomized prostate-cancer screening trial. N Engl J Med 360:1310–1319
29. De Koning HJ, Auvinen A, Berenguer Sanchez A et al (2002) Large-scale randomised prostate cancer screening trials: program performances in the European randomised screening for prostate cancer trial and the prostate, lung, colorectal and ovary cancer trial. Int J Cancer 97:237–244
30. Barry M (2009) Screening for prostate cancer, the controversy that refused to die. N Engl J Med 13:1351–1354
31. Schröder FH (2012) Landmarks in prostate cancer screening. BJU Int 110(Suppl 1):3–7
32. Andriole GL, Crawford ED, Grubb RL 3rd, Buys SS, Chia D, Church TR, Fouad MN, Isaacs C, Kvale PA, Reding DJ, Weissfeld JL, Yokochi LA, O'Brien B, Ragard LR, Clapp JD, Rathmell JM, Riley TL, Hsing AW, Izmirlian G, Pinsky PF, Kramer BS, Miller AB, Gohagan JK, Prorok PC, PLCO Project Team (2012) Prostate cancer screening in the randomized prostate, lung, colorectal, and ovarian cancer screening trial: mortality results after 13 years of follow-up. J Natl Cancer Inst 104:125–132
33. Schröder FH, Hugosson J, Roobol MJ, Tammela TL, Ciatto S, Nelen V, Kwiatkowski M, Lujan M, Lilja H, Zappa M, Denis LJ, Recker F, Páez A, Määttänen L, Bangma CH, Aus G, Carlsson S, Villers A, Rebillard X, van der Kwast T, Kujala PM, Blijenberg BG, Stenman UH, Huber A, Taari K, Hakama M, Moss SM, de Koning HJ, Auvinen A (2012) ERSPC investigators. Prostate-cancer mortality at 11 years of follow-up. N Engl J Med 15(366):981–990
34. Moyer VA, U.S. Preventive Services Task Force (2012) Screening for prostate cancer: U.S. Preventive Services Task Force recommendation statement. Ann Intern Med 157:120–134
35. Semjonow A, Albrecht W, Bialk P, Gerl A, Lamerz R, Schmid HP et al (1999) Tumor markers in prostate cancer: EGTM recommendations. Anticancer Res 19:2785–2820
36. Sturgeon CM, Duffy MJ, Stenman UK, Lilja H, Brünner N, Chan DW et al (2008) National academy of clinical biochemistry laboratory medicine practice guidelines for use of tumor markers in testicular, prostate, colorectal, breast and ovarian cancers. Clin Chem 54:e11–e79
37. Horwich A, Hugosson J, de Reijke T, Wiegel T, Fizazi K, Kataja V, Panel Members (2013) Prostate cancer: ESMO consensus conference guidelines 2012. Ann Oncol 24:1141–1162
38. Romero I, Bast RC Jr (2012) Minireview: human ovarian cancer: biology, current management, and paths to personalizing therapy. Endocrinology 153:1593–1602
39. Hensley ML, Castiel M, Robson ME (2000) Screening for ovarian cancer: what we know, what we need to know. Oncology 14:1601–1616
40. Clarke-Pearson DL (2009) Screening for ovarian cancer. N Engl J Med 361:170–176
41. Rosenthal AN, Jacobs IJ (1998) The role of CA 125 in screening for ovarian cancer. Int J Biol Markers 13:216–220
42. Bast RC Jr, Urban N, Shridhar V (2002) Early detection of ovarian cancer: promise and reality. Cancer Treat Res 107:61–97
43. Jacobs I, Davies AP, Bridges J, Stabile I, Fay T, Lower A et al (1993) Prevalence screening for ovarian cancer in postmenopausal women by CA 125 measurements and ultrasonography. Br Med J 306:1030–1034
44. Jacobs I, Skates SJ, MacDonald N, Menon U, Rosenthal AN, Davies AP et al (1999) Screening for ovarian cancer: a pilot randomised controlled trial. Lancet 353:1207–1210
45. Menon U, Skates SJ, Lewis S, Rosenthal AN, Rufford B, Sibley K et al (2005) Prospective study using the risk of ovarian cancer algorithm to screen for ovarian cancer. J Clin Oncol 23:7919–7926

46. Menon U, Jacobs I (2002) Screening for ovarian cancer. Best Pract Res Clin Obstet Gynaecol 16:469–482
47. Skates SJ, Xy F-J, Yu Y-H, Sjövall K, Einhorn N, Chang Y et al (1995) Towards an optimal algorithm for ovarian cancer screening with longitudinal tumor markers. Cancer 76:2004–2010
48. Skates SJ, Menon U, MacDonald N, Rosenthal AN, Oram DH, Knapp RC et al (2003) Calculation of the risk of ovarian cancer from serial CA 125 values for preclinical detection in postmenopausal women. J Clin Oncol 21:206s–210s
49. Buys SS, Partridge E, Greene MH, Prorok PC, Reading D et al (2005) Ovarian cancer screening in the Prostate, Lung, Colorectal and Ovarian (PLCO) cancer screening trial. Am J Obstet Gynecol 193:1630–1639
50. Partridge E, Kreimer AR, Greenlee RT, Williams C, Xu JL, Church TR et al (2009) Results from four rounds of ovarian cancer screening in a randomized trial. Obstet Gynecol 113:775–782
51. Buys SS, Partridge E, Black A, Johnson CC, Lamerato L, Isaacs C, Reding DJ, Greenlee RT, Yokochi LA, Kessel B, Crawford ED, Church TR, Andriole GL, Weissfeld JL, Fouad MN, Chia D, O'Brien B, Ragard LR, Clapp JD, Rathmell JM, Riley TL, Hartge P, Pinsky PF, Zhu CS, Izmirlian G, Kramer BS, Miller AB, Xu JL, Prorok PC, Gohagan JK, Berg CD, PLCO Project Team (2011) Effect of screening on ovarian cancer mortality: the Prostate, Lung, Colorectal and Ovarian (PLCO) cancer screening randomized controlled trial. JAMA 305:2295–2303
52. Menon U, Gentry-Maharaj A, Hallett R, Ryan A, Burnell M, Sharma A, Lewis S et al (2009) Sensitivity and specificity of multimodal and ultrasound screening for ovarian cancer, and stage distribution of detected cancers: results of the prevalence screen of the UK Collaborative Trial of Ovarian Cancer Screening (UKCTOCS). Lancet Oncol 10:327–340
53. Duffy MJ, Bonfrer JM, Kulpa J, Rustin GJS, Soletormos G, Torre GC et al (2005) CA 125 in ovarian cancer: European Group on Tumor Markers (EGTM) guidelines for clinical use. Int J Gynecol Cancer 15:679–691
54. Lambert M (2012) ACS releases updated guidelines on cancer screening. Am Fam Physician 86(571):576–577
55. Morgan RJ, Alvarez RD, Armstrong DK, Burger RA, Castells M, Chen LM, Copeland L, Crispens MA, Gershenson D, Gray H, Hakam A, Havrilesky LJ, Johnston C, Lele S, Martin L, Matulonis UA, O'Malley DM, Penson RT, Remmenga SW, Sabbatini P, Santoso JT, Schilder RJ, Schink J, Teng N, Werner TL, Hughes M, Dwyer MA (2012) Ovarian cancer, version 3.2012. J Natl Compr Canc Netw 10:1339–1349
56. Rosenthal AN, Fraser L, Manchanda R, Badman P, Philpott S, Mozersky J, Hadwin R, Cafferty FH, Benjamin E, Singh N, Evans DG, Eccles DM, Skates SJ, Mackay J, Menon U, Jacobs IJ (2013) Results of annual screening in phase i of the United Kingdom familial ovarian cancer screening study highlight the need for strict adherence to screening schedule. J Clin Oncol 31:49–57
57. Cunningham D, Atkin W, Lenz HJ, Lynch HT, Minsky B, Nordlinger B, Starling N (2010) Colorectal cancer. Lancet 375:1030–1047
58. Fearon ER (2011) Molecular genetics of colorectal cancer. Annu Rev Pathol 6:479–507
59. Levin B, Lieberman DA, McFarland B, Smith RA, Brooks D, Andrews KS et al (2008) Screening and surveillance for the early detection of colorectal cancer and adenomatous polyps, 2008: a joint guideline from the American Cancer Society, the US multi-society task force on colorectal cancer, and the American College of Radiology. CA Cancer J Clin 58:130–160
60. Allison JE, Fraser CG, Halloran SP, Young GP (2012) Comparing fecal immunochemical tests: improved standardization is needed. Gastroenterology 142:422–424
61. Mandel JS (2007) Which colorectal cancer screening test is best? J Natl Cancer Inst 99:1424–1425
62. Allison JE, Tekawa IS, Ransom LJ, Adrain AL (1996) A comparison of fecal occult-blood tests for colorectal-cancer screening. N Engl J Med 334:155–159
63. Allison JE, Sakoda LC, Levin TR, Tucker JP, Tekawa IS, Cuff T et al (2007) Screening for colorectal neoplasms with new fecal occult blood tests: update on performance characteristics. J Natl Cancer Inst 99:1462–1470
64. Fraser CG (2012) A future for faecal haemoglobin measurements in the medical laboratory. Ann Clin Biochem 49:518–526
65. Hewitson P, Glasziou P, Irwig L, Towler B, Watson E (2007) Screening for colorectal cancer using fecal the occult blood test, Hemoccult. Cochrane Database Syst Rev (1):CD001216. doi:10.1002/14651858.CD001216.pub2
66. National Comprehensive Cancer Network Clinical Practice Guidelines in Oncology, Colorectal Cancer Screening. (2008). Version 2. Available at http://www.nccn.org/physician_gls?PDF/colorectal_screening.pdf. Accessed 12 Nov 2008
67. Duffy MJ, van Dalen A, Haglund C, Hansson L, Holinski-Feder E, Klapdor R et al (2007) Tumor markers in colorectal cancer: European Group on Tumor Markers (EGTM) guidelines for clinical use. Eur J Cancer 43:1348–1360
68. US Prevenntive Services Task Force (2008) Screening for colorectal cancer: U.S. Preventive Services Task Force recommendation statement. Ann Int Med 149:627–637
69. Duffy MJ, van Rossum LG, van Turenhout ST, Malminiemi O, Sturgeon C, Lamerz R, Nicolini A, Haglund C, Holubec L, Fraser CG, Halloran SP

(2011) Use of faecal markers in screening for colorectal neoplasia: a European group on tumor markers position paper. Int J Cancer 128:3–11
70. Seckl MJ, Sebire NJ, Berkowitz RS (2010) Gestational trophoblastic disease. Lancet 376:717–729
71. Schmid P, Nagai Y, Agarwal R, Hancock B, Savage PM, Sebire NJ, Lindsay I, Wells M, Fisher RA, Short D, Newlands ES, Wischnewsky MB, Seckl MJ (2009) Prognostic markers and long-term outcome of placental-site trophoblastic tumours: a retrospective observational study. Lancet 374:48–55
72. FIGO Oncology Committee (2002) FIGO staging for gestational trophoblastic neoplasia 2000. FIGO Oncology Committee. Int J Gynaecol Obstet 77:285–287
73. Srivastava S (2013) The early detection research network: 10-year outlook. Clin Chem 59:60–67
74. Leng S, Do K, Yingling CM, Picchi MA, Wolf HJ, Kennedy TC, Feser WJ, Baron AE, Franklin WA, Brock MV, Herman JG, Baylin SB, Byers T, Stidley CA, Belinsky SA (2012) Defining a gene promoter methylation signature in sputum for lung cancer risk assessment. Clin Cancer Res 18:3387–3395
75. Kanthan R, Senger JL, Kanthan SC (2012) Fecal molecular markers for colorectal cancer screening. Gastroenterol Res Pract 2012:184343

The Role of Metabolomics in the Study of Cancer Biomarkers and in the Development of Diagnostic Tools

4

Jean-Pierre Trezzi, Nikos Vlassis, and Karsten Hiller

Abstract

This chapter introduces the emerging field of metabolomics and its application in the context of cancer biomarker research. Taking advantage of modern high-throughput technologies, and enhanced computational power, metabolomics has a high potential for cancer biomarker identification and the development of diagnostic tools. This chapter describes current metabolomics technologies used in cancer research, starting with metabolomics sample preparation, elaborating on current analytical methodologies for metabolomics measurement and introducing existing software for data analysis. The last part of this chapter deals with the statistical analysis of very large metabolomics datasets and their relevance for cancer biomarker identification.

Keywords

Analysis of body fluids • Biomarkerdetermination • Cerebrospinal fluid (CSF) • Data normalization • Diagnostic tool • Feces analysis • Gas chromatography • High-performance liquid chromatography (HPLC) • Liquid chromatography • Mass spectrometry • Metabolite extraction • Metabolites • Metabolomics • Metabolomics data analysis tools • Metabolomicsdatasets • Metabolomicstechnologies • Metabolomicsworkflow • NMR spectroscopy • Plasma analysis • Primary metabolites • Saliva analysis • Secondary metabolites • Serum analysis • Statistical analysis • Urine analysis

J.-P. Trezzi • K. Hiller (✉)
Luxembourg Centre for Systems Biomedicine, University of Luxembourg, 7, avenue des Hauts-Fourneaux, 4362 Esch-sur-Alzette, Luxembourg
e-mail: karsten.hiller@uni.lu

N. Vlassis
Adobe Research, San Jose, CA (USA)

R. Scatena (ed.), *Advances in Cancer Biomarkers*, Advances in Experimental Medicine and Biology 867, DOI 10.1007/978-94-017-7215-0_4

4.1 Introduction to Metabolomics

Cancer is one of the most prevailing causes for death in developed countries. In order to meet all the necessary requirements and facilitate uncontrolled cell proliferation, tumor cells are forced to alter their metabolism. First approaches in cancer metabolism date back to the 1920s, when Otto Warburg showed an alteration of the cancer cell metabolism. He observed that cancer cells show an increase in glucose uptake and lactic acid production combined with reduced oxygen consumption. Even in sufficient presence of oxygen, cancer cells seem to prefer metabolizing glucose into lactic acid instead of pursuing oxidative phosphorylation [1, 2]. However, not much is known about the underlying metabolic mechanisms of the "Warburg effect", which is still highly discussed in the research community [3]. Therefore, the ultimate goal of cancer metabolomics is to understand its "biochemical fingerprint" and to take this information for diagnostic, prognostic and predictive purposes.

In the last decades, much effort was put into the optimization of sensitive high-throughput metabolomics technologies, the development of sophisticated computational algorithms and statistical data analysis pipelines. This chapter highlights the potential of metabolomics for cancer biomarker identification and the development of diagnostic tools.

The emerging field of metabolomics involves the comprehensive analysis of the metabolome (the total set of metabolites or small molecules) of a given cell, tissue or organism and can be seen as the integrated output of cellular reactions involving its genome, its transcriptome, its proteome as well as environmental influences. All components of these different "omics" levels have a strong interaction within a biological system (Fig. 4.1). Analyzing the metabolome may provide the most sensitive approach for detecting cellular and environmental changes in a biological system. As an example, an enzyme perturbation generally remains undetected on the level of the genome, transcriptome or proteome, but is detectable at the metabolomics level. On the other hand, a genetic perturbation (e.g. mutation) can also be detected by analyzing the metabolome. As metabolomics is depicting the final phenotype of a given cell or organism, it has a very high potential as a suitable cancer biomarker discovery and analysis tool.

Metabolomics studies can basically be divided into two classes: Targeted and non-targeted. A targeted analysis is used for the identification and quantification of pre-defined metabolites [4, 5]. A non-targeted study consists of analyzing all accessible metabolites in a given sample. Although non-targeted approaches are by far not as specific and sensitive as targeted approaches, in cancer biomarker discovery studies, non-targeted approaches are the first choice as the whole metabolic profile including unknown compounds is screened. Thus, differentiation of the different experimental classes (case vs. control) becomes possible by statistical analysis of the different metabolic profiles. Later on, targeted approaches may further elaborate the cancer biomarker study by more specific analysis of the previously determined biomarkers.

One of the most important characteristics of every metabolism is its very fast turnover. Many metabolites have a very limited half-life as they are constantly produced and degraded by biochemical reactions [6]. This characteristic is one of the major challenges for any metabolomics study as processing time can easily become a limiting factor in terms of sensitivity and reproducibility. In addition to constant dynamic changes, physical and chemical properties of metabolites are further complicating their analysis. In contrast to the analytical accessibility of the relatively homogeneous macromolecules of the genome (4 nucleotides), the transcriptome and the proteome (20 amino acids), the metabolome represents a vast diversity of chemical structures.

Formally, **metabolites** or small molecules are defined as molecules with a molecular mass below 1500 Da and are involved in thousands of enzyme-catalyzed biochemical processes. They

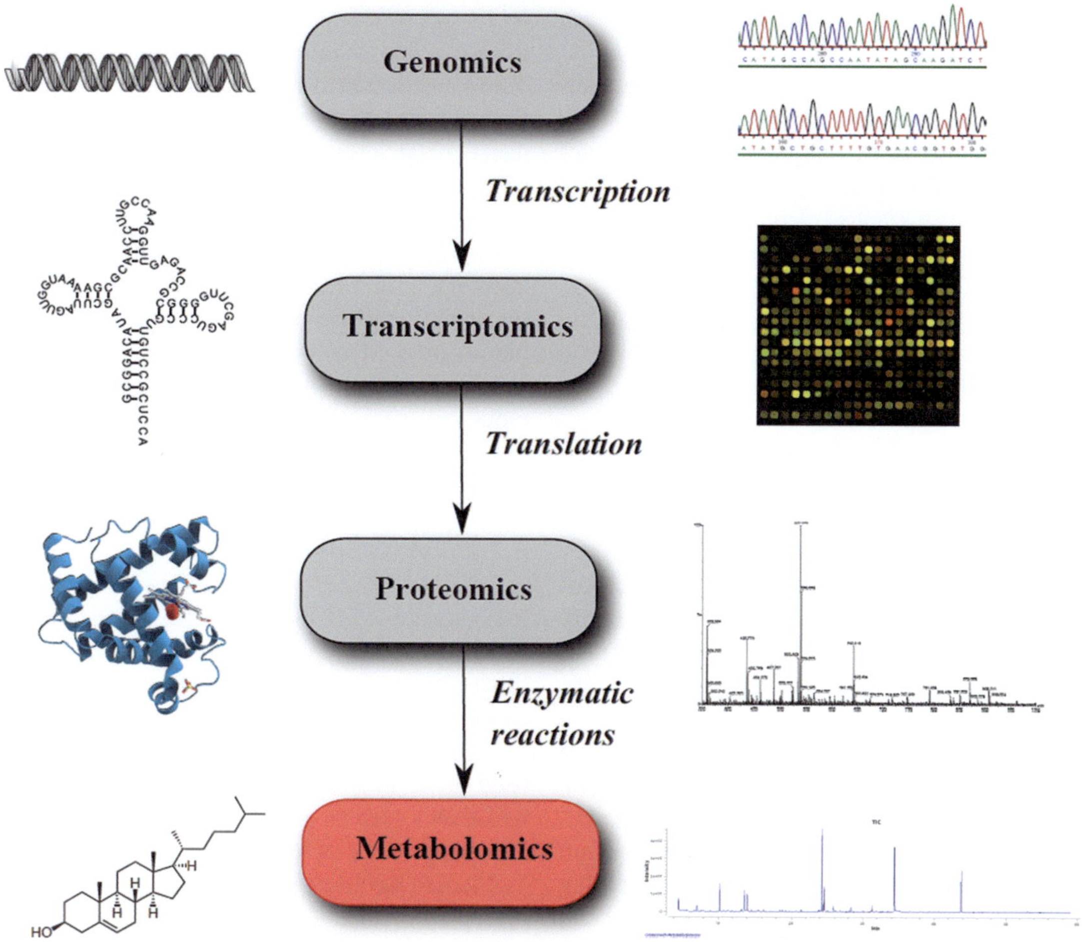

Fig. 4.1 Position of metabolomics in Systems Biology. Metabolomics is downstream of all other '-omes' and thus probably the most sensitive approach for detecting cellular and environmental changes in a biological system

link intra- and extracellular biochemical reactions to metabolic pathways crucial for a well-coordinated functioning within a cell. Therefore, metabolites are directly linked to the actual in vivo state of a given organism. Up till now, the total number of metabolites participating in human metabolism is still unknown. The human metabolome database (http://www.hmdb.ca) lists over 7900 metabolites that had been measured and identified in humans, whereas only 2000 of them are of direct human origin [7].

Metabolites can be divided in two main groups: primary metabolites and secondary metabolites. The former are essential metabolites involved in fundamental life processes, such as reproduction or growth. This group consists of a multitude of metabolites corresponding to different substance classes e.g. sugars, organic acids, amino acids, lipids, nucleotides etc. Without these metabolites, the organism would not be viable. Secondary metabolites are mostly non-essential metabolites that appear to play important roles in very specific pathways or under special conditions and are not directly involved in essential life processes. Plant-derived secondary metabolites, such as quinones (e.g. plumbagin, juglone and thymoquinone) have been shown to possess anti-metastasis and anti-proliferation effects in different in vitro and in vivo cancer models [8].

4.2 Analytical Technologies

Although many analytical techniques for metabolite measurement have been developed, mainly three technologies are applied: liquid chromatography coupled to mass spectrometry (LC/MS), gas chromatography coupled to mass spectrometry (GC/MS) and nuclear magnetic resonance (NMR) spectroscopy.

4.2.1 NMR

NMR spectroscopy is a quantitative high-throughput technology based on the magnetic properties of metabolite atom nuclei. Nuclear energy levels are defined by "spin states", characterizing the spinning behavior of the electrical charge of a nucleus. In metabolomics, primarily ^{1}H and ^{13}C NMR spectroscopy are applied. These atoms are of high interest as they can only have two spin states: spin-up (+½) and spin-down (−½). In a given metabolite, there will also be a mixture of different ^{1}H or ^{13}C spin states [9]. Applying a strong electromagnetic field makes the magnetic nuclei move from a low-energy spin level to a high-energy spin level by absorbing electromagnetic radiation coming from a second electromagnetic field (radiofrequency). After a certain time, the nuclei emit electromagnetic radiation and move back to a low-energy state. Each chemical group is characterized by the range of frequencies (chemical shift, showing the electron density around nuclei) applied on the electromagnetic field [9]. As an example, in $-CH_3$ (methyl) groups the chemical shift will be lower than for –CHO (aldehyde) groups because of the higher electronegativity of the oxygen atom that forces the electrons to move in its direction instead of staying nearby the H atoms.

The main advantages of NMR spectroscopy are that it is non-destructive (non-invasive), there is normally no prior metabolite separation or chemical modification required and the metabolites are easily quantifiable. NMR can also be considered as a non-biased method, as every metabolite containing atoms with an odd number of electrons (^{1}H, ^{13}C) can be detected. Therefore, NMR spectroscopy represents an effective quantification and identification method. However, due to the low sensitivity compared to mass spectrometry approaches (e.g. LC/MS), low abundance metabolites cannot be detected and signal overlaps can occur when measuring complex samples, such as human blood serum. Ludwig et al. [5] proposed a targeted NMR metabolomics approach to reduce this issue and could detect a metabolic signature in colorectal cancer in human blood serum. Many other promising NMR cancer studies have been published, e.g. for oral squamous cell carcinoma, breast cancer, colorectal cancer and pancreatic cancer [10–13].

4.2.2 Mass Spectrometry

In contrast to NMR-based studies, mass spectrometric analyses typically rely on a metabolite separation prior to MS measurement, especially for complex samples such as human blood serum or plasma. Therefore, mass spectrometry is rarely used alone and is often coupled to separation techniques such as gas chromatography (GC) or liquid chromatography (LC).

Modern **liquid chromatography** devices, like high-performance liquid chromatography (HPLC) instruments are equipped with an HPLC column operating under high pressure which has shown great potential in enhancing the chromatographic separation [14, 15]. Applying high pressures, the metabolites are forced through the column and provide a better resolution compared to conventional LC methods. After separation, metabolites need to be ionized prior to detection. Ionization techniques such as electrospray ionization (ESI) have to be performed [16].

However, soft ESI methods do not provide much compound characterization information due to the absence of compound fragmentation during ionization. To circumvent this problem, several methods are used in LC/MS studies. Tandem mass spectrometry (MS/MS) is the combination of two mass analyzers, e.g. quadrupole (Q) and time-of-flight (TOF) analyzers (Fig. 4.2). In the quadrupole analyzer (MS1), specific ions (precursor ions) are selected and subsequently

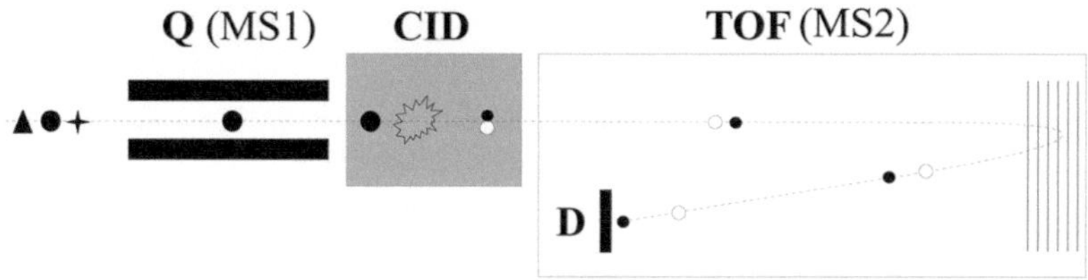

Fig. 4.2 Schematic overview of a Q-TOF analyser. After ionization, target ions are selected by the quadrupole analyser (Q/MS1) and deviated into a collision cell (CID) where they collide with gas molecules and thereby get fragmented. Finally, the fragment ions reach the TOF analyser (MS2) in which their complete mass spectrum is recorded based on flight time (Courtesy of Dr. Christian Jäger)

fragmented in a collision cell (CID). The product ions are transmitted to a time-of-flight analyzer (MS2) to obtain a complete mass spectrum of the dissociated precursor ion.

Several other techniques follow this principle: (1) ionization, (2) precursor ion selection, (3) collision-induced dissociation (CID), (4) mass analysis, (5) Detection (D). These techniques are highly relevant in targeted approaches due to their specific ion filtering. The most common techniques are triple quadrupole analyzers (QqQ) or quadrupole ion trap analyzers (QTRAP). Besides the measurement of ion mass over charge ratio (m/z), QTRAPs are able to confine ions of interest by electrostatic attraction [17]. For metabolomics purposes, QTRAP analyzers, Orbitraps [18] and Fourier transform mass spectrometers [19] provide good accurate masses.

Using LC-MS/MS metabolomics strategies, Zhang et al. found that epoxy docosapentaenoic acid, which is synthesized from the omega-3 fatty acid docosahexaenoic acid, is inhibiting angiogenesis in vivo and in vitro. Apart from inhibiting angiogenesis, the authors show that EDP is also inhibiting VEGF Receptor 2 signaling, the primary tumor growth and tumor metastasis [20].

In most cases and in contrast to GC/MS, LC/MS does not need any chemical modification on the initial sample. Compared to NMR spectroscopy, LC/MS-based studies usually require significantly smaller sample volumes.

Gas chromatography coupled to mass spectrometry (GC/MS) is a metabolite separation and analysis technique that can only cope with volatile metabolites. For that reason, the metabolites have to be chemically modified. The volatility of a metabolite depends directly on its physicochemical properties. Thus, the chemical modification has to act on the polarity of the molecule. This is done by a process called derivatization consisting of a chemical substitution which replaces the active protons of functional groups, e.g. –OH, –COOH etc. with non-polar groups. The most widely used derivatization is N-methyl-N-(trimethylsilyl) trifluoroacetamide (MSTFA) in combination with methoxyamine hydrochloride. Methoxyamine hydrochloride derivatizes aldehydes or ketones by adding methoxyamine (MOX) groups. In sugars, for example, this derivatization prevents the formation of cyclic forms and open-chain forms will be conserved to reduce the complexity of the chromatogram (Fig. 4.3).

After injection of the derivatized sample into the GC, metabolites are transported by an inert carrier gas (generally helium or hydrogen) through a fused silica column coated with a liquid stationary phase on which the actual separation takes place. Gas chromatographs can be operated in either a temperature-gradient or an isothermal modus. For more complex metabolomics samples, such as blood plasma, a temperature-gradient is used. Consequently, the metabolites are interacting with the liquid stationary phase inside the column. Metabolites have different retention times due to the different boiling points, molecular structure and polarities. The retention time is defined as the time that the metabolite needs to pass through the GC column before reaching the MS and depends on the applied temperature gradient, installed column

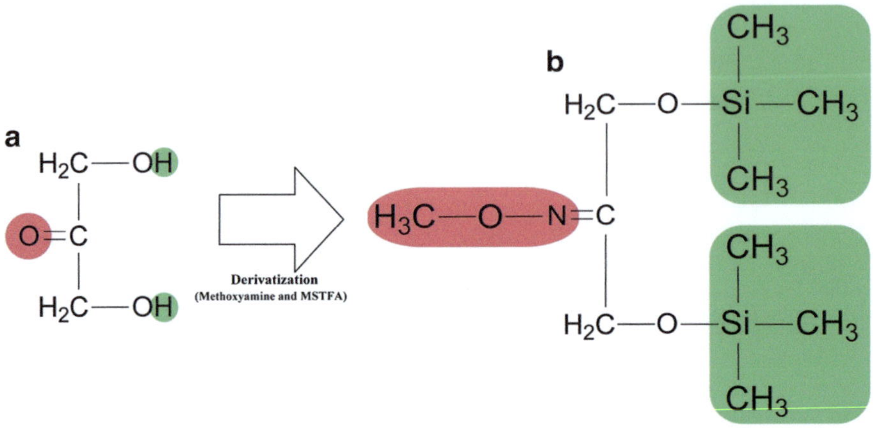

Fig. 4.3 Chemical derivatization. GC only separates hydrophobic and volatile compounds. Therefore, metabolites have to be modified via chemical derivatization. In the case of the illustrated derivatization of dihydroxyacetone (*a*), methoxyamine substitutes carbonyl groups (*red*). N-Methyl-N-trimethylsilyl-trifluoroacetamide (MSTFA) is used to replace active protons of functional groups such as carboxyl, hydroxyl, amines, amides and thiol groups by trimethylsilyl groups (*green*). The derivatized metabolite (*b*) can then be separated by GC and measured by MS

and carrier gas flow. Once entered the mass spectrometer through the GC/MS interface, the metabolites are ionized. Typically, electron ionization (EI), chemical ionization (CI) or atmospheric pressure chemical ionization (APCI) are performed in combination with GC. CI and APCI belong to soft ionization techniques in which the molecular ion remains intact. This provides useful information for structure elucidation. In contrast to CI and APCI, EI is a hard ionization technique but provides reproducible metabolite fragmentation patterns. The fragmentation pattern of each metabolite is unique and can be used for reliable and unambiguous compound identification. The resulting ions are continuously scanned by the mass analyzer according to their m/z ratio before reaching the detector.

Although GC/MS measurements have many advantages over NMR, such as low sample volumes, low cost and separation prior to MS, a drawback of GC/MS measurements is that the derivatized metabolites have a higher molecular weight than the initial metabolites. Furthermore, derivatization complicates metabolite identification since it "masks" the true metabolite structure [14]. In contrast to GC/MS, LC/MS techniques usually have a wider range of detectable metabolites and do not require chemical derivatization of the samples. However, GC/MS techniques enable better compound identification than LC/MS techniques. Furthermore, both techniques use different ionization modes. Whereas GC/MS devices are most often equipped with EI sources, LC/MS are generally equipped with ESI sources. Hard EI provides better fragmentation patterns than soft ESI. In destructive LC and GC/MS techniques losses of analytes occur due to several physicochemical factors which is not the case in NMR spectroscopy.

4.3 Sample Collection and Processing

Due to the fast turnover rates and the high sensitivity of certain metabolites, biological samples have to be delicately treated to obtain the best possible readout. The correct sample handling and processing is without any doubt a very crucial step in every metabolomics analysis. For metabolomics studies, it is of great importance to maintain the collected samples as close to the in vivo state as possible. Previous studies on pre-analytical handling of human blood and urine have shown that the processing temperature and time have a high impact on the stability of these samples [21]. After blood collection, biochemical reactions for example in erythrocytes continue and thereby change the metabolic profile of the plasma sample.

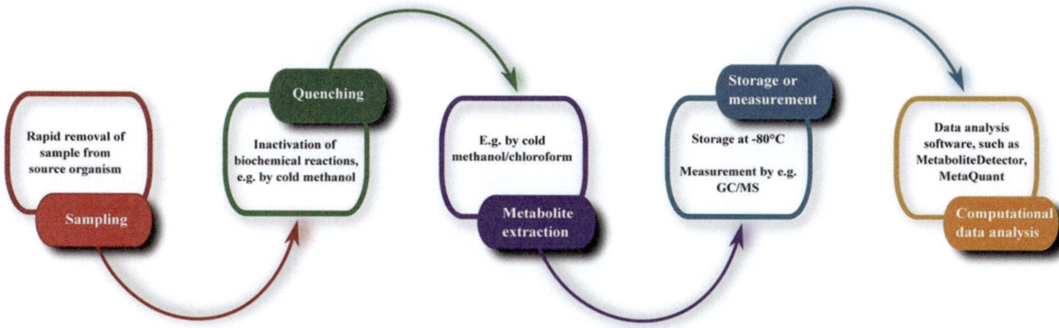

Fig. 4.4 **A classical metabolomics workflow**. After sampling, the metabolism has to be stopped (quenched) as quickly as possible prior to metabolite extraction. Extracted metabolites can be either stored at −80 °C or directly be measured using methods like NMR or mass spectrometry. Finally, a computational data analysis is applied on the obtained raw data to extract information relevant for the experiment

Metabolomics sample processing procedures depend on the aim of the study and the nature of the biological sample. However, almost every metabolomics experiment includes the following crucial steps (Fig. 4.4):

- Quick sample collection
- Quenching (Stopping any metabolic activity in the sample)
- Metabolite extraction

A quick and standardized sample withdrawal is essential to maintain the sample quality as close as possible to the in vivo state. As most biochemical reactions will still remain active in freshly collected samples, a quick handling and low storage temperatures are crucial to stabilize the sample. Ideally, the sample preparation should be performed immediately after sample collection. However, especially in clinical studies, it is often not possible to process the samples immediately. Therefore, there is an urgent need for highly controlled and standardized protocols to assure optimal sample quality.

Quenching is a rapid procedure by which biochemical processes are stopped and the metabolism is instantly inactivated. Classic quenching methods are performed by extreme changes in temperature or pH of the sample. Perchloric acid is mainly used for pH-dependent quenching. Quenching by cold methanol is widely used in metabolomics due to its high quenching effectiveness. Quenching can be either performed with pure methanol or methanol/water mixtures. In cell culture based metabolomics conventional quenching methods are problematic due to metabolite leakage from cells. It has been shown that reducing the methanol proportion in such mixtures reduces cellular metabolite leakage. The longer the quenching step takes, the lower the accuracy of the measurement, because the delayed inactivation of biochemical reactions significantly contributes to variations in metabolite concentrations compared to the in vivo state [22].

Adequate **metabolite extraction** (Box 4.1) has a high impact on the outcome quality of a metabolomics study. For human body fluids, such as blood plasma, saliva and urine, metabolite extraction and quenching are performed together in one step by directly adding an ice-cold methanol/water mixture to the sample. This mixture is firstly homogenized by soft shaking and then centrifuged. These steps should preferably be performed at lower temperatures (e.g. on ice, 4 °C). After centrifugation, the obtained pellet is composed of all kinds of macromolecules, such as DNA, RNA and proteins whereas the supernatant contains polar metabolites. In a GC/MS based study, different metabolite extraction protocols for cells in culture cells were compared and it was found that methanol/water mixtures were the most reproducible in terms of metabolite recovery, although this method could not be universally used [23].

Box 4.1: Metabolite Extraction from Human Body Fluids for MS Analysis

In cancer metabolomics, proper and standardized sample handling is crucial to guarantee high quality samples and adequate results. The metabolite extraction from human body fluids, such as blood plasma and serum, saliva and cerebrospinal fluid requires a quick inactivation of all biochemical processes (quenching). One example for a classical metabolite extraction protocol for human body fluids involves the following steps:

1. Add 1 volume sample in 9 volumes ice-cold Methanol/Water mixture (8:1). Typically, not more than 5–20 μl of sample volume is needed for an MS measurement.
2. Homogenize the mix by shaking at 4 °C for 5 min
3. Centrifuge the homogenized mix at 16,000 *g* for 5 min at 4 °C
4. Pipet the supernatant in analytical vials
5. Dry the samples by centrivap at −4 °C
6. The dried metabolite extracts can either be stored at −80 °C or directly be prepared for mass spectrometric measurement. In the case of an LC/MS measurement the metabolites need to be dissolved in an appropriate solvent; in the case of GC/MS a two step derivatization using MSTFA and methoxyamine hydrochloride can be performed.

4.4 Metabolomics Analysis of Body Fluids

4.4.1 Blood

Human **blood** is one of the most sampled body fluids in research due to its direct contact to nearly every component of the human body and is, therefore, also widely used in cancer related metabolomics studies. In metabolomics, the blood collection tubes have to be carefully selected. Blood collection tubes for plasma often contain anticoagulants, such as EDTA or citrate. Whereas EDTA provides unwanted peaks in the chromatogram, citrate heavily interferes with endogenous peaks. For serum generation, the whole blood tubes have to clot for about half an hour at room temperature. This is problematic as during this time, biochemical processes continue and change the metabolic profile of the sample. It has been shown that plasma has a better reproducibility and is from a metabolomics point of view more stable than serum. On the other hand, serum shows higher metabolite concentrations than plasma which makes serum analysis attractive for biomarker studies [24].

In a large-scale LC/MS based study, the metabolic profiles of blood **plasma** from 120 healthy controls, 120 patients with adenomatous polyps and 120 patients with colorectal cancer has been analyzed. It was shown that choline-containing phospholipids decrease with the progression of colorectal cancer and are, therefore, highly relevant as colorectal cancer prognostic biomarkers [25]. Another GC/MS based study of human blood **serum** revealed that 2-hydroxybutyrate, aspartic acid, kynurenine and cystamine have the potential of being early colorectal cancer diagnostic biomarkers [26]. These studies show the high potential of human blood based metabolomics studies as cancer biomarker discovery tool for both diagnosis and prognosis.

4.4.2 Urine

Urine is an easily accessible body fluid. Sampling is very easy and non-invasive. However, urinary urea levels are high and tend to interfere with other endogenous metabolite peaks. In order to avoid this interference, urine is pre-treated with urease, which digests urea to ammonia and carbon dioxide.

Acylcarnitines might be considered as potential prognostic biomarkers of kidney cancer. Comparing metabolomics profiles of urine samples from early-stage kidney cancer patients with those from late-stage kidney cancer patients, acylcarnitines were found to be significantly increased in late-stage kidney cancer. Interestingly, acylcarnitine levels in early-stage kidney cancer were significantly lower compared to control samples. These findings complicate the use of acylcarnitines as early-stage diagnostic biomarkers of kidney cancer [27]. Surprisingly, urine analysis is also suitable for oral cancer biomarker research. Xie et al. [28] analyzed urine samples from 37 patients with oral squamous cell carcinoma (OSCC), 32 patients with oral leukoplakia (OLK) and 34 healthy controls. They found that OSCC samples have significantly changed levels of 6-hydroxynicotic acid and valine compared to healthy subjects. The difference between OSCC and OLK urine samples could be best explained by changes in 6-hydroxynicotic acid, cysteine and tyrosine levels [28]. Taken together, all these findings point to a promising tool of urine metabolomics for various forms of cancer.

4.4.3 Saliva

Saliva has a very high potential as diagnostic body fluid due the ease, rapidness and non-invasiveness of its collection. However, saliva shows a high variability across different samples. The salivary metabolite composition differs when the sampling is performed from different mouth regions. Also smoking habits, gender and the use of salivation stimulants shows significant changes in metabolite levels [29]. Saliva sampling can be performed by either simple spitting or swabbing. One swabbing method is the use of cotton rolls or "eye sponges" absorbing saliva when applied in the mouth of the donor. Given that cotton rolls give an uncomfortable sensation in the mouth, eye sponges showed to be best suited for saliva collection [30]. Due to the high number of bacterial colonies in the mouth region, it is required to rinse the mouth with water before sampling to reduce the number of bacteria-derived metabolic artifacts.

As an extension of the urine based study of Xie et al. [28] described above, saliva was tested on the same patients. It has been found that levels of lactic acid and valine were different when comparing OSCC to healthy controls [31]. Although this study demonstrates the potential of saliva as an adequate body fluid for cancer biomarker determination, its sampling is more complicated compared to urine and blood.

4.4.4 Cerebrospinal Fluid (CSF)

CSF is not only providing a protective environment for the brain but is also in direct contact with all components of the central nervous system. This characteristic makes CSF a very attractive body fluid for analyzing the metabolic changes in the central nervous system. The sampling itself is a limiting factor for such studies, as it is painful and needs hospitalization of the patient. In comparison to human blood plasma, CSF has a lower biological variation. Although metabolite levels in plasma are higher as in CSF, the number of detectable metabolites is similar [32].

In a study based on glioma biomarker discovery, CSF of 32 glioma patients has been analyzed in three groups: grades I–II (early-stage), grade III (invasive) and glioblastomas (grade IV). Primarily, two metabolites were significantly altered when comparing the different groups: Citric acid and isocitric acid. Both metabolites were significantly lower in grade I–II than in the glioblastoma group. Similarly, the levels of citric acid and isocitric acid were lower in grade III samples compared to gliobastoma samples [33].

4.4.5 Feces

An NMR-based study of **fecal water** extracts from patients with colorectal cancer showed a complementary analysis to fecal metabolomics studies. The authors showed that acetate and butyrate levels are lower in colorectal cancer patients compared to healthy controls whereas proline and cysteine levels were higher [11].

In conclusion, all described body fluids are suitable for profiling the metabolome. Although blood is one of the most sampled biospecimen, its sampling is invasive and needs a trained person for sampling. On the other hand, urine sampling is non-invasive but needs special treatment before MS analysis. Saliva collection is extremely easy and non-invasive, but results can be more variable, and thus less predictive.

4.5 Data Analysis

During a typical GC or LC/MS measurement, mass spectra are continuously recorded resulting in a 3 dimensional dataset. This means that a mass spectrum exists for every time-point of the chromatographic separation. An example of a small GC/MS dataset is depicted in Fig. 4.5.

The challenge of every MS based metabolomics study is to determine metabolite abundances within this complex dataset and align those across many measurements to make them accessible for further statistical analyses. Typically, a metabolomics data analysis consists of the following steps: (1) peak detection, (2) peak alignment, (3) deconvolution and detection of compound spectra, (4) mapping of deconvoluted mass spectra across several chromatograms, (5) quantification of metabolite amounts, (6) statistical analysis (Fig. 4.6).

4.5.1 Raw Data Processing

After raw data acquisition by mass spectrometry, sophisticated bioinformatics tools are needed for proper data processing. Most of modern MS instruments enable the conversion of the vendor-specific data formats into vendor-neutral formats, such as netCDF or mzXML, which can be imported into metabolomics data analysis software programs [34].

Depending on the instrument, MS data can be recorded in two different modes: centroid or profile. In centroid mode, each ion is represented as a discrete m/z, intensity pair. In profile mode the ions are represented by peaks each containing a collection of points. Although a profile mass spectrum is useful to better evaluate the quality of the measurement, it needs to be converted to a centroid spectrum before further analyses can be performed.

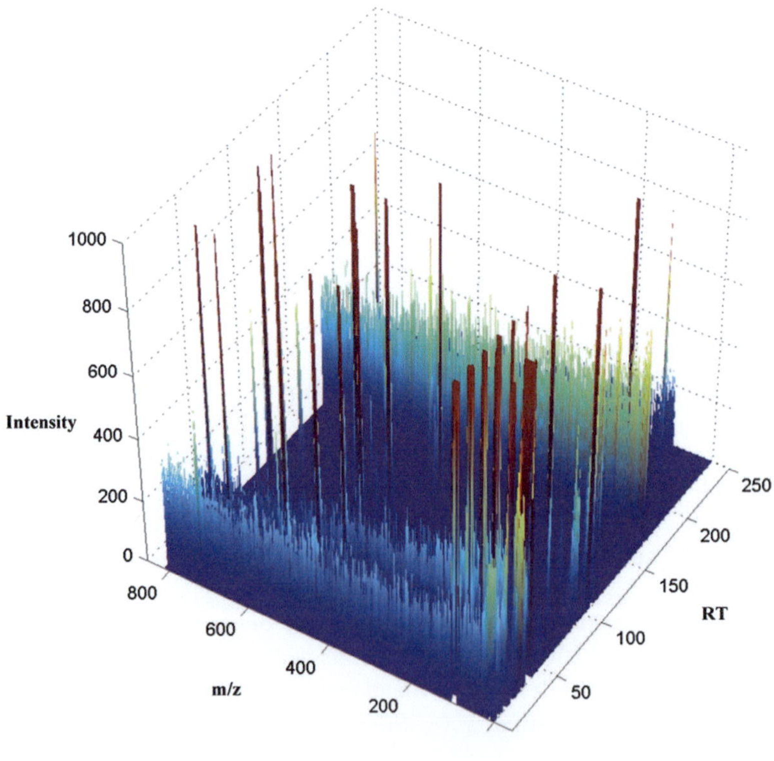

Fig. 4.5 3D representation of a GC/MS data-set. Due to the complexity of GC/MS data, sophisticated data analysis algorithms have to be applied. Every data point represents an intensity (ion count) for a specific m/z value at a specific retention time

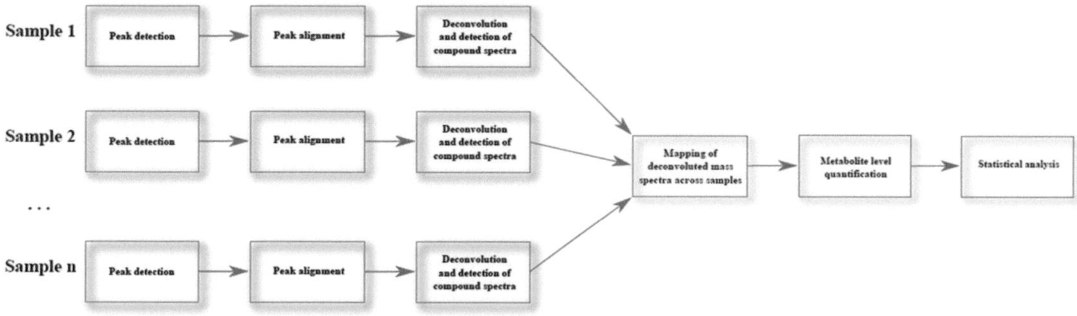

Fig. 4.6 Typical metabolomics data analysis pipeline

The next step involves the detection of all ion-chromatographic peaks. This means, for every detected ion (m/z value), exact maximizations over time are determined. Since ions originating from one compound maximize at the same retention time, all peaks with an identical maximization time are combined to a mass spectrum. This procedure is known as **ion-chromatographic deconvolution** and allows to obtain pure mass spectra even for co-eluting compounds. This process is very important as pure compound mass spectra are the basis for compound identification and chromatogram alignment. In summary, ion-chromatographic deconvolution filters out individual peaks to make them accessible for analysis [14]. Many deconvolution algorithms are already included in vendor-provided software but can also be performed by freely available software [35, 36].

Over time, instrumental variations, such as changes in pressure, column aging and temperature can occur which directly affects the retention time of a given metabolite over different runs [14]. To circumvent this problem, an **alignment** of the same metabolite detected in different samples has to be performed. Compound alignment algorithms are generally based on time correlation optimized warping, parametric time warping and dynamic time warping [37]. Since the mass spectrum of a compound serves as its specific fingerprint, the best alignment is obtained if these data are included in the alignment algorithm [35, 36].

In the case of a gas chromatographic separation (as in GC/MS), the retention time of a compound depends on the installed GC column, the applied temperature profile as well as other instrument specific factors. To make the time axis of GC/MS chromatograms which have been acquired under different conditions or by different labs compatible, a retention index calibration is often performed. This calibration transforms the retention time of every detected metabolite to a defined retention index based on the measurement of reference compounds. For that purpose, an internal or external alkane solution containing a mixture of n-alkanes is measured and the retention times of known and unknown metabolites are related to the retention times of the n-alkanes acquired under the same GC conditions. This procedure provides a very effective way of calibrating all raw data according to pre-defined retention indexes [38].

4.5.2 Metabolomics Data Analysis Software and Databases

Due to the complexity of raw data processing, high-throughput metabolomics data has to be analyzed by specific software. Apart from commercial vendor-specific software (e.g. Sieve, ThermoFischer and Markerlynx, Waters), adequate software is also freely available as stand-alone or plugin for other software (Table 4.1).

Many metabolomics data analysis R packages are freely available, such as the "Metabonomics Package" for the statistical analysis of NMR data [39] and "XCMS2 package" for LC/MS raw data processing [40]. Besides R-based software, free web-based software such as MetDAT can be applied for mass spectrometric data processing,

Table 4.1 Metabolomics data analysis tools

Name	Platform	User interface	Link
MAVEN	LC/MS	Standalone application	http://maven.princeton.edu/
XCMS2	LC-MS/MS	R and Web	http://metlin.scripps.edu/xcms/
MetaboliteDetector	GC/MS	Standalone application	http://md.tu-bs.de
MetAlign	GC/MS and LC/MS	Standalone application	http://www.metalign.nl
MetaQuant	GC/MS	Standalone application	http://bioinformatics.org/metaquant
MSFACTs	GC/MS	Standalone application	http://www.noble.org/plantbio/sumner/msfacts/
Met-Idea	GC/MS	Standalone application	http://bioinfo.noble.org/download/
COLMAR	NMR	Web	http://spinportal.magnet.fsu.edu/
MetaboID	NMR	Standalone application	http://rams.biop.lsa.umich.edu/research/metabolomics
MZMine2	LC/MS	Standalone application	http://mzmine.sourceforge.net/
tagfinder	GC/MS	Standalone application	http://www-en.mpimp-golm.mpg.de/03-research/researchGroups/01-dept1/Root_Metabolism/smp/TagFinder

analysis and visualization [41]. Furthermore, there exist numerous open-source standalone programs mainly based on C++ or Java programming language. MetAlign [42], MetaboliteDetector [35], MetaQuant [43] and MAVEN [44] are freely available standalone applications for mass spectrometry-based data processing and analysis.

The MetAlign software program (http://www.metalign.nl) allows the analysis of GC/MS and LC/MS-based data by the application of sophisticated data pre-processing algorithms. The most relevant features of this software are the calculation of accurate masses, baseline correction and mass-peak artifact filtering. Furthermore, the data pre-processing output is compatible with most statistical software programs [42]. The MetaboliteDetector software (http://metabolitedetector.tu-bs.de) was designed for GC/MS data analysis. The main features of this software include ion-chromatographic deconvolution, peak detection and compound identification [35] as well as the alignment of chromatograms derived from different measurements. Compound identification requires a GC/MS reference compound library which can be created by the MetaboliteDetector software itself or by importing existing libraries, such as the NIST library [45].

MetaQuant (http://bioinformatics.org/metaquant/) is a Java-based GC/MS data analysis software. The MetaQuant software enables automatic peak recognition, calibration and quantification. Furthermore, compound classification options are available and compatible with databases, such as KEGG. Build-in regression algorithms facilitate GC/MS data analysis. The MAVEN software (http://maven.princeton.edu) allows LC/MS-based data analysis by sophisticated computational algorithms. Besides peak detection, sum formula prediction and natural isotope abundance calculation, the software enables pathway visualization and isotope flux animation.

In addition to compound detection and alignment, compound identification is requested by most metabolomics studies. Due to the combination of superior chromatographic separation and compound fragmentation during EI ionization, GC/MS derived compound spectra can easily be identified by matching against a compound library. Currently, there are several libraries available: The commercial NIST library http://www.nist.gov/srd/nist1a.cfm contains more than 200 k entries [45] and the commercial Fiehn library (http://fiehnlab.ucdavis.edu/projects/FiehnLib/) contains more than 1000 entries [46]. In addition, there exist the freely available Golm database (http://gmd.mpimp-golm.mpg.de/) containing more than 500 entries [47]. Although there already exist reference spectra libraries for LC/

MS as for example Metlin (http://metlin.scripps.edu/) [48], compound identification is in most cases more challenging and mostly more than 90 % of the detected compounds remain unidentified. However, taking benefit of the high mass accuracy of most current mass spectrometers, it is easily possible to derive potential sum formulas for unidentified metabolites of interest.

4.5.3 Data Normalization

Data normalization is the process by which meaningful and hidden information is extracted from raw data. In most cases, this step is required to perform adequate statistical analysis. Metabolomics data normalization can be divided in three main classes: centering, scaling and transformations.

Centering is subtracting the mean of the total number of variables (metabolite intensities) in each sample. Thereby, metabolite levels can be compared to fluctuations around 0 which is an adjustment of the differences between low and high metabolite levels. Normalization based on **scaling** divide each variable by the scaling factor which can be the standard deviation or the mean calculated from the total metabolite intensities in the sample. In autoscaling, the centered metabolite intensity is divided by the standard deviation. Autoscaling thereby enables the comparison of metabolite levels across samples as all metabolite levels are equally important. However, this method also increases the measurement-dependent errors. In contrast to autoscaling, paretoscaling uses the square root of the standard deviation and is thereby closer to the original not normalized data than autoscaled data. However, this method is very sensitive to large fold changes that are not as dominant as in the raw data. The last class of normalization, **transformations**, is often based on log transformation which reduces heteroscedasticity. However, when approaching a value close to zero, the transformed value tends to approach minus infinity which is problematic for the analysis of low abundant metabolites [49].

For a more detailed and complete review of metabolomics data normalization, the reader should consult the excellent review of van den Berg et al. [49] which also highlights the importance of choosing the correct normalization method for the biological question to be answered.

4.6 Statistical Analysis/Biomarker Determination

High-throughput metabolomics technologies generate very large amounts of data. In a typical metabolomics experiment, the number N of observations (i.e., samples) can be in the order of a few dozens, while the number p of variables (e.g., metabolite concentrations) can be in the order of hundreds or more. This is known in the statistical literature as the $p \gg N$ scenario, which often calls for novel statistical analysis methods that go beyond the classical t-test and ANOVA [50].

In general, there are two classical approaches to the statistical analysis of multivariate data. In the first approach, known as *unsupervised learning*, each observation $x = (x_1, \ldots, x_p)$ is treated as a point in a high-dimensional space and the analysis attempts to find patterns or regularities among all points in the data set. The latter may involve projecting the data to a low-dimensional subspace for visualization, estimating the probability density function of the data, or clustering the data. A classical unsupervised learning method is *principal component analysis* (PCA). This is a linear dimension reduction method aiming to reduce the number p of variables in the dataset, while still maintaining as much variation of the original data as possible [51]. PCA is the most widely used method in metabolomics studies for providing a rapid overview of the data [52]. However, PCA is a linear projection method that may fail to capture possible non-linear structure in the data. Recently, several powerful *nonlinear dimension reduction* methods have appeared in the machine learning literature, which are better suited to visualizing high-dimensional data [53, 54].

The second main approach to multivariate data analysis is known as *supervised learning*. Here, each observation x_n is labelled with an extra 'class' variable $y_n \in \{-1,1\}$ that indicates the context or condition, e.g., cancer patients vs. healthy controls, different cell types, etc. The archetypal supervised learning problem is *classification*, which amounts to computing a function or rule that helps predicting the unknown class of an observation. Two popular classification methods are *logistic regression* and the *support vector machine (SVM)*. Their popularity mainly stems from their good theoretical properties and the existence of efficient solvers [55–57]. In the $p \gg N$ scenario we consider, both logistic regression and SVM aim at finding a *separating hyperplane* of the data. Formally, this amounts to estimating $p+1$ parameters

$$\omega = (\omega_0, \omega_1, \ldots, \omega_p)$$

such that the linear projection of the input data to the vector ω, i.e., the function

$$f(x;\omega) = \sum_{i=1}^{p} \omega_i x_i + \omega_0$$

minimizes a certain misclassification 'loss'. In the simplest two-class case (e.g., cases vs. controls), both logistic regression and SVM can be shown to solve the following *convex optimization* problem:

$$\min_{\omega} \sum_{n=1}^{N} L(y_n, f(x_n;\omega)) + \lambda \omega_2^2$$

Where $L(y,f)$ is a *loss function*, $\|\omega\|_2$ denotes the Euclidean norm of ω, and λ is a nonnegative constant (possibly zero). The only difference between logistic regression and SVM is the choice of loss function:

$$L(y,f) = \max\{1 - yf, 0\} (SVM)$$

$$L(y,f) = \log[1 + \exp(-yf)] (Logistic\, regression).$$

Both methods are 'margin maximization' methods, which means that, in the case of separable data and at the limit $\lambda \to 0$, they compute an optimal separating hyperplane.

Another supervised learning problem, which is of major interest for knowledge discovery and data interpretation in the context of cancer metabolomics, is *variable selection*. This involves choosing a subset of the original set of p variables that discriminate well the different classes. In our context, that could amount to finding a subset of metabolites that are responsible for significant changes in the metabolic profile, and that allow predicting cases from controls [58]. In the $p \gg N$ scenario of interest, variable selection is typically obtained as a byproduct of sparse regularization, as we explain next. Guyon and Elisseeff [59] discuss different approaches to variable selection.

An important issue that has to be carefully addressed in all above methods is the problem of *overfitting*, i.e., the tendency of a learned classifier to model noise instead of the real signal in the data. In theory, overfitting can be avoided if a learning algorithm is tuned to optimize the *generalization error* of the classifier, i.e., the average prediction error that the classifier makes on independent, off-sample data. However, directly estimating the generalization error is not easy. A simple and practical approximation is obtained via *K-fold cross-validation*: The dataset is randomly split into K equally sized subsets, and each of the K subsets is held out as a test set while the classifier is trained on the remaining $K-1$ subsets. The average prediction error of the classifier on the K held-out subsets is then used to assess the generalization performance of the classifier. Cross-validation is a simple procedure, which, if done properly, allows for efficient model selection and parameter tuning. We refer to Hastie et al. [50] and Ambroise and McLachlan [60] for detailed discussions, including common pitfalls.

In the $p \gg N$ scenario, the suggested way to tackle overfitting is by a combined use of cross-validation and *regularization* [50]. Regularization amounts to adding a penalty term to the objective function of the optimization problem (as in the optimization problems for logistic regression and SVM above), as a way to constrain the search towards the most useful (signal-wise) model parameters. A popular regularization approach is *Lasso* [61], in which the penalty term involves the L1-norm of the model parameters (instead of the Euclidean norm as above), thereby encouraging *sparse* models, i.e., models that have only few (e.g., N or less) nonzero parameters. Sparse regularization automatically selects a good subset of variables that increase the signal-to-noise ratio in classification.

Ideally, the regularization penalty should be defined in a way that leverages domain knowledge. Recent work by the authors demonstrates how to incorporate contextual biological knowledge that is given in the form of pairwise similarities between variables, e.g., a molecular network. This can be regarded as a generalization of the *fused Lasso* approach [62] to more general *structured sparsity induced priors*, which have recently attracted much attention by the statistical machine learning community (see Bach et al. [63] and references therein). More generally, a challenging problem in metabolomics research for cancer is how to best capture existing biomedical knowledge into mathematical models for learning.

Acknowledgments The authors thank Dr. Christian Jäger for the critical review of the book chapter.

References

1. Koppenol WH, Bounds PL, Dang CV (2011) Otto Warburg's contributions to current concepts of cancer metabolism. Nat Rev Cancer 11:325–337
2. Warburg O (1956) On the origin of cancer cells. Science 123:309–314
3. Vander Heiden MG, Cantley LC, Thompson CB (2009) Understanding the Warburg effect: the metabolic requirements of cell proliferation. Science 324:1029–1033
4. Lu W, Bennett BD, Rabinowitz JD (2008) Analytical strategies for LC-MS-based targeted metabolomics. J Chromatogr B Analyt Technol Biomed Life Sci 871:236–242
5. Ludwig C, Ward DG, Martin A, Viant MR, Ismail T, Johnson PJ, Wakelam MJ, Gunther UL (2009) Fast targeted multidimensional NMR metabolomics of colorectal cancer. Magn Reson Chem 47(Suppl 1):S68–S73
6. Villas-Boas SG, Mas S, Akesson M, Smedsgaard J, Nielsen J (2005) Mass spectrometry in metabolome analysis. Mass Spectrom Rev 24:613–646
7. Wishart DS, Tzur D, Knox C, Eisner R, Guo AC, Young N, Cheng D, Jewell K, Arndt D, Sawhney S et al (2007) HMDB: the human metabolome database. Nucleic Acids Res 35:D521–D526
8. Lu J-J, Bao J-L, Wu G-S, Xu W-S, Huang M-Q, Chen X-P, Wang Y-T (2013) Quinones derived from plant secondary metabolites as anti-cancer agents. Anticancer Agents Med Chem 13:456–463
9. Bothwell JH, Griffin JL (2011) An introduction to biological nuclear magnetic resonance spectroscopy. Biol Rev Camb Philos Soc 86:493–510
10. Bathe OF, Shaykhutdinov R, Kopciuk K, Weljie AM, McKay A, Sutherland FR, Dixon E, Dunse N, Sotiropoulos D, Vogel HJ (2011) Feasibility of identifying pancreatic cancer based on serum metabolomics. Cancer Epidemiol Biomarkers Prev 20:140–147
11. Monleon D, Morales JM, Barrasa A, Lopez JA, Vazquez C, Celda B (2009) Metabolite profiling of fecal water extracts from human colorectal cancer. NMR Biomed 22:342–348
12. Tiziani S, Lopes V, Gunther UL (2009) Early stage diagnosis of oral cancer using 1H NMR-based metabolomics. Neoplasia 11:269–276, 264p following 269
13. Weljie AM, Bondareva A, Zang P, Jirik FR (2011) 1H NMR metabolomics identification of markers of hypoxia-induced metabolic shifts in a breast cancer model system. J Biomol NMR 49:185–193
14. Villas-Boas SG, Nielsen J, Smedsgaard J, Hansen MA, Roessner-Tunali U (2007) Metabolome analysis: an introduction, vol 24. Wiley, Hoboken
15. Wilson ID, Plumb R, Granger J, Major H, Williams R, Lenz EM (2005) HPLC-MS-based methods for the study of metabonomics. J Chromatogr B 817:67–76
16. Smith RD, Loo JA, Edmonds CG, Barinaga CJ, Udseth HR (1990) New developments in biochemical mass spectrometry: electrospray ionization. Anal Chem 62:882–899
17. March RE (1997) An introduction to quadrupole ion trap mass spectrometry. J Mass Spectrom 32:351–369
18. Hu Q, Noll RJ, Li H, Makarov A, Hardman M, Graham Cooks R (2005) The Orbitrap: a new mass spectrometer. J Mass Spectrom 40:430–443
19. Amster IJ (1996) Fourier transform mass spectrometry. J Mass Spectrom 31:1325–1337
20. Zhang G, Panigrahy D, Mahakian LM, Yang J, Liu JY, Stephen Lee KS, Wettersten HI, Ulu A, Hu X, Tam S et al (2013) Epoxy metabolites of docosahexaenoic acid (DHA) inhibit angiogenesis, tumor growth, and metastasis. Proc Natl Acad Sci U S A 110:6530–6535
21. Bernini P, Bertini I, Luchinat C, Nincheri P, Staderini S, Turano P (2011) Standard operating procedures for pre-analytical handling of blood and urine for metabolomic studies and biobanks. J Biomol NMR 49:231–243
22. de Jonge LP, Douma RD, Heijnen JJ, van Gulik WM (2012) Optimization of cold methanol quenching for quantitative metabolomics of *Penicillium chrysogenum*. Metabolomics 8:727–735
23. Sellick CA, Knight D, Croxford AS, Maqsood AR, Stephens GM, Goodacre R, Dickson AJ (2010) Evaluation of extraction processes for intracellular metabolite profiling of mammalian cells: matching

extraction approaches to cell type and metabolite targets. Metabolomics 6:427–438
24. Yu Z, Kastenmüller G, He Y, Belcredi P, Möller G, Prehn C, Mendes J, Wahl S, Roemisch-Margl W, Ceglarek U (2011) Differences between human plasma and serum metabolite profiles. PLoS One 6:e21230
25. Li S, Guo B, Song J, Deng X, Cong Y, Li P, Zhao K, Liu L, Xiao G, Xu F (2013) Plasma choline-containing phospholipids: potential biomarkers for colorectal cancer progression. Metabolomics 9:202–212
26. Nishiumi S, Kobayashi T, Ikeda A, Yoshie T, Kibi M, Izumi Y, Okuno T, Hayashi N, Kawano S, Takenawa T (2012) A novel serum metabolomics-based diagnostic approach for colorectal cancer. PLoS One 7:e40459
27. Ganti S, Taylor SL, Kim K, Hoppel CL, Guo L, Yang J, Evans C, Weiss RH (2012) Urinary acylcarnitines are altered in human kidney cancer. Int J Cancer 130:2791–2800
28. Xie GX, Chen TL, Qiu YP, Shi P, Zheng XJ, Su MM, Zhao AH, Zhou ZT, Jia W (2012) Urine metabolite profiling offers potential early diagnosis of oral cancer. Metabolomics 8:220–231
29. Takeda I, Stretch C, Barnaby P, Bhatnager K, Rankin K, Fu H, Weljie A, Jha N, Slupsky C (2009) Understanding the human salivary metabolome. NMR Biomed 22:577–584
30. de Weerth C, Jansen J, Vos MH, Maitimu I, Lentjes EG (2007) A new device for collecting saliva for cortisol determination. Psychoneuroendocrinology 32:1144–1148
31. Wei J, Xie G, Zhou Z, Shi P, Qiu Y, Zheng X, Chen T, Su M, Zhao A, Jia W (2011) Salivary metabolite signatures of oral cancer and leukoplakia. Int J Cancer 129:2207–2217
32. Crews B, Wikoff WR, Patti GJ, Woo H-K, Kalisiak E, Heideker J, Siuzdak G (2009) Variability analysis of human plasma and cerebral spinal fluid reveals statistical significance of changes in mass spectrometry-based metabolomics data. Anal Chem 81:8538–8544
33. Nakamizo S, Sasayama T, Shinohara M, Irino Y, Nishiumi S, Nishihara M, Tanaka H, Tanaka K, Mizukawa K, Itoh T (2013) GC/MS-based metabolomic analysis of cerebrospinal fluid (CSF) from glioma patients. J Neuro Oncol 113(1):65–74
34. Pedrioli PG, Eng JK, Hubley R, Vogelzang M, Deutsch EW, Raught B, Pratt B, Nilsson E, Angeletti RH, Apweiler R (2004) A common open representation of mass spectrometry data and its application to proteomics research. Nat Biotechnol 22:1459–1466
35. Hiller K, Hangebrauk J, Jäger C, Spura J, Schreiber K, Schomburg D (2009) MetaboliteDetector: comprehensive analysis tool for targeted and nontargeted GC/MS based metabolome analysis. Anal Chem 81:3429–3439
36. Stein SE (1999) An integrated method for spectrum extraction and compound identification from gas chromatography/mass spectrometry data. J Am Soc Mass Spectrom 10:770–781
37. Sugimoto M, Kawakami M, Robert M, Soga T, Tomita M (2012) Bioinformatics tools for mass spectroscopy-based metabolomic data processing and analysis. Curr Bioinform 7:96
38. Kovàts ES (1961) Zusammenhänge zwischen Struktur und gasehromatographischen Daten organischer Verbindungen. Fresenius J Anal Chem 181:351–364
39. Izquierdo-García J, Rodríguez I, Kyriazis A, Villa P, Barreiro P, Desco M, Ruiz-Cabello J (2009) A novel R-package graphic user interface for the analysis of metabonomic profiles. BMC Bioinformatics 10:363
40. Benton H, Wong D, Trauger S, Siuzdak G (2008) XCMS2: processing tandem mass spectrometry data for metabolite identification and structural characterization. Anal Chem 80:6382–6389
41. Biswas A, Mynampati KC, Umashankar S, Reuben S, Parab G, Rao R, Kannan VS, Swarup S (2010) MetDAT: a modular and workflow-based free online pipeline for mass spectrometry data processing, analysis and interpretation. Bioinformatics 26:2639–2640
42. Lommen A (2009) MetAlign: interface-driven, versatile metabolomics tool for hyphenated full-scan mass spectrometry data preprocessing. Anal Chem 81:3079–3086
43. Bunk B, Kucklick M, Jonas R, Münch R, Schobert M, Jahn D, Hiller K (2006) MetaQuant: a tool for the automatic quantification of GC/MS-based metabolome data. Bioinformatics 22:2962–2965
44. Melamud E, Vastag L, Rabinowitz JD (2010) Metabolomic analysis and visualization engine for LC–MS data. Anal Chem 82:9818–9826
45. Babushok V, Linstrom P, Reed J, Zenkevich I, Brown R, Mallard W, Stein S (2007) Development of a database of gas chromatographic retention properties of organic compounds. J Chromatogr A 1157:414–421
46. Kind T, Wohlgemuth G, Lee DY, Lu Y, Palazoglu M, Shahbaz S, Fiehn O (2009) FiehnLib: mass spectral and retention index libraries for metabolomics based on quadrupole and time-of-flight gas chromatography/mass spectrometry. Anal Chem 81:10038–10048
47. Kopka J, Schauer N, Krueger S, Birkemeyer C, Usadel B, Bergmüller E, Dörmann P, Weckwerth W, Gibon Y, Stitt M (2005) GMD@ CSB. DB: the Golm metabolome database. Bioinformatics 21:1635–1638
48. Smith CA, O'Maille G, Want EJ, Qin C, Trauger SA, Brandon TR, Custodio DE, Abagyan R, Siuzdak G (2005) METLIN: a metabolite mass spectral database. Ther Drug Monit 27:747–751
49. van den Berg RA, Hoefsloot HC, Westerhuis JA, Smilde AK, van der Werf MJ (2006) Centering, scaling, and transformations: improving the biological information content of metabolomics data. BMC Genomics 7:142
50. Hastie T, Tibshirani R, Friedman J (2009) The elements of statistical learnin. Springer, New York

51. Jolliffe IT (2002) Principal component analysis, 2nd edn. Springer, New York
52. Katajamaa M, Orešič M (2007) Data processing for mass spectrometry-based metabolomics. J Chromatogr A 1158:318–328
53. Lee JJA, Verleysen M (2007) Nonlinear dimensionality reduction. Springer, New York/London
54. Van der Maaten, LJP (2013) Barnes-Hut SNE. In: Proceedings of the international conference on learning representations, Scottsdale, Arizona (USA)
55. Bottou L (2010) Large-Scale machine learning with stochastic gradient descent. In: Proceedings of the 19th international conference on computational statistics, Paris (France)
56. Koh K, Kim S-J, Boyd SP (2007) An interior-point method for large-scale l1-regularized logistic regression. J Mach Learn Res 8:1519–1555
57. Vapnik V (1995) The nature of statistical learn theory. Springer, New York
58. Goodacre R, Broadhurst D, Smilde AK, Kristal BS, Baker JD, Beger R, Bessant C, Connor S, Capuani G, Craig A (2007) Proposed minimum reporting standards for data analysis in metabolomics. Metabolomics 3:231–241
59. Guyon I, Elisseeff A (2003) An introduction to variable and feature selection. J Mach Learn Res 3:1157–1182
60. Ambroise C, McLachlan G (2002) Selection bias in gene extraction on the basis of microarray gene-expression data. Proc Natl Acad Sci 99:6562–6566
61. Tibshirani R (1996) Regression shrinkage and selection via the lasso. J R Stat Soc Series B Stat Methodol 58(1):267–288
62. Tibshirani R, Saunders M, Rosset S, Zhu J, Knight K (2005) Sparsity and smoothness via the fused lasso. J R Stat Soc Series B Stat Methodol 67:91–108
63. Bach F, Jenatton R, Mairal J, Obozinski G (2012) Structured sparsity through convex optimization. Stat Sci 27:450–468

The Role of Epigenomics in the Study of Cancer Biomarkers and in the Development of Diagnostic Tools

5

Mukesh Verma

Abstract

Epigenetics plays a key role in cancer development. Genetics alone cannot explain sporadic cancer and cancer development in individuals with no family history or a weak family history of cancer. Epigenetics provides a mechanism to explain the development of cancer in such situations. Alterations in epigenetic profiling may provide important insights into the etiology and natural history of cancer. Because several epigenetic changes occur before histopathological changes, they can serve as biomarkers for cancer diagnosis and risk assessment. Many cancers may remain asymptomatic until relatively late stages; in managing the disease, efforts should be focused on early detection, accurate prediction of disease progression, and frequent monitoring. This chapter describes epigenetic biomarkers as they are expressed during cancer development and their potential use in cancer diagnosis and prognosis. Based on epigenomic information, biomarkers have been identified that may serve as diagnostic tools; some such biomarkers also may be useful in identifying individuals who will respond to therapy and survive longer. The importance of analytical and clinical validation of biomarkers is discussed, along with challenges and opportunities in this field.

M. Verma (✉)
Epidemiology and Genomics Research Program, Division of Cancer Control and Population Sciences, National Cancer Institute (NCI), National Institutes of Health (NIH), Suite# 4E102. 9609 Medical Center Drive, MSC 9763, Bethesda, MD 20892-9726, USA
e-mail: vermam@mail.nih.gov

R. Scatena (ed.), *Advances in Cancer Biomarkers*, Advances in Experimental Medicine and Biology 867, DOI 10.1007/978-94-017-7215-0_5

Keywords

Biomarker • Bladder cancer • Blood cancer • Brain cancer • Breast cancer • Cancer • Cancer epigenetics • Cervical cancer • Chromatin • Colorectal cancer • Diagnosis • Early detection • Endometrial cancer • Epigenetic inhibitors • Epigenetics • Epigenomic biomarkers • Gastric cancer • Genomic instability • Glioma • Head and neck cancer • Histone • Kidney cancer • Leukemia and lymphoma • Liver cancer • Lung cancer • Methylation • microRNA • Ovarian cancer • Pancreatic cancer • Prognosis • Prostate cancer • Skin cancer • Surveillance • Validation

5.1 Introduction

The need to identify and characterize biomarkers for cancer diagnosis is critical, because cancer is a heterogeneous disease and patients' individual molecular profiling—which results from the tumor microenvironment—determines disease development and response to treatment. The tumor microenvironment is affected by all of the epigenomic components in the cell. In addition, epigenetics is an integral part of cancer initiation, development, and recurrence [1–7]. Epigenetics involves alterations in promoters, histones, microRNA (miRNA) expression, and chromatin structure (sometimes called "epimutations") [8–10]. Cancer-specific methylation alterations are hallmarks of different cancers [11] and may cause genomic instability, genomic alterations, and changes in gene expression [11–13]. Polycomb group (PcG) protein loci that are targeted by tumor suppressors also are regulated by methylation during stem cell differentiation into different types of cells [14]. A systematic approach to following epigenetic changes in tumor development may lead to the identification of diagnostic biomarkers for cancer. Baylin's group has suggested that integration of the genome and hypermethylome may provide insights into major pathways in cancer development and enable the identification of new biomarkers for cancer diagnosis and prognosis [15]. Functional methylation analysis of clinical samples from individuals diagnosed with breast cancer and controls identified early epigenetic biomarkers for diagnosis and prognosis [16]. In addition, a recent characterization of the methylome by age may be useful in studying disease-associated changes in the methylome [17].

5.2 Technological Advancements

Next-generation sequencing and other technological advancements in the epigenomic field have made it possible to conduct epigenomic analysis at the genomic level [4, 8, 15, 18, 19]. As an example, epigenome-wide analysis of 215 adult B-cell acute lymphoblastic leukemia (ALL) patients and matched controls identified hypomethylation of selected genes and overexpression of fusion proteins [19]. A microarray-based methylated CpG island recovery assay followed by bisulfite sequencing was used to identify cervical cancer-specific genes that could distinguish cervical squamous cell carcinoma (SCC)/CIN2-3 from CIN1/normal [20]. Polymorphisms of the miRNA coding region also have been utilized in cancer diagnosis [21]. Diagnostic dendrograms created with a combination of hypermethylated markers and CpG island microarrays, and similar to those generated in gene-expression analyses, are complementary to gene-expression profiles and can be developed from archived material. Genome-wide methylation analysis of gastric cancer patients with *Helicobacter pylori* (*H. pylori*) infection indicated that inflammatory pathways are involved in gastric cancer development [22]. Genome-wide methylation analysis also has been completed for renal cancer

[23], and global histone profiling was conducted in lung cancer to identify disease-associated biomarkers [24].

An ideal diagnostic biomarker should have high sensitivity and specificity. To determine the sensitivity and specificity of biomarkers, the area under the curve (AUC) of a receiver operating characteristic (ROC) curve is measured. The AUC of an ROC curve is a measure of the ability of a continuous marker to accurately classify tumor and nontumor tissue. Such a curve is a plot of sensitivity versus 1 minus specificity (1—specificity) values associated with all dichotomous markers that can be formed by varying the value threshold used to designate a marker as "positive" [25]. An AUC of 1 corresponds to a marker with perfect accuracy, whereas an AUC of 0.5 corresponds to an uninformative marker. Most of the epigenetic diagnostic biomarkers described below are methylation biomarkers; however, in a few cancers, histone and miRNA biomarkers also have been identified.

5.3 Epigenomic Markers in Cancer Diagnosis

The complexity and heterogeneity of cancer progression suggests that a single biomarker and/or a small panel of biomarkers is needed to characterize cancer [26–37]. Biomarkers also may distinguish between indolent and aggressive forms of cancer. Vogelstein et al. proposed 12 pathways for pancreatic cancer that may distinguish between normal and cancer patients [38]. In breast cancer, different molecular subtypes exist that are difficult to distinguish by morphology alone [18, 26, 39]. In invasive ductal carcinoma, diverse phenotypes with distinct characteristics have been reported [40, 41]. Further analysis suggests that different subtypes can be identified by different epigenetic biomarkers. Diagnosis of such disease and its subtypes can be conducted using CpG island methylation phenotype (CIMP) biomarkers [11]. Methylation markers also are useful in determining the response to treatment. In the next section, examples of different epigenetic biomarkers in a variety of tumor types are discussed. A summary of epigenetic biomarkers useful in diagnosing different cancer types is provided in Table 5.1.

5.3.1 Bladder Cancer

Among genitourinary neoplasms, bladder cancer incidence and prevalence are surpassed only by prostate cancer [42]. Those biomarkers that have implications for diagnosis and prognosis include DNA methylation of *APC, RARB2, RASSF1A, JUP, DAL1, APAF1*, and *DAPK1* [9, 43–46]; histone modifications in the coding regions of *RASSF1A, PTGS2, PTEN*, and *CDH1* (H3K4me2, H3K18Ac, H3K4m31, H3K4me2, H3K4me3, H3K18Ac) [47]; and abnormal expression of miRNAs (miR-141, miR-155, miR-1233, and miR-32 [48]. Mutations were not detected in those genes that were hypermethylated during bladder cancer development. *TIMP3* methylation was associated with disease-free survival [49]. Compared to using routine sonogram examination and cystoscopy (an invasive and expensive technology) to detect bladder cancer, epigenetic biomarkers may provide a better alternative that uses noninvasive technologies to collect samples and an easy assay method to diagnose bladder cancer, including identification of different bladder cancer subtypes [9, 50]. The concept of field effect (an area of tissue that is susceptible to transformation) also has been proposed for detecting bladder cancer that may lead to cancer recurrence [49].

5.3.2 Blood Cancer (Leukemia and Lymphoma)

Hypomethylation and overexpression of the *IL2RA(CD25)* and *E2aPBX1* fusion proteins were observed in adult B-cell precursor ALL [19]. Ishihara et al. reported overexpression of plasma miR-155 and underexpression of miR-126 in adult T-cell leukemia (ATL) [51]. A profile of miRNAs overexpressed in chronic lymphocytic leukemia (CLL) was reported by Moussay et al. [52]. Methylation patterns of *p16*

Table 5.1 Epigenomic biomarkers as diagnostic tools in different cancers

Cancer type	Biomarker
Bladder cancer	Methylation of *APC, RARB2, RASSF1A, JUP, DAL1, APAF1,* and *DAPK1* [45, 46]; histone modifications in the coding regions of *RASSF1A, PTGS2, CDH1,* and *PTEN* [47]; overexpression of miR-141, miR155, miR-1233, and miR-32 [48]
Blood cancer (leukemia and lymphoma)	Overexpression of plasma miR-155 and underexpression of miR-126 in ATL [51]; p16 and MGMT hypermethylation in AML [53]; overexpression of *IL2RA(CD25)* and E2aPBX1 fusion protein [19]; miRNA profile in CLL [52]
Brain cancer	*p16INK4, p14ARF, RARbeta,* and *TIMP3* hypermethylation in glioblastoma [56, 58]; *ANKDD1A, GAD1, HIS1H3E, PCDHA8, PHOX2B, SIX3*, and *SST* hypermethylation in glioma [60]
Breast cancer	Methylation of *NDRG2* and *HOXD1* for diagnosis [16]; methylation of *CDO1, CKM, CRIP1, KL,* and *TAC1* for prognosis [16]; functional hypermethylation of a combination of *KL* and *TAC1* for survival [16]; breast cancer CpG island methylator phenotype for detection [11]; abnormal expression of EZH2 and polycomb repressor 2 [62]
Cervical cancer	*SOX9* hypermethylation [20]; HPV *L1* gene and LCR methylation status [65, 66]; *DKK3* methylation [67]; *CDH1* methylation [68]; *p16(INK4a), p15(INK4b)* methylation [70]; PCTH methylation [71]; *PCTH* [71]; *TIMP-3* [71, 72]; *SFRP1, SFRP2,* and *SFRP4* methylation [73]; *vimentin* methylation [74]
Colorectal cancer (CRC)	Methylation of *EBN2* [80]; *p14 ARF, RASSF1A,* and *APC1a* [81]; *EBN2* [80]; *p14 ARF, RASSF1A,* and *APC1a* [81]; *Kiss-1* [82]; *MLH1, MSH2, SLIT2, HIC1, MGMT, SFRP1,* and *CDKN2A* [76]; miRNA expression and polycomb repressor complex [76]; histone modification [85, 86]
Endometrial cancer	Methylation of *APC, CHFR, Sprouty 2, RASSF1A, GPR54, CDH1,* and *RSK4* [87], *CDH1, MGMT, hMLH1, p16, PR-B, PTEN,* and *RARb2* [90]; miRNA profiling [89]
Gastric cancer (stomach cancer)	Histone profiles [102]; CIMP [103]; methylation of *NGRD2* [104]; *RASGRF1* [105]; *vimentin* [109]; *CDH1* [106]; *Helicobacter pylori* infection [100]; miRNA expression [108]
Head and neck cancer	Methylation of *FOXM1* [111]; *p16(INK4a)* [112]; *DAPK1, CDH1,* and *ADAM23* [115]; microsatellite instability at 3 loci and hypermethylation of *hMLH1, hMSH2* [117]; histone methyltransferase expression [118]

Kidney cancer (renal cancer)	Higher levels of histone deacetylase 1 and 2 [123]; hypomethylation of LINE-1 [122]; methylation of CpGs in the promoter of *GATA5* [119], *HIC1* [120], and *SFRP1* [121]
Liver cancer (hepatocellular carcinoma)	miRNA polymorphism [21]; methylation of *RASSF1A* [14]; *RASSF1A, GSTP1, CHRNA3*, and *DOK1* [128]; H3K4me3 [129]
Lung cancer	Histone profiling (H3K9Ac, H3K9TriMe, and H4K16Ac) [24]; methylation of *p16(INK4a)* [134]; GDNF, MTHFR, OPCML, TNFRSF25, TCF21, PAX8, PTPRN2, and PITX2 [135]; PAX5alpha, GATA5, and SULF2 [136]; RUNX-3 [137]; SHOX2 [138, 139]; APC, CDH1, MGMT, DCC, RASSF1A, and AIM1 [140]
Oral cancer	Overexpression of miR-155 [196]; hypermethylation of FHL1 [197]; p16(INK4A), cytoglobin, E-cadherin, and TMEFF2 [198, 199]; tropomyoson receptor kinase (TRK) [200, 201]; p15(INK4b) [201]; mirR-9 [202]; IL-6 [203]; NID2, HOX9 [204]; histone profiling (H3K27me3 and H4K20me1) [205]
Ovarian cancer	NKIRAS1/RPL15, THRB, RBPS3 (CTDSPL), IQSEC1, NBEAL2, ZIC4, LOC285205, FOXP1, LOC285205, CGGBP1, EPHB1, and NKIRAS1/RPL15 [142]; MLH1, RASSF1A, HIC1, DAPK, OPCML, CCBE1, FZD4, DVL1, NFATC3, ROCK1, LRP5, AXIN1, NDK1, and FBXO32 [141]
Pancreatic cancer	p16 [144]; hMLH1 and hMLH2 [145]; cyclin D2 [147]; TFP1, BN1P3, and RELN [148]; PcG proteins and chromatin remodeling (PcG) [149]
Prostate cancer	GSTP1, APC, MDR1, GPX3, 14-3-3 sigma TDRD1, IGF2, DICER1, ADARB1, HILS1, GLMN, and TRIM27, TNRC6A, and DGCR8, IGFBP7, KLK6, KLK10 [151–154]; acetylated histones H3K9, H3K18, and H4K12, and dimethylated H4R3 and H3K4 [150]; miRNA profiling [157]; miR-16, miR-195, miR-26a [158]
Skin cancer	AKAP12 methylation [160]; 5- hydroxymethycytosine (5hmC) [163]; miR-29c and DNMT3B [164]
Testicular cancer	miR-199a [206]; methylation of imprinting gene SNRPN [207]; MAEL [208]; VASA [209]

and *MGMT* correlated with disease stratification in acute myeloid leukemia (AML) [53]. In genome-wide methylation analyses, specific CpG island methylation was reported in classical Hodgkin lymphoma, an atypical germinal center-derived B cell lymphoma that has lost its B cell identity [54]. *p16 (INK4A)* hypermethylation was found to be a negative prognostic marker in B cell lymphoma [55].

5.3.3 Brain Cancer

Glioblastoma Promoter hypermethylation of *BEX1, BEX2, p16INK4, p14ARF, GATA6, EMP3, RAR-beta, TES,* and *TIMP3* was observed in glioblastoma [56, 57]. The *p16INK/Rb* pathway is the most frequently altered pathway in this tumor type. *Rb* is considered a tumor suppressor gene as it functions as an inhibitor of cell cycle regulation. The protein product of this gene, pRB, binds with the E2 family of transcription factors to repress the target gene by epigenetic mechanisms (which is achieved by recruitment of a co-repressor that affects chromatin compaction) [58]. In terms of histone modifications, the loss of H3K9 acetylation and H3K9 methylation, loss of H4K16 acetylation, and H4K20 trimethylation were reported in glioblastoma [59].

Glioma Genes that are inactivated by hypermethylation in glioma include *ANKDD1A, GAD1, HIS1H3E, PCDHA8, PHOX2B, SIX3,* and *SST*; and miR-185 expression that resulted in activation of DNA methyltransferase-1 (*DNMT1*) in tissue samples from a case–control study [60]. DiVinci et al. reported correlation of methylation status of *HOXA* genes and subgroups of glioma and proposed therapeutic implications for this research [61].

5.3.4 Breast Cancer

Enhancer of Zeste 2 (EZH2) and polycomb repressor complex 2 contribute to the alteration of histones, especially the trimethylation of H3K27 in breast cancer. This results in genomic instability and the inactivation of several genes [62]. Breast cancer methylation markers include *BRCA1, RASSFA, APC,* and *RAR-beta* [63]. Other epigenetic regulation of breast cancer includes methylation of *NDRG2* and *HOXD1,* used for diagnosis [16]; methylation of *CDO1, CKM, CRIP1, KL,* and *TAC1,* used for prognosis [16]; functional hypermethylation of the combination of *KL* and *TAC1,* used for survival [16]; and CIMP, used for detection [11]. miRNA profiling of miR-122 and miR-375 helped in distinguishing breast cancer patients from controls [64]. Levels of these miRNAs were determined in blood (the collection of which is considered a noninvasive process, as opposed to tissue biopsies).

5.3.5 Cervical Cancer

SOX9 hypermethylation status could distinguish cervical SCC/CIN2-3 from CIN1/normal and was proposed as a diagnostic marker for cervical cancer [20]. The methylation status of different genes of the human papillomavirus (HPV) was proposed to be useful in cervical cancer diagnosis and disease stratification [65, 66]. *DKK3* methylation status correlated with disease-free survival in cervical cancer [67]. Abudukadeer et al. proposed using the hypermethylation of *CDH1* in cervical cancer prognosis [68]. The reactivation of tumor suppressor genes in cervical cancer has been achieved by trichostatin treatment [69]. Jha et al. reported methylation of *p16(INK4a)* and *p15(INK4b)* in cervical cancer patient samples and found an association between passive smoking and contraceptive use with the methylation levels of these two genes [70]. Other genes found to be hypermethylated in cervical cancer include *PCTH* [71]; *TIMP-3* [71, 72]; *SFRP1, SFRP2,* and *SFRP4* [73]; and *vimentin* [74].

5.3.6 Colorectal Cancer (CRC)

Both the candidate gene approach and genome-wide association studies have been conducted to identify genes associated with CRC [75–79]. Some of the genes regulated by methylation in CRC include *EBN2* [80]; *p14 ARF, RASSF1A,* and *APC1a* [81]; *Kiss-1* [82]; and *MLH1, MSH2, SLIT2, HIC1, MGMT, SFRP1,* and *CDKN2A* [76]. Methylation analysis of 111 primary CRC patients and 46 matched normal colorectal mucosa controls was followed for 20 years to evaluate the role of *p14 ARF, RASSF1A,* and *APC1a* in survival. The methylation of these genes was found to be a prognostic factor in CRC [81]. The role of long interspersed nuclear elements 1 (LINE-1) in familial CRC was evaluated by Ogino et al. in a retrospective study, and heritable predisposition of LINE-1 methylation was observed [83]. The prognostic impact of CIMP and microsatellite instability (MSI) on the response to CRC treatment also has been studied [75]. Methylation of genes targeted by the CRC of suppressor proteins was demonstrated by Dallol et al. [76]. The development of CRC involves interaction between a network of miRNA expressions and methylation of specific genes [84]. Histone modifications also contribute to CRC development; Tamagawa et al. recently demonstrated a correlation between global histone modifications and overall survival in metachronous liver metastases in CRC [85]. In addition, H3K9me2 showed chromatin remodeling in CRC [86].

5.3.7 Endometrial Cancer

The involvement of methylation and miRNA expression in endometrial cancer has been demonstrated [87–89]. Selected genes that become inactivated by hypermethylation in endometrial cancer include *APC, CHFR, Sprouty 2, RASSF1A, GPR54, CDH1,* and *RSK4* [87]; as well as *CDH1, MGMT, hMLH1, p16, PR-B, PTEN,* and *RARb2* [90].

5.3.8 Gastric Cancer (Stomach Cancer)

A number of genes, such as *GATA4* [91]; *SOX9* [92]; *MDM2, DYRK2,* and *LYZ* [93]; *TSPYL5* [94]; and *TPEF/HPP1* [95], are regulated epigenetically and may be biomarkers of stomach cancer. Another group demonstrated an association between mutations in selected genes and CIMP in gastric cancer [96]. *H. pylori* infection is a risk factor for gastric cancer and induces an epigenetically regulated inflammatory pathway [97, 98]. miRNAs have been proposed as a bridge from *H. pylori* infection to gastritis to gastric cancer [99]. Other groups also observed similar results [100]. Histone markers for gastric cancer diagnosis also have been proposed [101, 102]. ChIP-on-chip analyses indicated higher levels of H3K9 acetylation, H4K16 acetylation, and H3K9me3 correlation of H3K9me3 with tumor stage and recurrence [102]. Genome-wide CpG island profiles in more than 200 samples showed CIMP in gastric cancer patients [103]. Hypermethylation of *N-myc downstream regulated gene 2* (*NDRG2*) was correlated with higher metastasis of gastric cancer in tissue samples from patients [104]. Hypermethylation of *RASGRF1* was observed in intestinal or diffuse type gastric cancer in mucosa from patients as compared with mucosa from healthy individuals [105]. *CDH1* hypermethylation indicated poor prognosis in gastric cancer [106]. Alves et al. reported inactivation of *COX2, CDKN2A,* and *HLMH1* by hypermethylation in *H. pylori-positive* patient samples [107]. Ando et al. observed miRNA-mediated inactivation of selected genes in previously infected or currently infected gastric cancer patients and reported an epigenetic field effect in some cases [108]. In addition, *vimentin* hypermethylation in serum samples was reported as a diagnostic marker for this cancer [109].

5.3.9 Head and Neck Cancer

Hypermethylation of several genes was observed in saliva and tissue samples; some of these genes could be good candidates for use in diagnosing head and neck cancer [110–116]. Genes that are methylated in head and neck cancer include *FOXM1* [111]; *p16(INK4a)* [112]; and *DAPK1, CDH1,* and *ADAM23* [115]. Genomic instability and hypermethylation of mismatch repair genes (*hMLH1, hMSH2*) in head and neck cancer were reported by Demokan et al. [117]. Histone methyltransferase is another biomarker that has potential in diagnosing head and neck cancer [118].

5.3.10 Kidney Cancer (Renal Cancer)

Methylation of a number of genes, such as CpGs in the promoter of *GATA5* [119], *HIC1* [120], and *SFRP1* [121], was found to be associated with renal cancer [42, 47]. LINE-1 methylation also has been shown to contribute to the development of renal cancer [122]. Histone deacetylases 1 and 2 were found in higher quantities in specimens from renal cancer patients compared to healthy people, indicating the presence of aggressive cancer [123]. Hildebrandt et al. demonstrated the involvement of miRNA in renal cancer development [124]. In addition, genome-wide methylation analysis indicated hypermethylation of a large number of genes that could be potential diagnostic biomarkers for renal cancer [23].

5.3.11 Liver Cancer (Hepatocellular Carcinoma)

Zhou et al. demonstrated the contribution of single nucleotide polymorphisms in miRNA coding regions to the development of liver cancer [21]. They reported finding miR-146a (rs2910164 G>C) and miR-499 (rs3746444T>C) polymorphisms in a Chinese population while analyzing tissue from 186 primary liver cancer patients and 483 controls. The methylation status of genes targeted by CRC suppressor proteins was studied for markers that were involved in stem cell differentiation to liver cells, and *RASSF1A* was found to be involved in the early stages of liver carcinogenesis [14]. Liver cancer etiology involves infection with hepatitis viruses (HBV, HCV, and HDV) and other factors, resulting in chronic liver disease such as cirrhosis [125]. An abnormal gene expression profile, high genomic instability, and overall hypomethylation were observed in liver cancer samples compared to samples from healthy participants [126, 127]. Abnormal methylation was reported in liver cancer associated with HBV and HCV infection [128]. Selected genes regulated by abnormal methylation include *RASSF1A, GSTP1, CHRNA3*, and *DOK1* [128]. Histone H3K4me3 also has been used in diagnosing liver cancer [129].

5.3.12 Lung Cancer

miRNAs are excellent tools for use in diagnosing lung cancer [130–133]. These miRNAs were collected from tissue or serum [132] or in free-circulating form [131]. Global histone modification analysis was performed on lung cancer patient samples (non-small cell lung carcinoma, NSCLC). H3K9Ac, H3K9TriMe, and H4K16Ac were found to be associated with cancer recurrence; H4K20triMe was not found to be associated with lung cancer recurrence or survival [24]. Methylation markers for lung cancer diagnosis include *p16(INK4a)* [134]; *GDNF, MTHFR, OPCML, TNFRSF25, TCF21, PAX8, PTPRN2*, and *PITX2* [135]; *PAX5alpha, GATA5*, and *SULF2* [136]; *RUNX-3* [137]; *SHOX2* [138, 139]; and *APC, CDH1, MGMT, DCC, RASSF1A*, and *AIM1* [140]. It is known that half of all new lung cancer cases belong to former smokers and never smokers; therefore, proper representation of lung cancer from never smokers should be included in any screening analyses.

5.3.13 Ovarian Cancer

Ovarian cancer is one of the deadliest cancers because it frequently is asymptomatic until it has reached advanced stages [141]. A set of methylation biomarkers was identified for diagnosing ovarian cancer with 72 % sensitivity and 94 % specificity. These markers were *NKIRAS1/RPL15, THRB, RBPS3 (CTDSPL), IQSEC1, NBEAL2, ZIC4, LOC285205*, and *FOXP1* [142]. These investigators also characterized additional biomarkers and identified *LOC285205, CGGBP1,*

EPHB1, and *NKIRAS1/RPL15* as able to distinguish between stage I and II and stage III and IV ovarian cancer with a sensitivity of 80 % and specificity of 88 % [142]. Additional potential epigenetic markers for ovarian cancer include: *MLH1, RASSF1A, HIC1, DAPK, OPCML, CCBE1, FZD4, DVL1, NFATC3, ROCK1, LRP5, AXIN1, NDK1*, and *FBXO32* [141].

5.3.14 Pancreatic Cancer

No effective therapeutic strategies have been developed for pancreatic ductal adenocarcinoma, an aggressive tumor, because it is diagnosed late. Epigenetic markers might improve early diagnosis of this tumor type. *KRAS* mutations generally are present in pancreatic cancer. Therefore, in many studies methylation markers are selected in *KRAS*-positive samples [143]. *p16* methylation has been reported in pancreatic cancer [144]; and Li et al. reported hypermethylation of mismatched repair genes (*hMLH1* and *hMLH2*) in a population-based study [145]. In an exploratory study, cell-free DNA from pancreatic cancer patients and pancreatitis patients was analyzed by methylation and a distinct pattern of methylation was observed [146]. Methylation of *cyclin D2* also was reported by investigators [147]. Other genes that have been shown by their methylation status to be involved in pancreatic cancer include *TFP1, BN1P3*, and *RELN* [148]. In addition, it has been proposed that the chromatin-modeling PcG proteins could contribute to the development of pancreatic cancer [149].

5.3.15 Prostate Cancer

A number of genes, such as *GSTP1, cyclin D2, IGFBP7, KLK6,* and *KLK10*, have been reported to be methylated in prostate cancer [150–153]. Based on the clustering analysis of expressed genes in moderately and poorly differentiated prostate glands and normal glands using whole genome oligonucleotide microarrays, 12 epigenetically regulated genes were identified [154]. In prostate cancer, *TDRD1, IGF2, DICER1, ADARB1, HILS1, GLMN,* and *TRIM27* were upregulated; and *TNRC6A* and *DGCR8* were downregulated. Based on levels of the acetylated histones H3K9, H3K18, and H4K12, and dimethylated H4R3 and H3K4, low-grade prostate cancer (Gleason score of 6 or less) was shown to be divided into two prognostically separate groups [150]. miRNAs can function as oncomirs or tumor suppressor miRs, and miRNA profiling was reported to be altered during prostate cancer development [155, 156]. miR-34 has been shown to modulate chromatin in prostate cancer cells via the AKT pathway [157]. Circulating miRNAs miR-16, miR-195, and miR-26a were shown to distinguish between prostate cancer and benign prostate hyperplasia with a sensitivity of 78.4 % and a specificity of 66.7 % [158]. Global methylation profiling also was shown to predict prostate cancer [159].

5.3.16 Skin Cancer (Melanoma)

When 195 samples (basal cell carcinoma, squamous cell carcinoma, and active keratosis) were analyzed by methylation-specific, high-resolution melting, the *AKAP12* gene showed differential methylation levels that correlated with the advancement of skin cancer [160]. Methylation of arsenic in drinking water causes the formation of mono- and dimethylated arsenite and contributes to skin cancer [161, 162]. 5-hydroxymethylcytosine (5hmC) is an intermediate of DNA demethylation, and its low levels have been observed in melanoma [163]. Its gradual loss was correlated with the advancement of skin cancer. In addition, miR-29c and DNMT3B were reported to be involved in melanoma disease outcome [164].

5.3.16.1 Suitable Samples to Assay Epigenomic Biomarkers

Table 5.2 summarizes different types of samples that were used to assay epigenetic diagnostic markers. Blood and tissue samples were the most commonly used samples. In a few examples, multiple epigenetic markers were analyzed in the same sample [165]. In some cases, samples are

Table 5.2 Sample types commonly used in cancer epigenetics

Samples	Comments
Blood	Methylation analysis in bladder cancer [192, 210]; gliomas [211]; breast cancer [17, 212]; leukemia [213]; deacetylation of different proteins in breast cancer after vorinostat treatment [184]
Buccal cells/buccal swabs	Methylation analysis of LINE-1 in bladder cancer [192]; methylation-specific PCR in laryngeal cancer [214] and cervical cancer [215]
Cerebrospinal fluid	Methylation pattern of several genes in gliomas [211]; leukemia [213]
Circulating DNA and miRNA	Plasma-circulating DNA in prostate cancer [216]; circulating DNA in methylation analysis in breast cancer [194]; miR-143, miR-221, miR-423, and miR-608 in plasma of CRC patients [217]; miR-121 in plasma of prostate cancer patients, and miR-141, miR-200b, and miR-375 in serum of prostate cancer patients [218]; miR-375 and miR-122 in serum of breast cancer patients [64]
Exfoliated cells from the cervix	LINE-1 methylation patterns in cervical cancer [219, 220]; methylation in the HPV genome in cervical cancer [220]; methylation profiling for cervical cancer screening [221]
Exfoliated cells from urine	LINE-1 methylation patterns were compared in exfoliated cells, tissues, and blood from bladder cancer patients [168]; methylation levels of laminin genes in bladder cancer [222]
Nipple aspirate	Methylation analysis in breast cancer [169, 223]
Paraffin-embedded tissues	Methylation levels in breast cancer [212], bladder cancer [192]
Sputum	Methylation signature of lung cancer [224, 225]; methylation levels of different genes in lung cancer and chronic obstructive pulmonary diseases [226]
Stool	miRNA profiling in CRC [166, 227]; methylation patterns in CRC [166, 167]
Tissue samples	Genome-wide methylation analysis in breast cancer [228], cervical cancer [229], and CRC [77]; candidate gene approach to follow methylation levels in breast cancer [230]; methylation-specific PCR in laryngeal cancer [214], gliomas [211], and hepatocellular carcinoma [129]; histone ChIP-on-chip analysis in oropharyngeal squamous carcinoma [205]; histone gene expression in colon cancer [231]; global histone analysis in lung cancer [24]; multiple biomarkers from the same sample in breast cancer [165]
Urine	Methylation-specific PCR in prostate cancer [232]; methylation analysis in bladder cancer [192, 233]

stored for long periods of time before epigenetic changes are assayed, and sample stability must be assessed before studies are conducted. One such study assessed the stability of stool samples and analyzed and validated methylation results to evaluate potential markers for CRC diagnosis [166]. In another study, Elliott et al. compared methylation results from DNA isolated from stool with mucosa biopsies and observed similar results [167]. LINE-1 methylation patterns were compared in exfoliated cells, tissues, and blood from bladder cancer patients, and it was concluded that exfoliated cells are suitable for detecting cancer and for screening high-risk populations [168]. For detecting breast cancer, matched samples of nipple aspirate and mammary ductoscopy were analyzed by quantitative methylation analysis and comparable results were obtained [169]. Dulaimi et al. observed that during methylation analysis, if some genes are unmethylated in tissue samples, they also are unmethylated in matched serum samples [170]. All of these examples indicate that noninvasively collected samples can be used for epigenetic analysis.

5.3.16.2 Epidemiologic Studies in Cancer Epigenetics

Epigenetic alterations are a common event in cancer, and their identification can provide insights into the carcinogenic process and suggest clinically relevant biomarkers [28, 37]. Research focused on biomarker-based early detection has the potential to reduce mortality rates. After potential epigenetic biomarkers are identified, they should be validated for potential use in screening to identify those who are at risk of developing cancer. Examples of the use of epidemiology and epigenetics in cancer are described below in which biomarkers played a significant role in cancer diagnosis, disease stratification, outcome, and prognosis.

Based on high-density microarray analysis, Nelson et al. identified methylation profiling that could distinguish between lung cancer subtypes and controls in three populations with hundreds of participants [171]. These investigators suggested including these genes in translational studies aimed at developing a screening method to detect early lung cancer. In a case–control study (92 head and neck squamous cell carcinoma [HNSCC] cases and 92 cancer-free controls), blood DNA methylation profiling of the *FGD4, SERPING1, WDR39, IL27, HYAL2*, and *PLEKHA6* genes was used to generate ROC curves. After adjusting for age, gender, smoking, and alcohol consumption, results indicated that hypermethylation of these six genes was associated with HNSCC [172]. In renal cell carcinoma (RCC), methylation of *HIC1* was associated with disease stratification [120]. Tissues used in this study consisted of clear cell RCC, papillary RCC, and mixed histologies. Tumor-free tissues from areas at least 2 cm away from the primary tumor site were obtained from the same patients. In another study, Marsit et al. identified methylated markers associated with the aggressiveness of bladder cancer in two independent, nonconsecutive, population-based bladder cancer series (tumors from 344 individuals involved in a case–control study of incident bladder cancer diagnosed between 1994–1998 in the first series; and tumors from 264 individuals diagnosed between 2002 and 2004 in the second series) [173]. *HOXB2* hypermethylation alone was found to be associated with invasive bladder cancer; whereas hypermethylation of *HOXB2, KRT13*, and *FRZB* together was associated with the prediction of high-grade, noninvasive disease. These studies may suggest genes with potential as clinical markers of disease and genes and pathways with potential as targets for therapeutic treatment. In another study of bladder cancer, *RUNX3* hypermethylation was found to be correlated with disease progression (increased tumor stage and grade) in bladder cancer [174]. In this study, primary tumors from non-muscle invasive bladder cancer (NMIBC) patients with histologically verified cell carcinoma who underwent transurethral resection at Chungbuk National University, Korea, were collected between 1995 and 2009.

A study in Tunisian women (tissue from 117 breast cancer patients and 65 paired normal breast tissues, and 16 fibroadenomas and five mastopathies from women without carcinoma used as controls) found that patients with methylated *BRCA1* and/or *BRCA2* showed significantly longer survival compared to those with unmethylated tumors [175]. Participants in this study had no family history of breast cancer. *BRCA1* methylation correlated well with patient age and triple-negative phenotype (ER^-, PR^-, $HER2^-$). Poage's group developed a novel approach to CpG grouping (based on genomic features and PcG target genes) to identify a classifier that is associated with survival in HNSCC [176]. Biospecimens were obtained from an ongoing population-based, case-control study in the Boston area (Head and Neck Oncology Programs in Brigham and Women's Hospital, Beth Israel Deaconess Medical Center, Boston Medical Center, Dana Farber Cancer Institute, Massachusetts General Hospital, and New England Medical Center) [176, 177]. This study demonstrated the integration of genetic and epigenetic information. Ling et al. conducted a population-based study in esophageal squamous cell carcinoma (ESCC) (209 specimens were collected prospectively from ESCC patients in Zhejiang Province Cancer Hospital between 2004 and 2010, and matching morphologically normal esophageal epithelium tissues were collected 6–10 cm away from tumors during surgery) and observed that MSH2 promoter methylation levels were associated with disease survival [178]. Plasma-circulating DNA was used to follow up disease-free survival.

In another epidemiologic study, histone profiling in 408 patient samples (tissues) was performed by tissue microarray and immunohistochemical analysis. In this case-control study of NSCLC, histone profiling of H3 (H3K9Ac, H3K9TriMeth), and H4 (H4K16Ac, H4K20TriMeth) was determined to evaluate its association with disease recurrence and survival [24]. After the analysis, subjects were grouped into different categories based on profile: acetylation dominant, methylation dominant, co-dominant, and modification-deficient. Compared to other groups, the acetylation-dominant group showed better prognosis in survival analysis [24]. Previously, histone profiling was studied in regard to recurrence and survival in liver cancer and gastric cancer [85, 102].

In another study of NSCLC, circulating miRNA levels were associated with survival [179]. Serum miRNA signatures were identified in a genome-wide serum miRNA profiling of patients with stages I to IIIa lung adenocarcinoma and squamous carcinoma (treated with both surgery and adjuvant chemotherapies). Four specific miRNA signatures were identified that might be markers for following survival in lung cancer. A total of 303 patients were included in this analysis: 60 patients were selected for the discovery stage for Solexa sequencing—30 patients who survived more than 30 months on the last follow-up were classified as the longer survival group, and 30 patients who survived less than 25 months were classified as the shorter survival group. The remaining 243 participants were in the training or testing groups. Another group of investigators reported similar results in tissue samples, with the additional information that histology was associated with miRNA expression [180]. To repress transcription, miRNA binds to the messenger RNA (mRNA) of the transcribed gene. If the binding site of miRNA is mutated or has a polymorphism, gene transcription continues. In a case-control study of more than 700 cases of bladder cancer (undergoing radiotherapy) and more than 700 controls, polymorphisms in an miRNA-binding site were evaluated, and correlations with therapy outcome were observed [181]. These investigators are applying a similar approach in breast cancer patients undergoing treatment.

These examples indicate the role of the epigenome in cancer diagnosis as well as processes involved in carcinogenesis.

5.3.16.3 Epigenetic Inhibitors in Cancer Treatment

Four epigenetic inhibitors have been approved by the U.S. Food and Drug Administration (FDA) for the treatment of specific cancers [182]. DNA demethylating agents azacitidine (Vidaza®, sold by Celgene, New Jersey), and decitabine (Dacogen®, sold by Eisai, Japan) are used to treat myelodysplastic syndrome, which is the precursor of AML. Histone deacetylase inhibitors (sold by Celgene and Merck, New Jersey) are used to treat cutaneous lymphoma. Yan et al. treated AML with decitabine and performed methylome analysis [183]. The results indicated the feasibility of methylome analysis as a pharmacodynamic endpoint in methylating agent therapy [183]. In another study, the deacetylating agent vorinostat was used in combination with paclitaxel and bevacizumab for breast cancer therapy in a small group of patients to assess the efficacy of the treatment [184]. A clinical study conducted at The Johns Hopkins University showed that the combination of a demethylating agent and a histone deacetylase inhibitor lead to reduced lung tumor size [185]. Based on his results, Baylin has suggested that including epigenetic drugs in regular cancer treatment leads cells to become susceptible to routine drugs and improves drug efficacy. Challenges remain, however, in the field of epigenetic inhibitors, including a lack of predictive markers, relatively unclear mechanisms of response and resistance to treatment, and low response in solid tumors.

5.4 Potential Challenges and Opportunities

Clinical validation of identified epigenetic biomarkers is the key challenge in the field of cancer diagnosis. Pepe et al. have proposed five phases of biomarker validation [186]. Analytical validity is defined as the ability of an assay to accurately and reliably measure an analyte in the laboratory as well as in clinical samples. Clinical validation requires the detection or prediction of the associated disease (cancer) in specimens from targeted patients. After epigenetic biomarkers are identified, the assay and biomarker must be approved by the FDA before these biomarkers can be utilized in clinical samples. The FDA has provided guidelines for this process, including specific analytical and clinical validation tests that biomarkers must pass. If biomarkers, assays, or devices are intended for clinical use in patient samples, they should be reviewed by the FDA's Center for Devices and Radiological Health for their ability to analytically measure the biomarker. Biomarkers and devices for quantification are expected to yield equivalent results. Biomarker qualification by the FDA enables collaboration among stakeholders, reduces costs for individual stakeholders, and provides biomarkers that are useful for the general public and the private sector.

Another challenge in the field of epigenetic biomarkers is identifying which epigenetic alterations are the "drivers" and which are the "passengers" during cancer progression. "Driver" epimutations may appear as low-frequency alterations, requiring many samples to be screened before tumor-specific "driver" epimutations can be identified. Integrating genomic information with epigenomic information presents another challenge. In addition, limitations exist in identifying morphometric biomarkers (in vivo imaging), such as in chromatin remodeling during cancer progression. These changes occur much earlier than any phenotypic changes are observed in tumor development.

Combining multiple markers may increase the sensitivity and specificity of biomarkers [4, 28, 32, 37, 187–191]. Integrating genomic and proteomic markers with epigenetic markers may facilitate distinguishing between different cancer subtypes and cancer stages [15, 26, 37], as has been accomplished for breast cancer by the integration of genomic DNA copy number arrays, exome sequencing, methylation profiling, mRNA arrays, miRNA sequencing, and reverse-phase protein arrays [18].

The results of methylation profiling from blood and tissues often differ [192]. Koestler et al. conducted a systematic epigenome-wide methylation analysis and demonstrated that shifts in leukocyte subpopulations may account for a considerable proportion of variability in these patterns [193]. Sturgeon et al. could not distinguish breast cancer cases and controls in a clinical setting when serum or plasma DNA methylation patterns of selected genes were evaluated [194]. Insufficient material, technical shortcomings, or lack of experience are other challenges faced by investigators in diagnosing different cancers, including brain cancer [195]. Industrial partnerships in major projects may produce useful outcomes in these areas. Proper sharing of views and dissemination of knowledge, and collaborations among investigators in different disciplines, are the key to the successful identification and validation of candidate epigenetic biomarkers for cancer diagnosis.

Routine technologies for cancer diagnosis cannot detect low-grade cancers or cancers at the premalignant stage. Epigenetic markers may be useful in these situations. Cost-effective technologies are needed that have high sensitivity and specificity and can be used with samples that are collected through noninvasive means. The availability of genome-wide methylation, histone, and miRNA analysis technologies, and our rapidly accumulating knowledge regarding the epigenome, may make the translation of findings discussed in this article possible in the near future. Epigenetic biomarkers also may be useful in identifying patients who will benefit from drug therapy without developing a resistance to the drugs being taken. Recently developed drugs for cancer treatment are based on specific pathways and may be useful for individuals in whom these pathways are altered. This approach can be designed for personalized medicine and precision medicine. Epigenetic biomarkers may be useful in such approaches.

Acknowledgements I am thankful to Joanne Brodsky of SCG, Inc., for reading the manuscript and providing suggestions.

References

1. Jones PA (2005) Overview of cancer epigenetics. Semin Hematol 42:S3–S8
2. Khare S, Verma M (2012) Epigenetics of colon cancer. Methods Mol Biol 863:177–185
3. Mishra A, Verma M (2012) Epigenetics of solid cancer stem cells. Methods Mol Biol 863:15–31
4. Kumar D, Verma M (2009) Methods in cancer epigenetics and epidemiology. Methods Mol Biol 471:273–288
5. Verma M, Maruvada P, Srivastava S (2004) Epigenetics and cancer. Crit Rev Clin Lab Sci 41:585–607
6. Verma M, Dunn BK, Ross S, Jain P, Wang W, Hayes R et al (2003) Early detection and risk assessment: proceedings and recommendations from the workshop on epigenetics in cancer prevention. Ann N Y Acad Sci 983:298–319
7. Verma M (2003) Viral genes and methylation. Ann N Y Acad Sci 983:170–180
8. Baylin SB, Jones PA (2011) A decade of exploring the cancer epigenome—biological and translational implications. Nat Rev Cancer 11:726–734
9. Han H, Wolff EM, Liang G (2012) Epigenetic alterations in bladder cancer and their potential clinical implications. Adv Urol 2012:546917
10. Peltomaki P (2012) Mutations and epimutations in the origin of cancer. Exp Cell Res 318:299–310
11. Fang F, Turcan S, Rimner A, Kaufman A, Giri D, Morris LG et al (2011) Breast cancer methylomes establish an epigenomic foundation for metastasis. Sci Transl Med 3:75ra25
12. Jones PA, Baylin SB (2007) The epigenomics of cancer. Cell 128:683–692
13. Melichar B, Kroupis C (2012) Cancer epigenomics: moving slowly, but at a steady pace from laboratory bench to clinical practice. Clin Chem Lab Med 50:1699–1701
14. Chen YL, Ko CJ, Lin PY, Chuang WL, Hsu CC, Chu PY et al (2012) Clustered DNA methylation changes in polycomb target genes in early-stage liver cancer. Biochem Biophys Res Commun 425:290–296
15. Yi JM, Dhir M, Van Neste L, Downing SR, Jeschke J, Glockner SC et al (2011) Genomic and epigenomic integration identifies a prognostic signature in colon cancer. Clin Cancer Res 17:1535–1545
16. Jeschke J, Van Neste L, Glockner SC, Dhir M, Calmon MF, Deregowski V et al (2012) Biomarkers for detection and prognosis of breast cancer identified by a functional hypermethylome screen. Epigenetics 7:701–709
17. Heyn H, Li N, Ferreira HJ, Moran S, Pisano DG, Gomez A et al (2012) Distinct DNA methylomes of newborns and centenarians. Proc Natl Acad Sci U S A 109:10522–10527
18. Cancer Genome Atlas Network (2012) Comprehensive molecular portraits of human breast tumours. Nature 490:61–70
19. Geng H, Brennan S, Milne TA, Chen WY, Li Y, Hurtz C et al (2012) Integrative epigenomic analysis identifies biomarkers and therapeutic targets in adult B-acute lymphoblastic leukemia. Cancer Discov 2:1004–1023
20. Wu JH, Liang XA, Wu YM, Li FS, Dai YM (2013) Identification of DNA methylation of SOX9 in cervical cancer using methylated-CpG island recovery assay. Oncol Rep 29:125–132
21. Zhou J, Lv R, Song X, Li D, Hu X, Ying B et al (2012) Association between two genetic variants in miRNA and primary liver cancer risk in the Chinese population. DNA Cell Biol 31:524–530

22. Shin CM, Kim N, Jung Y, Park JH, Kang GH, Park WY et al (2011) Genome-wide DNA methylation profiles in noncancerous gastric mucosae with regard to Helicobacter pylori infection and the presence of gastric cancer. Helicobacter 16:179–188
23. Ricketts CJ, Morris MR, Gentle D, Brown M, Wake N, Woodward ER et al (2012) Genome-wide CpG island methylation analysis implicates novel genes in the pathogenesis of renal cell carcinoma. Epigenetics 7:278–290
24. Song JS, Kim YS, Kim DK, Park SI, Jang SJ (2012) Global histone modification pattern associated with recurrence and disease-free survival in non-small cell lung cancer patients. Pathol Int 62:182–190
25. Anglim PP, Alonzo TA, Laird-Offringa IA (2008) DNA methylation-based biomarkers for early detection of non-small cell lung cancer: an update. Mol Cancer 7:81
26. Kelloff GJ, Sigman CC (2012) Cancer biomarkers: selecting the right drug for the right patient. Nat Rev Drug Discov 11:201–214
27. Srinivas PR, Verma M, Zhao Y, Srivastava S (2002) Proteomics for cancer biomarker discovery. Clin Chem 48:1160–1169
28. Verma M (2012) Epigenetic biomarkers in cancer epidemiology. Methods Mol Biol 863:467–480
29. Banerjee HN, Verma M (2006) Use of nanotechnology for the development of novel cancer biomarkers. Expert Rev Mol Diagn 6:679–683
30. Verma M, Manne U (2006) Genetic and epigenetic biomarkers in cancer diagnosis and identifying high risk populations. Crit Rev Oncol Hematol 60:9–18
31. Verma M, Seminara D, Arena FJ, John C, Iwamoto K, Hartmuller V (2006) Genetic and epigenetic biomarkers in cancer: improving diagnosis, risk assessment, and disease stratification. Mol Diagn Ther 10:1–15
32. Verma M (2004) Biomarkers for risk assessment in molecular epidemiology of cancer. Technol Cancer Res Treat 3:505–514
33. Wagner PD, Verma M, Srivastava S (2004) Challenges for biomarkers in cancer detection. Ann N Y Acad Sci 1022:9–16
34. Verma M, Srivastava S (2003) New cancer biomarkers deriving from NCI early detection research. Recent Results Cancer Res 163:72–84, discussion 264–6
35. Negm RS, Verma M, Srivastava S (2002) The promise of biomarkers in cancer screening and detection. Trends Mol Med 8:288–293
36. Srivastava S, Verma M, Henson DE (2001) Biomarkers for early detection of colon cancer. Clin Cancer Res 7:1118–1126
37. Verma M, Khoury MJ, Ioannidis JP (2013) Opportunities and challenges for selected emerging technologies in cancer epidemiology: mitochondrial, epigenomic, metabolomic, and telomerase profiling. Cancer Epidemiol Biomarkers Prev 22:189–200
38. Gerstung M, Eriksson N, Lin J, Vogelstein B, Beerenwinkel N (2011) The temporal order of genetic and pathway alterations in tumorigenesis. PLoS One 6:e27136
39. Jones S, Zhang X, Parsons DW, Lin JC, Leary RJ, Angenendt P et al (2008) Core signaling pathways in human pancreatic cancers revealed by global genomic analyses. Science 321:1801–1806
40. Ni Y, Xie X, Bu H, Zhang Z, Wei B, Yin L et al (2013) Concurrent primary angiosarcoma and invasive ductal carcinoma in the same breast. J Clin Pathol 66:263–264
41. Blaichman J, Marcus JC, Alsaadi T, El-Khoury M, Meterissian S, Mesurolle B (2012) Sonographic appearance of invasive ductal carcinoma of the breast according to histologic grade. AJR Am J Roentgenol 199:W402–W408
42. Henrique R, Luis AS, Jeronimo C (2012) The epigenetics of renal cell tumors: from biology to biomarkers. Front Genet 3:94
43. Hoque MO, Begum S, Topaloglu O, Jeronimo C, Mambo E, Westra WH et al (2004) Quantitative detection of promoter hypermethylation of multiple genes in the tumor, urine, and serum DNA of patients with renal cancer. Cancer Res 64:5511–5517
44. Brait M, Begum S, Carvalho AL, Dasgupta S, Vettore AL, Czerniak B et al (2008) Aberrant promoter methylation of multiple genes during pathogenesis of bladder cancer. Cancer Epidemiol Biomarkers Prev 17:2786–2794
45. Hoque MO, Begum S, Topaloglu O, Chatterjee A, Rosenbaum E, Van Criekinge W et al (2006) Quantitation of promoter methylation of multiple genes in urine DNA and bladder cancer detection. J Natl Cancer Inst 98:996–1004
46. Peters I, Rehmet K, Wilke N, Kuczyk MA, Hennenlotter J, Eilers T et al (2007) RASSF1A promoter methylation and expression analysis in normal and neoplastic kidney indicates a role in early tumorigenesis. Mol Cancer 6:49
47. Costa VL, Henrique R, Ribeiro FR, Pinto M, Oliveira J, Lobo F et al (2007) Quantitative promoter methylation analysis of multiple cancer-related genes in renal cell tumors. BMC Cancer 7:133
48. Jung M, Mollenkopf HJ, Grimm C, Wagner I, Albrecht M, Waller T et al (2009) MicroRNA profiling of clear cell renal cell cancer identifies a robust signature to define renal malignancy. J Cell Mol Med 13:3918–3928
49. Friedrich MG, Chandrasoma S, Siegmund KD, Weisenberger DJ, Cheng JC, Toma MI et al (2005) Prognostic relevance of methylation markers in patients with non-muscle invasive bladder carcinoma. Eur J Cancer 41:2769–2778
50. Rini BI, Campbell SC, Escudier B (2009) Renal cell carcinoma. Lancet 373:1119–1132
51. Ishihara K, Sasaki D, Tsuruda K, Inokuchi N, Nagai K, Hasegawa H et al (2012) Impact of miR-155 and

miR-126 as novel biomarkers on the assessment of disease progression and prognosis in adult T-cell leukemia. Cancer Epidemiol 36:560–565

52. Moussay E, Wang K, Cho JH, van Moer K, Pierson S, Paggetti J et al (2011) MicroRNA as biomarkers and regulators in B-cell chronic lymphocytic leukemia. Proc Natl Acad Sci U S A 108:6573–6578
53. Kraguljac Kurtovic N, Krajnovic M, Bogdanovic A, Suvajdzic N, Jovanovic J, Dimitrijevic B et al (2012) Concomitant aberrant methylation of p15 and MGMT genes in acute myeloid leukemia: association with a particular immunophenotype of blast cells. Med Oncol 29:3547–3556
54. Ammerpohl O, Haake A, Pellissery S, Giefing M, Richter J, Balint B et al (2012) Array-based DNA methylation analysis in classical Hodgkin lymphoma reveals new insights into the mechanisms underlying silencing of B cell-specific genes. Leukemia 26:185–188
55. Zainuddin N, Kanduri M, Berglund M, Lindell M, Amini RM, Roos G et al (2011) Quantitative evaluation of p16(INK4a) promoter methylation using pyrosequencing in de novo diffuse large B-cell lymphoma. Leuk Res 35:438–443
56. Alelu-Paz R, Ashour N, Gonzalez-Corpas A, Ropero S (2012) DNA methylation, histone modifications, and signal transduction pathways: a close relationship in malignant gliomas pathophysiology. J Signal Transduct 2012:956958
57. Alaminos M, Davalos V, Ropero S, Setien F, Paz MF, Herranz M et al (2005) EMP3, a myelin-related gene located in the critical 19q13.3 region, is epigenetically silenced and exhibits features of a candidate tumor suppressor in glioma and neuroblastoma. Cancer Res 65:2565–2571
58. Nakamura M, Yonekawa Y, Kleihues P, Ohgaki H (2001) Promoter hypermethylation of the RB1 gene in glioblastomas. Lab Invest 81:77–82
59. Fraga MF, Ballestar E, Villar-Garea A, Boix-Chornet M, Espada J, Schotta G et al (2005) Loss of acetylation at Lys16 and trimethylation at Lys20 of histone H4 is a common hallmark of human cancer. Nat Genet 37:391–400
60. Zhang Z, Tang H, Wang Z, Zhang B, Liu W, Lu H et al (2011) MiR-185 targets the DNA methyltransferases 1 and regulates global DNA methylation in human glioma. Mol Cancer 10:124
61. Di Vinci A, Casciano I, Marasco E, Banelli B, Ravetti GL, Borzi L et al (2012) Quantitative methylation analysis of HOXA3, 7, 9, and 10 genes in glioma: association with tumor WHO grade and clinical outcome. J Cancer Res Clin Oncol 138:35–47
62. Yoo KH, Hennighausen L (2012) EZH2 methyltransferase and H3K27 methylation in breast cancer. Int J Biol Sci 8:59–65
63. Buhmeida A, Merdad A, Al-Maghrabi J, Al-Thobaiti F, Ata M, Bugis A et al (2011) RASSF1A methylation is predictive of poor prognosis in female breast cancer in a background of overall low methylation frequency. Anticancer Res 31:2975–2981
64. Wu X, Somlo G, Yu Y, Palomares MR, Li AX, Zhou W et al (2012) De novo sequencing of circulating miRNAs identifies novel markers predicting clinical outcome of locally advanced breast cancer. J Transl Med 10:42
65. Clarke MA, Wentzensen N, Mirabello L, Ghosh A, Wacholder S, Harari A et al (2012) Human papillomavirus DNA methylation as a potential biomarker for cervical cancer. Cancer Epidemiol Biomarkers Prev 21:2125–2137
66. Das Ghosh D, Bhattacharjee B, Sen S, Premi L, Mukhopadhyay I, Chowdhury RR et al (2012) Some novel insights on HPV16 related cervical cancer pathogenesis based on analyses of LCR methylation, viral load, E7 and E2/E4 expressions. PLoS One 7:e44678
67. Kang WS, Cho SB, Park JS, Lee MY, Myung SC, Kim WY et al (2013) Clinico-epigenetic combination including quantitative methylation value of DKK3 augments survival prediction of the patient with cervical cancer. J Cancer Res Clin Oncol 139:97–106
68. Abudukadeer A, Bakry R, Goebel G, Mutz-Dehbalaie I, Widschwendter A, Bonn GK et al (2012) Clinical relevance of CDH1 and CDH13 DNA-methylation in serum of cervical cancer patients. Int J Mol Sci 13:8353–8363
69. Huang Y, Song H, Hu H, Cui L, You C, Huang L (2012) Trichosanthin inhibits DNA methyltransferase and restores methylation-silenced gene expression in human cervical cancer cells. Mol Med Rep 6:872–878
70. Jha AK, Nikbakht M, Jain V, Capalash N, Kaur J (2012) p16(INK4a) and p15(INK4b) gene promoter methylation in cervical cancer patients. Oncol Lett 3:1331–1335
71. Lof-Ohlin ZM, Levanat S, Sabol M, Sorbe B, Nilsson TK (2011) Promoter methylation in the PTCH gene in cervical epithelial cancer and ovarian cancer tissue as studied by eight novel Pyrosequencing(R) assays. Int J Oncol 38:685–692
72. Jeong DH, Youm MY, Kim YN, Lee KB, Sung MS, Yoon HK et al (2006) Promoter methylation of p16, DAPK, CDH1, and TIMP-3 genes in cervical cancer: correlation with clinicopathologic characteristics. Int J Gynecol Cancer 16:1234–1240
73. Chung MT, Sytwu HK, Yan MD, Shih YL, Chang CC, Yu MH et al (2009) Promoter methylation of SFRPs gene family in cervical cancer. Gynecol Oncol 112:301–306
74. Jung S, Yi L, Kim J, Jeong D, Oh T, Kim CH et al (2011) The role of vimentin as a methylation biomarker for early diagnosis of cervical cancer. Mol Cells 31:405–411
75. Han SW, Lee HJ, Bae JM, Cho NY, Lee KH, Kim TY et al (2013) Methylation and microsatellite status and recurrence following adjuvant FOLFOX in colorectal cancer. Int J Cancer 132:2209–2216

76. Dallol A, Al-Maghrabi J, Buhmeida A, Gari MA, Chaudhary AG, Schulten HJ et al (2012) Methylation of the polycomb group target genes is a possible biomarker for favorable prognosis in colorectal cancer. Cancer Epidemiol Biomarkers Prev 21:2069–2075
77. Fang WJ, Zheng Y, Wu LM, Ke QH, Shen H, Yuan Y et al (2012) Genome-wide analysis of aberrant DNA methylation for identification of potential biomarkers in colorectal cancer patients. Asian Pac J Cancer Prev 13:1917–1921
78. Khamas A, Ishikawa T, Mogushi K, Iida S, Ishiguro M, Tanaka H et al (2012) Genome-wide screening for methylation-silenced genes in colorectal cancer. Int J Oncol 41:490–496
79. Coppede F (2011) Epigenetic biomarkers of colorectal cancer: focus on DNA methylation. Cancer Lett 342(2):238–247
80. Hibi K, Mizukami H, Saito M, Kigawa G, Nemoto H, Sanada Y (2012) FBN2 methylation is detected in the serum of colorectal cancer patients with hepatic metastasis. Anticancer Res 32:4371–4374
81. Nilsson TK, Lof-Ohlin ZM, Sun XF (2013) DNA methylation of the p14ARF, RASSF1A and APC1A genes as an independent prognostic factor in colorectal cancer patients. Int J Oncol 42:127–133
82. Moya P, Esteban S, Fernandez-Suarez A, Maestro M, Morente M, Sanchez-Carbayo M (2012) KiSS-1 methylation and protein expression patterns contribute to diagnostic and prognostic assessments in tissue specimens for colorectal cancer. Tumour Biol 34:471–479
83. Ogino S, Nishihara R, Lochhead P, Imamura Y, Kuchiba A, Morikawa T et al (2013) Prospective study of family history and colorectal cancer risk by tumor LINE-1 methylation level. J Natl Cancer Inst 105:130–140
84. Li BQ, Yu H, Wang Z, Ding GH, Liu L (2013) MicroRNA mediated network and DNA methylation in colorectal cancer. Protein Pept Lett 20:352–363
85. Tamagawa H, Oshima T, Shiozawa M, Morinaga S, Nakamura Y, Yoshihara M et al (2012) The global histone modification pattern correlates with overall survival in metachronous liver metastasis of colorectal cancer. Oncol Rep 27:637–642
86. Nakazawa T, Kondo T, Ma D, Niu D, Mochizuki K, Kawasaki T et al (2012) Global histone modification of histone H3 in colorectal cancer and its precursor lesions. Hum Pathol 43:834–842
87. Banno K, Kisu I, Yanokura M, Masuda K, Kobayashi Y, Ueki A et al (2012) Endometrial cancer and hypermethylation: regulation of DNA and MicroRNA by epigenetics. Biochem Res Int 2012:738274
88. Banno K, Kisu I, Yanokura M, Masuda K, Ueki A, Kobayashi Y et al (2012) Epigenetics and genetics in endometrial cancer: new carcinogenic mechanisms and relationship with clinical practice. Epigenomics 4:147–162
89. Cohn DE, Fabbri M, Valeri N, Alder H, Ivanov I, Liu CG et al (2010) Comprehensive miRNA profiling of surgically staged endometrial cancer. Am J Obstet Gynecol 202:656 e1–656 e8
90. Tao MH, Freudenheim JL (2010) DNA methylation in endometrial cancer. Epigenetics 5:491–498
91. Varier RA, Vermeulen M (2012) Differential epigenetic regulation of GATA4 in gastric adenocarcinomas. Epigenomics 4:367
92. Jazirehi AR, Arle D, Wenn PB (2012) Role of epigenetic modifications of SOX 9 in gastric carcinoma. Epigenomics 4:253
93. Park JH, Park J, Choi JK, Lyu J, Bae MG, Lee YG et al (2011) Identification of DNA methylation changes associated with human gastric cancer. BMC Med Genomics 4:82
94. Jung Y, Park J, Bang YJ, Kim TY (2008) Gene silencing of TSPYL5 mediated by aberrant promoter methylation in gastric cancers. Lab Invest 88:153–160
95. Ebert MP, Mooney SH, Tonnes-Priddy L, Lograsso J, Hoffmann J, Chen J et al (2005) Hypermethylation of the TPEF/HPP1 gene in primary and metastatic colorectal cancers. Neoplasia 7:771–778
96. Kim JG, Takeshima H, Niwa T, Rehnberg E, Shigematsu Y, Yoda Y et al (2013) Comprehensive DNA methylation and extensive mutation analyses reveal an association between the CpG island methylator phenotype and oncogenic mutations in gastric cancers. Cancer Lett 330:33–40
97. Nanjo S, Asada K, Yamashita S, Nakajima T, Nakazawa K, Maekita T et al (2012) Identification of gastric cancer risk markers that are informative in individuals with past H. pylori infection. Gastric Cancer 15:382–388
98. Ushijima T, Hattori N (2012) Molecular pathways: involvement of helicobacter pylori-triggered inflammation in the formation of an epigenetic field defect, and its usefulness as cancer risk and exposure markers. Clin Cancer Res 18:923–929
99. Zabaleta J (2012) MicroRNA: a bridge from H. pylori infection to gastritis and gastric cancer development. Front Genet 3:294
100. Huang FY, Chan AO, Rashid A, Wong DK, Cho CH, Yuen MF (2012) Helicobacter pylori induces promoter methylation of E-cadherin via interleukin-1beta activation of nitric oxide production in gastric cancer cells. Cancer 118:4969–4980
101. Ziogas D, Roukos D (2009) Epigenetics in gastric cancer: challenges for clinical implications. Ann Surg Oncol 16:2077–2078
102. Park YS, Jin MY, Kim YJ, Yook JH, Kim BS, Jang SJ (2008) The global histone modification pattern correlates with cancer recurrence and overall survival in gastric adenocarcinoma. Ann Surg Oncol 15:1968–1976
103. Zouridis H, Deng N, Ivanova T, Zhu Y, Wong B, Huang D et al (2012) Methylation subtypes and large-scale epigenetic alterations in gastric cancer. Sci Transl Med 4:156ra40

104. Chang X, Li Z, Ma J, Deng P, Zhang S, Zhi Y et al (2013) DNA methylation of NDRG2 in gastric cancer and its clinical significance. Dig Dis Sci 58:715–723
105. Takamaru H, Yamamoto E, Suzuki H, Nojima M, Maruyama R, Yamano HO et al (2012) Aberrant methylation of RASGRF1 is associated with an epigenetic field defect and increased risk of gastric cancer. Cancer Prev Res (Phila) 5:1203–1212
106. Yu QM, Wang XB, Luo J, Wang S, Fang XH, Yu JL et al (2012) CDH1 methylation in preoperative peritoneal washes is an independent prognostic factor for gastric cancer. J Surg Oncol 106:765–771
107. Alves MK, Ferrasi AC, Lima VP, Ferreira MV, de Moura Campos Pardini MI, Rabenhorst SH (2011) Inactivation of COX-2, HMLH1 and CDKN2A gene by promoter methylation in gastric cancer: relationship with histological subtype, tumor location and helicobacter pylori genotype. Pathobiology 78:266–276
108. Ando T, Yoshida T, Enomoto S, Asada K, Tatematsu M, Ichinose M et al (2009) DNA methylation of microRNA genes in gastric mucosae of gastric cancer patients: its possible involvement in the formation of epigenetic field defect. Int J Cancer 124:2367–2374
109. Shirahata A, Sakuraba K, Kitamura Y, Yokomizo K, Gotou T, Saitou M et al (2012) Detection of vimentin methylation in the serum of patients with gastric cancer. Anticancer Res 32:791–794
110. Demokan S, Dalay N (2011) Role of DNA methylation in head and neck cancer. Clin Epigenetics 2:123–150
111. Teh MT, Gemenetzidis E, Patel D, Tariq R, Nadir A, Bahta AW et al (2012) FOXM1 induces a global methylation signature that mimics the cancer epigenome in head and neck squamous cell carcinoma. PLoS One 7:e34329
112. Demokan S, Chuang A, Suoglu Y, Ulusan M, Yalniz Z, Califano JA et al (2012) Promoter methylation and loss of p16(INK4a) gene expression in head and neck cancer. Head Neck 34:1470–1475
113. Yalniz Z, Demokan S, Suoglu Y, Ulusan M, Dalay N (2011) Simultaneous methylation profiling of tumor suppressor genes in head and neck cancer. DNA Cell Biol 30:17–24
114. Righini CA, de Fraipont F, Timsit JF, Faure C, Brambilla E, Reyt E et al (2007) Tumor-specific methylation in saliva: a promising biomarker for early detection of head and neck cancer recurrence. Clin Cancer Res 13:1179–1185
115. Calmon MF, Colombo J, Carvalho F, Souza FP, Filho JF, Fukuyama EE et al (2007) Methylation profile of genes CDKN2A (p14 and p16), DAPK1, CDH1, and ADAM23 in head and neck cancer. Cancer Genet Cytogenet 173:31–37
116. Hasegawa M, Nelson HH, Peters E, Ringstrom E, Posner M, Kelsey KT (2002) Patterns of gene promoter methylation in squamous cell cancer of the head and neck. Oncogene 21:4231–4236
117. Demokan S, Suoglu Y, Demir D, Gozeler M, Dalay N (2006) Microsatellite instability and methylation of the DNA mismatch repair genes in head and neck cancer. Ann Oncol 17:995–999
118. Biron VL, Dort JC (2008) Epigenetic perspective into head and neck cancer through in silico gene expression profiling of histone lysine methyltransferases. J Otolaryngol Head Neck Surg 37:366–372
119. Peters I, Eggers H, Atschekzei F, Hennenlotter J, Waalkes S, Trankenschuh W et al (2012) GATA5 CpG island methylation in renal cell cancer: a potential biomarker for metastasis and disease progression. BJU Int 110:E144–E152
120. Eggers H, Steffens S, Grosshennig A, Becker JU, Hennenlotter J, Stenzl A et al (2012) Prognostic and diagnostic relevance of hypermethylated in cancer 1 (HIC1) CpG island methylation in renal cell carcinoma. Int J Oncol 40:1650–1658
121. Atschekzei F, Hennenlotter J, Janisch S, Grosshennig A, Trankenschuh W, Waalkes S et al (2012) SFRP1 CpG island methylation locus is associated with renal cell cancer susceptibility and disease recurrence. Epigenetics 7:447–457
122. Liao LM, Brennan P, van Bemmel DM, Zaridze D, Matveev V, Janout V et al (2011) LINE-1 methylation levels in leukocyte DNA and risk of renal cell cancer. PLoS One 6:e27361
123. Fritzsche FR, Weichert W, Roske A, Gekeler V, Beckers T, Stephan C et al (2008) Class I histone deacetylases 1, 2 and 3 are highly expressed in renal cell cancer. BMC Cancer 8:381
124. Hildebrandt MA, Gu J, Lin J, Ye Y, Tan W, Tamboli P et al (2010) Hsa-miR-9 methylation status is associated with cancer development and metastatic recurrence in patients with clear cell renal cell carcinoma. Oncogene 29:5724–5728
125. Varier RA, Vermeulen M (2012) Epigenetics and the prognosis of hepatocellular carcinoma. Epigenomics 4:368
126. Lee JS, Chu IS, Heo J, Calvisi DF, Sun Z, Roskams T et al (2004) Classification and prediction of survival in hepatocellular carcinoma by gene expression profiling. Hepatology 40:667–676
127. Calvisi DF, Ladu S, Gorden A, Farina M, Lee JS, Conner EA et al (2007) Mechanistic and prognostic significance of aberrant methylation in the molecular pathogenesis of human hepatocellular carcinoma. J Clin Invest 117:2713–2722
128. Lambert MP, Paliwal A, Vaissiere T, Chemin I, Zoulim F, Tommasino M et al (2011) Aberrant DNA methylation distinguishes hepatocellular carcinoma associated with HBV and HCV infection and alcohol intake. J Hepatol 54:705–715
129. He C, Xu J, Zhang J, Xie D, Ye H, Xiao Z et al (2012) High expression of trimethylated histone H3 lysine 4 is associated with poor prognosis in hepatocellular carcinoma. Hum Pathol 43:1425–1435
130. Gao W, Xu J, Shu YQ (2011) miRNA expression and its clinical implications for the prevention and

diagnosis of non-small-cell lung cancer. Expert Rev Respir Med 5:699–709
131. Lin PY, Yang PC (2011) Circulating miRNA signature for early diagnosis of lung cancer. EMBO Mol Med 3:436–437
132. Keller A, Leidinger P, Gislefoss R, Haugen A, Langseth H, Staehler P et al (2011) Stable serum miRNA profiles as potential tool for non-invasive lung cancer diagnosis. RNA Biol 8:506–516
133. Xie Y, Todd NW, Liu Z, Zhan M, Fang H, Peng H et al (2010) Altered miRNA expression in sputum for diagnosis of non-small cell lung cancer. Lung Cancer 67:170–176
134. Belinsky SA, Nikula KJ, Palmisano WA, Michels R, Saccomanno G, Gabrielson E et al (1998) Aberrant methylation of p16(INK4a) is an early event in lung cancer and a potential biomarker for early diagnosis. Proc Natl Acad Sci U S A 95:11891–11896
135. Anglim PP, Galler JS, Koss MN, Hagen JA, Turla S, Campan M et al (2008) Identification of a panel of sensitive and specific DNA methylation markers for squamous cell lung cancer. Mol Cancer 7:62
136. Leng S, Do K, Yingling CM, Picchi MA, Wolf HJ, Kennedy TC et al (2012) Defining a gene promoter methylation signature in sputum for lung cancer risk assessment. Clin Cancer Res 18:3387–3395
137. Yu GP, Ji Y, Chen GQ, Huang B, Shen K, Wu S et al (2012) Application of RUNX3 gene promoter methylation in the diagnosis of non-small cell lung cancer. Oncol Lett 3:159–162
138. Dietrich D, Kneip C, Raji O, Liloglou T, Seegebarth A, Schlegel T et al (2012) Performance evaluation of the DNA methylation biomarker SHOX2 for the aid in diagnosis of lung cancer based on the analysis of bronchial aspirates. Int J Oncol 40:825–832
139. Schmidt B, Liebenberg V, Dietrich D, Schlegel T, Kneip C, Seegebarth A et al (2010) SHOX2 DNA methylation is a biomarker for the diagnosis of lung cancer based on bronchial aspirates. BMC Cancer 10:600
140. Begum S, Brait M, Dasgupta S, Ostrow KL, Zahurak M, Carvalho AL et al (2011) An epigenetic marker panel for detection of lung cancer using cell-free serum DNA. Clin Cancer Res 17:4494–4503
141. Gloss BS, Samimi G (2012) Epigenetic biomarkers in epithelial ovarian cancer. Cancer Lett 342(2):257–263
142. Kashuba V, Dmitriev AA, Krasnov GS, Pavlova T, Ignatjev I, Gordiyuk VV et al (2012) NotI microarrays: novel epigenetic markers for early detection and prognosis of high grade serous ovarian cancer. Int J Mol Sci 13:13352–13377
143. Kisiel JB, Yab TC, Taylor WR, Chari ST, Petersen GM, Mahoney DW et al (2012) Stool DNA testing for the detection of pancreatic cancer: assessment of methylation marker candidates. Cancer 118:2623–2631
144. Kumari A, Srinivasan R, Vasishta RK, Wig JD (2009) Positive regulation of human telomerase reverse transcriptase gene expression and telomerase activity by DNA methylation in pancreatic cancer. Ann Surg Oncol 16:1051–1059
145. Li M, Zhao ZW (2012) Clinical implications of mismatched repair gene promoter methylation in pancreatic cancer. Med Oncol 29:970–976
146. Liggett T, Melnikov A, Yi QL, Replogle C, Brand R, Kaul K et al (2010) Differential methylation of cell-free circulating DNA among patients with pancreatic cancer versus chronic pancreatitis. Cancer 116:1674–1680
147. Matsubayashi H, Sato N, Fukushima N, Yeo CJ, Walter KM, Brune K et al (2003) Methylation of cyclin D2 is observed frequently in pancreatic cancer but is also an age-related phenomenon in gastrointestinal tissues. Clin Cancer Res 9:1446–1452
148. Omura N, Goggins M (2009) Epigenetics and epigenetic alterations in pancreatic cancer. Int J Clin Exp Pathol 2:310–326
149. Grzenda A, Ordog T, Urrutia R (2011) Polycomb and the emerging epigenetics of pancreatic cancer. J Gastrointest Cancer 42:100–111
150. Cooper CS, Foster CS (2009) Concepts of epigenetics in prostate cancer development. Br J Cancer 100:240–245
151. Dobosy JR, Roberts JL, Fu VX, Jarrard DF (2007) The expanding role of epigenetics in the development, diagnosis and treatment of prostate cancer and benign prostatic hyperplasia. J Urol 177:822–831
152. Sullivan L, Murphy TM, Barrett C, Loftus B, Thornhill J, Lawler M et al (2012) IGFBP7 promoter methylation and gene expression analysis in prostate cancer. J Urol 188:1354–1360
153. Olkhov-Mitsel E, Van der Kwast T, Kron KJ, Ozcelik H, Briollais L, Massey C et al (2012) Quantitative DNA methylation analysis of genes coding for kallikrein-related peptidases 6 and 10 as biomarkers for prostate cancer. Epigenetics 7:1037–1045
154. Shaikhibrahim Z, Lindstrot A, Ochsenfahrt J, Fuchs K, Wernert N (2013) Epigenetics-related genes in prostate cancer: expression profile in prostate cancer tissues, androgen-sensitive and -insensitive cell lines. Int J Mol Med 31:21–25
155. Paone A, Galli R, Fabbri M (2011) MicroRNAs as new characters in the plot between epigenetics and prostate cancer. Front Genet 2:62
156. Alshalalfa M (2012) MicroRNA response elements-mediated miRNA-miRNA interactions in prostate cancer. Adv Bioinformatics 2012:839837
157. Majid S, Dar AA, Saini S, Shahryari V, Arora S, Zaman MS et al (2013) MiRNA-34b inhibits prostate cancer through demethylation, active chromatin modifications, and AKT pathways. Clin Cancer Res 19:73–84
158. Mahn R, Heukamp LC, Rogenhofer S, von Ruecker A, Muller SC, Ellinger J (2011) Circulating microRNAs (miRNA) in serum of patients with prostate cancer. Urology 77:1265 e9–1265 e16
159. Mahapatra S, Klee EW, Young CY, Sun Z, Jimenez RE, Klee GG et al (2012) Global methylation profiling

for risk prediction of prostate cancer. Clin Cancer Res 18:2882–2895
160. Wu W, Zhang J, Yang H, Shao Y, Yu B (2011) Examination of AKAP12 promoter methylation in skin cancer using methylation-sensitive high-resolution melting analysis. Clin Exp Dermatol 36:381–385
161. Chen YC, Guo YL, Su HJ, Hsueh YM, Smith TJ, Ryan LM et al (2003) Arsenic methylation and skin cancer risk in southwestern Taiwan. J Occup Environ Med 45:241–248
162. Yu RC, Hsu KH, Chen CJ, Froines JR (2000) Arsenic methylation capacity and skin cancer. Cancer Epidemiol Biomarkers Prev 9:1259–1262
163. Burgess DJ (2012) Epigenetics: melanoma insights written in the DNA. Nat Rev Cancer 12:738–739
164. Nguyen T, Kuo C, Nicholl MB, Sim MS, Turner RR, Morton DL et al (2011) Downregulation of microRNA-29c is associated with hypermethylation of tumor-related genes and disease outcome in cutaneous melanoma. Epigenetics 6:388–394
165. Xu X, Jin H, Liu Y, Liu L, Wu Q, Guo Y et al (2012) The expression patterns and correlations of claudin-6, methy-CpG binding protein 2, DNA methyltransferase 1, histone deacetylase 1, acetyl-histone H3 and acetyl-histone H4 and their clinicopathological significance in breast invasive ductal carcinomas. Diagn Pathol 7:33
166. Bosch LJ, Mongera S, Terhaar Sive Droste JS, Oort FA, van Turenhout ST, Penning MT et al (2012) Analytical sensitivity and stability of DNA methylation testing in stool samples for colorectal cancer detection. Cell Oncol (Dordr) 35:309–315
167. Elliott GO, Johnson IT, Scarll J, Dainty J, Williams EA, Garg D et al (2013) Quantitative profiling of CpG island methylation in human stool for colorectal cancer detection. Int J Colorectal Dis 28:35–42
168. Patchsung M, Boonla C, Amnattrakul P, Dissayabutra T, Mutirangura A, Tosukhowong P (2012) Long interspersed nuclear element-1 hypomethylation and oxidative stress: correlation and bladder cancer diagnostic potential. PLoS One 7:e37009
169. Zhu W, Qin W, Hewett JE, Sauter ER (2010) Quantitative evaluation of DNA hypermethylation in malignant and benign breast tissue and fluids. Int J Cancer 126:474–482
170. Dulaimi E, Hillinck J, Ibanez de Caceres I, Al-Saleem T, Cairns P (2004) Tumor suppressor gene promoter hypermethylation in serum of breast cancer patients. Clin Cancer Res 10:6189–6193
171. Nelson HH, Marsit CJ, Christensen BC, Houseman EA, Kontic M, Wiemels JL et al (2012) Key epigenetic changes associated with lung cancer development: results from dense methylation array profiling. Epigenetics 7:559–566
172. Langevin SM, Koestler DC, Christensen BC, Butler RA, Wiencke JK, Nelson HH et al (2012) Peripheral blood DNA methylation profiles are indicative of head and neck squamous cell carcinoma: an epigenome-wide association study. Epigenetics 7:291–299
173. Marsit CJ, Houseman EA, Christensen BC, Gagne L, Wrensch MR, Nelson HH et al (2010) Identification of methylated genes associated with aggressive bladder cancer. PLoS One 5:e12334
174. Yan C, Kim YW, Ha YS, Kim IY, Kim YJ, Yun SJ et al (2012) RUNX3 methylation as a predictor for disease progression in patients with non-muscle-invasive bladder cancer. J Surg Oncol 105:425–430
175. Ben Gacem R, Hachana M, Ziadi S, Amara K, Ksia F, Mokni M et al (2012) Contribution of epigenetic alteration of BRCA1 and BRCA2 genes in breast carcinomas in Tunisian patients. Cancer Epidemiol 36:190–197
176. Poage GM, Butler RA, Houseman EA, McClean MD, Nelson HH, Christensen BC et al (2012) Identification of an epigenetic profile classifier that is associated with survival in head and neck cancer. Cancer Res 72:2728–2737
177. Marsit CJ, McClean MD, Furniss CS, Kelsey KT (2006) Epigenetic inactivation of the SFRP genes is associated with drinking, smoking and HPV in head and neck squamous cell carcinoma. Int J Cancer 119:1761–1766
178. Ling ZQ, Zhao Q, Zhou SL, Mao WM (2012) MSH2 promoter hypermethylation in circulating tumor DNA is a valuable predictor of disease-free survival for patients with esophageal squamous cell carcinoma. Eur J Surg Oncol 38:326–332
179. Hu Z, Chen X, Zhao Y, Tian T, Jin G, Shu Y et al (2010) Serum microRNA signatures identified in a genome-wide serum microRNA expression profiling predict survival of non-small-cell lung cancer. J Clin Oncol 28:1721–1726
180. Landi MT, Zhao Y, Rotunno M, Koshiol J, Liu H, Bergen AW et al (2010) MicroRNA expression differentiates histology and predicts survival of lung cancer. Clin Cancer Res 16:430–441
181. Teo MT, Landi D, Taylor CF, Elliott F, Vaslin L, Cox DG et al (2012) The role of microRNA-binding site polymorphisms in DNA repair genes as risk factors for bladder cancer and breast cancer and their impact on radiotherapy outcomes. Carcinogenesis 33:581–586
182. Boumber Y, Issa JP (2011) Epigenetics in cancer: what's the future? Oncology (Williston Park) 25:220–226
183. Yan P, Frankhouser D, Murphy M, Tam HH, Rodriguez B, Curfman J et al (2012) Genome-wide methylation profiling in decitabine-treated patients with acute myeloid leukemia. Blood 120:2466–2474
184. Ramaswamy B, Fiskus W, Cohen B, Pellegrino C, Hershman DL, Chuang E et al (2012) Phase I-II study of vorinostat plus paclitaxel and bevacizumab in metastatic breast cancer: evidence for vorinostat-induced tubulin acetylation and Hsp90 inhibition in vivo. Breast Cancer Res Treat 132:1063–1072

185. Juergens RA, Wrangle J, Vendetti FP, Murphy SC, Zhao M, Coleman B et al (2011) Combination epigenetic therapy has efficacy in patients with refractory advanced non-small cell lung cancer. Cancer Discov 1:598–607
186. Pepe MS, Etzioni R, Feng Z, Potter JD, Thompson ML, Thornquist M et al (2001) Phases of biomarker development for early detection of cancer. J Natl Cancer Inst 93:1054–1061
187. Khoury MJ, Freedman AN, Gillanders EM, Harvey CE, Kaefer C, Reid BC et al (2012) Frontiers in cancer epidemiology: a challenge to the research community from the epidemiology and genomics research program at the national cancer institute. Cancer Epidemiol Biomarkers Prev 21:999–1001
188. Verma M (2009) Proteomics and cancer epidemiology. Methods Mol Biol 471:197–215
189. Verma M, Kumar D (2007) Application of mitochondrial genome information in cancer epidemiology. Clin Chim Acta 383:41–50
190. Verma M, Naviaux RK, Tanaka M, Kumar D, Franceschi C, Singh KK (2007) Meeting report: mitochondrial DNA and cancer epidemiology. Cancer Res 67:437–439
191. Verma M (2005) Pancreatic cancer epidemiology. Technol Cancer Res Treat 4:295–301
192. van Bemmel D, Lenz P, Liao LM, Baris D, Sternberg LR, Warner A et al (2012) Correlation of LINE-1 methylation levels in patient-matched buffy coat, serum, buccal cell, and bladder tumor tissue DNA samples. Cancer Epidemiol Biomarkers Prev 21:1143–1148
193. Koestler DC, Marsit CJ, Christensen BC, Accomando W, Langevin SM, Houseman EA et al (2012) Peripheral blood immune cell methylation profiles are associated with nonhematopoietic cancers. Cancer Epidemiol Biomarkers Prev 21:1293–1302
194. Sturgeon SR, Balasubramanian R, Schairer C, Muss HB, Ziegler RG, Arcaro KF (2012) Detection of promoter methylation of tumor suppressor genes in serum DNA of breast cancer cases and benign breast disease controls. Epigenetics 7:1258–1267
195. von Deimling A, Korshunov A, Hartmann C (2011) The next generation of glioma biomarkers: MGMT methylation, BRAF fusions and IDH1 mutations. Brain Pathol 21:74–87
196. Rather MI, Nagashri MN, Swamy SS, Gopinath KS, Kumar A (2013) Oncogenic microRNA-155 downregulates tumor suppressor CDC73 and promotes oral squamous cell carcinoma cell proliferation: implications for cancer therapeutics. J Biol Chem 288:608–618
197. Koike K, Kasamatsu A, Iyoda M, Saito Y, Kouzu Y, Koike H et al (2013) High prevalence of epigenetic inactivation of the human four and a half LIM domains 1 gene in human oral cancer. Int J Oncol 42:141–150
198. Shaw RJ, Hobkirk AJ, Nikolaidis G, Woolgar JA, Triantafyllou A, Brown JS et al (2013) Molecular staging of surgical margins in oral squamous cell carcinoma using promoter methylation of p16(INK4A), cytoglobin, E-cadherin, and TMEFF2. Ann Surg Oncol 20(8):2796–2802
199. Zhou J, Cao J, Lu Z, Liu H, Deng D (2011) A 115-bp MethyLight assay for detection of p16 (CDKN2A) methylation as a diagnostic biomarker in human tissues. BMC Med Genet 12:67
200. Sasahira T, Ueda N, Yamamoto K, Bhawal UK, Kurihara M, Kirita T et al (2013) Trks are novel oncogenes involved in the induction of neovascularization, tumor progression, and nodal metastasis in oral squamous cell carcinoma. Clin Exp Metastasis 30:165–176
201. Kordi-Tamandani DM, Ladies MA, Hashemi M, Moazeni-Roodi AK, Krishna S, Torkamanzehi A (2012) Analysis of p15INK4b and p16INK4a gene methylation in patients with oral squamous cell carcinoma. Biochem Genet 50:448–453
202. Minor J, Wang X, Zhang F, Song J, Jimeno A, Wang XJ et al (2012) Methylation of microRNA-9 is a specific and sensitive biomarker for oral and oropharyngeal squamous cell carcinomas. Oral Oncol 48:73–78
203. Gasche JA, Hoffmann J, Boland CR, Goel A (2011) Interleukin-6 promotes tumorigenesis by altering DNA methylation in oral cancer cells. Int J Cancer 129:1053–1063
204. Guerrero-Preston R, Soudry E, Acero J, Orera M, Moreno-Lopez L, Macia-Colon G et al (2011) NID2 and HOXA9 promoter hypermethylation as biomarkers for prevention and early detection in oral cavity squamous cell carcinoma tissues and saliva. Cancer Prev Res (Phila) 4:1061–1072
205. Biron VL, Mohamed A, Hendzel MJ, Alan Underhill D, Seikaly H (2012) Epigenetic differences between human papillomavirus-positive and -negative oropharyngeal squamous cell carcinomas. J Otolaryngol Head Neck Surg 41(Suppl 1):S65–S70
206. Cheung HH, Davis AJ, Lee TL, Pang AL, Nagrani S, Rennert OM et al (2011) Methylation of an intronic region regulates miR-199a in testicular tumor malignancy. Oncogene 30:3404–3415
207. Lee SH, Appleby V, Jeyapalan JN, Palmer RD, Nicholson JC, Sottile V et al (2011) Variable methylation of the imprinted gene, SNRPN, supports a relationship between intracranial germ cell tumours and neural stem cells. J Neurooncol 101:419–428
208. Xiao L, Wang Y, Zhou Y, Sun Y, Sun W, Wang L et al (2010) Identification of a novel human cancer/testis gene MAEL that is regulated by DNA methylation. Mol Biol Rep 37:2355–2360
209. Sugimoto K, Koh E, Sin HS, Maeda Y, Narimoto K, Izumi K et al (2009) Tissue-specific differentially methylated regions of the human VASA gene are potentially associated with maturation arrest phenotype in the testis. J Hum Genet 54:450–456
210. Marsit CJ, Karagas MR, Andrew A, Liu M, Danaee H, Schned AR et al (2005) Epigenetic inactivation of

SFRP genes and TP53 alteration act jointly as markers of invasive bladder cancer. Cancer Res 65:7081–7085
211. Liu BL, Cheng JX, Zhang W, Zhang X, Wang R, Lin H et al (2010) Quantitative detection of multiple gene promoter hypermethylation in tumor tissue, serum, and cerebrospinal fluid predicts prognosis of malignant gliomas. Neuro Oncol 12:540–548
212. Sebova K, Zmetakova I, Bella V, Kajo K, Stankovicova I, Kajabova V et al (2011) RASSF1A and CDH1 hypermethylation as potential epimarkers in breast cancer. Cancer Biomark 10:13–26
213. Kishi T, Tanaka Y, Ueda K (2000) Evidence for hypomethylation in two children with acute lymphoblastic leukemia and leukoencephalopathy. Cancer 89:925–931
214. Szaumkessel M, Richter J, Giefing M, Jarmuz M, Kiwerska K, Tonnies H et al (2011) Pyrosequencing-based DNA methylation profiling of Fanconi anemia/BRCA pathway genes in laryngeal squamous cell carcinoma. Int J Oncol 39:505–514
215. Virmani AK, Muller C, Rathi A, Zoechbauer-Mueller S, Mathis M, Gazdar AF (2001) Aberrant methylation during cervical carcinogenesis. Clin Cancer Res 7:584–589
216. Cortese R, Kwan A, Lalonde E, Bryzgunova O, Bondar A, Wu Y et al (2012) Epigenetic markers of prostate cancer in plasma circulating DNA. Hum Mol Genet 21:3619–3631
217. Tokarz P, Blasiak J (2012) The role of MiRNA in metastatic colorectal cancer and its significance in cancer prognosis and treatment. Acta Biochim Pol 59:467–474
218. Selth LA, Tilley WD, Butler LM (2012) Circulating microRNAs: macro-utility as markers of prostate cancer? Endocr Relat Cancer 19:R99–R113
219. Piyathilake CJ, Macaluso M, Alvarez RD, Chen M, Badiga S, Siddiqui NR et al (2011) A higher degree of LINE-1 methylation in peripheral blood mononuclear cells, a one-carbon nutrient related epigenetic alteration, is associated with a lower risk of developing cervical intraepithelial neoplasia. Nutrition 27:513–519
220. Sun C, Reimers LL, Burk RD (2011) Methylation of HPV16 genome CpG sites is associated with cervix precancer and cancer. Gynecol Oncol 121:59–63
221. Apostolidou S, Hadwin R, Burnell M, Jones A, Baff D, Pyndiah N et al (2009) DNA methylation analysis in liquid-based cytology for cervical cancer screening. Int J Cancer 125:2995–3002
222. Sathyanarayana UG, Maruyama R, Padar A, Suzuki M, Bondaruk J, Sagalowsky A et al (2004) Molecular detection of noninvasive and invasive bladder tumor tissues and exfoliated cells by aberrant promoter methylation of laminin-5 encoding genes. Cancer Res 64:1425–1430
223. Antill YC, Mitchell G, Johnson SA, Devereux L, Milner A, Di Iulio J et al (2010) Gene methylation in breast ductal fluid from BRCA1 and BRCA2 mutation carriers. Cancer Epidemiol Biomarkers Prev 19:265–274
224. Miyake M, Gomes Giacoia E, Aguilar Palacios D, Rosser CJ (2012) Lung cancer risk assessment for smokers: gene promoter methylation signature in sputum. Biomarker Med 6:512
225. Flores KG, Stidley CA, Mackey AJ, Picchi MA, Stabler SP, Siegfried JM et al (2012) Sex-specific association of sequence variants in CBS and MTRR with risk for promoter hypermethylation in the lung epithelium of smokers. Carcinogenesis 33:1542–1547
226. Guzman L, Depix MS, Salinas AM, Roldan R, Aguayo F, Silva A et al (2012) Analysis of aberrant methylation on promoter sequences of tumor suppressor genes and total DNA in sputum samples: a promising tool for early detection of COPD and lung cancer in smokers. Diagn Pathol 7:87
227. Kunte DP, DelaCruz M, Wali RK, Menon A, Du H, Stypula Y et al (2012) Dysregulation of microRNAs in colonic field carcinogenesis: implications for screening. PLoS One 7:e45591
228. Faryna M, Konermann C, Aulmann S, Bermejo JL, Brugger M, Diederichs S et al (2012) Genome-wide methylation screen in low-grade breast cancer identifies novel epigenetically altered genes as potential biomarkers for tumor diagnosis. FASEB J 26:4937–4950
229. Lendvai A, Johannes F, Grimm C, Eijsink JJ, Wardenaar R, Volders HH et al (2012) Genome-wide methylation profiling identifies hypermethylated biomarkers in high-grade cervical intraepithelial neoplasia. Epigenetics 7:1268–1278
230. Botla SK, Gholami AM, Malekpour M, Moskalev EA, Fallah M, Jandaghi P et al (2012) Diagnostic values of GHSR DNA methylation pattern in breast cancer. Breast Cancer Res Treat 135:705–713
231. Sporn JC, Jung B (2012) Differential regulation and predictive potential of MacroH2A1 isoforms in colon cancer. Am J Pathol 180:2516–2526
232. Dimitriadis E, Kalogeropoulos T, Velaeti S, Sotiriou S, Vassiliou E, Fasoulis L et al (2013) Study of genetic and epigenetic alterations in urine samples as diagnostic markers for prostate cancer. Anticancer Res 33:191–197
233. Kim YK, Kim WJ (2009) Epigenetic markers as promising prognosticators for bladder cancer. Int J Urol 16:17–22

Efficient, Adaptive Clinical Validation of Predictive Biomarkers in Cancer Therapeutic Development

6

Robert A. Beckman and Cong Chen

Abstract

Predictive biomarkers, defined as biomarkers that can be used to identify patient populations who will optimally benefit from therapy, are an important part of the future of oncology. They have the potential to reduce the size and cost of clinical development programs for oncology therapy, while increasing their probability of success and the ultimate value of cancer medicines. But predictive biomarkers do not always work, and under these circumstances they add cost, complexity, and time to drug development. This chapter describes Phase 2 and 3 development methods which efficiently and adaptively evaluate the ability of the biomarker to predict clinical outcomes. In the end, the biomarker is emphasized to the extent that it is actually predictive. This allows clinical cancer drug developers to manage uncertainty in the validity of biomarkers, leading to maximal value for predictive biomarkers and their associated oncology therapies.

Keywords

Clinical outcome • Clinical performance • Clinical practice • Clinical validation • Linearity • Oncology personalized medicine • Oncology therapies • Phase 1 clinical studies • Phase 2 clinical studies • Phase 3 clinical studies • Predictive biomarker • Reproducibility • Sensitivity • Specificity • Stratification • The multiple comparisons problem • Translational medicine

R.A. Beckman (✉)
Departments of Oncology and of Biostatistics, Bioinformatics, and Biomathematics, Lombardi Comprehensive Cancer Center and Innovation Center for Biomedical Informatics, Georgetown University Medical Center, 2115 Wisconsin Avenue, Suite 110, Washington, DC 2007, USA

1551 33rd Street NW, Washington, DC 2007, USA
e-mail: eniac1915@gmail.com

C. Chen
Biostatistics and Research Decision Sciences, Merck Research Laboratories, Rahway, NJ, USA

R. Scatena (ed.), *Advances in Cancer Biomarkers*, Advances in Experimental Medicine and Biology 867, DOI 10.1007/978-94-017-7215-0_6

6.1 Introduction: Biomarkers, Promise and Pitfalls

Predictive biomarkers, or "responder identification" biomarkers, are molecular or other characteristics of a patient or a patient's malignancy which predict increased benefit (or toxicity) from a particular drug. Predictive classifiers, which may be constructed from one biomarker or a composite of biomarkers, identify patients more likely to benefit (or experience toxicity). With increasing knowledge of the molecular biology of cancer, the number and potential of these predictive biomarkers and classifiers is increasing.

Currently, the risk of cancer drug development is high due to a high failure rate of clinical trials. This may be due to heterogeneity between patients' tumors, leading to trials where most of the patients cannot benefit from the drug. In this situation, the "signal" from the patients who benefit may be lost in the "noise" from the patients who do not benefit. By applying predictive biomarkers, we can select the patients who will benefit more precisely, ultimately leading to a greater chance of detection of the signal of benefit. For example, trastuzumab was studied in metastatic breast cancer patients whose tumors overexpressed its target, the Her2-neu protein [14, 26]. This therapy has been very successful in benefiting approximately 20 % of metastatic breast cancer patients, but if the clinical trial had been done in an unselected metastatic breast cancer population it almost certainly would have been negative. Thus, predictive biomarkers offer an increased probability of success of oncology trials.

Clinical trials which are performed in an unselected population have a small average benefit because patients who cannot benefit contribute to the average. The number of patients required to detect a small benefit in a randomized trial is much higher than that required to detect a large benefit. In fact, the size of the trial is proportional to the *inverse square* of the benefit size. For example, by doubling the size of the average benefit, you can reduce the required size of the randomized trials to detect it by a factor of 4. This also can lead to a decreased cost of clinical development.

National health authorities and payors are increasingly demanding value for medicines. Value is measured in cost per quality adjusted life year (QALY), and the UK National Institute for Clinical Excellence (NICE) generally expects this cost to be 30,000 British pounds or less. Most cancer medicines exceed this cost because of the high cost of their development and the low average benefit. The high cost is driven by low probabilities of success and high cost of clinical development programs, and the low average benefit by treatment of many patients who will not benefit.

Clearly, predictive biomarkers have the potential to increase the value of cancer medicines and decrease their cost. Examples of successful applications of predictive biomarkers include her2neu expression for trastuzumab therapy of breast cancer [14, 26], sensitizing mutations in the epidermal growth factor receptor (EGFR) gene for gefitinib and erlotinib therapy of non-small cell lung cancer [20, 21], ras wild type status for therapy of colorectal cancer with anti-EGFR therapy using cetuximab or panitumumab [1, 7, 19, 28], alk translocations for crizotinib therapy of lung cancer [24], and V600E mutations for vemurafenib therapy of melanoma [8].

However, predictive biomarkers do not always work. A notable exception was found when patients without measurable EGFR receptor expression were found to benefit from anti-EGFR antibody therapy in colorectal cancer. This may have been due to insufficient assay sensitivity, loss of EGFR antigen on storage of clinical specimens, sampling error within a heterogeneous tumor, or evolution of the tumor between when the specimen was obtained (often at diagnosis) and the time of treatment (frequently ar relapse) [22, 29]. These practical pitfalls affect the real clinical performance of every predictive biomarker. Thus, the value of a predictive biomarker can only be measured by its clinical performance, not by its theoretical value or value in the laboratory. Although it seemed self-evident that anti-EGFR antibody therapy should require measured EGFR expression, this was not the case in actual clinical practice.

In addition to the reasons cited above, predictive biomarkers may fail if they represent an overly simplified summary of very complex and partially understood cancer biology. In the laboratory, animal models may be designed to highlight simple biological features. But in the patient, more complex and varied mechanisms will often be at play. Importantly, members of drug development teams may have contributed to the development of leading predictive biomarker hypotheses. These same members may have difficulty objectively assessing the uncertainty in the clinical application of the hypotheses, leading to drug development programs which overemphasize predictive biomarkers.

When predictive biomarkers fail, they can lead to an unnecessary narrowing of the treated population, or to narrowing it in the wrong way (for colorectal cancer treated with anti-EGFR therapy, EGFR expression was the wrong predictive biomarker, whereas k-ras mutation, the right predictive biomarker, was discovered much later).

The use of predictive biomarkers involves various costs and challenges. Significant resources must be invested in order to discover biomarkers, develop assays for biomarkers, and formally develop a "companion diagnostic assay" which meets regulatory requirements for co-approval with the therapy as a means of selecting patients [18]. Patient selection requires the availability of suitable diagnostic tissue, and patients who have insufficient diagnostic tissue will be ineligible for the trial, leading to recruitment difficulties.

The great promise of predictive biomarkers, together with inconsistent results, and the significant investment of time and money required, have led to variable attitudes ranging from uncritical enthusiasm to harsh skepticism [15, 23]. The skepticism is well expressed by Ratain and Glassman [23]: "Whereas 'wins' have occurred here,… most attempts to identify such biomarkers have been nothing more than expensive fishing expeditions. Drug response is multifactorial; patient populations are heterogeneous; potential markers are innumerable; and scientific underpinnings to marker development are imperfect."

These issues and legitimate concerns may hinder the development of a field which is increasing in promise with increasing molecular understanding of cancer. The lack of consensus on interdisciplinary drug development teams about if, when, and how to apply predictive classifiers is manifest in the many clinical trials we still observe today which lack a meaningful use of these classifiers.

Key dilemmas include:

- When and to what degree to invest in predictive biomarkers
- When to select only for patients who are "positive" for the predictive biomarkers and when to include some patients who are "negative" for the biomarker.

An approach for predictive biomarker integration into oncology clinical development is presented in this chapter. It was developed after extensive cross functional discussions among discovery scientists, translational medicine experts, clinicians, statisticians, regulatory affairs experts, and commercial experts from several pharmaceutical and biotechnology firms, and is inspired by a broad consensus from these discussions, although not representing the official position of the firms [5]. This chapter will first outline the principles behind the recommended approach, then describe key tactics, and finally discuss the significance as well as new developments in the personalized strategies for cancer therapy.

6.2 Central Principle

The central principle is validation of predictive biomarkers through documentation of their predictive value in the clinic. This implies early investment in preclinical predictive biomarker discovery programs and assay development, and in early phase clinical studies involving biomarkers in every case. However, the degree of emphasis of predictive biomarkers in Phase 3 will depend on how well they have predicted clinical data in earlier trials.

This central principle has two corollaries: (1) "biomarker negative" patients must be included in some of the early studies to demonstrate that the predictive biomarker can distinguish between patients who benefit and those who don't. (2) the predictive biomarker hypothesis must undergo formal statistical testing. This implies that a single predictive biomarker hypothesis must be prioritized prospectively (ideally before the start of Phase 2). Statistical testing cannot be effective for multiple candidate predictive biomarker hypotheses.

The inclusion of "biomarker negative" patients can create ethical issues. If we believe, based on understanding of cancer biology or on preclinical data, that biomarker negative patients may not benefit, is it ethical to treat them? Ethicists generally use the term *equipoise* as a criterion for treatment in this case. That is, in a randomized controlled trial, there must be a level of uncertainty about which arm is better, which in this case corresponds to an uncertainty about whether the experimental therapy will benefit biomarker negative patients. As discussed in the introduction, equipoise tends to be underestimated in many instances. Members of the drug development team may be biased in favor of their discoveries and hypotheses. The complexity of the human setting compared to the simple preclinical models may be underestimated. Publication bias, which leads to more frequent and prominent publication of biomarker success stories than cautionary tales, can also lead to underestimation of equipoise. Because of equipoise, there may be an ethical concern with denying an experimental therapy to a "biomarker negative" patient when the truth of the predictive biomarker hypothesis is unknown and the patient has few other options. Some anti-EGFR therapies, such as gefitinib and erlotinib, offer benefit to biomarker negative patients although it is less than that offered biomarker positive patients. Other anti-EGFR therapies such as cetuximab offer benefit in patients in whom EGFR expression cannot be detected.

Nonetheless, we do not favor single agent treatment of biomarker negative patients with an experimental therapy designed for biomarker positive patients in instances where the mechanism of the therapy is well understood and the scientific rationale behind the predictive biomarker hypothesis is strong. As an alternative, we propose combination therapy by a randomized add-on design: background therapy ± experimental therapy. Ordinarily, the background therapy will be the standard of care therapy for that clinical cancer scenario. However, in some instances the standard of care therapy and the proposed experimental therapy may antagonize each other. Preclinical work should attempt to determine if this is a risk. In such cases, it may be necessary to develop a combination of experimental agents, where one experimental agent is the background therapy and the other is the test therapy to which the predictive biomarker hypothesis applies. In both cases, there should be the expectation that biomarker negative patients may benefit from the background therapy.

The second corollary of the central principle is that one predictive biomarker or classifier must be prioritized for formal statistical testing in Phase 2 clinical studies. This predictive biomarker hypothesis must be chosen in advance of the Phase 2 data being available. The hypothesis is also termed a "clinical benefit identification hypothesis" [5], where clinical benefit can be defined in a variety of ways depending on the Phase 2 study, and the hypothesis is that "biomarker positive" patients will have more clinical benefit than "biomarker negative" patients. It is all too common for multiple candidate predictive biomarkers to be used and for teams to retrospectively examine the data looking for a predictive biomarker hypothesis that "works". This is precisely what Ratain and Glassman call "a fishing expedition" [23]. Testing a large number of predictive biomarker hypotheses increases the false positive rate in nearly direct proportion to the number of hypotheses tested, a phenomenon called *the multiple comparisons problem.* If the team looks for additional hypotheses after data is available, the chance of finding something that "works" coincidentally is even higher. This then leads to failed phase 3 studies.

Often it is unclear which biomarker hypothesis should be prioritized for formal statistical testing, due to the complexity of the biology.

Although the prioritized hypothesis is formally tested in Phase 2, other candidate hypotheses can be examined in an exploratory fashion. If the primary prioritized hypothesis fails, and one of the exploratory hypothesis appears to work, this is a lower level of evidence, and needs to be confirmed in a second Phase 2 study wherein the former exploratory hypothesis is prospectively chosen as the primary biomarker hypothesis. Repeating phase 2 may seem like a setback, but in fact it is progress. Such an iterative process may often be required, and reflects evolving understanding. It is common for a lead drug candidate to have backups, and similarly we should expect a lead biomarker hypothesis to have backups.

Choosing the primary predictive biomarker hypothesis should be based on scientific evidence from in vitro and in vivo models, Phase 1 clinical studies, Phase 2a exploratory unrandomized studies, neoadjuvant studies where tissue for exploratory biomarker work can be readily obtained, and where applicable, experimental medicine studies in patients or volunteers. Moreover, studies of tissue banks should have determined the expected prevalence of biomarker positive and negative subgroups in the proposed PoC indications. If the biomarker positive subgroup is too small, it may be difficult to enroll a suitable trial, and if the biomarker negative subgroup is too small, it may not be cost effective to screen when the error rate of the assay is considered.

Ideally, the primary predictive biomarker hypothesis should be chosen prior to the beginning of the Phase 2 study. This will allow *stratification* for the predictive biomarker status in phase 2, ensuring that the experimental and control groups have equal proportions of biomarker negative patients and reducing confounding of conclusions in Phase 2 due to imbalances in other factors that may influence clinical benefit.

If the primary predictive biomarker hypothesis is chosen prior to Phase 2, the drug developer may choose to begin formal development of an in vitro diagnostic (IVD) candidate assay. This assay must be sufficiently robust and well characterized to be independently approved by health authorities. This includes full analytic validation for linearity, sensitivity, specificity, and reproducibility, and understanding of pre-analytical variables such as sample preparation and age, to allow the assurance that patients can be reliably selected under actual clinical practice conditions. Development of an IVD candidate is a substantial investment. However, as the process can take 1–2 years, it must be begun early to avoid delay in starting Phase 3. Generally, phase 3 is expected to be performed with an IVD candidate assay since it is that assay which must be clinically validated by the Phase 3 result.

If the primary predictive biomarker hypothesis cannot be chosen in advance of Phase 2, it is possible to delay the specification of the hypothesis until just before the Phase 2 samples are analyzed, the so-called "prospective retrospective approach" [25]. The analysis is still prospective if the hypothesis is stated and documented prior to sample analysis. The most rigorous way to document the primary predictive biomarker hypothesis is to amend the clinical study to incorporate it into the Phase 2 primary endpoint. For internal decision making by a drug development team, amending the statistical analysis plan may be sufficient.

The prospective-retrospective approach will have disadvantages. Failure to stratify for the predictive biomarker hypothesis means the biomarker positive and negative subgroups may be imbalanced with respect to other factors that affect clinical benefit. Development of an IVD candidate assay may well delay the start of Phase 3 in this scenario.

6.3 Other Fundamental Principles

A second fundamental principle is maximization of the efficiency of clinical development. This is very important given the need to develop both a therapy and a predictive biomarker hypothesis simultaneously while controlling the numbers of patients required and the costs.

Efficiency is defined by a benefit-cost ratio (BCR). Chen and Beckman [9–11] examined the optimal size for a randomized Phase 2 proof of concept (PoC) study that maximizes the BCR. Benefit is defined as the risk adjusted number of "true positives" identified by a Phase 2 program: i.e. therapies that truly work for the indications. Cost is defined as the risk adjusted number of patients that will be used in the Phase 2 and Phase 3 programs combined. "Risk adjusted" accounts for the possibility of wrong decisions due to the statistical limitations of Phase 2 studies. For example, if the Phase 2 study is false positive, the drug development team will spend money on a Phase 3 study which will be negative, increasing the cost. Conversely, if a Phase 2 study is falsely negative, the drug development team will not choose to do a Phase 3 study even though the therapy actually works, reducing the benefit.

The false positive (Type I) and false negative (Type II) error rates can be reduced by doing a larger Phase 2 trial. However, this increases the cost of the Phase 2 trial. Chen and Beckman [9] modeled the realistic scenario in which there is a limited budget for Phase 2 PoC studies. This is universally true both in pharmaceutical and biotech settings and in academic programs funded by public sources. The number of potential PoC studies is always large given multiple available therapies, therapeutic combinations, and indications. At any given time, on the order of 1000 therapies are under development for oncology, creating a number of possible PoC studies well exceeding available budgets.

In this scenario, a larger Phase 2 study will have lower Type I and Type II error rates but consume more of the resources. If the Phase 2 PoC study budget is not sufficient to pay for all the PoC studies of interest, the larger study will result in an opportunity cost. There will be a PoC study of interest which is not funded. If this study would have been successful, that opportunity is lost. Chen and Beckman termed this opportunity cost "*Type III error*" [5].

Statisticians traditionally require a study large enough to lower the type I and II errors to 10 % and 20 % respectively. However, Chen and Beckman [9–11] showed that it is 10–30 % more efficient as judged by the BCR to reduce the size of a PoC study and increase the Type II error to 40 %, but allow more hypotheses to be tested. This is true because of the important effect of Type III error. The resulting non-traditional, but optimally efficient PoC powering scheme is termed *"Chen-Beckman powering"* or *"Chen-Beckman power"*.

The above results assume a variety of hypotheses to be tested, of equal merit. However, based on preclinical information or other considerations, the drug development team may judge some hypotheses to have greater value and/or probability of success than others. The same mathematics can be used to find the corresponding optimal Type I error rate and Type II error rate for each hypothesis, and the optimal allocation of resources, in which PoC trials based on particularly strong hypotheses get more than their share of resources, PoC trials based on weaker hypotheses get less resources, and still other PoC trials based on the weakest hypotheses are not done. In the case of two hypotheses, if one is much stronger than the other, the algorithm may recommend devoting all of the resources to the stronger hypothesis, mirroring the traditional paradigm.

Maximizing efficiency and utility of clinical development will be evident in the tactics described below, including the Phase 2 study, the decision of what type of Phase 3 study to perform, and the design of an adaptive Phase 3 study when the truth of the predictive biomarker hypothesis is uncertain after Phase 2.

Two other principles were considered fundamental. Firstly, decision making must be adaptive. Secondly, there must be continuous integration of biomarker and clinical data. These principles are demonstrated in the tactics elucidated below.

6.4 Tactics

6.4.1 The Efficiency Optimized Biomarker Stratified Randomized Phase 2 Study

Three options exist for randomized Phase 2 designs incorporating predictive biomarkers. In the enrichment design, only biomarker positive patients are studied. In the biomarker strategy design, patients are randomized either to (a) randomly chosen therapy, or (b) predictive biomarker directed therapy. In the biomarker stratified design, both biomarker positive and biomarker negative patients are randomly assigned to either control or experimental therapy. Thus, the study has four groups: biomarker positive experimental, biomarker positive control, biomarker negative experimental, and biomarker negative control. Stratification means that the positive and negative groups are independent strata and are randomized independently to ensure that there is no accidental confounding by other factors that might affect clinical benefit. It has been demonstrated that, when there is equipoise, the most efficient design is the biomarker stratified design [17].

A randomized biomarker stratified Phase 2 PoC study is essentially testing two hypotheses at once: the hypothesis that the therapy works in biomarker positive patients, and the hypothesis that the therapy works in biomarker negative patients. This may alternately be formulated as the trial is testing a hypothesis about the drug and a hypothesis about the predictive biomarker. In any case, testing two hypotheses at once would ordinarily imply a doubling of the Phase 2 sample size and cost. However, one can reduce the cost and optimize the efficiency by powering each hypothesis test at the Chen-Beckman power [5].

In judging clinical benefit, we recommend using a continuous endpoint like progression free survival (PFS, the time to tumor worsening or death, whichever comes first) as opposed to a discrete endpoint such as response rate (RR, percentage of patients whose tumors shrink a standard minimum percentage), since the former is informative for all patients even when RR is low (as is the case for some targeted therapies). In addition, PFS is more highly correlated with the outcome variable of greatest interest, overall survival (OS, time to death) [27]. Mathematical techniques exist for adjusting for the imperfect correlation between PFS and OS [13]. Drug developers rarely wait for definitive OS data from phase 2 to make a decision about whether or not to proceed with Phase 3, as that would significantly slow development.

6.4.2 Decision Analysis Guided Phase 2–3 Predictive Biomarker Transition

At the end of the biomarker stratified randomized phase 2 study, there are four possible outcomes, which can be graphed as regions on a two dimensional graph [5]:

- Region 1: the therapy does not work in either biomarker negative or positive patients. This results in a "No Go" decision to not perform Phase 3 studies.
- Region 2: the therapy works in biomarker positive patients only. Proceed to a Phase 3 study enriched for biomarker positive patients only.
- Region 3: the therapy works equally well in biomarker positive and biomarker negative patients. That is, the therapy works, but the predictive biomarker hypothesis does not. Proceed to a traditional phase 3 study in an unselected patient population.
- Region 4: the therapy works in biomarker positive patients, and there is a trend towards efficacy in biomarker negative patients which is insufficient to reach statistical significance. Nonetheless, there may be some ambiguity due to the limited statistical power of phase 2. Proceed to collect more information in an adaptive Phase 3 design described in the next section.

Drawing the exact borders between these four regions in order to make a quantitative decision requires decision analysis. Each possible course of action has a certain benefit or utility if it is the correct decision and a certain harm or negative utility if it is the wrong one. Assigning these utilities is a subjective process that is done with the aid of experts on the drug development team. For example, if we decide to perform an unselected Phase 3 study when in fact the therapy works only in biomarker positive patients, we may have a falsely negative Phase 3 study. However, if we perform an enriched study when the therapy works in the entire population, we have narrowed the potential population that would benefit unnecessarily.

Once utility values are assigned to each possible outcome of each possible action, the probabilities of different outcomes are calculated as a function of the Phase 2 study data (each point on the two dimensional graph represents a possible Phase 2 outcome). The borders between the regions on the graph are then drawn to optimize the risk adjusted utility, subject to the constraint that the false positive rate of proceeding to Phase 3 is controlled to be less than a specified level.

6.4.3 Adaptive, Predictive Performance-Based Hypothesis Prioritization in Phase 3

In region 4 of the graph in the previous section, there is still some ambiguity regarding the clinical benefit afforded by the therapy in biomarker negative patients. Thus, the Phase 3 study must test two hypotheses:

- Hypothesis 1: The therapy works in an unselected population
- Hypothesis 2: The therapy works in a biomarker-defined subset of the unselected population

Chen and Beckman [12] developed a Phase 3 study which tests both hypotheses simultaneously. According to health authority regulations, the total false positive rate (Type I error) of a Phase 3 trial must be 5 % or less. However, this Type I error may be apportioned or "split" between more than one hypothesis. It is possible to define a fixed split of the Type I error, for example 4 % to hypothesis 1 and 1 % to hypothesis 2 [16]. However, in the method we suggest, the split is optimized, based on the Phase 2 data and the Phase 3 data up to an interim analysis point, to maximize the power of the Phase 3 study.

The optimized Type I error split has the effect of emphasizing Hypothesis 2 above to the exact degree that the predictive biomarker hypothesis has been predictive to that point in development. It is a data-driven adaptation which maximizes development efficiency.

While some adaptations within Phase 3 can be controversial for national health authorities, in this case the adaptation does not affect patient selection or management, or Type I error. The data-driven rules for choosing the Type I error split can be defined in advance and given to an independent Data Monitoring Committee for automatic execution. These safeguards make it highly likely that the design would be acceptable to both national health authorities and local ethics committees.

6.4.4 The Phase 2+ Method for Allowing Phase 2 Data to Influence Adaptation Within Phase 3

Continuous adaptation is a cornerstone of our approach. Yet real-time adaptation is not optimal in oncology in that the endpoint of greatest interest, OS, is delayed relative to other endpoints. This means that real-time adaptation is often based on other endpoints which do not correlate perfectly with OS.

In the typical late development oncology program, the PFS result in the Phase 2 PoC study is used to make a decision to proceed to Phase 3. The primary endpoint of the Phase 3 study is typically OS, as this is the most significant endpoint for patients and is critical for approval by national health authorities.

If the Phase 3 is itself adaptive, as in the preceding section, the adaptation is typically made based on Phase 3 interim data. At this time, there is very little OS data available, and therefore the adaptation must be made based on PFS even though the primary endpoint of the study is OS. Moreover, unblinding the Phase 3 study at the interim analysis to make an adaptation may inflate the Type I error.

We have proposed an alternative: the use of maturing phase 2 data to influence the Phase 3 adaptation [5]. Maturing OS data from the Phase 2 study provides a way for the Phase 3 study to adapt based on OS, which is also its primary endpoint. By refraining from using data within the Phase 3 study for adaptation, there will be no issue with Type I error control. Thus, the effectiveness and rigor of the adaptation are improved.

6.5 Conclusion and Future Directions in Oncology Personalized Medicine

This chapter has outlined an approach to integrating predictive biomarkers into oncology clinical development programs. Key principles are formal validation of a single prioritized predictive biomarker hypothesis against clinical benefit endpoints, optimization of development efficiency, and continuous adaptation. The result is a program which is demanding and may occasionally reject putative predictive biomarkers, but which will ultimately result in maximum value from biomarkers. The program allows drug developers to manage the risk of uncertain therapies and uncertain predictive biomarkers optimally.

The current oncology personalized medicine paradigm is based on matching patients to therapies based on the use of predictive biomarkers. This approach generally types patients based on the consensus properties of a bulk sample obtained either right before treatment or at some time in the past.

However, tumors are genetically unstable, and this is the most efficient way for them to evolve [2–4]. As a consequence, heterogeneity not only exists *between* patients, but *within* patients, such that no two tumor cells are alike within a single patient. Minor sub-clones may have clinical consequences, and continued evolution under therapy suggests limitations of a strategy which is reactive to the present state rather than attempting to anticipate the future.

A recent simulation study [6] demonstrates that non-standard personalized medicine strategies which account for minor sub-clones (including the risk that they may exist below the detection limit) and tumor evolution (by anticipating future states) can greatly enhance median survival and cure rates for almost all tumor types. Ideal application of these non-standard strategies requires detailed molecular understanding of drug sensitivity phenotypes and their evolution, as well as non-invasive tumor sampling methods which have not yet been perfected. However, both non-invasive techniques for tumor measurement and our molecular understanding of cancer are continuously improving.

Non-standard personalized medicine strategies might be likened to a chess master that thinks several moves ahead, compared to our current state of the art which reacts one move at a time. However, in order to play like a master, one must first know the chess pieces and how they move. Predictive biomarkers and their clinical validation defines these rules for the large number of moves and pieces which make up the very serious strategic contest of cancer therapy.

Acknowledgments The authors wish to thank Jason Clark for contributing the decision analysis guided Phase 2-Phase 3 predictive biomarker transition, and Donald Bergstrom, Robert Phillips, Richard M. Simon, and Linda Sun for helpful discussions.

References

1. Amado RG, Wolf M, Peeters M et al (2008) Wild-type KRAS is required for panitumumab efficacy in patients with metastatic colorectal cancer. J Clin Oncol 26:1626–1634
2. Beckman RA (2009) Mutator mutations enhance tumorigenic efficiency across fitness landscapes. PLoS One 4:e5860
3. Beckman RA (2010) Efficiency of carcinogenesis: in the mutator phenotype inevitable? Semin Cancer Biol 20:340–352
4. Beckman RA, Loeb LA (2006) Efficiency of carcinogenesis with and without a mutator mutation. Proc Natl Acad Sci U S A 103:14410–14415
5. Beckman RA, Clark J, Chen C (2011) Integrating predictive biomarkers and classifiers into oncology clinical development programs. Nat Rev Drug Discov 10:735–748
6. Beckman RA, Schemmann GS, Yeang CH (2012) Impact of genetic dynamics and single-cell heterogeneity on development on nonstandard personalized medicine strategies for cancer. Proc Natl Acad Sci U S A 109:14586–14591
7. Bokemeyer C, Bondarenko I, Hartmann JT et al (2008) KRAS status and efficacy of first-line treatment of patients with metastatic colorectal cancer (mCRC) with FOLFOX with or without cetuximab: the OPUS experience. J Clin Oncol 26(Suppl):15S, abstract

8. Chapman PD, Hauschild A, Robert C et al (2011) Improved survival with vemurafenib in melanoma with BRAF V600E mutation. N Engl J Med 364:2507–2516
9. Chen C, Beckman RA (2007) Optimal cost effective designs of proof of concept trials and associated Go-No Go decisions. In: Proceedings of the American Statistical Association, biometrics section
10. Chen C, Beckman RA (2009) Optimal cost-effective Go-No Go decisions in late stage oncology drug development. Stat Biopharm Res 1:159–169
11. Chen C, Beckman RA (2009) Optimal cost-effective phase II proof of concept and associated Go-No Go decisions. J Biopharm Stat 1:424–436
12. Chen C, Beckman RA (2009) Hypothesis testing in a confirmatory phase III trial with a possible subset effect. Stat Biopharm Res 1:431–440
13. Chen C, Sun L, Chih C (2013) Evaluation of early efficacy endpoints for proof-of-concept trials. J Biopharm Stat 23:413–424
14. Cobleigh MA, Vogel CL, Tripathy D et al (1999) Multinational study of the efficacy and safety of humanized anti-HER2 monoclonal antibody in women who have HER2-overexpressing metastatic breast cancer that has progressed after chemotherapy for metastatic disease. J Clin Oncol 17:2639–2648
15. Dalton WS, Friend SH (2006) Cancer biomarkers – an invitation to the table. Science 312:1165–1168
16. Freidlin B, Simon RM (2005) Adaptive signature design: an adaptive clinical trial design for generating and prospectively testing a gene expression signature for sensitive patients. Clin Cancer Res 11:7872–7878
17. Freidlin B, McShane L, Korn EL (2010) Randomized clinical trials with biomarkers: design issues. J Natl Cancer Inst 102:152–160
18. Kelloff GJ, Sigman CC (2012) Cancer biomarkers: selecting the right drug for the right patient. Nat Rev Drug Discov 11:201–214
19. Lievre A, Bachet JB, Le Corre D et al (2006) KRAS mutation status is predictive of response to cetuximab therapy in colorectal cancer. Cancer Res 66:3992–3995
20. Paez JG, Janne PA, Lee JC et al (2004) EGFR mutations in lung cancer: correlation with clinical response to gefitinib therapy. Science 30:1497–1500
21. Pao W, Miller V, Zakowski M et al (2004) EGF receptor gene mutations are common in lung cancers from "never smokers" and are associated with sensitivity of tumors to gefitinib and erlotinib. Proc Natl Acad Sci U S A 101:13306–13311
22. Ransohoff DF, Gourlay ML (2010) Sources of bias in specimens for research about molecular markers for cancer. J Clin Oncol 28:698–704
23. Ratain MJ, Glassman RH (2007) Biomarkers in phase I oncology trials: signal, noise, or expensive distraction? Clin Cancer Res 13:6545–6548
24. Shaw AT, Kim DW, Nakagawa K et al (2013) Crizotinib versus chemotherapy in advanced alk-positive lung cancer. N Engl J Med 368:2385–2394
25. Simon RM, Paik S, Hayes DF (2009) Use of archived specimens in evaluation of prognostic and predictive biomarkers. J Natl Cancer Inst 101:1446–1452
26. Slamon DJ, Leyland-Jones B, Shak S et al (2001) Use of chemotherapy plus a monoclonal antibody against HER2 for metastatic breast cancer that overexpresses HER2. N Engl J Med 344:783–792
27. Tang PA, Bentsen SM, Chen EX, Siu LL (2007) Surrogate endpoints for median overall survival in metastatic colorectal cancer: literature-based analysis from 39 randomized controlled trials of first-line chemotherapy. J Clin Oncol 25:4562–4568
28. Van Cutsem E, Lang I, D'haens G et al (2008) KRAS status and efficacy in the first-line treatment of patients with metastatic colorectal cancer (mCRC) treated with FOLFIRI with or without cetuximab: the CRYSTAL experience. J Clin Oncol 26(Suppl):15S, abstract
29. Yan L, Beckman RA (2005) Pharmacogenetics and pharmacogenomics in oncology therapeutic antibody development. Biotechniques 39:565–568

Part II

Tumor Markers – A Critical Revision: Enzymes

Prostate Specific Antigen as a Tumor Marker in Prostate Cancer: Biochemical and Clinical Aspects

7

J.W. Salman, I.G. Schoots, S.V. Carlsson, G. Jenster, and M.J. Roobol

Abstract

In this chapter the use of prostate specific antigen (PSA) as a tumor marker for prostate cancer is discussed. The chapter provides an overview of biological and clinical aspects of PSA. The main drawback of total PSA (tPSA) is its lack of specificity for prostate cancer which leads to unnecessary biopsies. Moreover, PSA-testing poses a risk of overdiagnosis and subsequent overtreatment. Many PSA-based markers have been developed to improve the performance characteristics of tPSA. As well as different molecular subforms of tPSA, such as proPSA (pPSA) and free PSA (fPSA), and PSA derived kinetics as PSA-velocity (PSAV) and PSA-doubling time (PSADT). The prostate health index (phi), PSA-density (PSAD) and the contribution of non PSA-based markers such as the urinary transcripts of PCA3 and TMPRSS-ERG fusion are also discussed. To enable further risk stratification tumor markers are often combined with clinical data (e.g. outcome of DRE) in so-called nomograms. Currently the role of magnetic resonance imaging (MRI) in the detection and staging of prostate cancer is being explored.

Keywords

Diagnostic tools in prostate cancer • Free PSA • Molecular forms of PSA • mpMRI • PCA3 • Percent free PSA • ProPSA • Prostate • Prostate cancer • Prostate health index • PSA biology • PSA cut-off value • PSA derived parameters • PSAkinetics • PSA physiology • PSA-assays • PSA-density • PSA-doubling time • PSA-velocity • TMPRSS2:ERG gene fusion

J.W. Salman (✉) • I.G. Schoots • S.V. Carlsson
G. Jenster • M.J. Roobol
Department of Urology, Erasmus Medical Centre,
Na-1710, P.O. Box 2040, 3000 CA Rotterdam,
Netherlands
e-mail: jolandasalman@gmail.com

R. Scatena (ed.), *Advances in Cancer Biomarkers*, Advances in Experimental Medicine and Biology 867, DOI 10.1007/978-94-017-7215-0_7

Abbreviations

% (−2)pPSA	Percent (−2)proPSA (= (−2) pPSA/ fPSA)
%fPSA	Percent free PSA (= fPSA/ tPSA × 100 %)
(−2)pPSA	(−2)proPSA (precursor form of prostate specific antigen)
(−4)pPSA	(−4)proPSA (precursor form of prostate specific antigen)
(−5)pPSA	(−5)proPSA (precursor form of prostate specific antigen)
(−7)pPSA	(−7)proPSA (precursor form of prostate specific antigen)
Aa	Amino-acids
ADC	Apparent diffusion coefficient
AUA	American Urological Association
BCR	Biochemical recurrence
BPH	Benign prostatic hyperplasia
BPSA	Benign prostate specific antigen
cPSA	Complexed prostate specific antigen
DCE	Dynamic contrast-enhanced imaging
DD3	Differential display clone 3 gene
DRE	Digital rectal examination
DWI	Diffusion weighted imaging
e.g.	Exempli gratia (for example)
EAU	European Association of Urology
ERSPC	European randomized study of screening for prostate cancer
FDA	United States Food and Drug Administration
fPSA	Free prostate specific antigen
hK1	Human kallikrein 1
hK2	Human kallikrein 2
hK3	Human kallikrein 3
hK4	Human kallikrein 4
i.e.	id est (that is)
iPSA	Intact prostate specific antigen
LR	Likelihood ratio
mpMRI	Multiparametric MRI
MRI	Magnetic resonance imaging
mRNA	Messenger ribonucleic acid
MRSI	Magnetic resonance spectroscopic imaging
PC	Prostate cancer
PCA3	Prostate cancer antigen 3
PCPT	Prostate cancer prevention trial
PFS	Progression free survival rate
Phi	Prostate health index ((−2)pPSA/ fPSA) × $\sqrt{tPSA}$)
PLCO	Prostate, lung, colorectal and ovarian screening trial
pPSA	Pro prostate specific antigen
PPV	Positive predictive value
PSA	Prostate specific antigen
PSAD	PSA-density
PSADT	PSA-doubling time
PSAV	PSA-velocity
RP	Radical prostatectomy
RT	Radiation therapy
T2WI	T2- weighted images
TMPRRS2	Transmembrane protease serine 2
tPSA	Total prostate specific antigen
TRUS	Transrectal ultrasound

7.1 Introduction

7.1.1 The Prostate

The prostate is an exocrine gland located beneath the urinary bladder in men. The prostate envelopes the proximal urethra and ejaculatory ducts. The main function is the production of an alkaline fluid that is part of the semen. About 25–30 % of the total volume of the ejaculate is produced by the prostate. The prostate consist of five zonal components: one third of the prostate consist of a non-glandular anterior zone and the other two third of the prostate is divided in four glandular zones: the peripheral zone (70 % of the glandular prostate), central zone (25 %), transition zone (5 %) and periurethral tissue (<1 %). In younger men the prostate is about the size of a walnut, however in older men the prostate usually enlarges. Mainly the transition zone starts growing, resulting in compression of the central zone and stretching of the peripheral zone [1]. About 65–70 % of the prostate cancers arise in the peripheral zone of the prostate.

7.1.2 ProstateCancer

Prostate cancer is the second most frequently diagnosed cancer and the sixth leading cause of cancer death in men worldwide, with an estimated 913,000 new cases and 258,000 deaths in 2008 [2]. In the USA and Europe it is even the most common cancer type in men in terms of new cases and the second respectively third in terms of mortality in the USA and Europe [3, 4]. In the USA men have about a 1 in 6 lifetime risk (16 %) of being diagnosed with prostate cancer [4]. There is a great geographic variety in prostate cancer incidence and mortality rates [5]. A major factor of influence is the use of prostate specific antigen (PSA) as a diagnostic tool, a blood test that has been available since the early 1990s. In addition factors such as cancer registrations, genetics, diet, lifestyle and environment play a role in prostate cancer incidence and mortality rates. The highest prostate cancer incidence rates are found in the highest income regions of the world since the practice of PSA-testing and subsequent biopsy is common there [2, 5]. Mortality rates tend to be higher in low to middle income countries of the world including parts of South America, the Caribbean, and sub-Saharan Africa as compared to high income countries.

7.1.3 Diagnostic Tools in ProstateCancer

Early prostate cancer usually causes no clinical symptoms. For a long time the only way to examine the prostate was by digital rectal examination (DRE), which is still an important diagnostic tool today. A DRE is considered abnormal if a change in texture of the prostate gland is palpated, e.g. nodularity or induration. A suspicious DRE is related with a higher risk of prostate cancer, but the findings between medical examiners are moderately reproducible [6], and still many malignancies are missed. Ultimately, DRE fails to detect a significant number of malignancies, and of those detected a significant number are at an advanced stage. Around the year 1930, needle aspiration was introduced to remove prostatic cells for microscopic examination. The first techniques involved transperineal needle aspiration assisted by a finger in the rectum to guide the needle in the prostate. The next step involved a digital guided transrectal biopsy procedure. Digital guidance has been replaced by image guidance. The transrectal ultrasound (TRUS) was introduced end 1960s. TRUS was initially used to direct the biopsies, later on also for identifying possible cancer foci in the prostate seen as hypo-echoic defects on the ultrasound. In 1989, Hodge et al. showed that in men with a suspicious DRE the ultrasound guided random (sextant) systematic prostate biopsies were more effective in detecting prostate cancer compared to biopsies just directed to the lesion [7]. Over time biopsy protocols have been extended to allow lateral sampling and increase the sample density. Since late 1980s – early 1990s, the use of PSA as an early detection tool has become a main topic in the prostate cancer research field. Multiple studies have been conducted to assess the use of PSA, DRE and TRUS, separately or in different combinations, for the use of early detection of prostate cancer. During the last decade magnetic resonance imaging (MRI) of the prostate has shown promising initial results in detecting, localizing and possibly staging prostate cancer. In addition MRI can be of use in guiding the prostate biopsy. Despite all these currently used modalities (PSA, DRE and TRUS) to estimate the risk of prostate cancer, histological assessment of prostate tissue is still the golden standard to confirm the presence and the characteristics of prostate cancer. In 1966, an American Pathologist, D.F. Gleason, developed a grading system 'the Gleason Score' for evaluating architecture changes in prostate cancer, which is still the system used today [8]. The Gleason grading system remains the strongest predictor of outcome for men diagnosed with prostate cancer [9]. In 2005, modifications to the Gleason grading system for prostate carcinoma were established on the International Society of Urologic Pathology (ISUP) meeting, with the aim to help pathologists use the Gleason grading system in a more uniform manner worldwide [10].

7.2 PSA

7.2.1 PSA: Biology and Physiology

PSA is a glycoprotein with a molecular mass of 33-kD, also known as human kallikrein 3. PSA belongs to the tissue kallikrein family. The cluster of genes for the family of tissue kallikreins is located on human chromosome 19q13.3–4 [11]. PSA was first isolated and defined in the 1970s [12–14]. In 1980, PSA was measured quantitatively in the serum by Papsidero et al. and the protein PSA purified from prostatic tissue was shown to be identical to PSA in human serum [15]. Until the beginning of this century, only three human tissue kallikreins were identified: human kallikrein 1 (hK1, the pancreatic/renal kallikrein), human kallikrein 2 (hK2, glandular kallikrein) and human kallikrein 3 (hK3, PSA). Now a total of 15 tissue kallikrein genes have been revealed [16]. Kallikreins are serine proteases that cleave certain high molecular weight proteins that can result in the formation of bioactive peptides such as kinins. Many kallikreins are regulated by steroid hormones. PSA, hK2 and hK4 seem to be expressed primarily in prostate tissue [17]. Transcription of the PSA gene is positively and directly regulated by the androgen receptor. PSA is produced almost exclusively by the luminal epithelial cells of all types of prostatic glandular tissue, benign and malignant. The majority of glandular tissue in the prostate is located in the peripheral zone. The fluid produced by glandular tissue is excreted to the excretory ducts and then into the urethra [17]. Most of the produced PSA will be excreted into the seminal fluid. The biological function of PSA is to cleave the high molecular weight gel-forming proteins semenogelin I and II into smaller polypeptides. This seminal vesicle specific proteins semenogelin I and II are involved in the seminal coagulum (clot) formation. The action of cleaving these proteins by PSA results in liquefaction of the coagulum [18], thereby decreasing its viscosity and increasing motility of spermatozoa [19]. In normal prostate tissue the tight and ordered prostatic glandular architecture keeps PSA confined to the prostate gland. Only very small amounts of active and inactive PSA produced in the prostate end up in the circulation (Fig. 7.1). Normally the PSA concentration in serum is a million-fold lower than in the seminal fluid [20]. The calculated half-life of serum PSA ranges between 2.2 and 3.2 days [21, 22]. In prostate cancer PSA-levels in serum are about ten times higher per gram of tissue than from benign hyperplasia tissue, potentially due to the loss of the architecture of the prostate tissue in prostate cancer [21].

7.2.2 Molecular Forms of PSA

In normal prostate luminal epithelial cells PSA is initially synthesized as a preproprotein containing 261 amino acids. In the prostatic ducts, a 244 amino acid precursor is formed after removal of the 17 amino acid proleader sequence. This inactive precursor enzyme containing a seven amino N-terminal-pro-leader peptide is named (−7)proPSA ((−7)pPSA). Active, mature PSA is generated when the pro-leader peptide is removed mainly by hK2, but also by hK4 (Fig. 7.1) [23].

The active PSA can become inactive PSA after proteolysis. Active PSA in serum is bound by protease inhibitors to form complexes (cPSA). Inactive PSA does not form complexes and circulates in an unbound state as free PSA (fPSA). The function of protease inhibitors is to prevent potentially damaging protease activity of PSA. The serum total PSA (tPSA) is equal to fPSA plus cPSA. About 70–90 % of tPSA is bound to alpha-1-antichymotrypsin or other proteins such as alpha-2-macroglobulin, alpha-1-proteaseinhibitor, or protein C inhibitor [17]. fPSA represents only 10–30 % of the tPSA [17]. Enzymatically inactive fPSA has three distinct molecular forms (Fig. 7.2). The first form is benign PSA (BPSA) which is expressed preferentially in the transitional zone of the prostate gland. BPSA is associated with benign prostatic hyperplasia (BPH) [24]. The second form is intact PSA (iPSA) which is similar to native active PSA except that it is enzymatically inactive. The third from is proPSA (pPSA) which is expressed mostly in the peripheral zone of the

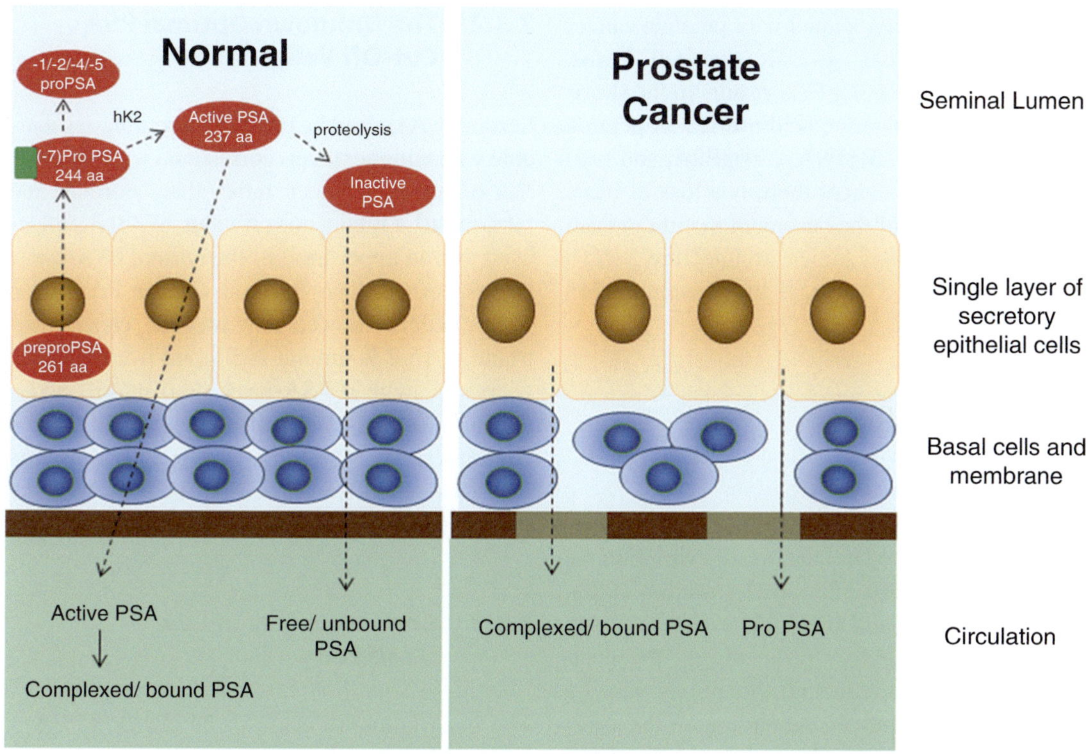

Fig. 7.1 Model of prostate specific antigen (PSA) synthesis in normal prostate tissue versus prostate cancer. In normal secretory epithelial cells inactive preproPSA is produced, containing 261 amino-acids (aa). The removal of a 17 amino-acid leader sequence results in the inactive (−7)proPSA, containing 244 amino-acids. The produced proPSA (pPSA) is secreted into the seminal lumen were mainly hK2 removes the pro-leader peptide to form mature, active PSA, containing 237 amino-acids. Also truncated forms of pPSA are formed, which are all enzymatically inactive. A small fraction of the active PSA can diffuse into the serum were it is bound to protease inhibitors. The largest fraction of active PSA in the lumen undergoes proteolysis to generate inactive PSA which in small portions enters the blood stream were it circulates as free/ unbound PSA (fPSA). In prostate cancer disruption of the basal cell layer and basement membrane leads to a decrease in luminal processing resulting in increasing levels of complexed PSA (cPSA) and pPSA in serum, and decreasing levels of serum fPSA. Figure adapted from Balk et al. [17]

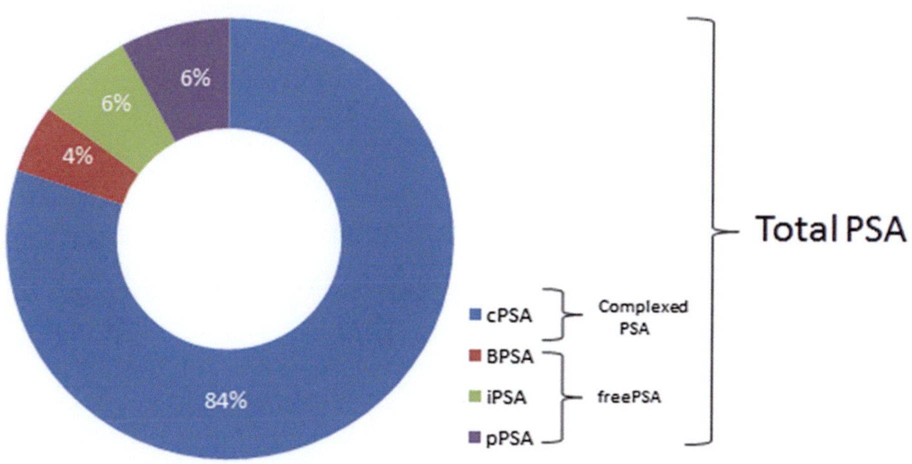

Fig. 7.2 Overview of molecular forms of PSA

prostate. pPSA is associated with prostate cancer [25, 26]. pPSA has several truncated forms. Partial cleavage of (−7)pPSA results in the shortening of the seven amino acid pro-leader peptide into respectively (−5)pPSA, (−4)pPSA, and (−2) pPSA. In prostate cancer there is a loss of basal cells, disordering of the basement membrane and disruption of normal lumen architecture, which appears to allow PSA release into the circulation (Fig. 7.1) [17].

7.3 PSA-Test

7.3.1 PSA-Assays

It is important to be aware of variation in tPSA. This includes biological variation (PSA, renal elimination) and analytical variation (assay performance, laboratory processing). The measurements of tPSA concentrations may vary by two in identical samples depending on the assay used [27–29]. Since the United States Food and Drug Administration (FDA) approval of the PSA-test as a diagnostic marker, numerous PSA-assays are commercially available. The first widely available PSA-test was the Hybritech Tandem-R PSA- assay. Many studies and thresholds for PSA are based on this Hybritech standard. Because of many differences in PSA-assays the WHO adopted a mixture of 90 % cPSA and 10 % fPSA as one of the new standards in 1999 (the WHO 90:10 PSA-standard) [30]. The variation between assays for tPSA measurements declined from 10 % to 15 % in the early nineties to 3–5 % today [31]. The detection limit improved from 0.3–0.5 ng/mL to 0.01–0.02 ng/mL [31]. Although the differences are small nowadays, the use of different PSA-assays may affect the result of tPSA-measurements. Many clinicians are unaware of the issue that different PSA-assays are used, and the possible effect on the PSA-measurements. Despite influences of biological an analytical variations on measured PSA-levels, higher serum PSA is generally associated with increased specificity and decreased sensitivity.

7.3.2 The Unknown Optimal PSA Cut-Off Value

Serum PSA should be regarded a continuous variable where higher levels correspond with a greater risk of prostate cancer, rather than 'normal' and 'abnormal'. Often a cut-off value of 4.0 ng/mL is used, but an upper limit of the normal PSA-range is unspecified. The Prostate Cancer Prevention Trial (PCPT) showed that prostate cancer was found in 15.2 % among 2950 men from 62 to 91 years old, with a PSA-level ≤4.0 ng/mL and a normal DRE. 14.9 % of these cancers had a Gleason score ≥7 (Table 7.1) [32]. These data show that there is no threshold below which the risk for (high grade) prostate cancer is zero.

7.3.3 Consequences of Low Specificity

The most common cause of an elevated PSA is BPH. Other benign conditions that could affect the serum PSA-level are urinary retention, prostatitis, and ejaculation. Furthermore medication (e.g. finasteride, dutasteride) and prostate manipulation (e.g. cystoscopy, catheterisation, prostate massage, TURP, biopsy) are known to influence the PSA-level [33, 34]. As indicated, serum PSA has a low specificity for prostate cancer. This is especially true in the diagnostic grey zone of PSA between 2 and 10 ng/mL. In this grey zone benign and malignant prostate diseases frequently co-exist. PSA is a continuum; no single

Table 7.1 Prevalence of prostate cancer in men with a PSA ≤ 4.0 ng/mL. Results of the study by Thompson et al. in 2004. Out of the 2950 men, 449 had prostate cancer of which 67 where Gleason score ≥ 7 [32]

PSA-level (ng/mL)	Men with prostate cancer (%)	Men with Gleason score ≥ 7 (%)
0–0.5	6.6	12.5
0.6–1.0	10.1	10.0
1.1–2.0	17.0	11.8
2.1–3.0	23.9	19.1
3.1–4.0	26.9	25.0

PSA prostate specific antigen

cut-off point yields a high specificity and sensitivity for prostate cancer simultaneously. Because of the low specificity of PSA many men are undergoing unnecessary biopsies. Furthermore a significant number of indolent tumors are detected (overdiagnosis), because PSA is not able to differentiate between potentially aggressive and indolent prostate cancers. Table 7.2 shows the continuum of prostate cancer risk for different PSA ranges in the PCPT. In the placebo-group of the PCPT, a total of 5587 (65.2 %) men received at least one biopsy procedure during the 7-year study period if PSA was >4 ng/mL or in case of a suspicious DRE. A total of 1225 (21.9 %) men were diagnosed with prostate cancer [35]. The sensitivity, specificity and likelihood ratio (LR) of prostate cancer detection for all PSA ranges in relation to Gleason grade are shown. Table 7.3 shows similar results for the distribution of PSA and prostate cancer detection in the European randomized study of screening for prostate cancer (ERSPC) [36]. A total of 9779 men aged 55–74 years were included and biopsied (2267 men) if they presented with a PSA ≥4 ng/mL and/ or an abnormal DRE or TRUS.

Draisma et al. developed a simulation model to predict overdiagnosis in the ERSPC trial. With annual screening from age 55–67 years the estimated overdiagnosis rate was 50 %. With a 4 year screening interval this was still 48 % [37]. Overdiagnosis poses the burden of living a life with cancer of no consequence to the patient. Moreover, overdiagnosis can lead to overtreatment which can subsequently cause unnecessary side effects such as sexual dysfunction, urinary incontinence and bowel problems. Not to forget that unnecessary biopsies, overdiagnosis and overtreatment contributes to healthcare costs.

Table 7.2 Sensitivity, specificity, and likelihood ratio associated with serum PSA-levels for prostate cancer detection: calculated from PCPT data (Adapted from Thompson et al. [35])

	PC vs. no PC (all grades)			PC Gleason grade ≥8 vs. Gleason grade <8 or no PC		
PSA-level (ng/mL)	Sensitivity (%)	Specificity (%)	LR	Sensitivity (%)	Specificity (%)	LR
1.1	83.4	38.9	1.4	94.7	35.9	1.5
2.1	52.6	72.5	1.9	86.0	65.9	2.5
2.6	40.5	81.1	2.1	78.9	75.1	3.2
3.1	32.2	86.7	2.4	68.4	81.0	3.6
4.1	20.5	93.8	3.3	50.9	89.1	4.7
6.1	4.6	98.5	3.1	26.3	97.5	10.5
10.1	0.9	99.7	3.0	5.3	99.5	10.6

PC prostate cancer, *PSA* prostate specific antigen, *LR* likelihood ratio, *PCPT* prostate cancer prevention trial

Table 7.3 Positive predictive value of different PSA values: calculated from ERSPC data (Adapted from Schröder et al. [36])

PSA-level (ng/mL)	Men (n)	% of total	Prostate cancer diagnosis (n)	Proportion of total prostate cancers (%)	PPV	Biopsies (n) per cancer detected
0.0–0.09	3559	36.4	4	0.8	2.2	45.8
1.0–1.9	3051	31.2	45	9.5	8.8	11.4
2.0–2.9	1198	12.3	30	6.3	13.6	7.4
3.0–3.9	702	7.2	44	9.3	25.3	3.9
4.0–9.9	1063	10.9	241	51.0	24.5	4.1
≥10	206	2.1	109	23.0	56.5	1.8
Total	9779	100.0	100.0	100.0	20.9	4.8

PSA prostate specific antigen, *ERSPC* European randomized study of screening for prostate cancer, *PPV* positive predictive value

7.4 PSA Modifications

Serum tPSA is still the most commonly used cancer biomarker for prostate cancer. Several molecular forms of PSA and their ratios, as well as PSA-derived parameters and dynamics have been developed and tested, all with the goal to improve specificity for both the distinction between men with and without prostate cancer, and between aggressive and indolent prostate cancer.

7.4.1 Free PSA and Percent Free PSA

The decreased luminal proteolytic processing of PSA produced by tumor cells causes an increase in cPSA and a concomitant decrease in fPSA, resulting in a lower ratio of serum percent free PSA (%fPSA, synonym to f:t PSA-ratio, is free/total PSA × 100) [38]. After the identification of fPSA [39], it was approved by the FDA in 1998 as an aid to prostate cancer detection in men with total PSA-levels of 4–10 ng/mL. This was decided after the study by Catalona et al. which showed that %fPSA can reduce unnecessary biopsies with 20 %, while keeping a 95 % detection rate for prostate cancer [40]. A %fPSA cut-off of ≤25 % was recommended for patients with a tPSA-level 4–10 ng/mL and a normal DRE. The %fPSA significantly improved the predictive accuracy with an area under the curve (AUC) of 0.72 as compared to 0.53 for tPSA alone. Above findings have been confirmed in several studies and reviews [41–43]. %fPSA is used to distinguish between prostate cancer and BPH as a cause of elevated PSA. An increase in %fPSA correlates with a lower risk of prostate cancer and vice versa. %fPSA is most useful at extreme values. Although there is no optimum cut-off, in most studies %fPSA is called low when <10 % and high when >25 % [41, 42]. A multi-centre study by Catalona et al. showed that 56 % of men with <10 % fPSA had prostate cancer, compared with only 8 % of men with >25 % fPSA [43]. In the Finnish arm of the ERSPC the use of %fPSA was evaluated in a screening setting in screen-negative men (tPSA < 3 ng/mL) [44]. The median follow-up was 5.8 years. Men with a %fPSA in the lowest quartile (<14.2 %) had a 6.9-fold risk of being diagnosed with prostate cancer compared with men in the highest quartile group (>23.7 %). In summary %fPSA improves cancer detection over tPSA alone, while reducing unnecessary prostate biopsies. This is especially true in men with a tPSA between 4 and 10 ng/mL, the diagnostic grey zone, where the clinician is unsure whether the PSA-elevation is due to BPH or prostate cancer. A limitation is that %fPSA lacks clear thresholds balancing specificity and sensitivity for the early detection of prostate cancer. As in tPSA, %fPSA should be considered as a continuum of risk. The lower the %fPSA, the higher the probability of prostate cancer. Noteworthy is the fact that fPSA and tPSA should be measured using kits obtained from the same supplier and that fPSA is less stable than cPSA causing a greater analytic variability.

7.4.2 ProPSA, Its Derivatives and the Prostate Health Index

Different precursor isoforms of PSA (−2, −4, −5 and −7 pPSA) have been evaluated to improve prostate cancer detection, especially in men presenting with a tPSA-level of 2–10 ng/mL [45–47]. Particularly (−2)pPSA, a molecular isoform of fPSA, has shown a higher specificity for the prediction of prostate cancer and detection over tPSA or %fPSA. Also its derivatives %(−2)pPSA (calculated by (−2)pPSA divided by fPSA) and the prostate health index (phi), which is a mathematical combination of tPSA, fPSA and (−2)pPSA, has shown promising results in identifying prostate cancer in men with a PSA-level between 2 and 10 ng/mL. In a review, Hori et al. concluded that most studies have found no improvement in prostate cancer detection by using (−5, or −7) pPSA rather than fPSA or other current PSA-based measurements [48–51]. The included studies evaluating (−2)pPSA and its derivatives have shown promising results [52, 53]. Both phi and %(−2)pPSA substantially improve the predictive value of PSA in the detection of early stage prostate cancer and are also able to predict prostate cancer aggressiveness [54, 55]. A study by Jansen et al. retrospectively evaluated the value of (−2)pPSA and phi, with the goal to improve diagnostic accuracy in prostate cancer detection. In two centres a total of 756 European men, with a tPSA-level of 2–10 ng/mL with histologically proven prostate cancer on biopsy or no biopsy detectable malignancy were included. In both centres the highest predictive value for prostate cancer was found with phi (AUC's 0.709 and 0.750 respectively), closely followed by %(−2)pPSA (AUC's of 0.695 and 0.716 respectively). At 95 % sensitivity, phi and %(−2)pPSA also both improved specificity (23 % resp. 31 % for phi and 20 resp. 22 % for %(−2)pPSA), compared to tPSA (10 % resp. 8 %) [54]. A study by Lazzeri et al. confirmed the positive findings regarding phi and (−2)pPSA. In patients with a tPSA of 2–10 ng/mL, phi and %(−2)pPSA were the most significant and accurate individual predictors for prostate cancer detection at first biopsy (AUC's both 0.67) [55]. (−2)pPSA and phi were also positively correlated with Gleason scores. The subforms (−2)pPSA and phi were studied in a case–control trial by Stephan et al. in 2013 [56]. The aim of this multicentre study was to reduce unnecessary biopsy and improve detection of aggressive cancer by the use of (−2)pPSA and phi. A total of 1362 patients (694 men having prostate cancer) with a tPSA-level of 1.6–8.0 ng/mL who underwent initial or repeat TRUS guided core biopsy were included (≥10 biopsies). %(−2)pPSA and phi were superior in predicting prostate cancer when used separately, but also when used in a model including age, prostate volume, DRE, tPSA and %fPSA. In addition phi was significantly higher in patients with Gleason ≥7 tumors. In conclusion both phi and (−2)pPSA improve specificity over tPSA, in prostate cancer detection in the PSA range 2–10 ng/mL.

7.4.3 PSA Derived Parameters and Kinetics

Several calculated parameters and kinetics based on PSA have been developed and studied, with the goal to increase specificity of tPSA-based testing. PSA-density (PSAD), PSA-velocity (PSAV), and PSA-doubling time (PSADT) will be discussed briefly.

7.4.3.1 PSA-Density

The concept of PSAD is to evaluate PSA-level in relation to prostate volume and is calculated by dividing the tPSA-level by the prostate volume, expressed in ng/mL/mL. PSAD was first introduced in 1992 to make a distinction between an elevated PSA-level being caused by BPH or prostate cancer [57], again crucial in men with a tPSA in the grey-zone [58]. One of the practical problems with PSAD is the volume assessment [59]. DRE assessed volume can be unreliable. TRUS is more accurate but here also the problem of inter-examiner differences exists. Another disadvantage is that a TRUS is an invasive procedure and mostly performed at the time of the TRUS guided biopsy. Therefore PSAD is less useful in determining the need for prostate biopsy. PSAD could be of use in prognostication of prostate cancer aggressiveness to determine which treatment to employ [43]. However, %fPSA provides comparable results to PSAD in terms of prostate cancer detection and prediction of aggressiveness, and a blood test is not as inconvenient as a TRUS and is performed anyway when the PSA is obtained [43].

7.4.3.2 PSA-Velocity

PSAV is the rate of change in PSA over time. There are several methods to calculate PSAV with different outcomes [60]. It is used as a pre-treatment and post-treatment indicator. First the pre-treatment use will be discussed. In 1992, Carter et al. introduced PSAV and reported that in men with a tPSA 4–10 ng/mL a PSAV of >0.75 ng/mL/year was found as a significant predictor of prostate cancer diagnosis with a sensitivity of 72 % and a specificity of 95 % [61].

In 2006 another study by Carter et al. showed that in 980 men (124 men with prostate cancer) with a PSAV >0.35 ng/mL/year at 10–15 years before diagnosis, were significantly more likely to die from prostate cancer than men with a PSAV ≤0.35 ng/mL/year (RR 4.7, 95 % CI 1.3–16.5; $p = 0.02$) [62]. In 2009, in the Swedish and Dutch arm of the ERSPC trial, it was found that PSAV only marginally enhanced the predictive accuracy of baseline models including tPSA, age and %fPSA [63]. Also in the ERPSC and PCPT studies, PSAV was not found to be an independent predictor for detecting (significant) prostate cancer on biopsy and when PSAV is used as a biopsy indicator, a large number of clinically significant prostate cancers would be missed. When using a PSAV cut-off ≥0.15, a number of 69 (11.1 %) significant prostate cancers would have been missed [64, 65]. All the men in the ERSPC and PCPT had undergone biopsy, minimizing the verification bias. In many other studies, especially those reporting additional value of PSAV, not all men were biopsied. Men not biopsied were assumed not to have prostate cancer, resulting in a biased estimate of the predictive value of PSAV. A recent study in 2013 found that long-term PSAV in addition to baseline PSA-levels could improve classification of prostate cancer risk and mortality [66]. A systematic review on the use of PSAV before definitive treatment by Vickers et al. in 2009, concluded about pre-treatment PSAV that many studies had deficiencies and that there is little evidence that measurement of PSAV in untreated men provided predictive information beyond that available from tPSA alone [67]. Despite this observation, the National Cancer Center Comprehensive Network recommends PSAV for the use in early prostate cancer detection. Men with a high PSAV (>0.35 ng/mL/year) are recommended to be biopsied, even in the absence of other indications. Vickers et al. evaluated the guidelines and again did not found evidence that supported this recommendation [68]. PSAV is also evaluated for post-treatment use. D'Amico et al. reported in two studies about the association between PSAV and prostate cancer mortality after treatment [69, 70]. In the first study, 1095 men with localized prostate cancer treated with radical prostatectomy were included. In 262 men the year prior to diagnosis the PSAV increased by more than 2 ng/mL/year. In this group 24 events of prostate cancer deaths were reported, compared to 3 events in the group of 833 men with a PSAV ≤2.0 ng/mL/yr (relative risk 20.4, 95 % CI (6.2–67.9), $p<0.001$). Men with a PSAV >2.0 ng/mL/yr had a significantly higher risk of dying from prostate cancer despite radical prostatectomy [69]. In the second study 358 men with localized prostate cancer treated with radiation therapy were evaluated with the same purpose. Also in these men the >2 ng/mL/year increase in PSAV the year prior to diagnosis was significantly associated with a higher risk of death due to prostate cancer [70]. Out of the 150 men with a PSAV >2.0 ng/mL/yr, 28 men died of prostate cancer compared to 2 events in the group of 208 men with a PSAV ≤2.0 ng/mL/yr. Problems with PSAV are a lack of a standardized method for its determination. How many measurements are optimal to use, and what time interval is the best between the measurements [60]? There is also no optimum PSAV cut-off value for separating men at low and high risk. Finally there is the problem of lead time when PSAV is used in a population based screening. Screening allows the diagnosis to be made many years earlier than its clinical detection. At that time PSAV is in the same range for men with and without prostate cancer. The European Association of Urology (EAU) guidelines state that PSAV and PSADT (discussed in next paragraph) have limited use in the diagnosis of prostate cancer [71]. In summary, there is evidence that PSAV can be useful post-treatment, and to distinguish the more aggressive tumors from indolent tumors. The use of PSAV in the detection of prostate cancer (pre-treatment) is an ongoing discussion.

7.4.3.3 PSA-Doubling Time

PSADT demonstrates the time period (in months/years) for a certain level of PSA to increase by a factor of two. PSADT can be measured and used before and after treatment of prostate cancer. Post-treatment PSADT is associated with clinical progression, recurrence, development of metastasis and prostate cancer mortality. Post radical prostatectomy (RP) PSA is usually zero if the surgery was successful, so all men start at the same level which makes it easier to use and assess. PSADT has been used in monitoring recurrence after RP for localized prostate cancer by Pound et al. They showed that a PSADT <10 months is predictive for risk and time to the development of metastatic disease [72]. Freedland et al. also investigated the use of PSADT in risk assessment for biochemical recurrence (BCR) after RP in 379 patients, and concluded that the shorter the postoperative PSADT, the higher the risk of dying from prostate cancer [73]. With a PSADT <15 months, prostate cancer accounted for an estimated 90 % of all deaths by 15 years after recurrence. The majority of prostate cancer deaths occurred among patients with an intermediate PSADT 3.0–8.9 months [74]. PSADT is also used in the pre-treatment setting. For example in a large active surveillance cohort (PRIAS) a PSADT of <3 years is used as one of the parameters to decide if active treatment is recommended [75]. A systematic review by Vickers et al. analysed the use of pre-treatment PSADT as a prognostic factor in prostate cancer and concludes as for pre-treatment PSAV that there is little evidence for the use of PSADT in untreated patients in predicting information beyond that provided by tPSA alone [67]. A problem with PSADT in a pre-treatment setting is that men start out with very different PSA-levels. PSADT is strongly influenced by baseline PSA-level, and in an untreated prostate the PSA-level can be influenced by benign and malignant conditions. Overall PSADT is more of use post-treatment and in assessing tumor aggressiveness than in detection of prostate cancer or pre-treatment use.

7.5 Other Promising Biomarkers in ProstateCancer

To improve accuracy of diagnosis many other biomarkers are being developed. These include urine, blood and genetic biomarkers. One of the advantages with urine markers is that they are easy and non-invasive to collect. We will discuss two of the most promising urine markers which are most advanced in development: the PCA3 (prostate cancer antigen 3) and the TMPRSS2:ERG gene fusion.

7.5.1 PCA3

In 1999, Bussemakers et al. identified and characterized the differential display clone 3 (DD3), later called PCA3 [76]. PCA3 is a segment of non-coding messenger ribonucleic acid (mRNA) mapped to chromosome 9q21-22. It does not encode a protein and its biologic role is unknown. PCA3 mRNA is overexpressed in 95 % of the prostatic tumors evaluated as compared to benign tissue [76]. The PCA3-test involves collection of a urine sample after DRE to mobilise prostatic (cancer) cells and extracellular vesicles (including RNA-containing prostasomes) into the urethra. This urine test is a non-invasive method, which makes it highly suitable for clinical purposes. The first urine test was developed by Hessels et al. in 2003 [77]. In 2006, a simpler and faster urine test was brought on the market [78]. Since then several assays have been developed, and the clinical use of PCA3 has been studied extensively. Usually a cut-off value of PCA3 ≥ 35 is adopted, resulting in a 47–69 % sensitivity and 72–79 % specificity [78–81]. Also PCA3 has shown to be an independent predictor for prostate cancer risk, so it can be used for PCA3-based nomograms [82]. PCA3 has shown to be independent of age, prostate volume and tPSA, for predicting prostate cancer [81]. The PCA3-test has also been analysed in the ERSPC trial for potential use as a first-line diagnostic test. A total of 721 pre-screened men, aged 63–75 years, were invited for re-screening. Participants underwent biopsy if serum PSA ≥ 3.0 ng/mL and/ or the PCA3 score was ≥10. In total, 122 prostate cancers were detected. A PCA3-score ≥35 showed a 68 % sensitivity and 56 % specificity. With this cut-off for PCA3, five cases of serious prostate cancer (stage ≥T2a and/ or Gleason score >3 + 3) were missed, but 52 % biopsies were saved, compared to tPSA ≥ 3.0 ng/mL which yields a sensitivity of 35 %, specificity of 69 %, number of serious cancers missed 11 %, and 68 % biopsies saved [83]. A recent review by Bradley et al. assessed the role of PCA3 in biopsy and treatment decision making [84]. The most important conclusion was that PCA3 had a higher diagnostic accuracy than tPSA increase, but with a low strength of evidence.

7.5.2 TMPRSS2:ERG Gene Fusion

In 2005, chromosomal rearrangements were identified in prostate cancer that fuse the 5' region of the androgen-regulated gene TMPRSS2 (transmembrane protease, serine 2) with ERG or ETV1 (erythroblastosis virus E26 transformation specific (ETS) transcription factor family members) [85]. The ERG oncogene is the most common ETS family member involved in such fusions. As a result of this rearrangement, the ERG gene becomes androgen-regulated and overexpressed as a TMPRSS2:ERG fusion or truncated ERG product. The fusion transcript and ERG protein overexpression are close to 100 % specific for the presence of prostate cancer in tissue-based studies. Approximately 50 % of PSA-screened prostate cancers harbour a TMPRSS2:ERG gene fusion [85]. Reverse transcription-polymerase chain reaction (RT-PCR)-based assays have been developed to detect TMPRSS2:ERG mRNA in urine [86, 87]. A sensitivity of 37 % and specificity of 93 % to predict prostate cancer was reported, resulting in a positive predictive value of 94 % [88]. Tomlins et al. reported recently about a new TMPRSS2:ERG urine test. Urine TMPRSS2:ERG was associated with indicators of clinically significant prostate cancer at biopsy and prostatectomy. Adding TMPRSS2:ERG and PCA3 to the PCPT risk calculator improved performance for predicting prostate cancer risk on biopsy (AUC 0.79, $p<0.001$) [89].

In conclusion, the performance characteristics of measuring urinary PCA3 and TMPRSS2:ERG fusion transcripts are encouraging and represent new methods for the development and expansion of prostate cancer-specific tests.

7.6 PSA in Clinical Management

PSA is used as a marker at all stages of prostate cancer; from detection until management. A short overview of the clinical use of PSA is presented here.

7.6.1 Monitoring of Therapeutic Response and Recurrence with PSA

The first work on the clinical use of PSA as a tumor marker of prostate cancer was carried out in the 1980s [21, 90]. In 1986, PSA was approved by the United States FDA as a marker to monitor treatment in patients with prostate cancer. PSA is used in clinical medicine to monitor therapeutic response and as an early indicator for recurrence of prostate cancer after therapy, e.g. RP or radiation therapy (RT). An elevation in PSA (biochemical recurrence, BCR) is found before clinical relapse. Pound et al. showed that no patients who were followed up for >5 years after RP, developed a recurrence without a concomitant rise in PSA [72]. Post-RP PSA-levels should become undetectable. A PSA-level ≥0.2 ng/mL confirmed by a second measurement is defined as BCR after RP by the American Urological Association (AUA) [91], and a similar definition is also used in the European guideline by the European Association of Urology (EAU). PSA is also used to assess responses on and recurrence after RT. In contrast to post-RP, this is more difficult because there is still prostate tissue in situ and the PSA-level is still detectable after treatment. In 2005, the Phoenix criteria were established in which BCR after RT is defined as a PSA rise by ≥2 ng/mL above the post-radiation nadir value, regardless of serum concentration of the nadir [92].

7.6.2 Prediction of Future Risk

tPSA-levels correlate strongly with the presence of prostate cancer and also with the aggressiveness of the disease. A study of Antenor et al. in 2005 reported about 2804 men with stage T1c prostate cancer treated with radical prostatectomy. The main endpoint was to try to find a relation between preoperative PSA-levels and the presence of organ-confined disease, pathologic Gleason grade ≥7, and the 10 year progression free survival rates (PFS) [93]. Results are listed in Table 7.4. Men with preoperative PSA-levels

Table 7.4 Results of the study by Antenor et al. in 2005. All results are statistically significant [93]

Preoperative PSA-level (ng/mL)	Organ-confined disease (%)	Gleason grade ≥7 (%)	10-year PFS (%)
2.6–4.0	81	23	88
4.1–7.0	74	28	80
7.1–10.0	72	35	76
>10	60	47	61

PSA prostate specific antigen, *PFS* progression free survival rate

between 2.6 and 4.0 ng/mL had the greatest rate of organ confined disease, the highest 10-year PFS rate, and lowest pathologic Gleason grade.

A study by Vickers et al. showed that the PSA at age 60 years is a strong predictor of developing aggressive prostate cancer, metastasis and disease-specific mortality at age 85 [94]. In men with a PSA-level greater than the median of 1 ng/mL at age 60, the benefits of screening seem to outweigh the harms. Baseline serum PSA-levels at young age have been analysed as a marker for predicting prostate cancer occurrence in the future. Several studies and reviews on the literature about baseline PSA-testing concluded that higher baseline levels of serum PSA were found to be associated with a greater risk of prostate cancer diagnosis during the next 20–30 years [95–97]. Lilja et al. reported that baseline PSA-measurement at or before age 50 predicts (advanced) prostate cancer diagnosis up to 30 years later. In the age group 44–50 years, 81 % of the prostate cancers that were advanced at diagnosis were found in men with a PSA-level above the median of 0.63 ng/mL. Recently a case–control study was published, showing that PSA concentration can be used to predict long term risk of metastasis or death from prostate cancer [98]. PSA is used in several prediction models and nomograms to predict for example the likelihood of a positive biopsy, aggressiveness of the prostate cancer and future risk of developing prostate cancer [99].

7.6.3 PSA in Screening

In the late 1980s and early 1990s, PSA was analysed for the use of early detection of prostate cancer. One of the first large clinical studies was conducted by Catalona et al. [100–102]. They concluded that the use of measurement of serum PSA in combination with DRE enhances early prostate cancer detection over DRE alone. Prostatic biopsy was considered in case of a PSA cut-off of 4 ng/mL or a suspicious DRE. The study showed that PSA-based screening led to cancer detection in an earlier and curable stage. In 1994, PSA was approved by the FDA as an aid in the early detection of prostate cancer, using a cut-off value of 4 ng/mL as the threshold for biopsy. Large scale screening for prostate cancer remained however controversial. To date, six randomized controlled trails are ongoing aiming to analyze the possible advantages and harms of PSA-based screening [103–108]. The two largest trails comparing the difference in prostate cancer mortality in men invited to regular PSA-testing versus controls will be discussed briefly. The first study is the Prostate, Lung, Colorectal and Ovarian cancer screening trial (PLCO) in the U.S.A. [103]. Between 1993 and 2001 a total of 76.693 men, aged 55–74 years, were randomized to either annual screening (annual PSA for 6 years and annual DRE for 4 years) or usual care (including opportunistic screening). A cut-off point for PSA of 4 ng/mL was used, based on the Hybritech/Beckman Coulter assay. A total of 57 % had complete follow-up to 13 years after randomization. A 12 % relative increase in prostate cancer incidence in the intervention arm was found. After 13 years of follow-up there was no evidence of a prostate cancer mortality benefit for annual screening (RR 1.09, 95 % CI: 0.87–1.36). A limitation of this trial is that 52 % of the men in the control group underwent screening during the study period, so the study was merely a comparison between intense screened men and less intense screened men rather than screening versus non-screening. In addition, 45 % of men had at least one PSA-test in the 3 years preceding randomization. The second, and worldwide the largest trial is the European Randomized Study of Screening for Prostate Cancer (ERSPC) [104]. Between 1991 and 2003, a total of 182.160 men aged 55–74 years, were included in eight European countries. A core age group of 162.388 men, aged 55–69 years, was predefined in the power calculation.

Men in the screening group underwent PSA-testing every 2–4 years. A cut-off value for PSA of ≥3 ng/mL was used in five centers and two centers used a cut-off value of ≥4 ng/mL, also based on the Hybritech/ Beckman Coulter assay. After a median follow-up of 11 years in the core age group the relative reduction in the risk of death form prostate cancer was 21 % in the screening group as compared to the control group (RR 0.79, 95 % CI 0.68–0.91; p=0.001), and even 29 % after adjustment for noncompliance [104]. A limitation of this study which could also be regarded as a strength, is that there are different study protocols per participating center. For example, different PSA cut-off values are used ranging from 2.5 to 4 ng/mL. There is a fine balance between choosing a higher PSA cut-off value which will improve biopsy specificity but with the risk that more (significant) cancers will be missed. On the other hand using a lower PSA cut-off improves sensitivity because of a higher detection rate but this also leads to more unnecessary biopsies and the identification of more indolent cancers (overdiagnosis). Before the introduction of PSA-based screening in the USA the prostate cancer mortality had been rising steadily for decades. Between 1990 and 2009 prostate cancer death rates have decreased by 40 % [4]. This can be ascribed to early detection but also improvement in treatment of prostate cancer. PSA-testing has also led that fewer men present with metastatic disease [109]. However, screening has both benefits and harms. Recently the U.S. Preventive Service Task Force (USPSTF) recommended against serum PSA-based screening for prostate cancer because of the uncertain ratio between harms and benefits (grade D recommendation) [110, 111]. However, one can raise questions about the justification of this recommendation [112]. The PLCO and ERSPC trials are still ongoing, so conclusions may be preliminary. Meta-analysis combining the different PSA-screening studies concluded that there is no effect of screening on prostate cancer mortality [113, 114]. These meta-analyses can be criticized since the trials included are very heterogeneous and not all designed to address prostate cancer mortality reduction [115].

7.6.4 Individual Risk Assessment by Nomograms

Despite contradictory results about the use of PSA-testing in population-based screening, with no doubt PSA has benefits on an individual base. Knowledge about the use of predictions based on PSA and other risk factors associated with prostate cancer, could be used in individual risk stratification and for the development of tailored screening programs to maximize benefits and minimize health care costs and prevent potential harm of screening: unnecessary tests, overdiagnosis, overtreatment, anxiety, decreased quality of life. A risk calculator combines multiple predictive factors to try to predict the probability of an outcome: e.g. the chance of prostate cancer risk on biopsy, risk of significant cancer, or the risk of metastasis. The use of risk calculators allows for a more individual assessment of prostate cancer risk instead of the one size fits all approach, and provides better predictive accuracy compared to PSA alone [116]. Two frequently used calculators are the PCPT and ERSPC risk calculators. The PCPT prostate cancer risk calculator is a predictive model of prostate cancer based on serum PSA, PSAV, DRE result, age, family history of prostate cancer, ethnicity and prior biopsy [65]. Individualized assessment of prostate cancer risk and risk of high-grade disease for men undergoing prostate biopsy is possible. The second is the ERSPC prostate cancer risk calculator. Six types of calculators have been developed to help indicate whether further investigation is required or to predict prostate cancer risk or the aggressiveness of prostate cancer. Variables used are age, family history of prostate cancer, serum PSA, DRE result, TRUS findings, prior biopsy and prostate volume [99, 117]. Comparisons between the calculators are published and show that overall, the ERSPC risk calculator has better discriminatory capability [118, 119]. In conclusion risk calculators and nomograms can be helpful in making individual decisions in daily practice about all aspects of prostate cancer; screening, treatment and follow-up.

7.7 Future Perspectives: Multiparametric MRI in ProstateCancer

Elevated PSA and abnormal DRE demonstrate poor performance characteristics in prostate cancer detection. Despite recent improvements in identifying novel prostate cancer biomarkers, it is still a long way to use these biomarkers individually or in a combination panel in clinical practice. The last decennium multiparametric MRI (mpMRI) has been evaluated extensively in the research field of prostate cancer.

7.7.1 Role of mpMRI in ProstateCancer Detection

A combination of PSA and DRE, together with Magnetic Resonance Imaging (MRI) in the detection of prostate cancer has been evaluated in numerous patient populations. The use of multiparametric MRI (mpMRI) in prostate cancer detection is recommended [120]. mpMRI includes a combination of high-resolution T2-weighted images (T2WI), and at least two functional MRI sequences. T2WI provides high-resolution morphologic information of the prostate gland. Functional techniques are Diffusion Weighted Imaging (DWI), Dynamic Contrast-Enhanced imaging (DCE), and Magnetic Resonance Spectroscopic Imaging (MRSI). DWI measures the diffusion properties of tissue, which is related to the amount of interstitial free water molecules and their permeability. Cancerous tissue, with higher cell densities and abundance of intra- and intercellular membranes, tends to have more restricted diffusion than normal tissue. Assessment of relative tissue signal attenuation at DWI is used for tumor detection and characterization. A more quantitative analysis of DWI is achieved by calculating the apparent diffusion coefficient (ADC) for each pixel of the image, which is displayed as a parametric ADC map. DCE-MRI is based on repetitive acquisition of sequential images during the passage of a contrast agent within a tissue of interest. Pharmacodynamics of the contrast agent within the tissue can be achieved qualitatively, semi-quantitatively and quantitatively. Cancerous tissue, with increased vascularity and permeability due to neo-angiogenesis, tends to have higher contrast enhanced parameters than normal tissue. MRSI assesses chemical composition of the metabolites citrate, creatine, and choline, which have characteristic resonance frequencies that can be measured. Prostate cancer shows a high level of choline and a low level of citrate relative to the normal peripheral zone. The sensitivity and specificity of mpMRI for prostate cancer detection in different patient populations demonstrate a range from 69 % to 95 % and 74 % to 94 %, respectively [121–126]. mpMRI improves the diagnostic accuracy in prostate cancer detection compared to T2WI alone, or in combination with only one functional technique [123–126]. The variety of sensitivity and specificity is due to the significant variability in the patient populations, coil designs, magnet strengths, gold standard correlation methodologies (biopsy vs. surgery), and level of expertise used in different studies, but also due to selection bias, verification bias and the absence of blinded study design. Therefore, there is an urgent need for randomized controlled trials to prove the additional value of mpMRI. However, the combination of elevated PSA, abnormal DRE, and subsequently the mpMRI may demonstrate a better performance than the combination of elevated PSA and DRE alone. To implement the mpMRI as a cornerstone of prostate cancer clinical work-up, still some other limitations have to be overcome. The availability and reading experience of mpMRI should be increased and cost-effective studies should become available. Recently, important improvements have been made to standardize imaging parameters and scoring systems for the interpretation and reporting of mpMRI [120, 127, 128].

7.7.2 Role of mpMRI in Targeted Image Guided Prostate Biopsy

As mpMRI may be valuable in detecting significant prostate cancer, consequently MRI guidance of prostate biopsies has been performed [129]. MRI-derived lesions can be targeted by

(1) cognitive targeting, (2) by the use of registration or fusion software to allow a lesion defined on MRI to be identified on ultrasound during a TRUS-guided biopsy procedure, either with or without a tracking device, and by (3) targeting within the MRI magnet (in-bore targeting). A recent published systematic review on image guided prostate biopsy using MRI derived targets, demonstrates that in men with at least one negative prior biopsy, 69 % (328 of 479 men) had an MRI abnormality with a similar positive biopsy rate of 70 % (229 of 328 men) [129]. In pooled analysis of biopsy-naive cohorts, where targeted and systematic cores were reported independently, 62 % (374 of 599) had suspicious findings on MRI, and 66 % (248 of 374) had prostate cancer on biopsy. This review concludes that the efficiency of the targeted sampling appeared superior to the standard systematic TRUS biopsy approach (70 % vs. 40 %). A targeted biopsy approach by MRI guidance may appear to aid in decreasing the number of men biopsied overall, increasing the proportion of men with clinically significant prostate cancer biopsied, and to lower the detection of insignificant prostate cancer. However, this review also concludes that these estimations are based on relatively few studies, using different thresholds for declaring a target, a variety of methods for targeting and a host of definitions of disease.

7.7.3 Role of mpMRI in PCa Risk Stratification

Instead of radical prostatectomy or radiation therapy, active surveillance of prostate cancer is a viable option for the management of low-risk disease. Nomograms may stratify patients into low-risk, mediate-risk or high-risk disease. Few nomograms for prostate cancer have been reported to discriminate low-risk disease from clinically significant disease in different patient cohorts [130, 131]. mpMRI can provide information about the risk of prostate cancer presence and prostate cancer aggressiveness. This could be used in combination with clinical variables for risk stratification. mpMRI is not included in standard clinical decision-making algorithms or in nomograms. Recently, T2WI-MRI and MRSI were incorporated into Kattan's nomogram and reported an improved prediction of insignificant prostate cancer [132]. Obviously, further studies should be undertaken, and these results need to be validated in larger patient populations and in multiple centers. However, these results are encouraging.

In conclusion, the mpMRI has emerged as a promising tool for the evaluation of the prostate by morphologic assessment, and can display altered cellularity, provide metabolic information, and aid in non-invasive characterization of tissue and tumor vascularity abnormalities, associated with prostate cancer. Subsequently, image guided prostate biopsy using MRI derived targets may appear to decrease the number of men biopsied overall, increase the detection of clinically significant prostate cancer, and lower the detection of insignificant prostate cancer. In individual risk stratification, the mpMRI may contribute to improve prostate cancer detection, in combination with PSA and many other clinical and biological variables.

References

1. Villeirs GM, LV K, De Neve WJ, De Meerleer GO (2005) Magnetic resonance imaging anatomy of the prostate and periprostatic area: a guide for radiotherapists. Radiother Oncol 76(1):99–106
2. Ferlay J, Shin HR, Bray F, Forman D, Mathers C, Parkin DM (2010) Estimates of worldwide burden of cancer in 2008: GLOBOCAN 2008. Int J Cancer 127(12):2893–2917
3. Ferlay J, Steliarova-Foucher E, Lortet-Tieulent J, Rosso S, Coebergh JW, Comber H et al (2013) Cancer incidence and mortality patterns in Europe: estimates for 40 countries in 2012. Eur J Cancer 49(6):1374–1403
4. Siegel R, Naishadham D, Jemal A (2013) Cancer statistics, 2013. CA Cancer J Clin 63(1):11–30
5. Center MM, Jemal A, Lortet-Tieulent J, Ward E, Ferlay J, Brawley O et al (2012) International variation in prostate cancer incidence and mortality rates. Eur Urol 61(6):1079–1092
6. Gosselaar C, Kranse R, Roobol MJ, Roemeling S, Schroder FH (2008) The interobserver variability of digital rectal examination in a large randomized trial for the screening of prostate cancer. Prostate 68(9):985–993

7. Hodge KK, McNeal JE, Terris MK, Stamey TA (1989) Random systematic versus directed ultrasound guided transrectal core biopsies of the prostate. J Urol 142(1):71–74, discussion 4–5
8. Gleason DF (1966) Classification of prostatic carcinomas. Cancer Chemother Rep 50(3):125–128
9. Mellinger GT, Gleason D, Bailar J 3rd (1967) The histology and prognosis of prostatic cancer. J Urol 97(2):331–337
10. Epstein JI, Allsbrook WC Jr, Amin MB, Egevad LL, Committee IG (2005) The 2005 International Society of Urological Pathology (ISUP) consensus conference on gleason grading of prostatic carcinoma. Am J Surg Pathol 29(9):1228–1242
11. Yousef GM, Luo LY, Diamandis EP (1999) Identification of novel human kallikrein-like genes on chromosome 19q13.3-q13.4. Anticancer Res 19(4B):2843–2852
12. Hara M, Koyanagi Y, Inoue T, Fukuyama T (1971) Some physico-chemical characteristics of " – seminoprotein", an antigenic component specific for human seminal plasma. Forensic immunological study of body fluids and secretion. VII. Nihon Hoigaku Zasshi 25(4):322–324
13. Wang MC, Valenzuela LA, Murphy GP, Chu TM (1979) Purification of a human prostate specific antigen. Invest Urol 17(2):159–163
14. Li TS, Beling CG (1973) Isolation and characterization of two specific antigens of human seminal plasma. Fertil Steril 24(2):134–144
15. Papsidero LD, Wang MC, Valenzuela LA, Murphy GP, Chu TM (1980) A prostate antigen in sera of prostatic cancer patients. Cancer Res 40(7):2428–2432
16. Yousef GM, Diamandis EP (2001) The new human tissue kallikrein gene family: structure, function, and association to disease. Endocr Rev 22(2):184–204
17. Balk SP, Ko YJ, Bubley GJ (2003) Biology of prostate-specific antigen. J Clin Oncol 21(2):383–391
18. Lilja H (1985) A kallikrein-like serine protease in prostatic fluid cleaves the predominant seminal vesicle protein. J Clin Invest 76(5):1899–1903
19. Lovgren J, Valtonen-Andre C, Marsal K, Lilja H, Lundwall A (1999) Measurement of prostate-specific antigen and human glandular kallikrein 2 in different body fluids. J Androl 20(3):348–355
20. Stephan C, Jung K, Lein M, Diamandis EP (2007) PSA and other tissue kallikreins for prostate cancer detection. Eur J Cancer 43(13):1918–1926
21. Stamey TA, Yang N, Hay AR, McNeal JE, Freiha FS, Redwine E (1987) Prostate-specific antigen as a serum marker for adenocarcinoma of the prostate. N Engl J Med 317(15):909–916
22. Oesterling JE, Chan DW, Epstein JI, Kimball AW Jr, Bruzek DJ, Rock RC et al (1988) Prostate specific antigen in the preoperative and postoperative evaluation of localized prostatic cancer treated with radical prostatectomy. J Urol 139(4):766–772
23. Kumar A, Mikolajczyk SD, Goel AS, Millar LS, Saedi MS (1997) Expression of pro form of prostate-specific antigen by mammalian cells and its conversion to mature, active form by human kallikrein 2. Cancer Res 57(15):3111–3114
24. Mikolajczyk SD, Millar LS, Wang TJ, Rittenhouse HG, Wolfert RL, Marks LS et al (2000) "BPSA," a specific molecular form of free prostate-specific antigen, is found predominantly in the transition zone of patients with nodular benign prostatic hyperplasia. Urology 55(1):41–45
25. Mikolajczyk SD, Millar LS, Wang TJ, Rittenhouse HG, Marks LS, Song W et al (2000) A precursor form of prostate-specific antigen is more highly elevated in prostate cancer compared with benign transition zone prostate tissue. Cancer Res 60(3):756–759
26. Mikolajczyk SD, Grauer LS, Millar LS, Hill TM, Kumar A, Rittenhouse HG et al (1997) A precursor form of PSA (pPSA) is a component of the free PSA in prostate cancer serum. Urology 50(5):710–714
27. Link RE, Shariat SF, Nguyen CV, Farr A, Weinberg AD, Morton RA et al (2004) Variation in prostate specific antigen results from 2 different assay platforms: clinical impact on 2304 patients undergoing prostate cancer screening. J Urol 171(6 Pt 1):2234–2238
28. Loeb S, Catalona WJ (2008) What to do with an abnormal PSA test. Oncologist 13(3):299–305
29. Blijenberg BG, Yurdakul G, Van Zelst BD, Bangma CH, Wildhagen MF, Schroder FH (2001) Discordant performance of assays for free and total prostate-specific antigen in relation to the early detection of prostate cancer. BJU Int 88(6):545–550
30. Rafferty B, Rigsby P, Rose M, Stamey T, Gaines DR (2000) Reference reagents for prostate-specific antigen (PSA): establishment of the first international standards for free PSA and PSA (90:10). Clin Chem 46(9):1310–1317
31. Bangma CH, van Schaik RH, Blijenberg BG, Roobol MJ, Lilja H, Stenman UH (2010) On the use of prostate-specific antigen for screening of prostate cancer in European randomised study for screening of prostate cancer. Eur J Cancer 46(17):3109–3119
32. Thompson IM, Pauler DK, Goodman PJ, Tangen CM, Lucia MS, Parnes HL et al (2004) Prevalence of prostate cancer among men with a prostate-specific antigen level<or =4.0 ng per milliliter. N Engl J Med 350(22):2239–2246
33. Oesterling JE (1991) Prostate specific antigen: a critical assessment of the most useful tumor marker for adenocarcinoma of the prostate. J Urol 145(5):907–923
34. Nadler RB, Humphrey PA, Smith DS, Catalona WJ, Ratliff TL (1995) Effect of inflammation and benign prostatic hyperplasia on elevated serum prostate specific antigen levels. J Urol 154(2 Pt 1):407–413
35. Thompson IM, Ankerst DP, Chi C, Lucia MS, Goodman PJ, Crowley JJ et al (2005) Operating

characteristics of prostate-specific antigen in men with an initial PSA level of 3.0 ng/ml or lower. JAMA 294(1):66–70
36. Schroder FH, Carter HB, Wolters T, van den Bergh RC, Gosselaar C, Bangma CH et al (2008) Early detection of prostate cancer in 2007. Part 1: PSA and PSA kinetics. Eur Urol 53(3):468–477
37. Draisma G, Boer R, Otto SJ, van der Cruijsen IW, Damhuis RA, Schroder FH et al (2003) Lead times and overdetection due to prostate-specific antigen screening: estimates from the European randomized study of screening for prostate cancer. J Natl Cancer Inst 95(12):868–878
38. Stenman UH, Leinonen J, Alfthan H, Rannikko S, Tuhkanen K, Alfthan O (1991) A complex between prostate-specific antigen and alpha 1-antichymotrypsin is the major form of prostate-specific antigen in serum of patients with prostatic cancer: assay of the complex improves clinical sensitivity for cancer. Cancer Res 51(1):222–226
39. Lilja H, Christensson A, Dahlen U, Matikainen MT, Nilsson O, Pettersson K et al (1991) Prostate-specific antigen in serum occurs predominantly in complex with alpha 1-antichymotrypsin. Clin Chem 37(9):1618–1625
40. Catalona WJ, Partin AW, Slawin KM, Brawer MK, Flanigan RC, Patel A et al (1998) Use of the percentage of free prostate-specific antigen to enhance differentiation of prostate cancer from benign prostatic disease: a prospective multicenter clinical trial. JAMA 279(19):1542–1547
41. Roddam AW, Duffy MJ, Hamdy FC, Ward AM, Patnick J, Price CP et al (2005) Use of prostate-specific antigen (PSA) isoforms for the detection of prostate cancer in men with a PSA level of 2–10 ng/ml: systematic review and meta-analysis. Eur Urol 48(3):386–399, discussion 98–9
42. Lee R, Localio AR, Armstrong K, Malkowicz SB, Schwartz JS, Free PSASG (2006) A meta-analysis of the performance characteristics of the free prostate-specific antigen test. Urology 67(4):762–768
43. Catalona WJ, Southwick PC, Slawin KM, Partin AW, Brawer MK, Flanigan RC et al (2000) Comparison of percent free PSA, PSA density, and age-specific PSA cutoffs for prostate cancer detection and staging. Urology 56(2):255–260
44. Finne P, Auvinen A, Maattanen L, Tammela TL, Ruutu M, Juusela H et al (2008) Diagnostic value of free prostate-specific antigen among men with a prostate-specific antigen level of <3.0 microg per liter. Eur Urol 54(2):362–370
45. Catalona WJ, Bartsch G, Rittenhouse HG, Evans CL, Linton HJ, Horninger W et al (2004) Serum pro-prostate specific antigen preferentially detects aggressive prostate cancers in men with 2 to 4 ng/ml prostate specific antigen. J Urol 171(6 Pt 1):2239–2244
46. Mikolajczyk SD, Catalona WJ, Evans CL, Linton HJ, Millar LS, Marker KM et al (2004) Proenzyme forms of prostate-specific antigen in serum improve the detection of prostate cancer. Clin Chem 50(6):1017–1025
47. de Vries SH, Raaijmakers R, Blijenberg BG, Mikolajczyk SD, Rittenhouse HG, Schroder FH (2005) Additional use of [−2] precursor prostate-specific antigen and "benign" PSA at diagnosis in screen-detected prostate cancer. Urology 65(5): 926–930
48. Bangma CH, Wildhagen MF, Yurdakul G, Schroder FH, Blijenberg BG (2004) The value of (−7, −5)pro-prostate-specific antigen and human kallikrein-2 as serum markers for grading prostate cancer. BJU Int 93(6):720–724
49. Hori S, Blanchet JS, McLoughlin J (2013) From prostate-specific antigen (PSA) to precursor PSA (proPSA) isoforms: a review of the emerging role of proPSAs in the detection and management of early prostate cancer. BJU Int 112(6):717–728
50. Lein M, Semjonow A, Graefen M, Kwiatkowski M, Abramjuk C, Stephan C et al (2005) A multicenter clinical trial on the use of (−5, −7) pro prostate specific antigen. J Urol 174(6):2150–2153
51. Miyakubo M, Ito K, Yamamoto T, Takechi H, Ohi M, Suzuki K (2009) Proprostate-specific antigen: its usefulness in the era of multiple-core prostate biopsy. Int J Urol 16(6):561–565
52. Sokoll LJ, Sanda MG, Feng Z, Kagan J, Mizrahi IA, Broyles DL et al (2010) A prospective, multicenter, National Cancer Institute Early Detection Research Network study of [−2]proPSA: improving prostate cancer detection and correlating with cancer aggressiveness. Cancer Epidemiol Biomarkers Prev 19(5):1193–1200
53. Rhodes T, Jacobson DJ, McGree ME, St Sauver JL, Girman CJ, Lieber MM et al (2012) Longitudinal changes of benign prostate-specific antigen and [−2] proprostate-specific antigen in seven years in a community-based sample of men. Urology 79(3):655–661
54. Jansen FH, van Schaik RH, Kurstjens J, Horninger W, Klocker H, Bektic J et al (2010) Prostate-specific antigen (PSA) isoform p2PSA in combination with total PSA and free PSA improves diagnostic accuracy in prostate cancer detection. Eur Urol 57(6):921–927
55. Lazzeri M, Haese A, de la Taille A, Palou Redorta J, McNicholas T, Lughezzani G et al (2013) Serum isoform [−2]proPSA derivatives significantly improve prediction of prostate cancer at initial biopsy in a total PSA range of 2–10 ng/ml: a multicentric European study. Eur Urol 63(6):986–994
56. Stephan C, Vincendeau S, Houlgatte A, Cammann H, Jung K, Semjonow A (2013) Multicenter evaluation of [−2]proprostate-specific antigen and the prostate health index for detecting prostate cancer. Clin Chem 59(1):306–314

57. Benson MC, Whang IS, Pantuck A, Ring K, Kaplan SA, Olsson CA et al (1992) Prostate specific antigen density: a means of distinguishing benign prostatic hypertrophy and prostate cancer. J Urol 147(3 Pt 2):815–816
58. Benson MC, McMahon DJ, Cooner WH, Olsson CA (1993) An algorithm for prostate cancer detection in a patient population using prostate-specific antigen and prostate-specific antigen density. World J Urol 11(4):206–213
59. Loeb S, Han M, Roehl KA, Antenor JA, Catalona WJ (2005) Accuracy of prostate weight estimation by digital rectal examination versus transrectal ultrasonography. J Urol 173(1):63–65
60. Connolly D, Black A, Murray LJ, Napolitano G, Gavin A, Keane PF (2007) Methods of calculating prostate-specific antigen velocity. Eur Urol 52(4):1044–1050
61. Carter HB, Pearson JD, Metter EJ, Brant LJ, Chan DW, Andres R et al (1992) Longitudinal evaluation of prostate-specific antigen levels in men with and without prostate disease. JAMA 267(16): 2215–2220
62. Carter HB, Ferrucci L, Kettermann A, Landis P, Wright EJ, Epstein JI et al (2006) Detection of life-threatening prostate cancer with prostate-specific antigen velocity during a window of curability. J Natl Cancer Inst 98(21):1521–1527
63. Vickers AJ, Wolters T, Savage CJ, Cronin AM, O'Brien MF, Pettersson K et al (2009) Prostate-specific antigen velocity for early detection of prostate cancer: result from a large, representative, population-based cohort. Eur Urol 56(5):753–760
64. Wolters T, Roobol MJ, Bangma CH, Schroder FH (2009) Is prostate-specific antigen velocity selective for clinically significant prostate cancer in screening? European randomized study of screening for prostate cancer (Rotterdam). Eur Urol 55(2):385–392
65. Thompson IM, Ankerst DP, Chi C, Goodman PJ, Tangen CM, Lucia MS et al (2006) Assessing prostate cancer risk: results from the prostate cancer prevention trial. J Natl Cancer Inst 98(8):529–534
66. Orsted DD, Bojesen SE, Kamstrup PR, Nordestgaard BG (2013) Long-term prostate-specific antigen velocity in improved classification of prostate cancer risk and mortality. Eur Urol 64(3):384–393
67. Vickers AJ, Savage C, O'Brien MF, Lilja H (2009) Systematic review of pretreatment prostate-specific antigen velocity and doubling time as predictors for prostate cancer. J Clin Oncol 27(3):398–403
68. Vickers AJ, Till C, Tangen CM, Lilja H, Thompson IM (2011) An empirical evaluation of guidelines on prostate-specific antigen velocity in prostate cancer detection. J Natl Cancer Inst 103(6):462–469
69. D'Amico AV, Chen MH, Roehl KA, Catalona WJ (2004) Preoperative PSA velocity and the risk of death from prostate cancer after radical prostatectomy. N Engl J Med 351(2):125–135
70. D'Amico AV, Renshaw AA, Sussman B, Chen MH (2005) Pretreatment PSA velocity and risk of death from prostate cancer following external beam radiation therapy. JAMA 294(4):440–447
71. Guideline Pc. Available from: http://www.uroweb.org/guidelines/online-guidelines/
72. Pound CR, Partin AW, Eisenberger MA, Chan DW, Pearson JD, Walsh PC (1999) Natural history of progression after PSA elevation following radical prostatectomy. JAMA 281(17):1591–1597
73. Freedland SJ, Humphreys EB, Mangold LA, Eisenberger M, Dorey FJ, Walsh PC et al (2005) Risk of prostate cancer-specific mortality following biochemical recurrence after radical prostatectomy. JAMA 294(4):433–439
74. Freedland SJ, Humphreys EB, Mangold LA, Eisenberger M, Dorey FJ, Walsh PC et al (2007) Death in patients with recurrent prostate cancer after radical prostatectomy: prostate-specific antigen doubling time subgroups and their associated contributions to all-cause mortality. J Clin Oncol 25(13):1765–1771
75. Bul M, Zhu X, Valdagni R, Pickles T, Kakehi Y, Rannikko A et al (2013) Active surveillance for low-risk prostate cancer worldwide: the PRIAS study. Eur Urol 63(4):597–603
76. Bussemakers MJ, van Bokhoven A, Verhaegh GW, Smit FP, Karthaus HF, Schalken JA et al (1999) DD3: a new prostate-specific gene, highly overexpressed in prostate cancer. Cancer Res 59(23): 5975–5979
77. Hessels D, Klein Gunnewiek JM, van Oort I, Karthaus HF, van Leenders GJ, van Balken B et al (2003) DD3(PCA3)-based molecular urine analysis for the diagnosis of prostate cancer. Eur Urol 44(1):8–15, discussion –6
78. Groskopf J, Aubin SM, Deras IL, Blase A, Bodrug S, Clark C et al (2006) APTIMA PCA3 molecular urine test: development of a method to aid in the diagnosis of prostate cancer. Clin Chem 52(6):1089–1095
79. Deras IL, Aubin SM, Blase A, Day JR, Koo S, Partin AW et al (2008) PCA3: a molecular urine assay for predicting prostate biopsy outcome. J Urol 179(4):1587–1592
80. Marks LS, Fradet Y, Deras IL, Blase A, Mathis J, Aubin SM et al (2007) PCA3 molecular urine assay for prostate cancer in men undergoing repeat biopsy. Urology 69(3):532–535
81. Haese A, de la Taille A, van Poppel H, Marberger M, Stenzl A, Mulders PF et al (2008) Clinical utility of the PCA3 urine assay in European men scheduled for repeat biopsy. Eur Urol 54(5):1081–1088
82. Auprich M, Haese A, Walz J, Pummer K, de la Taille A, Graefen M et al (2010) External validation of urinary PCA3-based nomograms to individually predict prostate biopsy outcome. Eur Urol 58(5):727–732
83. Roobol MJ, Schroder FH, van Leeuwen P, Wolters T, van den Bergh RC, van Leenders GJ et al (2010)

Performance of the prostate cancer antigen 3 (PCA3) gene and prostate-specific antigen in prescreened men: exploring the value of PCA3 for a first-line diagnostic test. Eur Urol 58(4):475–481
84. Bradley LA, Palomaki GE, Gutman S, Samson D, Aronson N (2013) Comparative effectiveness review: prostate cancer antigen 3 testing for the diagnosis and management of prostate cancer. J Urol 190(2):389–398
85. Tomlins SA, Rhodes DR, Perner S, Dhanasekaran SM, Mehra R, Sun XW et al (2005) Recurrent fusion of TMPRSS2 and ETS transcription factor genes in prostate cancer. Science 310(5748):644–648
86. Laxman B, Tomlins SA, Mehra R, Morris DS, Wang L, Helgeson BE et al (2006) Noninvasive detection of TMPRSS2:ERG fusion transcripts in the urine of men with prostate cancer. Neoplasia 8(10):885–888
87. Laxman B, Morris DS, Yu J, Siddiqui J, Cao J, Mehra R et al (2008) A first-generation multiplex biomarker analysis of urine for the early detection of prostate cancer. Cancer Res 68(3):645–649
88. Hessels D, Smit FP, Verhaegh GW, Witjes JA, Cornel EB, Schalken JA (2007) Detection of TMPRSS2-ERG fusion transcripts and prostate cancer antigen 3 in urinary sediments may improve diagnosis of prostate cancer. Clin Cancer Res 13(17):5103–5108
89. Tomlins SA, Aubin SM, Siddiqui J, Lonigro RJ, Sefton-Miller L, Miick S et al (2011) Urine TMPRSS2:ERG fusion transcript stratifies prostate cancer risk in men with elevated serum PSA. Sci Transl Med 3(94):94ra72
90. Kuriyama M, Wang MC, Papsidero LD, Killian CS, Shimano T, Valenzuela L et al (1980) Quantitation of prostate-specific antigen in serum by a sensitive enzyme immunoassay. Cancer Res 40(12): 4658–4662
91. Cookson MS, Aus G, Burnett AL, Canby-Hagino ED, D'Amico AV, Dmochowski RR et al (2007) Variation in the definition of biochemical recurrence in patients treated for localized prostate cancer: the American Urological Association Prostate Guidelines for Localized Prostate Cancer Update Panel report and recommendations for a standard in the reporting of surgical outcomes. J Urol 177(2):540–545
92. Roach M 3rd, Hanks G, Thames H Jr, Schellhammer P, Shipley WU, Sokol GH et al (2006) Defining biochemical failure following radiotherapy with or without hormonal therapy in men with clinically localized prostate cancer: recommendations of the RTOG-ASTRO phoenix consensus conference. Int J Radiat Oncol Biol Phys 65(4):965–974
93. Antenor JA, Roehl KA, Eggener SE, Kundu SD, Han M, Catalona WJ (2005) Preoperative PSA and progression-free survival after radical prostatectomy for stage T1c disease. Urology 66(1):156–160
94. Vickers AJ, Cronin AM, Bjork T, Manjer J, Nilsson PM, Dahlin A et al (2010) Prostate specific antigen concentration at age 60 and death or metastasis from prostate cancer: case-control study. BMJ 341:c4521
95. Loeb S, Carter HB, Catalona WJ, Moul JW, Schroder FH (2012) Baseline prostate-specific antigen testing at a young age. Eur Urol 61(1):1–7
96. Zhu X, Albertsen PC, Andriole GL, Roobol MJ, Schroder FH, Vickers AJ (2012) Risk-based prostate cancer screening. Eur Urol 61(4):652–661
97. Lilja H, Cronin AM, Dahlin A, Manjer J, Nilsson PM, Eastham JA et al (2011) Prediction of significant prostate cancer diagnosed 20 to 30 years later with a single measure of prostate-specific antigen at or before age 50. Cancer 117(6):1210–1219
98. Vickers AJ, Ulmert D, Sjoberg DD, Bennette CJ, Bjork T, Gerdtsson A et al (2013) Strategy for detection of prostate cancer based on relation between prostate specific antigen at age 40–55 and long term risk of metastasis: case-control study. BMJ 346:f2023
99. Available from: http://www.prostaatwijzer.nl/medical-risk-calculators
100. Catalona WJ, Richie JP, Ahmann FR, Hudson MA, Scardino PT, Flanigan RC et al (1994) Comparison of digital rectal examination and serum prostate specific antigen in the early detection of prostate cancer: results of a multicenter clinical trial of 6,630 men. J Urol 151(5):1283–1290
101. Catalona WJ, Smith DS, Ratliff TL, Dodds KM, Coplen DE, Yuan JJ et al (1991) Measurement of prostate-specific antigen in serum as a screening test for prostate cancer. N Engl J Med 324(17): 1156–1161
102. Catalona WJ, Smith DS, Ratliff TL, Basler JW (1993) Detection of organ-confined prostate cancer is increased through prostate-specific antigen-based screening. JAMA 270(8):948–954
103. Andriole GL, Crawford ED, Grubb RL 3rd, Buys SS, Chia D, Church TR et al (2012) Prostate cancer screening in the randomized prostate, lung, colorectal, and ovarian cancer screening trial: mortality results after 13 years of follow-up. J Natl Cancer Inst 104(2):125–132
104. Schroder FH, Hugosson J, Roobol MJ, Tammela TL, Ciatto S, Nelen V et al (2012) Prostate-cancer mortality at 11 years of follow-up. N Engl J Med 366(11):981–990
105. Hugosson J, Carlsson S, Aus G, Bergdahl S, Khatami A, Lodding P et al (2010) Mortality results from the Goteborg randomised population-based prostate-cancer screening trial. Lancet Oncol 11(8):725–732
106. Labrie F, Candas B, Cusan L, Gomez JL, Belanger A, Brousseau G et al (2004) Screening decreases prostate cancer mortality: 11-year follow-up of the 1988 Quebec prospective randomized controlled trial. Prostate 59(3):311–318
107. Kjellman A, Akre O, Norming U, Tornblom M, Gustafsson O (2009) 15-year followup of a population based prostate cancer screening study. J Urol 181(4):1615–1621, discussion 21

108. Sandblom G, Varenhorst E, Rosell J, Lofman O, Carlsson P (2011) Randomised prostate cancer screening trial: 20 year follow-up. BMJ 342:d1539
109. Jemal A, Ward E, Wu X, Martin HJ, McLaughlin CC, Thun MJ (2005) Geographic patterns of prostate cancer mortality and variations in access to medical care in the United States. Cancer Epidemiol Biomarkers Prev 14(3):590–595
110. Moyer VA, Force USPST (2012) Screening for prostate cancer: U.S. Preventive services task force recommendation statement. Ann Intern Med 157(2):120–134
111. Chou R, Croswell JM, Dana T, Bougatsos C, Blazina I, Fu R et al (2011) Screening for prostate cancer: a review of the evidence for the U.S. Preventive Services Task Force. Ann Intern Med 155(11):762–771
112. Carlsson S, Vickers AJ, Roobol M, Eastham J, Scardino P, Lilja H et al (2012) Prostate cancer screening: facts, statistics, and interpretation in response to the US Preventive Services Task Force review. J Clin Oncol 30(21):2581–2584
113. Ilic D, Neuberger MM, Djulbegovic M, Dahm P (2013) Screening for prostate cancer. Cochrane Database Syst Rev 1:CD004720
114. Djulbegovic M, Beyth RJ, Neuberger MM, Stoffs TL, Vieweg J, Djulbegovic B et al (2010) Screening for prostate cancer: systematic review and meta-analysis of randomised controlled trials. BMJ 341:c4543
115. Roobol MJ, Carlsson S, Hugosson J (2011) Meta-analysis finds screening for prostate cancer with PSA does not reduce prostate cancer-related or all-cause mortality but results likely due to heterogeneity – the two highest quality studies identified do find prostate cancer-related mortality reductions. Evid Based Med 16(1):20–21
116. Schroder F, Kattan MW (2008) The comparability of models for predicting the risk of a positive prostate biopsy with prostate-specific antigen alone: a systematic review. Eur Urol 54(2):274–290
117. van den Bergh RC, Roobol MJ, Wolters T, van Leeuwen PJ, Schroder FH (2008) The prostate cancer prevention trial and European randomized study of screening for prostate cancer risk calculators indicating a positive prostate biopsy: a comparison. BJU Int 102(9):1068–1073
118. Cavadas V, Osorio L, Sabell F, Teves F, Branco F, Silva-Ramos M (2010) Prostate cancer prevention trial and European randomized study of screening for prostate cancer risk calculators: a performance comparison in a contemporary screened cohort. Eur Urol 58(4):551–558
119. Oliveira M, Marques V, Carvalho AP, Santos A (2011) Head-to-head comparison of two online nomograms for prostate biopsy outcome prediction. BJU Int 107(11):1780–1783
120. Barentsz JO, Richenberg J, Clements R, Choyke P, Verma S, Villeirs G et al (2012) ESUR prostate MR guidelines 2012. Eur Radiol [Practice Guideline] 22(4):746–757
121. Park BK, Lee HM, Kim CK, Choi HY, Park JW (2008) Lesion localization in patients with a previous negative transrectal ultrasound biopsy and persistently elevated prostate specific antigen level using diffusion-weighted imaging at three Tesla before rebiopsy. Invest Radiol [Clinical Trial] 43(11):789–793
122. Sciarra A, Panebianco V, Ciccariello M, Salciccia S, Cattarino S, Lisi D et al (2010) Value of magnetic resonance spectroscopy imaging and dynamic contrast-enhanced imaging for detecting prostate cancer foci in men with prior negative biopsy. Clin Cancer Res [Clinical Trial Randomized Controlled Trial] 16(6):1875–1883
123. Iwazawa J, Mitani T, Sassa S, Ohue S (2011) Prostate cancer detection with MRI: is dynamic contrast-enhanced imaging necessary in addition to diffusion-weighted imaging? Diagn Interv Radiol [Comparative Study] 17(3):243–248
124. Tamada T, Sone T, Higashi H, Jo Y, Yamamoto A, Kanki A et al (2011) Prostate cancer detection in patients with total serum prostate-specific antigen levels of 4–10 ng/mL: diagnostic efficacy of diffusion-weighted imaging, dynamic contrast-enhanced MRI, and T2-weighted imaging. AJR Am J Roentgenol [Research Support, Non-US Gov't] 197(3):664–670
125. Kitajima K, Kaji Y, Fukabori Y, Yoshida K, Suganuma N, Sugimura K (2010) Prostate cancer detection with 3 T MRI: comparison of diffusion-weighted imaging and dynamic contrast-enhanced MRI in combination with T2-weighted imaging. J Magn Reson Imaging 31(3):625–631
126. Tanimoto A, Nakashima J, Kohno H, Shinmoto H, Kuribayashi S (2007) Prostate cancer screening: the clinical value of diffusion-weighted imaging and dynamic MR imaging in combination with T2-weighted imaging. J Magn Reson Imaging 25(1):146–152
127. Dickinson L, Ahmed HU, Allen C, Barentsz JO, Carey B, Futterer JJ et al (2013) Scoring systems used for the interpretation and reporting of multiparametric MRI for prostate cancer detection, localization, and characterization: could standardization lead to improved utilization of imaging within the diagnostic pathway? J Magn Reson Imaging 37(1):48–58
128. Moore CM, Kasivisvanathan V, Eggener S, Emberton M, Futterer JJ, Gill IS et al (2013) Standards of reporting for MRI-targeted biopsy studies (START) of the prostate: recommendations from an international working group. Eur Urol 64(4):544–552
129. Moore CM, Robertson NL, Arsanious N, Middleton T, Villers A, Klotz L et al (2013) Image-guided prostate biopsy using magnetic resonance imaging-derived targets: a systematic review. Eur Urol 63(1):125–140

130. Kattan MW, Eastham JA, Wheeler TM, Maru N, Scardino PT, Erbersdobler A et al (2003) Counseling men with prostate cancer: a nomogram for predicting the presence of small, moderately differentiated, confined tumors. J Urol 170(5):1792–1797
131. Roemeling S, Roobol MJ, Kattan MW, van der Kwast TH, Steyerberg EW, Schroder FH (2007) Nomogram use for the prediction of indolent prostate cancer: impact on screen-detected populations. Cancer [Randomized Controlled Trial Research Support, Non-US Gov't] 110(10):2218–2221
132. Shukla-Dave A, Hricak H, Akin O, Yu C, Zakian KL, Udo K et al (2012) Preoperative nomograms incorporating magnetic resonance imaging and spectroscopy for prediction of insignificant prostate cancer. BJU Int [Research Support, NIH, Extramural Validation Studies] 109(9):1315–1322

The Actual Role of LDH as Tumor Marker, Biochemical and Clinical Aspects

8

Vladimir Jurisic, Sandra Radenkovic, and Gordana Konjevic

Abstract

Lactate dehydrogenase (LDH) among many biochemical parameters represents a very valuable enzyme in patients with cancer with possibility for easy routine measurement in many clinical laboratories. Previous studies where mostly based on investigated LDH in serum of patients with cancer with aims to estimate their clinical significance. The new directions in investigation of LDH where based on the principle that tumor cells release intracellular enzymes trough damaged cell membrane, that is mostly consequence in intracellular mitochondrial machinery alteration, and apoptosis deregulation. This consideration can be used not only in-vitro assays, but also in respect to clinical characteristics of tumor patients. Based on new techniques of molecular biology it is shown that intracellular characteristics of LDH enzyme are very sensitive indicators of the cellular metabolic state, aerobic or anaerobic direction of glycolysis, activation status and malignant transformation. Using different molecular analyses it is very useful to analyzed intracellular LDH activity in different cell line and tumor tissues obtained from patients, not only to understanding complexity in cancer biochemistry but also in early clinical diagnosis. Based on understandings of the LDH altered metabolism, new therapy option is created with aims to blocking certain metabolic pathways and stop tumors growth.

V. Jurisic (✉)
Faculty of Medical Sciences, University of Kragujevac, Kragujevac, Serbia
e-mail: vdvd@lycos.com

S. Radenkovic
Institute of Oncology and Radiology of Serbia, Belgrade, Serbia

G. Konjevic
Institute of Oncology and Radiology of Serbia, Belgrade, Serbia

Faculty of Medicine, University of Belgrade, Belgrade, Serbia

R. Scatena (ed.), *Advances in Cancer Biomarkers*, Advances in Experimental Medicine and Biology 867, DOI 10.1007/978-94-017-7215-0_8

Keywords
Cancer glucose metabolism • Lactate dehydrogenase (LDH) • Lactate dehydrogenase-A (LDH-A) • LDH activity in clinical practice • LDH biochemistry • LDH in hematological diseases • LDH in lung cancer • LDH in melanoma • LDH isoenzymes • Spontaneously released LDH • Warburg effect

8.1 LDH Biochemistry in Cancer

Lactate dehydrogenase (LDH) among many biochemical parameters represents a very valuable enzyme in patients with cancer with possibility for easy routine measurement in many clinical and hospital laboratories [1, 2]. Previous studies where mostly based on investigated LDH in serum of patients with cancer with aims to estimate their clinical significance. Enormous clinical evidence indicates that LDH is an important prognostic factor for different tumor. Considering that the elevation of serum LDH level correlates with bulky tumor mass it represents an independent prognostic factor for hematological disease and for solid tumors including melanoma, lung cancer, breast and many other tumors and has been used following many years in routine clinical diagnosis [3–8].

LDH is a ubiquitous enzyme that is present in high concentrations in liver, kidney, myocardium, skeletal muscle and red blood cells. Recent findings show an important role LDH in tumor behavior [9, 10]. LDH plays a crucial role in the Warburg effect [11], which is the phenomenon that cancer cells switch from an aerobic to a predominantly anaerobic mechanism, in which glucose is converted to lactate. The Warburg effect seems to be a common feature of malignant cells that is important for their tumorigenic potential [12].

Many cancers show a strongly enhanced glycolytic metabolism of carbohydrates even in the presence of oxygen ('aerobic glycolysis'), a phenomenon firstly described by Otto Warburg ('Warburg effect'). Tumour cells need energy and nucleic acids for proliferation and growth [13]. For most of their energy needs, cancer cells depend on glycolysis. It has been suggested that the excessive glycolysis in tumors is required to support cell growth [12, 14, 15].

8.1.1 Glucose Metabolism in Cancer

Under normal oxygen concentrations (normoxia), timor tissues, but not adjacent normal tissues, exhibit a high rate of glucose consumption. This phenomen, known as aerobic glycolysis or the Warburg effect, has been widely exploited for the diagnosis and staging of human solid cancers [11, 16]. Today using FDG-PET ([(18)F] fluorodeoxyglucose positron emission tomography), it is possible to make an imaging technique for detecting increased glucose uptake by tumors [17].

Glycolysis is a ten step process that breaks down glucose to pyruvate, takes place in the cytoplasm of virtually all eukaryotic cells, and requires the presence of NAD+, but not oxygen, as an oxidizing agent. Under aerobic conditions, NAD+ is regenerated from NADH by oxidative phosphorylation, a five-step mitochondrial process in which a pair of electrons is transferred from electron donors, such as NADH and NADPH, to oxygen.

The energy released during this process is efficiently utilized to generate AT from ADP. In the absence of oxygen, NAD+ is regenerated in mammalian cells through the action of LDH-A, an enzyme that uses NADH as a cofactor to convert pyruvate to lactate. To sustain glycolysis under anaerobic conditions, known as anaerobic glycolysis, lactate is excreted from the cells as a waste product. Thus, in the absence of oxygen, the net cellular gain from glycolytic breakdown of one glucose molecule is two ATP molecules, which constitute less than 7 % of the total ATP generated by complete oxidation of glucose to CO_2 and H_20.

Cells normally switch from slow aerobic to rapid anaerobic consumption of glucose, a phenomenon first noted by Louis Pasteur in 1857, and known as Pasteur effect's. The avid consumption of glucose by tumor cells in the presence of oxygen (the Warburg effect) is associated with enhanced glycolytic flux, increased glucose oxidation in the pentose phosphate pathway (PPP), and down-regulation of mitochondrial respiration [13, 18]. Although such a mode of glucose utilization compromises ATP yields, it confers tumor cells a significant growth advantage by: (1) attenuating generation of reactive oxidative species (ROS) by oxidative phosphorylation, which are known to induce cellular senescence and/or apoptosis, and (2) providing a ready supply of NADH and other essential reagents for de novo biosynthesis of macromolecules needed for cell proliferation and invasion [19, 20].

Under the hypoxic conditions that prevail in many tumors, anaerobic glycolysis is often accompanied with significant acidosis of cellular microenvironment. By contrast, lactic acid produced under anaerobic conditions in normal tissues, as in over-worked skeletal muscles, is readily transported, via blood, to the liver for recycling. Thus, in tumor microenvironment the conversion of pyruvate to lactate is double-edged sword. On one hand, it facilitates anaerobic glycolysis by regenerating NAD+, but on the other it impairs the ability of the cells to sustain it, because of increased acid accumulation.

Recently, it has been shown that tumor cells that had lost functional p53 expression posses an increased tolerance to low intracellular and extracellular pH. It gives them growth advantage over neighboring normal p53 functional cells that undergo acid-induced p53-dependent apoptosis. Lowering external pH by these cells may lead to increased degradation of extracellular matrix that promotes angiogenesis and metastasis [21]. New data have linked the glycolytic and tumorigenic phenotype, the production of fructose-2-6-biphosphate, a well established tumor survival factor, is increased in the cytoplasm to enhance aerobic glycolysis and cell cycling.

8.1.2 LDH Isoenzymes

There are five LDH isoenzymes as a result of the five different combinations that are produced by two polypeptide chains (M and H) encoded by separate genes (A and B) [19, 22, 23]. The LDH1 is composed of four H-subunits, and the LDH5 of four M-subunits. As the number of the M- over H-chains increases, the LDH isoenzyme becomes more efficient in catalyzing the conversion of pyruvate to lactate (LDH5), while an increase of H- over M-chains (LDH1) favours the conversion of pyruvate to acetyl-CoA that enters into the citric acid cycle. The prevailing type of LDH depends upon the metabolic demands of a particular tissue [2, 6, 14, 24].

LDH is increased in the serum of a fraction of cancer patients, a feature closely related to prognosis [20, 25, 26]. It has been shown that LDH5 is the isoenzyme that is mainly overexpressed in cancer cells (Fig. 8.1), while LDH1 is often down-regulated in cancer cells compared to normal tissues [25, 26]. Although studies investigating the subtype of LDH enzyme in the serum of cancer patients are not available, it is postulated that M-subunit-containing isoenzymes, such as LDH5, are responsible for this rise, since LDH gene is strongly up-regulated in neoplasia in response to intratumoral hypoxia [20, 21, 27].

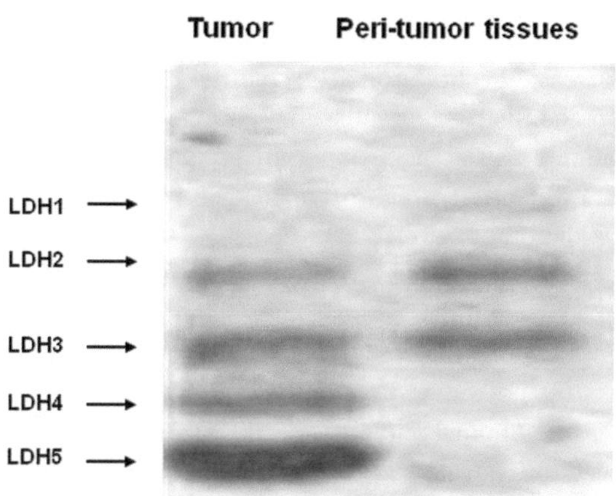

Fig. 8.1 Values of LDH isoenzymes activities in breast cancer tissue

8.2 Significance of Estimation of LDH and Their Isoenzymes in Tumor Tissues

Based on consideration that intracellular characteristics of LDH enzyme are very sensitive indicators of the cellular metabolic state [28], aerobic or anaerobic direction of glycolysis, activation status [29, 30], malignant transformation, it is also very useful to analyzed intracellular LDH activity in different cell line [31] and tumor tissues obtained from patients [32].

New techniques of molecular biology and proteomics research established in the last decade, enabled investigation of LDH in tumor tissues or histological specimens and give new view into the process of carcinogenesis [20, 24, 33]. Tissues for these analyses can be obtained after biopsy or surgery directly or after frozen storage of pathohistological specimens. Activity of LDH in tumor tissue can be determined using various methods including: classical biochemical methods and zymography, gel electrophoresis, two-dimensional electrophoresis immunohistochemisty, and Western blotting methods [34]. Tissues for our analyses usually where preserved during homogenization and after fixation or protection from proteolysis [35]. Based on developing and application new PCR techniques in cancer diagnosis, estimation of gene alteration and gene variation for LDH and LDH isoenzymes allow better understanding of anaerobic phenomena in cancer tissues [25, 26, 33]. Many clinical investigations regarding values of LDH has been based on easier estimation LDH activity by classical biochemistry methods in homogenized tissue sample using spectrophotometer and measuring the reduction of absorbance at 340 nm during oxidation of NADH.

In last period Western blotting analyses gives possibility for estimation the total protein amount in tissues using selected antibodies, but methods is semi quantitative [25, 26].

Immunohistochemistry is most common method for disease confirmation on tissues section for many tumours and also very used method for study LDH and LDH isoenzymes [20] expression in tumor tissues by commercially available monoclonal antibodies. Using immunehistochemistry it is possible to see localization and staining for LDH-A which is mainly cytoplasmic, although nuclear expression was also noted in many cancer cells.

It has been shown that that Lactate dehydrogenase-A (LDH-A) is one of the main isoforms of LDH expressed in breast tissue, prostate, colon cancer and it is a marker of altered intracellular anaerobic metabolism, which allows cancer cells to proliferate in hypoxic microenvironment [27, 33, 36]. However, the expression of LDH-A has been shown to have no relation to pathological subtypes of breast cancer classified by the status of Estrogen (ER), progesterone (PR), or Herceptin (Her-2). The Ki-67 positive cancer cells were significantly reduced in LDH-A deficiency tumor samples, while apoptosis ratio was enhanced. Our results suggested that LDH-A inhibition might offer a promising therapeutic strategy for breast cancer [37]. Interestingly, the new data that analyzed molecular aspect of LDH in terms of clinical significance, show that level of LDH-A enzyme in tumor tissue from breast cancer patients is increased with increasing BIRADS category on mammograms [32]. It was also recently shown that mammographically dense breast tissue (ACR3 or ACR4 by new classification, and ductal type of carcinoma) is associated with higher activity of LDH in tumor tissue of breast cancer patients. About 23.9 % higher activity of LDH enzyme was present in tissue (ratio malignant/adjacent) of breast cancer patients from radiologically dense tissue (ACR4) that have practical role in patients diagnosis [32]. LDH plays also an important role in mechanisms of Taxol resistance of breast cancer cells and higher levels of LDH in tumor tissue of breast cancer cell line are associated with high cell proliferation [37].

Malignant gliomas are one of the most aggressive cancers known. Previous studies on glycolysis and respiration in glioma cells have indicated that glioma cells have a high rate of aerobic glycolysis compared with other normal cells. This observation has led to the suggestion that gliomas derive most of their energy from glycolysis, regardless of whether their oxygen supply isadequate or low [38]. The gliomas show reliance on persistent aerobic glycolysis as their main source of ATP production, as exhibited by animal models, human glioma-derived cell cultures and in vivo human studies. Glioma cell lines have active different metabolic pathways that enable them to acquire a tolerance for nutrient deficiency. In addition, glioblastoma cell cultures show constitutive activation of the Akt oncogene, a frequent mutation in malignant tumours responsible for increasing cell proliferation results in a clear shift from normal aerobic respiration to abnormal, persistent aerobic glycolysis for cell survival [15]. Contrary to many other tumor cells that show up regulation of the LDH-A, that facilitates anaerobic metabolism of glucose and conversion of pyruvate to lactate, LDH-B isoform is more expressed in a different subsets of glioma cells or conversely that LDH-A expression is lost and could not be induced. The difference between normal glial cell and glioma cell metabolism has been exploited in last period as a potential new therapeutic strategy [39, 40] for malignant glioma (grades III and IV) which is non-responsive to aggressive radiotherapy and chemotherapy.

8.3 LDH Release from Cultured Cells In Vitro

For clinical application and prognosis, investigation of LDH release in-vitro from separated and cultured cells has a many advantages and superiority as a molecular biomarker in respect to determination of classical LDH from serum [6, 29]. For many types of cancer in early stages of disease and with small tumor mass below detectable values, for majority of them in early clinical stage, although serum LDH is useful for prognosis, it is not increases in all patients, especially when tumor cannot see by routine clinical diagnosis [41].

New directions in investigations were based on the principle that in-vitro cultured cells have provided more reliable results, much more in the early stages of disease that is not situation with serum LDH markers [6]. Cancer cells or cultured lymphocytes from tumor patients show difference to compared to healthy persons [42] and that they show significant membrane damage and consequently increased permeability and leakage of intracellular enzymes, including LDH [43, 44]. Mitochondria play an important role in cell survival and cell death, and its dysregulation of any form leads to diseases developing [38, 45]. This is a significant consequence altered mitochondria machinery [46] and abnormal mitochondrial apoptotic signaling in cancer cells that is accompanied with extensive release of intracellular enzymes [47, 48]. As LDH is much more increased intracellular enzyme in comparison to all other enzymes (Fig. 8.2), reflecting disturbance in anaerobic glycolysis in tumors cells [42] this makes it very suitable for evaluation in cultured cells. For clinical prognosis LDH release from in vitro cultured cells, can reflects presence

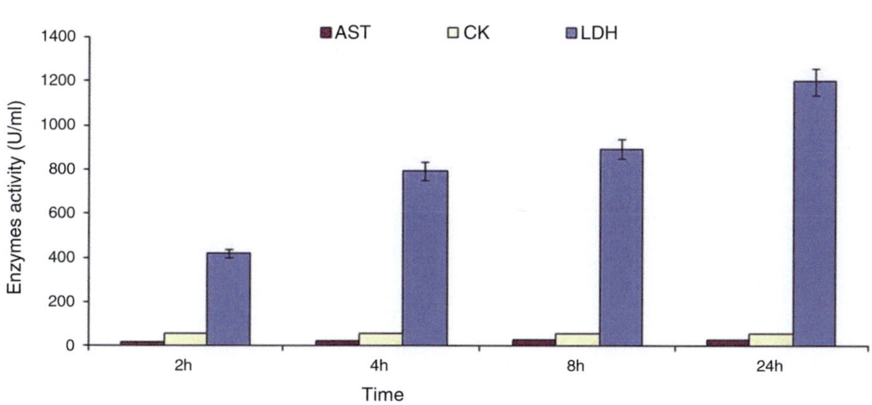

Fig. 8.2 Tumor cells released much more LDH in comparison to other enzymes after TNF-alpha treatment

circulated tumor cells or circulated tumor stem cells in blood very important for estimation of presence minimal residual diseases [29, 34, 45–47].

The phenomenon was described in literature as "spontaneously released LDH" from peripheral blood lymphocytes (PBL) or any cultured cells [47, 49–51]. It was shown that our cells posses without any stimulation or drug presence release of LDH enzymes trough cell membrane [6, 41]. For our investigation PBL population or other cells subsets it is need analyzed after separation on density gradient or by immunomagnetic sorting [34]. These analyses further requested short-time cell cultures in-vitro, usually following 2 h. Determination of released LDH enzymes can be possible measured by estimation of change in absorbance (Fig. 8.3) and using spectrophotometer reader. In biochemical reaction mixture substrate for LDH can be easy added and reaction was done in-vitro conditions in 96 micro-plate [47]. Analyses of the spontaneous LDH release activity can be also expressed in terms of total intracellular LDH activity [31]. The determination of LDH release as percentage is widely recognized to be a sensitive parameter for in-vitro drug evaluation, vaccine safety estimation or neural cell damage analyzed as well [52].

In view of this, Jurisic V et al. and Konjevic G et al., give novel and more complete evidence concerning the association of LDH PBL characteristics in different types of cancer [41]. These data indicates cell membrane damage in circulated PBL and that LDH release depending on clinical stage and bulky tumor mass much better then serum LDH [42]. In addition, correlation between decreased of NK cell activity in patients with advanced clinical stage of breast cancer patients with increased spontaneous LDH release indicated that circulating cells have membrane damage and that cells not only the release of intracellular enzymes, such as LDH but also released cytolytic protein perforin and granzymes from NK cells, necessary for the cytotoxic mechanism for tumor cell killing. Our studies indicated that PBL of breast cancer patients showed that significantly increased spontaneous LDH release was related to tumor mass and other clinical parameters as well clinically important Karnofski index, sex steroids hormones, and age of women, indicating role and significance of menopausal status [43]. Further, we showed significant positive correlation of spontaneous LDH release from circulating and cultured PBL with sera LDH. In many patients with lymphomas and breast cancer patients it was shown that spontaneous LDH is much more increased in comparison to serum LDH level and especially in patients where serum LDH is below referent values [6, 43].

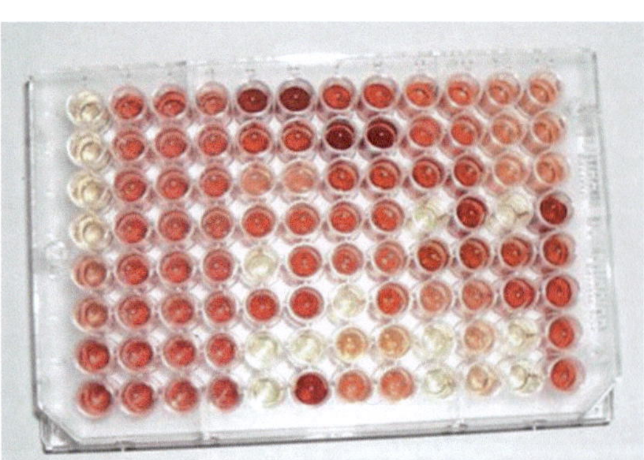

Fig. 8.3 Changes in absorbance reflect LDH activity. The measurements in 96 well plates during evaluation cell death in-vitro

8.4 Significance of Serum LDH Activity in Clinical Practice

8.4.1 Hematological Diseases

In lymphoid malignancies serum LDH has been investigated as a clinical biomarkers from earliest 60-th [53]. Its elevation is mostly associated with high tumor burden and with more aggressive clinical behavior [4, 14, 54]. In aggressive B-cell lymphomas, in mantle cell as well as in follicular lymphomas, LDH is strong adverse prognostic factor [1, 8, 55]. LDH level is analyzed in respect to the most useful clinical classification [56] and data is proposed that it is one of the most independent prognostic factor in International Non-Hodgkin's Lymphoma Prognostic Index (IPI). It has been verified that patients with NHL have high LDH level, but few reports have focused on LDH level of NHL patients with bone marrow involvement. The glycolytic enzyme system of tumor tissue in NHL patients with bone marrow involvement is more active than in those without bone marrow involvement, the LDH level is significantly higher in serum and body fluid that touched with tumor tissue. As the prognostic index of NHL, LDH rising often indicates the tendency of extranodal metastasis increase and it is a high-grade NHL. In addition, survival time in patients with high serum LDH was obviously shorter than in patients with normal serum LDH suggesting that a high LDH is a negative prognostic factor. Children with NHL serum LDH is a valuable parameter for defining patients with a markedly different prognosis: the poor prognosis of stage III patients with a serum LDH above 500 IU/L was much improved in successive studies when their treatment was intensified, primarily through a 10-fold increase in the dose of methotrexate. More recently, an additional LDH parameter (above or below 1000UI/L) has been used to further subdivide risk groups. One could argue that the word "extensive" has been replaced by an objective, if surrogate marker of tumor burden.

In a smaller series of patients with Walderstrom macroglobulinemia (WM), it has been shown that LDH may improve the discrimination ability of International Prognostic Scoring System [57]. In addition, LDH level by our score identified a subset of patients that have a very poor outcome, with a median survival of less than 3 years. Patients in high risk group without elevated LDH had a survival which was not very different from the outcome of patients who belonged to the intermediate risk group. Furthermore, for patients at high risk, LDH could also predict for cause of death: only 10 % of high risk patients with elevated LDH died from causes unrelated to WM, while 40 % of the high risk patients without elevated LDH died due to unrelated causes.

In patients with multiple myeloma elevated LDH is associated with high tumor mass, plasma cell leukemia or lymphoma-like clinical features [58, 59] and remains one of the most important adverse factors associated with poor progression free and overall survival even in patients with myeloma treated with tandem transplants with or without novel agents including thalidomide, lenalidomide or bortezomib. In patients with multiple myeloma serum LDH is also strongly associated with high level of pro-inflammatory cytokine especially with TNF-α and IL-6 [60].

Initial values of increased LDH, decreased fibrinogen levels and low platelet count were associated with an increased incidence of fatal bleeding and strongly correlated with death induced by bleeding, in patients with acute promyelocytic leukemia [61].

8.5 Solid Tumor

8.5.1 Melanoma

Serum lactate dehydrogenase (LDH) level is one of themost useful independent prognostic factors in metastatic melanoma [5]. Solid tumours require a blood supply to grow and metastasis. Increased serum LDH is believed to be related to the hypoxic environment of tumour cells. As LDH is not a secreted enzyme, the finding of elevated LDH in the serum of patients with advanced melanoma is probably due, party by melanoma-cell necrosis and apo-necrosis which likely occurs when part of a tumour outgrows its blood supply.

8.5.2 Lung Cancer

Several investigators concluded that LDH is an independent prognostic factor that correlates with disease stage, response to treatment and survival in lung cancer [3, 62]. Our studies showed that in patients with limited disease a significant correlation of LDH serum levels with tumor progression and survival exists. Patients with pretreatment LDH serum levels above 240 IU/L had a strongly increased risk of tumor recurrence and poor survival (2-year survival of 41 % in patients with LDH < 240 IU/L and of 8 % in patients with LDH > 240 IU/L). High LDH level also might indicate the presence of occult disease in those patients where no primary lesion could be found and it makes the detection of LDH elevations in the serum particularly relevant in cases with liver involvement [63]. However, do to its ubiquitous presence in tumors LDH is not suitable for tumor subtype. Moreover, in non-small cell lung cancer, LDH-5 expression was linked to high total serum LDH levels [64].

8.6 Conclusion

Together all of these data indicates that investigation of LDH as a tumor biomarkers, with the possibility to determined in sera, cultured cells and tumor tissues and that their measurement have an important role in early clinical tumor diagnosis. Based on new techniques it is possible to detect changes of LDH and their isoenzymes in tumor tissues and understanding complex biochemical processes. In last decade using radioactive techniques suck as PET, it is possible to measured energy in tissues sample and developing a new therapy with aims to blocking LDH metabolism.

Acknowledgement This work was supported by the grant No. 175056 of the Ministry of Science and Technology of the Republic of Serbia.

References

1. Benboubker L, Valat C, Linassier C et al (2000) A new serologic index for low-grade non-Hodgkin's lymphoma based on initial CA125 and LDH serum levels. Ann Oncol 11:1485–1491
2. Koukourakis MI, Kontomanolis E, Giatromanolaki A, Sivridis E, Liberis V (2009) Serum and tissue LDH levels in patients with breast/gynaecological cancer and benign diseases. Gynecol Obstet Invest 67(3):162–168
3. Sagman U, Feld R, Evans WK, Warr D, Shepherd FA, Payne D, Pringle J, Yeoh J, DeBoer G, Malkin A et al (1991) The prognostic significance of pretreatment serum lactate dehydrogenase in patients with small-cell lung cancer. J Clin Oncol 9:954–961
4. Coiffier B (1996) Advances in lymphoma research. Can prognostic factors be applied in treatment selection for aggressive lymphoma patients? Cancer Treat Res 85:53–77
5. Homsi J, Kashani-Sabet M, Messina JL, Daud A (2005) Cutaneous melanoma: prognostic factors. Cancer Control 12:223–229
6. Jurisic V, Bumbasirevic V, Konjevic G, Djuricic B, Spuzic I (2004) TNF-alpha induces changes in LDH isotype profile following triggering of apoptosis in PBL of non-Hodgkin's lymphomas. Ann Hematol 83(2):84–91, Epub 2003 Oct 28
7. Jurisic V, Terzic T, Pavlovic S, Colovic N, Colovic M (2008) Elevated TNF-alpha and LDH without parathormone disturbance is associated with diffuse osteolytic lesions in leukemic transformation of myelofibrosis. Pathol Res Pract 204(2):129–132
8. Ouyang QC, Wang PH (2001) The variation of the serum level of lactic dehydrogenace in 105 patients with non-Hodgkin's and its clinical significance. J Pract Oncol 16:111–113
9. De Berardinis RJ, Lum JJ, Hatzivassiliou G, Thompson CB (2008) The biology of cancer: metabolic reprogramming fuels cell growth and proliferation. Cell Metab 7:11–20
10. Luo J, Solimini NL, Elledge SJ (2009) Principles of cancer therapy: oncogene and non-oncogene addiction. Cell 136(5):823–837
11. Warburg O, Posener K, Negelein E (1924) U¨ ber den Stoffwechsel der Carcinomzelle. Biochem Z 152:309–344
12. Vander Heiden MG, Cantley LC, Thompson CB (2009) Understanding the Warburg effect: the metabolic requirements of cell proliferation. Science 324:1029–1033
13. Icard P, Lincet H (2012) A global view of the biochemical pathways involved in the regulation of the metabolism of cancer cells review. Biochim Biophys Acta (BBA) – Reviews on Cancer 1826(2):423–433
14. Lu R, Jiang M, Chen Z, Xu X, Hu H, Zhao X, Gao X, Guo L (2013) Lactate dehydrogenase 5 expression in non-hodgkin lymphoma is associated with the induced hypoxia regulated protein and poor prognosis. PLoS One 8(9):e74853. doi:10.1371/journal.pone.0074853
15. Shim H, Dolde C, Lewis B, Wu C, Dang G, Jungmann R, Dalla-Favera R, Dang C (1997) c-Myc transactivation of LDH-A: implications for tumor metabolism and growth. Proc Natl Acad Sci U S A 94: 6658–6663
16. Warburg O (1956) On respiratory impairment in cancer cells. Science 124:269–270
17. Chen JL, Appelbaum DE, Kocherginsky M, Cowey CL, Kimryn Rathmell W, McDermott DF, Stadler WM (2013) FDG-**PET** as a predictive biomarker for therapy with everolimus in metastatic renal cell cancer. Cancer Med 2(4):545–552. doi:10.1002/cam4.102
18. Kim J-W, Dang CV (2005) Multifaceted roles of glycolytic enzymes. Trends Biochem Sci 30(3):142–150
19. Harris AL (2002) Hypoxia: a key regulatory factor in tumour growth. Nat Rev Cancer 2:38–47
20. Kolev Y, Uetake H, Takagi Y, Sugihara K (2008) Lactate dehydrogenase-5 (LDH-5) expression in human gastric cancer: association with hypoxia-inducible factor (HIF-1alpha) pathway, angiogenic factors production and poor prognosis. Ann Surg Oncol 15:2336–2344

21. Greijer AE, van der Groep P, Kemming D, Shvarts A, Semenza GL, Meijer GA, van de Wiel MA, Belien JA, van Diest PJ, van der Wall E (2005) Up-regulation of gene expression by hypoxia is mediated predominantly by hypoxia- inducible factor 1. J Pathol 206:291–304
22. Huang D, Jungmann RA (1995) Transcriptional regulation of the lactate dehydrogenase A subunit gene by the phorbol ester 12-O-tetradecanoylphorbol-13-acetate. Mol Cell Endocrinol 108:87–94
23. Markert CL (1963) Lactate dehydrogenase isozymes: dissociation and recombination of subunits. Science 140:1329–1330
24. Grimm M, Alexander D, Munz A, Hoffmann J, Reinert S (2013) Increased LDH5 expression is associated with lymph node metastasis and outcome in oral squamous cell carcinoma. Clin Exp Metastasis 30(4):529–540. doi:10.1007/s10585-012-9557-2
25. Koukourakis MI, Giatromanolaki A, Sivridis E, Bougioukas G, Didilis V, Gatter KC, Harris AL (2003) Lactate dehydrogenase-5 (LDH-5) overexpression in non-small-cell lung cancer tissues is linked to tumour hypoxia, angiogenic factor production and poor prognosis. Br J Cancer 89(5):877–885. doi:10.1038/sj.bjc.6601205
26. Koukourakis MI, Giatromanolaki A, Sivridis E (2003) Lactate dehydrogenase isoenzymes 1 and 5: differential expression by neoplastic and stromal cells in non-small cell lung cancer and other epithelial malignant tumors. Tumour Biol 24:199–202
27. Langhammer S, Najjar M, Hess-Stumpp H, Thierauch KH (2011) LDH-A influences hypoxia-inducible factor 1alpha (HIF1 alpha) and is critical for growth of HT29 colon carcinoma cells in vivo. Target Oncol 6(3):155–162. doi:10.1007/s11523-011-0184-7
28. Rabinowitz Y, Dietz AA (1967) Malic and lactic dehydrogenase isoenzymes of normal and leukemic leukocytes separated on glass bead columns. Blood 29:182–195
29. Jurisic V, Konjevic G, Banicevic B, Djuricic B, Spuzic I (2000) Different alterations in lactate dehydrogenase (LDH) activity and profile of peripheral blood mononuclear cells in Hodgkin's and non-Hodgkin's lymphomas. Eur J Haematol 64:259–266
30. Wollberg P, Nelson BD (1992) Regulation of the expression of lactate dehydrogenase isozymes in human lymphocytes. Mol Cell Biochem 110:161–164
31. Jurisic V, Bogdanovic G, Kojic V, Jakimov D, Srdic T (2006) Effect of TNF-alpha on Raji cells at different cellular levels estimated by various methods. Ann Hematol 85(2):86–94
32. Radenkovic S, Milosevic Z, Konjevic G, Karadzic K, Rovcanin B, Buta M, Gopcevic K, Jurisic V (2013) Lactate dehydrogenase, catalase, and superoxide dismutase in tumor tissue of breast cancer patients in respect to mammographic findings. Cell Biochem Biophys 66(2):287–295. doi:10.1007/s12013-012-9482-7
33. Brown NJ, Higham SE, Perunovic B, Arafa M, Balasubramanian S, Rehman I (2013) Lactate dehydrogenase-B is silenced by promoter methylation in a high frequency of human breast cancers. PLoS One 8(2), e57697. doi:10.1371/journal.pone.0057697
34. Scatena R, Bottoni P, Giardina B (2013) Circulating tumour cells and cancer stem cells: a role for proteomics in defining the interrelationships between function, phenotype and differentiation with potential clinical applications. Biochim Biophys Acta (BBA) – Reviews on Cancer 1835(2):129–143
35. Gong G (2013) Local diffusion homogeneity (LDH): an inter-voxel diffusion MRI metric for assessing inter-subject white matter variability. PLoS One 8(6), e66366. doi:10.1371/journal.pone.0066366
36. Fantin VR, St-Pierre J, Leder P (2006) Attenuation of LDH-A expression uncovers a link between glycolysis, mitochondrial physiology, and tumor maintenance. Cancer Cell 9:425–434
37. Zhou M, Zhao Y, Ding Y, Liu H, Liu Z, Fodstad O, Riker AI, Kamarajugadda S, Lu J, Owen LB, Ledoux SP, Tan M (2010) Warburg effect in chemosensitivity: targeting lactate dehydrogenase-A re-sensitizes taxol-resistant cancer cells to taxol. Mol Cancer 9:33
38. Ordys BB, Launay S, Deighton RF, McCulloch J, Whittle IR (2010) The role of mitochondria in glioma pathophysiology. Mol Neurobiol 42:64–75
39. Folkins C, Man S, Xu P, Shaked Y, Hicklin DJ, Kerbel RS (2007) Anticancer therapies combining antiangiogenic and tumor cell cytotoxic effects reduce the tumor stem-like cell fraction in glioma xenograft tumors. Cancer Res 67:3560–3564
40. Pathania D, Millard M, Neamati N (2009) Opportunities in discovery and delivery of anticancer drugs targeting mitochondria and cancer cell metabolism. Adv Drug Deliv Rev 61(14):1250–1275. doi:10.1016/j.addr.2009.05.010
41. Konjević G, Jurisić V, Jakovljević B, Spuzić I (2002) Lactate dehydrogenase (LDH) in peripheral blood lymphocytes (PBL) of patients with solid tumors. Glas Srp Akad Nauka Med 47:137–147, Serbian
42. Jurisic V (2003) Estimation of cell membrane alteration after drug treatment by LDH release. Blood 101:2894
43. Konjević G, Jurisić V, Spuzić I (2001) Association of NK cell dysfunction with changes in LDH characteristics of peripheral blood lymphocytes (PBL) in breast cancer patients. Breast Cancer Res Treat 66(3):255–263
44. Weinberg F, Chandel NS (2009) Mitochondrial metabolism and cancer. Ann N Y Acad Sci 1177:66–73
45. Barbosa IA, Machado NG, Skildum AJ, Scott PM, Oliveira PJ (2012) Mitochondrial remodeling in cancer metabolism and survival: potential for new therapies. Biochim Biophys Acta 1826(1):238–254. doi:10.1016/j.bbcan.2012.04.005
46. Scatena R (2012) Mitochondria and cancer: a growing role in apoptosis, cancer cell metabolism and dedifferentiation. Review. Adv Exp Med Biol 942:287–308. doi:10.1007/978-94-007-2869-1_13

47. Jurisić V, Spuzić I, Konjević G (1999) A comparison of the NK cell cytotoxicity with effects of TNF-alpha against K-562 cells, determined by LDH release assay. Cancer Lett 138(1–2):67–72
48. Kroemer G, Galluzzi L, Brenner C (2007) Mitochondrial membrane permeabilization in cell death. Physiol Rev 87:99–163
49. Jurisić V, Konjević G, Jancić-Nedeljkov R, Sretenović M, Banicević B, Colović M, Spuzić I (2004) The comparison of spontaneous LDH release activity from cultured PBMC with sera LDH activity in non-Hodgkin's lymphoma patients. Med Oncol 21(2):179–185
50. Jurisic V, Kraguljac N, Konjevic G, Spuzic I (2005) TNF-alpha induced changes in cell membrane antigen expression on K-562 cells associated with increased lactate dehydrogenase (LDH) release. Neoplasma 52(1):25–31
51. Jurisic V, Srdic-Rajic T, Konjevic G, Bogdanovic G, Colic M (2011) TNF-α induced apoptosis is accompanied with rapid CD30 and slower CD45 shedding from K-562 cells. J Membr Biol 239(3):115–122. doi:10.1007/s00232-010-9309-7
52. Zhang P, Wang J, Wang D, Wang H, Shan F, Chen L, Hou Y, Wang E, Lu CL (2012) Dendritic cell vaccine modified by Ag85A gene enhances anti-tumor immunity against bladder cancer. Int Immunopharmacol 14(3):252–260. doi:10.1016/j.intimp.2012.07.014
53. Van der Helm HJ (1962) Interference of the measurement of lactate dehydrogenase (LDH) activity in human serum and plasma by LDH from blood cells. Clin Chim Acta 7:124–128
54. Korkolopoulou P, Thymara I, Kavantzas N, Vassilakopoulos TP, Angelopoulou MK, Kokoris SI, Dimitriadou EM, Siakantaris MP, Anargyrou K, Panayiotidis P, Tsenga A, Androulaki A, Doussis-Anagnostopoulou IA, Patsouris E, Pangalis GA (2005) Angiogenesis in Hodgkin's lymphoma: a morphometric approach in 286 patients with prognostic implications. Leukemia 19(6):894–900
55. Hoster E, Dreyling M, Klapper W, Gisselbrecht C, van Hoof A, Kluin-Nelemans HC et al (2008) A new prognostic index (MIPI) for patients with advanced-stage mantle cell lymphoma. Blood 111(2):558–565
56. Solal-Celigny P, Roy P, Colombat P, White J, Armitage JO, Arranz-Saez R et al (2004) Follicular lymphoma international prognostic index. Blood 104(5):1258–1265
57. Kastritis E, Zervas K, Repoussis P, Michali E, Katodrytou E, Zomas A et al (2009) Prognostication in young and old patients with Waldenstrom's macroglobulinemia: importance of the International Prognostic Scoring System and of serum lactate dehydrogenase. Clin Lymphoma Myeloma 9(1):50–52
58. Dimopoulos MA, Barlogie B, Smith TL, Alexanian R (1991) High serum lactate dehydrogenase level as a marker for drug resistance and short survival in multiple myeloma. Ann Intern Med 115(12):931–935
59. Maltezas D, Dimopoulos MA, Katodritou I, Repousis P, Pouli A, Terpos E, Panayiotidis P, Delimpasi S, Michalis E, Anargyrou K, Gavriatopoulou M, Stefanoudaki A, Tzenou T, Koulieris E, Sachanas S, Dimou M, Vassilakopoulos TP, Angelopoulou MK, Pangalis GA, Kyrtsonis MC (2013) Re-evaluation of prognostic markers including staging, serum free light chains or their ratio and serum lactate dehydrogenase in multiple myeloma patients receiving novel agents. Hematol Oncol 31(2):356–362. doi:10.1002/hon.2026
60. Jurisić V, Colović M (2002) Correlation of sera TNF-alpha with percentage of bone marrow plasma cells, LDH, beta2-microglobulin, and clinical stage in multiple myeloma. Med Oncol 19(3):133–139
61. Kim DY, Lee JH, Lee JH, Kim SD, Lim SN, Choi Y, Lee YS, Kang YA, Seol M, Jeon M, Kim JY, Lee KH, Lee YJ, Lee KH (2011) Significance of fibrinogen, D-dimer, and LDH levels in predicting the risk of bleeding in patients with acute promyelocytic leukemia. Leuk Res 35(2):152–158. doi:10.1016/j.leukres.2010.05.022
62. Stokkel MP, Van Eck-Smit BL, Zwinderman AH, Willems LN, Pauwels EK (1997) The diagnostic value of pretreatment serum LDH in patients with limited disease small-cell lung carcinoma. Int J Biol Markers 12:162–167
63. Stokkel MP, van Eck-Smit BL, Zwinderman AH, Willems LN, Pauwels EK (1998) Pretreatment serum LDH as additional staging parameter in small-cell lung carcinoma. Neth J Med 52:65–70
64. Koukourakis MI, Giatromanolaki A, Sivridis E, Gatter KC, Harris AL (2006) Lactate dehydrogenase 5 expression in operable colorectal cancer: strong association with survival and activated vascular endothelial growth factor pathway – a report of the Tumour Angiogenesis Research Group. J Clin Oncol 24:4301–4308

Neuron-Specific Enolase as a Biomarker: Biochemical and Clinical Aspects

9

Maria Antonietta Isgrò, Patrizia Bottoni, and Roberto Scatena

Abstract

Neuron-specific enolase (NSE) is known to be a cell specific isoenzyme of the glycolytic enzyme enolase. In vertebrate organisms three isozymes of enolase, expressed by different genes, are present: enolase α is ubiquitous; enolase β is muscle-specific and enolase γ is neuron-specific. The expression of NSE, which occurs as γγ- and αγ-dimer, is a late event in neural differentiation, thus making it a useful index of neural maturation.

NSE is a highly specific marker for neurons and peripheral neuroendocrine cells. As a result of the findings of NSE in specific tissues under normal conditions, increased body fluids levels of NSE may occur with malignant proliferation and thus can be of value in diagnosis, staging and treatment of related neuroendocrine tumours (NETs).

NSE is currently the most reliable tumour marker in diagnosis, prognosis and follow-up of small cell lung cancer (SCLC), even though increased levels of NSE have been reported also in non-small cell lung cancer (NSCLC). The level of NSE correlates with tumour burden, number of metastatic sites and response to treatment.

NSE can be also useful at diagnosis of NETs and gastroenteropancreatic (GEP)-NETs.

Raised serum levels of NSE have been found in all stages of neuroblastoma, although the incidence of increased concentration is greater in widespread and metastatic disease. Moreover, NSE determination in cord blood

M.A. Isgrò, MD (✉)
Institute of Biochemistry and Clinical Biochemistry, Catholic University of the Sacred Heart, Largo Agostino Gemelli 8, 00168 Rome, Italy

Department of Diagnostic and Molecular Medicine, Catholic University of the Sacred Heart, Largo Agostino Gemelli 8, 00168 Rome, Italy
e-mail: mariantoniettaisgro@yahoo.it

P. Bottoni • R. Scatena
Institute of Biochemistry and Clinical Biochemistry, School of Medicine, Catholic University, Largo Gemelli 8, 00168 Rome, Italy

R. Scatena (ed.), *Advances in Cancer Biomarkers*, Advances in Experimental Medicine and Biology 867, DOI 10.1007/978-94-017-7215-0_9

offers an early postnatal possibility of confirming the diagnosis of neuroblastoma in newborns.

NSE has been demonstrated to provide quantitative measures of brain damage and/or to improve the diagnosis and the outcome evaluation in ischaemic stroke, intracerebral hemorrhage, seizures, comatose patients after cardiopulmonary resuscitation for cardiac arrest and traumatic brain injury.

Increased NSE serum levels have also been found associated with melanoma, seminoma, renal cell carcinoma, Merkel cell tumour, carcinoid tumours, dysgerminomas and immature teratomas, malignant phaechromocytoma, Guillain-Barré syndrome and Creutzfeldt-Jakob disease.

Keywords
ENO1 • ENO2 • ENO3 • Neuron-specific enolase (NSE) • NSE as biomarker • NSE assays in body fluids • NSE biochemical properties • NSE clinical indications • NSE in brain damage • NSE in gastroenteropancreatic neuroendocrine tumours • NSE in lung cancer • NSE in melanoma • NSE in neuroblastoma • NSE in neuroendocrine tumours • NSE in seminoma • NSE mapping and gene function • Tissue NSE expression

9.1 Introduction

The rationale for studying cell specific proteins arises from the realization that proteins strictly localized or even greatly enriched in a given cell type are likely to be involved in biochemical pathways that are either specific to that cell type or performed in a different manner by that particular cell. This concept is further strengthened if the cell specific protein has an ontogenetic appearance parallel with the cell differentiation process. The structural and functional characterization of a given protein provides key insights regarding the function of specific cell types.

The elucidation and characterization of nervous system specific proteins is a particularly appropriate research strategy given the enormous cellular diversity and complexity of nervous system. Brain tissue contains a number of highly acidic soluble proteins that are not found in non-nervous tissues.

9.1.1 History

The highly acidic soluble brain protein 14-3-2 was first described by Moore and McGregor in 1965 [1]. Subsequent immunological studies demonstrated that it is characteristic of neurons; the 14-3-2 protein was therefore called neuron-specific protein [2]. Since the neuron-specific protein has been shown to exhibit enolase activity, it has been finally called neuron-specific enolase (NSE) [3, 4]. NSE is now known to be a cell specific isoenzyme of the glycolytic enzyme enolase (EC 4.2.1.11). It is not only a marker for all types of neurons, but also for all neuroendocrine or paraneuronal cells. The appearance of NSE is a late event in neural differentiation, thus making NSE a useful index of neural maturation.

9.2 Neuron-Specific Enolase (NSE)

9.2.1 Structure and Biochemical Properties

Enolase (2-phospho-D-glycerate hydrolyase; EC 4.2.1.11) is a "metal-activated metalloenzyme" that catalyzes the dehydration of 2-phospho-D-glycerate (PGA) to phosphoenolpyruvate (PEP) in the glycolytic pathway, and the reverse reaction, the hydration of PEP to PGA, in gluconeogenesis.

It is necessary for the anaerobic conversion of glucose to metabolites suitable for oxidation.

The catalytic activity of enolase requires as natural cofactor Mg^{2+} [5, 6]. Two types of metal-binding sites contribute to catalysis [7]. Metal binding in site I, traditionally called "conformational", induces a conformational change in the enzyme and enables binding of substrate or substrate analogues [8, 9]. Following binding of a substrate or a substrate analogue, the second metal ion, called "catalytic", can bind [10, 11] in site II and then the catalytic reaction occurs [7]. Release of the ligands is more complex. At the center of controversy is the observation that high metal ion concentrations inhibit enolase. Initially, the presence of a third, inhibitory, metal ion binding site was proposed [7]. In a recent study, data supporting an alternative explanation were obtained [12]. Two pathways for product release have been proposed. In the first, dominant at physiological conditions, the catalytic metal ion leaves first followed by product. However, even at very high metal ion concentrations the enzyme is not completely inhibited and it was proposed, as second possible pathway, that some product release takes place without metal ion dissociation from the complex.

In vertebrate organisms three isozymes of enolase, expressed by different genes, are present. Enolase α is ubiquitous; enolase β is muscle-specific and enolase γ is neuron-specific. All known eukaryotic enolases are dimeric. Tissue-specific isozymes (β and γ) readily form mixed dimers with enolase α; the intermediate form is a hybrid molecule containing an α and γ subunit; in vivo all possible dimers except βγ have been observed.

In the brain the isoenzymes non-neuronal enolase (NNE, αα-dimer) and NSE (γγ- and αγ-dimer) are expressed. NSE is the most acidic brain enolase, composed of two γ-subunits with a relative molecular mass of 39,000. NNE is the least acidic enolase isoenzyme, composed of two α-subunits with a relative molecular mass of 43,500 [13]. This form of enolase was designated non-neuronal enolase, since immunocytochemical studies have established its strict glial localization within nervous tissue [14]. The most marked difference between NSE and NNE is the apparently complete lack of immunological cross-reactivity between the two proteins [13, 15]. NNE is highly sensitive to chloride ions, urea and temperature. In contrast to this, NSE is markedly more stable towards chloride-induced inactivation. The relative insensitivity of NSE to chloride ions is particularly interesting, since this ion accumulates in nerve cells during periods of repeated depolarization. Possibly the relative resistance of NSE to chloride ions may have evolved to accommodate to the intracellular milieu in the neuron. A chloride sensitive enolase in the neuron would be inactivated and glycolysis would be interrupted at a time when metabolic energy is most needed [16].

Human NSE is a major brain protein that constitutes between 0.4 % and 2.2 % of the total soluble protein of brain, depending on the region. In some neurons NSE accounts for 3–4 % of the total soluble protein [16], which led to common use of NSE as a clinical marker for neuronal and neuroendocrine cells. This amount of the enzyme appears to be much more than is needed for its catalytic function and it is likely that NSE has other, as yet unknown roles.

The enzyme NSE has been purified, crystallized and its crystal structure determined [17]. In the crystals the enzyme forms the asymmetric complex $NSE \cdot Mg_2 \cdot SO_4/NSE \cdot Mg \cdot Cl$, where "/" separates the dimer subunits. The subunit that contains the sulfate (or phosphate) ion and two magnesium ions is in the closed conformation observed in enolase complexes with the substrate or its analogues; the other subunit is in the open conformation observed in enolase subunits without bound substrate or analogues. This indicates negative cooperativity for ligand binding between subunits. Electrostatic charge differences between isozymes α and γ, − 19 at physiological pH, are concentrated in the regions of the molecular surface that are negatively charged in α, i.e. surface areas negatively charged in α are more negatively charged in γ, while areas that are neutral or positively charged tend to be charge-conserved [17].

9.2.2 Amino Acid Sequence, Mapping and Gene Function

At least three genes encode the different isoforms of the enolase.

The complete amino acid sequence (433 residues) of the human neurone-specific γ isozyme of enolase was determined by a combination of direct amino acid sequencing and nucleotide sequencing of cloned cDNA in 1988 and compared [18] with the amino acid sequence of the human α isozymic form (433 amino acid protein) previously determined [19], concluding that the γ isozyme is more stringently conserved than is the α form. Three regions present significant differences (271–285, 298–316 and 416–433); these residues are mainly hydrophilic in character and are located on the surface of the three-dimensional structure of the enolase subunit [18], making them useful for immunization to raise antibodies specific for the neuron-specific form.

The gene of the γ subunit was isolated and the complete nucleotide sequence (from upstream to the 5' end to beyond the polyadenylation site) determined in 1991 [20]. The gene contains 12 exons (of which 11 coding exons) distributed over 9213 nucleotides, clustered in two groups: one including exons 2–7 and the other exons 9–12. Introns occur at positions identical to those reported for the homologous rat gene, as well as for the human α gene, supporting the existence of a single ancestor for the members of this gene family, with the exception of intron 1, which interrupts the 5'-untranslated sequence 13 bp upstream of the initiation methionine codon. The length of the noncoding exon 1 varies from 77 to 210 bp due to the presence of multiple start sites of transcription. The promoter region lacks canonical TATA and CAAT boxes, is very C+G-rich and contains several potential regulatory sequences. Furthermore, an inverted *Alu* sequence is present approximately 572 nucleotides upstream of the major start site. A comparison of the 5'-flanking region of the human γ-enolase gene with the same region of the rat gene revealed a high degree of sequence conservation [20]. Lack of TATA and CAAT boxes, heterogeneous start sites of transcription and the presence of C+G-rich sequences, all of which are found also in the rat γ-enolase gene [21], have been associated with mammalian "house-keeping" genes, whereas highly tissue-specific genes do not usually display these features [22]. As γ-enolase has been detected not only as a marker of neuronal differentiation [16], but also in a number of normal and transformed tissues of nonneuronal origin [23, 24], the tissue-specificity of this gene may be considered intermediate between that of constitutively expressed genes and that of specialized genes encoding proteins that are present only in determined cell types.

The human chromosome locations for the three gene loci (designated, in accordance with the guidelines for Human Gene Nomenclature, *ENO1*, *ENO2* and *ENO3* for the α-, γ-, and β-subunits, respectively) have been determined. *ENO1* has been mapped to the pter-p36.13 region of chromosome 1 [25, 26], *ENO2* was assigned to chromosome 12, in the distal region pter-p1205 [27–29] and *ENO3* to the short arm of chromosome 17 [30]. The regional assignment of *ENO2* to the short arm of chromosome 12 is particularly interesting. It is the fourth enzyme of the glycolytic pathway (after triose phosphate isomerase-I, glyceraldehydes-3-phosphate dehydrogenase and lactate dehydrogenase B) for which the gene has been assigned not only to the same chromosome, but also to the same arm. Even though these four genes are all separated by some distances and clearly not contiguous in the DNA sequences, the assignment of four genes related in a common pathway to a specific region of the chromosome may have some significance in evolution and possibly in gene regulation [28].

Muller et al. [31] proposed that homozygous deletions in passenger genes in cancer deletions can expose cancer-specific therapeutic vulnerabilities when the collaterally deleted gene is a member of a functionally redundant family of genes carrying out an essential function. The glycolytic gene ENO1 in the 1p36 locus is deleted in glioblastoma, which is tolerated by the expression of ENO2. Authors showed that short hairpin RNA-mediated silencing of ENO2 selectively inhibits growth, survival and the tumorigenic potential of ENO1-deleted GBM cells, and that the enolase inhibitor phosphonoacetohydroxamate is selectively toxic to ENO1-deleted GBM cells relative to ENO1-intact GBM cells or normal astrocytes. Authors also suggested that the principle of collateral vulnerability should be applicable to other passenger-deleted genes encoding functionally redundant essential activities and provide an effective treatment strategy for cancers containing such genomic events.

9.2.3 Tissue Protein Expression

In mammals the three isoforms of enolase are characterized by different tissue distributions as well as by distinct biochemical and immunological properties [32]. NNE is a nearly ubiquitous form, found in almost all tissues, and its expression precedes that of the other isoforms in the early stage of embryonic development; the β- or muscle-specific enolase (MSE) is present in adult skeletal muscle; NSE is the major form found in mature neurons and in cells of neuronal origin [16]. Many neurons express predominantly γ subunit, whereas some neurons and various neuroendocrine cells express a mixture of γ and α subunits. The transition from NNE to MSE or NSE in tissues such as muscle and nerve is developmentally regulated [33, 34].

In fetal rat brain, NNE is the dominant isoenzyme. NSE appears during neurogenesis and its amount increases during early neuronal differentiation [35]. These observations support a switch-over from α- to γ-subunit expression in neurons. Immunological studies are in favour of the assumption that neurons develop from proliferating NNE-immunoreactive cell populations without NSE-immunoreactivity [36]. The switch-over from NNE to NSE occurs after final cell division and migration and is therefore a good marker for neural differentiation and maturation.

9.3 NSE as a Biomarker

NSE is a highly specific marker for neurons, peripheral neuroendocrine tissue and APUD (Amine Precursor Uptake & Decarboxylation) cells and can therefore serve as a biochemical marker for tumours derived from these cells. Like chromogranin A (CgA), NSE as a general neuroendocrine marker cannot differentiate between different subtypes of neuroendocrine tumours (NETs); however, elevated NSE levels have been associated with poor tumour differentiation [37–40].

Using immunostaining techniques, NSE is seen in all types of neurons including granule cells, Purkinje cells, projection neurons and both sensory and autonomic neurons. NSE has also been demonstrated in a variety of normal cells including pinealocytes, pituitary glandular and peptide-secreting cells, thyroid parafollicular cells, adrenal medullary chromaffin cells, cells of the islets of Langerhans, Merkel's cells of the skin, neuroendocrine cells of the lung, erythrocytes. As a result of the findings of NSE in specific tissues under normal conditions, it was hypothesized that increased expression of NSE and increased serum levels of NSE could occur with malignant proliferation of these tissues and thus could be of value in diagnosis, staging and treatment of such cancers. The application of NSE determination in medical oncology can be assessed under various headings: determination of NSE content in tissue biopsies; serum measurements of NSE as a marker of tumour diagnosis, disease extent and response to therapy; determination of cerebrospinal fluid (CSF) NSE as an indicator of cranial and CNS metastases [41].

9.4 NSE Assays in Body Fluids

The specific localization of NSE in neurons and neuroendocrine cells suggests that assays of NSE levels in biological fluids such as spinal fluid, serum or urine might provide useful diagnostic information regarding disorders due to altered metabolism or turnover of these cell types. In addition, the histochemical detection and determination of NSE in biopsy material might be helpful in differential diagnosis. Importantly, the biological half-life of NSE in body fluids is approximately 24 h.

Solid phase radioimmunoassay (RIA) using ^{3}H-labelled antigen [42] and double antibody RIA have been described for NSE and NNE in brain tissue [43]. These procedures have also been used for the determination of NSE in other tissues. These assays were not sufficiently sensitive to measure nanogram amounts of each isoenzyme level in cell culture or in biological fluids such as CSF.

A RIA procedure adapted for measuring low amounts of enzyme proteins in body fluids was described by Parma et al. [44]. Increased sensitivity was achieved by labelling the antigen with ^{125}iodine, resulting in much higher specific activities relative to tritium-labelled NSE.

A simple kinetic method was described for the measurement of enzymatic activity of enolase in human serum and CSF [45]. The enzymatic activity was measured by a luminescent assay, making use of the luciferin-luciferase system.

It should be taken into account that the results obtained by enzymatic methods and immunoassays cannot be compared directly. The immunoassay measures the quantity of immunoreactive enolase protein regardless of its enzymatic activity. Results obtained by immunoassays are expressed in ng immunoreactive enzyme protein per mL, while results of enzymatic measurements are expressed in U/L.

A solid phase immunobioluminescent assay for NSE in human plasma was developed by Gerbitz et al. in 1984 [46].

A practicable sandwich-type enzyme immunoassay for NSE in human serum was established by the use of purified antibodies to bovine neuron-specific γγ-enolase [47].

A new enzyme immunoassay (galactosidase) for the rapid determination of NSE in serum was later developed by using monoclonal antibodies [48].

In 1986 Viallard and colleagues [49] proposed a new method for the determination of NSE. It consisted of two steps: first, an immunocapture of the γ-subunit containing isoenzymes was performed by adsorption on immobilized anti-γ-antibodies; second, enolase activity was determined by a bioluminescence assay in untreated control samples and in the supernatant of antibody treated samples. In the same year, Viallard and colleagues [50] described a rapid electrophoretic determination of NSE in serum. The assay procedure for each of the two neuron-specific enolases (αγ and γγ) and the NNE (αα) in serum involved two steps: electrophoretic separation of the isoenzymes on cellulose acetate and bioluminescence measurement of enolase activity.

In 1987 an enzyme-linked immunosorbent assay that used commercially available reagents was described [51]. The antibody used in this system reacted only with the γ-subunit and combined with the avidin-biotin conjugated peroxidase complex, provided a method that was both highly specific and sensitive for the measurements of NSE.

In 1989, monoclonal antibodies against neuron-specific enolase were used in an immunoradiometric assay (IRMA), with mono-disperse magnetizable particles as the solid phase [52]. The assay sensitivity was 0.4 μg/L and the inter-assay coefficient of variation (CV) was <5 % in the working range from 0.4 to 170 μg/L. Compared with RIA based on polyclonal antibodies, the incubation time was shorter, and precision and sensitivity were improved. The better sensitivity of the IRMA resulted from its ability to measure αγ- and γγ-enolase with equal response.

These data were also confirmed by Body et al. [53], with an improved sensitivity of the IRMA (93 %) over the RIA (83 %) in small cell lung cancer (SCLC) patients compared to healthy subjects, using an IRMA adapted from the method of Paus and Nustad [52].

After the first NSE enzyme immunoassay (EIA) as a two-step assay employing a specific monoclonal antibody against NSE in conjunction with a polyclonal (rabbit) antibody [54] and the further development of a one-step, solid-phase EIA employing two monoclonal antibodies to NSE [55], an international multicenter study was designated to evaluate the technical performance of the latter EIA transferred on a system which makes use of the electrochemiluminescence (ECL)-technology as the detection method [56]. The new test was shown to be a reliable and accurate diagnostic procedure for the measurement of NSE in serum samples, also presenting a wide measuring range and a fast throughput (incubation time of 18 min). In particular, intra- and inter-assay CVs, determined in six laboratories, ranged from 0.7 % to 5.3 % (inter-laboratory median: 1.3 %) and from 1.3 % to 8.5 % (inter-laboratory median: 3.4 %), respectively. Laboratory-to-laboratory comparability was excellent with respect to recovery and inter-assay CVs. The test was linear between 0.0 and 320 ng/mL (highest measured concentration). Based on a specificity of 95 % in comparison with the group suffering from benign lung diseases, the cut-off value for the discrimination between malignant and benign conditions was set at 21.6 ng/mL. NSE was raised in 73.4 % of SCLC patients and was significantly higher in extensive (ED, 87.8 %) as opposed to limited disease (LD, 56.7 %). NSE was also elevated in 16.0 % of the cases with non-small cell lung cancer (NSCLC) [56].

A new chemiluminescence enzyme immunoassay using magnetic nanoparticles was developed in 2012 for detection of NSE in human serum [57]: fluorescein isothiocyanate (FITC) labels NSE capture antibody connected with NSE and alkaline phosphatase labels NSE detection antibody in a sandwich-type detection manner. This immune complex is further reacted with anti-FITC coated magnetic beads and enriched in a magnetic field, thus enhancing the sensitivity. The limit of detection of this method was <0.2 ng/mL, the recovery >83.0 % and the CV <10.0 %. This immunoassay is highly selective and not interfered by hook effect [57].

In 2013 Torsetnes and colleagues [58] presented a new validated method for quantification of NSE in serum at both reference and elevated levels. The analytical approach utilizes selective sample preparation by immunoextraction of all forms of NSE (αγ, γγ and γ) followed by tryptic digestion, and separation and detection by LC-SRM-MS (Liquid Chromatography-Selected Reaction Monitoring/Mass Spectrometry). The quantification of NSE is performed through a signature peptide specific for the γ-subunit of NSE (tryptic peptide γ16; ELPLYR). The method shows linearity $r^2 > 0.999$ (range 5–500 ng/mL), intra-day precision <13 %, accuracy >95 % and a limit of quantification (of 38 pg/mL with a signal-to-noise ratio above 10) significantly lower than endogenous levels of healthy subjects. In addition, the method simultaneously allows determination of the αγ-heterodimer through a signature peptide specific for the α-subunit (tryptic peptide α12; TIAPALVSK) [58].

A new enzyme-free electrochemical immunoassay protocol was developed by Li and Tian in 2013 [59] for the sensitive electronic monitoring of NSE on a monoclonal mouse anti-human NSE antibody-modified glassy carbon electrode, using guanine-decorated graphene nanostructures (GGN) as nanotags. To construct such an enzyme-free immunoassay format, guanine and polyclonal rabbit anti-human NSE antibody (pAb) were co-immobilized on the graphene nanostructures through the carbodiimide coupling. Based on a sandwich-type immunoassay mode, the assay was carried out in 0.1 M pH 7.4 PBS containing 5 μM $Ru(bpy)_3^{2+}$ (bpy = 2,2′-bipyridine) through the catalytic oxidation of $Ru(bpy)_3^{2+}$ toward the guanine on the GGN. The presence of graphene nanostructures increases the immobilized amount of guanine, thus amplifying a detectable electronic signal. The covalent conjugation of guanine and pAb on the GGN results in a good repeatability and intermediate reproducibility down to 9.5 %. Under optimal conditions, the dynamic concentration range of the developed immunoassay spans from 0.005 to 80 ng/mL NSE with a detection limit of 1.0 pg/mL at a signal-to-noise ratio of 3σ (where σ is the standard deviation of the blank). In addition, the methodology was evaluated by assaying the spiking serum samples, and the relative standard deviation values between the electrochemical immunoassay and a commercialized enzyme-linked immunosorbent assay was 2.8–7.0 % [59].

The effects of storage conditions, lipemia, icterus and haemolysis on the stability of NSE in serum samples were evaluated by measuring NSE concentrations with a solid-phase EIA [60]. NSE stability was demonstrated for as long as 5 weeks in samples stored at 4 °C and −20 °C; but in samples stored at room temperature, NSE decreased 20 % after 2 weeks and 70 % after 5 weeks. The effect of hyperlipemia was negligible, at increased concentrations of cholesterol (up to 15.4 mmol/L) and triglyceride (up to 19.7 mmol/L); bilirubin (up to 0.84 mmol/L) had no effect on NSE. Unlike lipemia and icterus, haemolysis in serum significantly affected NSE results. This interference is caused by the high NSE content in erythrocytes [61]. Therefore, NSE concentrations should not be measured in visibly haemolyzed samples or in samples stored at room temperature.

Ramont et al. [62] evaluated the effects of haemolysis and storage condition on NSE both in CSF and serum. They found that the concentration of NSE in CSF decreased significantly (−27.6 %) when stored at −20 °C for 1 month. At −80 °C, the stability of NSE in CSF was better, but the NSE concentration still decreased progressively when samples were stored for more than 3 months. The decrease was 5 % of the initial level after 6 months, 19.5 % after 8 months and 21.9 % after 9 months. On the other hand, the NSE concentration in serum was stable at −80 °C for at least 9 months. These data show that NSE in CSF is very unstable. NSE stability might be influenced by the volume of the aliquot and by the protein concentration in the sample. In any case, the level of NSE measured depends on the temperature and duration of freezing. Authors also observed a significant increase in NSE concentration in all haemolyzed samples (serum and CSF) and a significant correlation between the increase in NSE concentration and the index of haemolysis. They concluded that all samples for NSE measurement should be stored at −80 °C and analyzed within 6 months after sampling in the case of CSF; serum may be kept frozen for longer periods (up to 9 months). Moreover, it is necessary to systematically evaluate the index of haemolysis before deciding whether or not to perform NSE measurement in either serum or CSF.

More recently, Planche and colleagues [63] confirmed an increase in serum NSE concentration parallel to the haemolytic index (about 150 % for an haemolytic index of 10), concluding that NSE determinations should be performed only for samples presenting an haemolytic index ≤10, in order to allow a good monitoring of kinetics of the marker.

No difference was found in serum NSE concentrations between men and women and in intra-individual variance between genders [64]. Within- and between-subject CVs were 13.6 % and 11.5 %, respectively (12.1 % and 11.7 %, respectively, according to Dittadi and Gion [65]); the low individuality allows the use of a single population-based reference interval. The reference change value (i.e. the minimal difference that must be exceeded for change in two consecutive marker results in the same individual to become clinically relevant) was 39 %. Desirable analytical goals for imprecision, bias and total error were <6.8 %, ±4.5 % and ±15.7 %, respectively [64].

9.5 Clinical Indications for NSE Determination

Since the original description of NSE by Moore and McGregor in 1965 [1] and its exploration as a marker for neuroendocrine neoplasms by Prinz and Marangos [66], there have been many accounts of its use in clinical medicine. NETs may originate in different organs, from cells embriologically different but expressing common phenotypic characteristics, such as: the immune-reactivity for markers of neuroendocrine differentiation (defined as "pan-neuroendocrine"), the capacity to secrete specific or aspecific peptides and hormones and the expression of some receptors, that are the basis of the current diagnostic and therapeutical approach, peculiar to these tumours [67]. The primitive tumour, not always identifiable, may originate from cells of the so-called diffuse neuroendocrine system (DNES) in various organs. The prevalent sites of origin are the digestive and respiratory tracts. One of the peculiar features of the DNES cells is their ability to secrete a wide spectrum of peptides. This was the basis of the first hypothesis of the APUD system, theorized by Pearse in 1969 [68] and later developed by the same Author in the concept of DNES. DNES cells have different embryological origins, but share common secretory and/or neuroendocrine markers. In clinical practice, the diagnosis of NETs can be actually based on the detection of tissue and/or circulating neuroendocrine markers. The secretory pattern of NETs may differ according to the site of origin and grade of differentiation. However, most of the currently available circulating neuroendocrine markers are relatively aspecific. Furthermore, significant variations of circulating levels of these markers may not only result from active secretory cellular process, but can also reflect cytolysis occurring during tumour growth or as a consequence of chemo-, radio- or radio-metabolic therapies.

The assessment of neuroendocrine markers may therefore play a role in different steps of

NETs management: diagnosis, prognostic significance, choice of therapy, follow-up and evaluation of the response to treatment.

NSE can be considered either a general marker of differentiation (pan-neuroendocrine tissue marker, crucial to evaluate the neuroendocrine differentiation of a tumour) or a general marker of secretion (the secretory pattern varying on the basis of the embryological origin and stage of the disease). As a marker of differentiation, NSE was reported to be more sensitive than CgA in large-cell as well as in SC poorly differentiated neuroendocrine carcinomas [69]. The role of enolase as marker of preferential glycolitic metabolism in proliferating cancer cell should be evaluated. The major weakness of this marker is represented by the low specificity of the currently commonly used antibodies anti-γ chain, which are unable to discriminate the homo-dimer γγ from the other hetero-dimers not specific for NETs. Even though anti-NSE monoclonal antibodies have been developed, those used at moment still show also low sensitivity. As a general marker of secretion, NSE showed a higher sensitivity and specificity in SCL neuroendocrine carcinomas, when compared to CgA (77 % and 85 % vs. 50 % and 71 %, respectively). In these patients, an inverse correlation between circulating levels and prognosis has been reported. Circulating NSE can, therefore, be used in the follow-up to evaluate responsiveness to therapy and to detect disease relapse early on. In all the other kinds of NETs, NSE shows a lower sensitivity and specificity when compared to CgA. NSE sensitivity in the diagnosis of gastroenteropancreatic (GEP)-NETs is about 40 %, but rises to 70 % in some studies [39, 70]. NSE tissue positivity is independent from the secretory activity of the tumour. In fact, NSE is not assumed to be a secretory protein, because it is located only in the cytoplasm of cells and the amount of NSE in tumour tissue does not seem to correlate with the circulating levels. During the follow-up, it should be considered that circulating NSE can be paradoxically increased in response to radio-metabolic treatment or chemo-therapy, as a consequence of a high death rate of cells with neuroendocrine differentiation, which can cause the release of this cytoplasmatic enzyme.

9.5.1 Lung Cancer

Lung cancer remains the most common and lethal human cancer, showing a continually rising incidence especially among women.

Lung cancers are classified into four major cell types by histology: SCLC (which accounts for around 20 % of lung cancers and has a neuroendocrine cellular origin), lung adenocarcinoma, squamous cell lung cancer (SQC) and large cell lung cancer, the last three types being grouped together as NSCLC [71]. Differentiation between SCLC and NSCLC is very important for prognostic and therapeutic reasons, due to their different behaviour. In addition to histology, an alternative diagnostic methodology may be useful, especially if the system is based on simple laboratory tests, performed on serum.

9.5.1.1 Small Cell Lung Cancer (SCLC)

SCLC is characterized by its rapid doubling time and propensity for early metastases. In essence, there are two clinical stages: LD, where the tumour is confined to one hemithorax and ED, when metastases occur in the contralateral chest and at distant sites. Metastases initially occur in the lymph nodes and thereafter in other organs such as other areas of the lung, liver, adrenal glands, brain, bone and bone marrow. Twenty to twenty-five percent of patients have LD, and though treatment is potentially curative, 5-year survival rates are poor (15–25 %, compared with <5 % in ED patients). SCLC is a malignancy associated with neuroendocrine differentiation; thus, neuroendocrine markers such as NSE and CgA have proven to be helpful in immunohistochemically characterizing these malignant lung tumours and can be used as tumour markers, being released into the circulation.

NSE is currently the most reliable tumour marker in SCLC, even though it is not an ideal biomarker; it is helpful when making the diagnosis (it is raised in 75 % of patients at diagnosis) [72] and in the prognosis and the follow-up of SCLC. However, its sensitivity is low, particularly in patients with LD.

The level of NSE has been correlated with tumour burden and number of metastatic sites and a good correlation was found between the initial decline in plasma concentration and response to treatment [73–75].

Spinazzi et al. [76] confirmed that NSE was elevated in the large majority of newly diagnosed patients with SCLC prior to treatment, but NSE did not appear a valid tool to differentiate SCLC from NSCLC, probably because of the relatively frequent neuroendocrine behaviour of the latter.

Giovanella et al. [77] investigated the role of tumour markers CEA, NSE, TPS and CYFRA 21.1 in lung cancer diagnosis and staging. In SCLC patients, NSE and CYFRA 21.1 showed the highest sensitivity (56 %), NSE was the most accurate single marker and the combination of NSE and CYFRA 21.1 (according to the principle "one or both positive") improved significantly the diagnostic accuracy of NSE from 67 % to 75 %. The cut-off value considered for NSE was 12.5 ng/mL. The sensitivity of NSE and CYFRA 21.1 in LD (39 % and 54 %) and ED (75 % and 57 %) was a remarkable finding. A better sensitivity of CYFRA 21.1 was demonstrated in early stages of SCLC. On the other hand, only NSE was a discriminant marker between LD and ED. An applicable model of biomarkers in SCLC could be the concurrent assay of NSE and CYFRA 21.1 in pretherapeutic assessment and therapy planning [78]. CYFRA 21.1 does not play an important role during therapy monitoring and follow-up; in these phases, NSE alone may be employed.

Paone and colleagues [79] used discriminant analysis as a method to optimize the discriminant power of serum tumour marker levels for differentiation between SCLC and NSCLC. They selected and considered together NSE and CYFRA 21.1, generating the following formula:

$$\text{canonic variable} = \text{LnNSE} \times 2.37032 - \text{LnCYFRA } 21.1 \times 0.37699 - 5.55988$$

which provided a good discrimination between the two types of lung cancer, with a 93 % rate of correct classification (NSE being the most powerful discriminant factor) [80]. A possible clinical target of the score described could be represented by those patients in whom lung cancer is diagnosed by means of clinical and radiological signs, but where the histological type cannot be recognized because cytology is negative and invasive diagnostic techniques cannot be applied, especially in elderly patients with poor cardiorespiratory functions.

Jørgensen et al. [81] evaluated the influence of pretreatment serum NSE in addition to more conventional prognostic factors on survival duration in SCLC patients. Increased values of NSE (>12.5 ng/mL) were observed in 81 % of the patients; NSE was the most powerful prognostic factor followed by poor performance status and extensive stage disease. The three prognostic factors NSE, performance status and stage of disease, enabled the establishment of a prognostic index (PI) based on a simple algorithm ($PI = z_{NSE} + z_{stage} + 2z_{performance\ status}$). This segregated the patients into four groups with clearly different prognosis. Based on these results, Authors recommended NSE and performance status, in addition to stage, for prognostic stratification in treatment trials on SCLC.

Considering the low specificity of NSE, due to a relatively high false-positive rate in patients with non-malignant lung diseases and NSCLC and increased levels by haemolysis [82], Takada et al. [83] attempted to clarify whether serum levels of a carboxy-terminal fragment of pro-gastrin-releasing peptide, ProGRP(31–98), could serve as a more accurate tumour marker in patients with SCLC than NSE. Sensitivity in SCLC patients was 72.3 % for ProGRP(31–98) and 62.4 % for NSE. Comparing the area under the receiver operating characteristic curve (AUC) of ProGRP(31–98) with that of NSE, ProGRP(31–98) was the most powerful marker (0.94 vs. 0.81, respectively).

The use of CgA can be proposed to enhance the sensitivity and accuracy of NSE in SCLC diagnosis, even though serum NSE remains the marker of choice for biochemical disease staging and monitoring of SCLC [84].

Petrović et al. [85] found that CgA, ProGRP and NSE levels were all significantly greater in patients with ED compared with LD. A worse performance status, the presence of ED and raised serum levels of ProGRP (>58 pg/mL), CgA (>56 ng/mL) and NSE (>19.0 ng/mL) were all associated with significantly shorter median survival times. Performance status, disease stage, NSE, CgA and ProGRP levels were each significant independent prognostic indicators for survival. Authors concluded that there is a potential role for ProGRP, NSE and CgA in both staging and prognosing survival of SCLC patients [85].

9.5.1.2 Non-small Cell Lung Cancer (NSCLC)

Even though NSE is the tumour marker of first choice for SCLC, increased serum NSE has been reported in 11.7–28 % of patients with NSCLC [78]. According to Broers et al. [86], neuroendocrine properties may be expressed in various histologic types of lung cancer, because both NSCLC and SCLC derive from a common cell lineage and their differentiation occurs at a later stage of oncogenetic development. NSE expression is an unfavourable sign, because NSCLC and in particular SQCs with neuroendocrine differentiation are more aggressive than others. At the same time, those patients may have a better response to chemotherapy. Kulpa et al. [87] found that, in SQC patients, despite diagnostic sensitivity of NSE was 0.275 at 0.95 specificity, its high pretreatment concentrations were associated with shorter survival. They concluded that NSE was an independent, but nonspecific, prognostic factor in SQC, in particular in patients with stages IIIB-IV, which may be treated with chemotherapy.

However, the predictive and prognostic role of NSE in NSCLC is still controversial, since several studies did not find a prognostic value [88, 89], while others reported that NSE is an important prognostic factor for NSCLC [90, 91]. Nevertheless, in a recent meta-analysis which included 2389 patients, Yan et al. [92] did not find any association of NSE concentration with prognosis for NSCLC.

9.5.2 Neuroendocrine Tumours (NETs)

The incidence of NETs is very low (0.1 % of all malignant neoplasms). These tumours show a low proliferation rate, which is particularly marked in NETs located in the GEP district. The symptoms may be related to biologically active substances hypersecretion rather than to neoplastic growth [40]. In these neoplasms, the presence of high specificity circulating biomarkers and the expression of somatostatin receptors have been demonstrated. NETs can be subdivided into two categories with respect to their capacity to release bioactive molecules. Biologically active NETs, or functioning tumours, are those tumours that release growth factors, hormones or other local mediators in a constitutive manner. Patients affected by such neoplasms suffer from a complex of symptoms related to the hypersecretory activity of the tumour itself. Given the low proliferation rate of NETs, these syndromes are the most disabling aspect of the disease and often can be fatal because of the severe disturbances they induce. Biologically inactive NETs and, in some cases, also carcinoids, gastrinomas, glucagonomas, somatostatinomas and neurotensinomas, are considered to be silent malignancies, because they are nonsecretory tumours. Mainly for this reason, patients with nonfunctioning NETs often are diagnosed late and in an already metastatic stage. No standard treatments are currently available for patients suffering from NETs. Hence, an early diagnosis and a thorough study of the biological characterization of the tumour may be fundamental to offer more tailored and timely therapies. In addition, the need for specific biomarkers also is related to the evaluation of response to treatment. Experimental data consider CgA and NSE the best biomarkers available today for NETs; their determination is particularly meaningful, because they are expressed by both functioning and nonfunctioning tumours. Bajetta et al. [40] examined a large cohort of patients with histopathologically assessed NETs (including hindgut, midgut, foregut and pancreatic islet cell tumours) and proved that CgA was the best marker (specificity of 85.7 % and sensitivity of 67.9 %). CgA and NSE levels were significantly higher in patients with disease compared with disease free patients; NSE showed a specificity of 100 % but a rather low sensitivity (32.9 %), with a cut-off level of 12.5 ng/mL. Authors concluded that only CgA and NSE could be used at diagnosis of NETs; the utility of NSE in clinical follow-up is likely to be limited to a few selected cases. Conversely, CgA measurement seems to be extremely useful for signalling recurrences, confirming stable disease status and assessing the response to therapy.

Also Nobels et al. [37] concluded that CgA was the best general neuroendocrine serum marker, with the highest specificity for the detection of NETs compared to the other neuroendocrine markers. Nevertheless, Authors found that NSE was more frequently elevated than CgA in subjects with SCLC, Merkel cell tumour, insulinoma, paraganglioma and neuroblastoma.

9.5.2.1 Gastroenteropancreatic Neuroendocrine Tumours (GEP-NETs)

NETs are either confined to specific organs (e.g. chromaffin cells of the adrenal glands) or can be found scattered throughout the digestive tract as part of DNES. Tumours that originate from gastrointestinal cells belonging to the DNES and from pancreatic islets comprise the GEP-NETs and are thought to evolve from a common precursor stem cell of ectodermic origin.

The best general biomarker for GEP-NETs, as well as for NETs, is CgA, even though it should be complemented with specific markers related to localization of the primary tumour and clinical symptoms. NSE has been found to be elevated in 31–44 % of patients with GEP-NETs [37]; the combination of CgA and NSE in GEP-NETs has a higher sensitivity than either parameter separately.

Recently, an early response in NSE has been found related to therapeutic response with the mTOR inhibitor everolimus in patients with pancreatic NETs [93].

9.5.3 Neuroblastoma

Neuroblastoma is a neuroblastic tumour of the primordial neural crest and is the most common extracranial solid tumour of childhood, comprising between 8 % and 10 % of all childhood cancers. It is predominantly a disease of the first decade with ~80 % of children presenting at <4 years old. The disease accounts for 15 % of all childhood cancer deaths. Children with I, II or IV-S disease, or presenting in the first year of life, have a good prognosis. In contrast, children (≥1 year of age) with stage III and IV disease have 3-year survival rates of 50 % and 15 %, respectively. Most children present over the age of 1 year with metastatic (stage IV) disease; this group has an overall survival of 10–20 % [94].

Zeltzer et al. [95] found that serum NSE levels greater than 100 ng/mL were associated with a poor outcome in children with widespread metastatic neuroblastoma (clinical stage IV). This relation was highly significant in the subgroup of infants less than 1 year old at diagnosis. They concluded that serum NSE could be a useful disease marker and a prognostic indicator in children with metastatic neuroblastoma.

It was later demonstrated that raised serum levels of NSE can be found in all stages of neuroblastoma, although the incidence of increased concentration is greater in widespread and metastatic disease [96]. Authors hypothesized that those patients with the smallest tumour burden at diagnosis (stage I and stage II) would have the lowest range of serum NSE values; by contrast, patients with stage III and IV would have the widest range and highest levels of NSE (>100 ng/mL). In general, a low level predicted a good outcome and a high level was associated with a bad prognosis. In patients with stage IV-S disease, serum NSE levels were significantly lower than those in stage IV, despite their extensive tumour burden, and reflected the more benign clinical behaviour of this stage. Serum NSE levels correlated with response to therapy; all patients with initial levels above 100 ng/mL had levels below 100 ng/mL during remission. However not all patients had a serum NSE above 100 ng/mL coincident with relapse.

Riley et al. [97] conducted a meta-analysis of molecular and biological tumour markers described in neuroblastoma, to establish an evidence-based perspective on their clinical value for the screening, diagnosis, prognosis and monitoring of patients. They found that patients with high serum levels of NSE have a significantly worse outcome in terms of disease-free survival (hazard ratio=5.56; 95 % CI, 2.11–14.7; $p=0.0005$) and overall survival (hazard ratio=5.22; 95 % CI, 3.12–8.73; $p<0.0001$), identifying NSE biomarker as a potentially important prognostic tool in neuroblastoma.

Kintzel and colleagues [98] proposed to measure NSE levels in cord blood, in comparison with their reference values, to offer an early postnatal possibility of confirming the diagnosis of neuroblastoma in newborns. The finding of a solid or cystic suprarenal mass or paraspinal cervical and thoracic tumour by prenatal ultrasonography suggests congenital neuroblastoma, the most common malignancy during infancy. For the initial evaluation and subsequent treatment plan, rapid postnatal identification of the tumour is necessary. The measurement of NSE in cord blood offers the earliest possibility of biochemical detection in cases with suspected tumours. Authors determined NSE concentrations in cord blood samples from healthy term newborns, by means of a solid phase EIA based on the sandwich technique (the assay utilizes a specific monoclonal antibody to NSE immobilized on a polystyrene bead in conjunction with a polyclonal -rabbit-antibody). Median NSE concentration was 8.0 μg/L and the 5–95th percentiles were 4.8–19.4 μg/L. No differences between male and female newborns were detected [98].

9.5.4 Brain Damage

Potential candidate biomarkers of cerebral tissue damage, such as NSE, glial fibrillary acidic protein, tau-protein, myelin-basic protein and S100-β are released into the blood following ischaemic stroke from neurons, myelin and glia. The level of these markers in blood may indicate the extent of brain infarction. Moreover, in early-phase of acute stroke, determination of blood markers would result more easily and cheaply than other surrogate endpoints, such as radiological measurements of tissue damage, in order to evaluate the effects of treatment. An excellent blood marker of the volume of cerebral tissue damage would be well correlated with the "true" volume of cerebral tissue damage due to ischaemic stroke. However, this "true" volume is difficult to measure. Different estimates may depend on brain imaging modality, imaging timing, the method used to calculate volume or whether the method differentiates lesion swelling from lesion extent. The true "level" of a blood marker is also difficult to define; potentially useful statistics for blood marker levels are: a single measurement, a peak measurement or an integral (AUC) of blood marker levels over time.

Various studies have shown a positive correlation between NSE levels and infarct volume in patients of acute ischaemic stroke [99–101], whereas some studies have failed to demonstrate such relationship [102]. Studies have also pointed out that there is a significant correlation between NSE levels and stroke severity on admission [100, 101]. On the other hand, few investigators have found no such relationship [103]. The ability of NSE levels to predict functional neurological outcome in stroke patients is also a matter of recent interest with some studies suggesting that NSE is useful in predicting functional outcome [100, 101], while the other studies suggesting otherwise [99]. In view of contradictory findings of these studies, Zaheer et al. [104] conducted a study on 75 patients with acute ischaemic stroke in order to determine: the correlation between NSE levels at admission and infarct volume, stroke severity and early functional neurological outcome. Authors found: a positive correlation between concentration of NSE on day 1 and infarct volume determined by computed tomography scan (the largest infarct volume had the highest mean NSE levels); a strong negative correlation between Glasgow coma scale at presentation and concentration of NSE on day 1 (patients with a lower Glasgow coma scale and, therefore, greater stroke severity, had a higher mean NSE level); a positive correlation between NSE levels at day 1 and early neurological outcome assessed by the modified Rankin scale at day 30 (the mean concentration of NSE in patients with worse outcome was significantly higher than in patients with better outcome). They concluded that serum levels of NSE in first few days of ischaemic stroke can serve as a useful marker to predict stroke severity and early functional outcome.

According to Ahmad et al. [105], peak and AUC levels of NSE and S100-β levels correlate with radiological measures of infarct volume obtained within the first week after stroke. Nevertheless, they concluded that plasma biomarker values taken within the first 6 h of stroke are unlikely to be good predictors of subacute infarct extent, as there has been insufficient time for the markers to enter the circulation, and many factors can influence changes in infarct extent at the subacute time.

On the other hand, NSE has been demonstrated to provide quantitative measures of brain damage and/or to improve the diagnosis and the outcome evaluation also in other clinical settings, such as intracerebral hemorrhage [106], seizures [107], comatose patients after cardiopulmonary resuscitation for cardiac arrest [108, 109] and traumatic brain injury [110–112].

9.5.5 Melanoma

Increased NSE serum levels in patients with metastatic melanoma have been reported to be associated with a large tumour burden, with a gradual rise indicating disease progression and a poor prognosis [113].

Tofani et al. [114] found that in stages I and II, NSE is clearly superior to S100-β as a marker and should be included in the routine follow-up, since elevated serum NSE levels are probably associated with progression of the disease. In patients in stages III and IV, both NSE and S100-β may be elevated, but not necessarily both in the same patient; in these stages, diagnostic sensitivity increased to 62 % if isolated elevation of each marker was considered; thus both NSE and S100-β should be assayed in patients with advanced stage disease.

In ophthalmology, high levels of NSE have been demonstrated in the serum and aqueous humour of patients with malignant melanoma or retinoblastoma [115].

9.5.6 Seminoma

Fosså et al. [116] evaluated NSE as a marker in 54 patients with seminoma. Before orchiectomy, NSE was raised in 6 out of 21 patients with stage I seminoma and 11 out of 16 patients with metastases. After orchiectomy, the NSE returned to normal in all the stage I cases, but remained high in 6 out of the 12 patients with metastatic disease. They concluded that NSE was a useful marker in seminoma with a sensitivity and specificity of the same order as human chorionic gonadotrophin (hCG).

Tandstad and Klepp [117] found the same sensitivity for NSE as for beta-hCG at diagnosis in seminoma, but they concluded that serum NSE is of no clinical value during follow-up in monitoring patients with testicular cancer.

9.5.7 Rare Tumours

Raised levels of NSE have been observed in adults with renal cell carcinoma, confirming a similar report in children [118].

Merkel cell tumour may be associated with a small rise in NSE [119].

Carcinoid tumours are a variant of NETs. In a study of 26 patients with carcinoids, 38.5 % had a raised NSE. However, in this group plus another 18 patients with various NETs, 55 % of whom had raised NSE concentrations in the serum, there was no correlation between NSE concentrations and the extent of metastases [120].

Dysgerminomas and immature teratomas can be accompanied by increased serum NSE levels [121].

Benign phaeochromocytoma does not cause a rise in NSE, but in malignant phaechromocytoma half of the patients have an elevated NSE [122].

NSE has also been observed to be raised in small cell undifferentiated tumours of the pancreas [123].

9.5.8 Other Pathological Conditions/Clinical Indications

Increases in CSF NSE have been reported in several forms of brain and spinal cord disease. These include: Guillain-Barré syndrome [124, 125], Creutzfeldt-Jakob disease [125, 126] and meningeal hemorrhage [125].

The reports on CSF NSE levels in schizophrenia are equivocal. Vermuyten et al. [125] recorded increased levels, but Egan and colleagues [127] examined 50 patients with acute and chronic schizophrenia and found that CSF NSE levels were not raised.

9.6 Conclusion

NSE has been confirmed as a reliable biomarker in SCLC and neuroblastoma. It has shown its potential in NETs, melanoma, seminoma, rare tumours of neuroendocrine origin, Guillain-Barré syndrome and Creutzfeldt-Jakob disease. Opinions differ about the contribution of NSE to NSCLC and schizophrenia. The growing evidence of the usefulness of NSE in providing quantitative measures of brain damage and/or in improving the diagnosis and the outcome evaluation in several related clinical settings, represents a promising perspective of proposing NSE as a reliable biomarker for brain injury assessment.

References

1. Moore BW, McGregor T (1965) Chromatographic and electrophoretic fractionation of soluble proteins of brain and liver. J Biol Chem 240:1647–1653
2. Pickel VM, Reis DJ, Marangos PJ et al (1976) Immunocytochemical localization of nervous system specific protein (NSP-R) in rat brain. Brain Res 105:184–187
3. Bock E, Dissing J (1975) Demonstration of enolase activity connected to the brainspecific protein 14-3-2. Scand J Immunol 4(suppl 2):31–36
4. Marangos PJ, Zomzely-Neurath C, York C (1976) Determination and characterization of neuron specific protein (NSP) associated enolase activity. Biochem Biophys Res Commun 68:1309–1316
5. Wold F, Ballou CE (1957) Studies on the enzyme enolase. II. Kinetic studies. J Biol Chem 227:313–328
6. Brewer JM (1985) Specificity and mechanism of action of metal ions in yeast enolase. FEBS Lett 182:8–14
7. Faller LD, Baroudy BM, Johnson AM et al (1977) Magnesium ion requirements for yeast enolase activity. Biochemistry 16:3864–3869
8. Brewer JM, Weber G (1966) The effect of magnesium on some physical properties of yeast enolase. J Biol Chem 241:2550–2557
9. Faller LD, Johnson AM (1974) Calorimetric studies of the role of magnesium ions in yeast enolase catalysis. Proc Natl Acad Sci U S A 71:1083–1087
10. Hanlon DP, Westhead EW (1969) Kinetic studies on the activation of yeast enolase by divalent cations. Biochemistry 8:4255–4260
11. Brewer JM (1971) The increase of yeast enolase fluorescence produced by substrates and competitive inhibitors in the presence of excess Mg 2+. Biochim Biophys Acta 250:251–257
12. Poyner RR, Cleland WW, Reed GH (2001) Role of metal ions in catalysis by enolase: an ordered kinetic mechanism for a single substrate enzyme. Biochemistry 40:8009–8017
13. Marangos PJ, Zis AP, Clark RL et al (1978) Neuronal, non-neuronal and hybrid forms of enolase in brain: structural, immunological and functional comparisons. Brain Res 150:117–133
14. Schmechel DE, Brightman MW, Marangos PJ et al (1978) Granule cell neurons in developing rat and monkey cerebellum change from glial to neuronal enolase. J Anat 4:126
15. Schmechel D, Marangos PJ, Zis AP et al (1978) Brain enolases as specific markers of neuronal and glial cells. Science 199:313–315
16. Marangos PJ, Schmechel DE (1987) Neuron specific enolase, a clinically useful marker for neurons and neuroendocrine cells. Annu Rev Neurosci 10:269–295
17. Chai G, Brewer JM, Lovelace LL et al (2004) Expression, purification and the 1.8 angstroms resolution crystal structure of human neuron specific enolase. J Mol Biol 341:1015–1021
18. McAleese SM, Dunbar B, Fothergill JE et al (1988) Complete amino acid sequence of the neurone-specific gamma isozyme of enolase (NSE) from human brain and comparison with the non-neuronal alpha form (NNE). Eur J Biochem 178:413–417
19. Giallongo A, Feo S, Moore R et al (1986) Molecular cloning and nucleotide sequence of a full-length

cDNA for human alpha enolase. Proc Natl Acad Sci U S A 83:6741–6745
20. Oliva D, Calì L, Feo S et al (1991) Complete structure of the human gene encoding neuron-specific enolase. Genomics 10:157–165
21. Sakimura K, Kushiya E, Takahashi Y et al (1987) The structure and expression of neuron-specific enolase gene. Gene 60:103–113
22. Bird AP (1986) CpG-rich islands and the function of DNA methylation. Nature 321:209–213
23. Haimoto H, Takahashi Y, Koshikawa T et al (1985) Immunohistochemical localization of gamma-enolase in normal human tissues other than nervous and neuroendocrine tissues. Lab Invest 52:257–263
24. Van Obberghen E, Kamholz J, Bishop JG 3rd et al (1988) Human gamma enolase: isolation of a cDNA clone and expression in normal and tumor tissues of human origin. J Neurosci Res 19:450–456
25. Meera Khan P, Doppert BA, Hagemeijer A et al (1974) The human loci for phosphopyruvate hydratase and guanylate kinase are syntenic with the PGD-PGM1 linkage group in man-Chinese hamster somatic cell hybrids. Cytogenet Cell Genet 13:130–131
26. Cook PJ, Hamerton JL (1979) Report of the committee on the genetic constitution of chromosome 1. Cytogenet Cell Genet 25:9–20
27. Grzeschik KH (1976) Assignment of human genes: beta-glucuronidase to chromosome 7, adenylate kinase-1 to 9, a second enzyme with enolase activity to 12, and mitochondrial IDH to 15. Birth Defects Orig Artic Ser 12:142–148
28. Law ML, Kao FT (1982) Regional mapping of the gene coding for enolase-2 on human chromosome 12. J Cell Sci 53:245–254
29. Craig SP, Day IN, Thompson RJ et al (1990) Localisation of neurone-specific enolase (ENO2) to 12p13. Cytogenet Cell Genet 54:71–73
30. Feo S, Oliva D, Barbieri G et al (1990) The gene for the muscle-specific enolase is on the short arm of human chromosome 17. Genomics 6:192–194
31. Muller FL, Colla S, Aquilanti E et al (2012) Passenger deletions generate therapeutic vulnerabilities in cancer. Nature 488:337–342
32. Rider CC, Taylor CB (1974) Enolase isoenzymes in rat tissues. Electrophoretic, chromatographic, immunological and kinetic properties. Biochim Biophys Acta 365:285–300
33. Schmechel DE, Brightman MW, Marangos PJ (1980) Neurons switch from non-neuronal enolase to neuron-specific enolase during differentiation. Brain Res 190:195–214
34. Tanaka M, Sugisaki K, Nakashima K (1985) Switching in levels of translatable mRNAs for enolase isozymes during development of chicken skeletal muscle. Biochem Biophys Res Commun 133:868–872
35. Marangos PJ, Schmechel DE, Parma AM et al (1980) Developmental profile of neuron-specific (NSE) and non-neuronal (NNE) enolase. Brain Res 190:185–193
36. Chen SH, Omenn GS (1984) Human neuron-specific enolase: genetic and developmental studies. J Neurogenet 1:159–164
37. Nobels FR, Kwekkeboom DJ, Coopmans W et al (1997) Chromogranin A as serum marker for neuroendocrine neoplasia: comparison with neuron-specific enolase and the alpha-subunit of glycoprotein hormones. J Clin Endocrinol Metab 82:2622–2628
38. Eriksson B, Oberg K, Stridsberg M (2000) Tumor markers in neuroendocrine tumors. Digestion 62(Suppl 1):33–38
39. Baudin E, Gigliotti A, Ducreux M et al (1998) Neuron-specific enolase and chromogranin A as markers of neuroendocrine tumours. Br J Cancer 78:1102–1107
40. Bajetta E, Ferrari L, Martinetti A et al (1999) Chromogranin A, neuron specific enolase, carcinoembryonic antigen, and hydroxyindole acetic acid evaluation in patients with neuroendocrine tumors. Cancer 86:858–865
41. Carney DN, Teeling M (1988) Neuron-specific enolase: how useful as a cancer marker? Eur J Cancer Clin Oncol 24:825–828
42. Marangos PJ, Zomzely-Neurath C, York C (1975) Immunological studies of a nerve specific protein. Arch Biochem Biophys 170:289–293
43. Marangos PJ, Schmechel D, Parma AM et al (1979) Measurement of neuron-specific (NSE) and non-neuronal (NNE) isoenzymes of enolase in rat, monkey and human nervous tissue. J Neurochem 33:319–329
44. Parma AM, Marangos PJ, Goodwin FK (1981) A more sensitive radioimmunoassay for neuron-specific enolase suitable for cerebrospinal fluid determinations. J Neurochem 36:1093–1096
45. Wevers RA, Jacobs AA, Hommes OR (1983) A bioluminescent assay for enolase (EC 4.2.1.11) activity in human serum and cerebrospinal fluid. Clin Chim Acta 135:159–168
46. Gerbitz KD, Summer J, Thallemer J (1984) Brain-specific proteins: solid-phase immunobioluminescence assay for neuron-specific enolase in human plasma. Clin Chem 30:382–386
47. Kimura S, Uchikawa H, Yamamoto R et al (1984) Practicable enzyme immunoassay for neuron-specific enolase in human serum. J Appl Biochem 6:319–324
48. Kimura S, Uchikawa H, Yamamoto R et al (1986) Two-site column enzyme immunoassay for neuron-specific enolase (NSE) in human serum using monoclonal antibodies. J Immunol Methods 94:51–55
49. Viallard JL, Murthy MR, Bétail G et al (1986) Determination of serum neuron-specific enolase by differential immunocapture. Clin Chim Acta 161:1–10
50. Viallard JL, Ven Murthy MR, Dastugue B (1986) Rapid electrophoretic determination of neuron-specific enolase isoenzymes in serum. Clin Chem 32:593–597
51. Anastasiades KD, Mullins RE, Conn RB (1987) Neuron-specific enolase. Assessment by ELISA in

patients with small cell carcinoma of the lung. Am J Clin Pathol 87:245–249
52. Paus E, Nustad K (1989) Immunoradiometric assay for alpha gamma- and gamma gamma-enolase (neuron-specific enolase), with use of monoclonal antibodies and magnetizable polymer particles. Clin Chem 35:2034–2038
53. Body JJ, Paesmans M, Sculier JP et al (1992) Monoclonal immunoradiometric assay and polyclonal radioimmunoassay compared for measuring neuron-specific enolase in patients with lung cancer. Clin Chem 38:748–751
54. Schmitt UM, Stieber P, Hasholzner U et al (1996) Methodological and clinical evaluation of two automated enzymatic immunoassays as compared with a radioimmunoassay for neuron-specific enolase. Eur J Clin Chem Clin Biochem 34:679–682
55. Ebert W, Muley T (1998) Analytical performance of the new single step COBAS Core NSE EIA II and its diagnostic utility in comparison with the established COBAS Core NSE EIA. Clin Lab 44:871–879
56. Muley T, Ebert W, Stieber P et al (2003) Technical performance and diagnostic utility of the new Elecsys neuron-specific enolase enzyme immunoassay. Clin Chem Lab Med 41:95–103
57. Fu X, Meng M, Zhang Y et al (2012) Chemiluminescence enzyme immunoassay using magnetic nanoparticles for detection of neuron specific enolase in human serum. Anal Chim Acta 722:114–118
58. Torsetnes SB, Løvbak SG, Claus C et al (2013) Immunocapture and LC-MS/MS for selective quantification and differentiation of the isozymes of the biomarker neuron-specific enolase in serum. J Chromatogr B Analyt Technol Biomed Life Sci 929:125–132
59. Li GZ, Tian F (2013) Guanine-decorated graphene nanostructures for sensitive monitoring of neuron-specific enolase based on an enzyme-free electrocatalytic reaction. Anal Sci 29:1195–1201
60. Mercer DW, Virji MA, Barry GE, Piper ML (1990) New solid-phase enzyme immunoassay of neuron-specific enolase in serum: effect of storage temperature, lipemia, icterus, and hemolysis. Clin Chem 36:1519
61. Gerbitz KD, Summer J, Schumacher I et al (1986) Enolase isoenzymes as tumour markers. J Clin Chem Clin Biochem 24:1009–1016
62. Ramont L, Thoannes H, Volondat A et al (2005) Effects of hemolysis and storage condition on neuron-specific enolase (NSE) in cerebrospinal fluid and serum: implications in clinical practice. Clin Chem Lab Med 43:1215–1217
63. Planche V, Brochet C, Bakkouch A et al (2010) Importance of hemolysis on neuron-specific enolase measurement. Ann Biol Clin 68:239–242
64. Braga F, Ferraro S, Mozzi R et al (2013) Biological variation of neuroendocrine tumor markers chromogranin A and neuron-specific enolase. Clin Biochem 46:148–151
65. Dittadi R, Gion M (2013) Re: biological variation of neuroendocrine tumor markers chromogranin A and neuron-specific enolase. Clin Biochem 46:1145
66. Prinz RA, Marangos PJ (1982) Use of neuron specific enolase as a serum marker for neuroendocrine neoplasms. Surgery 97:887–889
67. Ferolla P, Faggiano A, Mansueto G et al (2008) The biological characterization of neuroendocrine tumors: the role of neuroendocrine markers. J Endocrinol Invest 31:277–286
68. Pearse AG (1969) The cytochemistry and ultrastructure of polypeptide hormone-producing cells of the APUD series and the embryologic, physiologic and pathologic implications of the concept. J Histochem Cytochem 17:303–313
69. Jiang SX, Kameya T, Shoji M et al (1998) Large cell neuroendocrine carcinoma of the lung: a histologic and immunohistochemical study of 22 cases. Am J Surg Pathol 22:526–537
70. Baudin E, Bidart JM, Rougier P et al (1999) Screening for multiple endocrine neoplasia type 1 and hormonal production in apparently sporadic neuroendocrine tumors. J Clin Endocrinol Metab 84:69–75
71. World Health Organization (1982) The World Health Organization histological typing of lung tumours. Second edition. Am J Clin Pathol 77:123–136
72. Quoix E, Purohit A, Faller-Beau M et al (2000) Comparative prognostic value of lactate dehydrogenase and neuron-specific enolase in small-cell lung cancer patients treated with platinum-based chemotherapy. Lung Cancer 30:127–134
73. Cooper EH, Splinter TA, Brown DA et al (1985) Evaluation of a radioimmunoassay for neuron specific enolase in small cell lung cancer. Br J Cancer 52:333–338
74. Harding M, McAllister J, Hulks G et al (1990) Neurone specific enolase (NSE) in small cell lung cancer: a tumour marker of prognostic significance? Br J Cancer 61:605–607
75. Gronowitz JS, Bergström R, Nôu E et al (1990) Clinical and serologic markers of stage and prognosis in small cell lung cancer. A multivariate analysis. Cancer 66:722–732
76. Spinazzi A, Soresi E, Borghini U et al (1990) Clinical value of neuron specific enolase and tissue polipeptidic antigen for the management of patients with lung cancer. J Nucl Med Allied Sci 34:141–145
77. Giovanella L, Ceriani L, Bandera M et al (1995) Evaluation of the serum markers CEA, NSE, TPS and CYFRA 21.1 in lung cancer. Int J Biol Markers 10:156–160
78. Giovanella L, Piantanida R, Ceriani L et al (1997) Immunoassay of neuron-specific enolase (NSE) and serum fragments of cytokeratin 19 (CYFRA 21.1) as tumor markers in small cell lung cancer: clinical evaluation and biological hypothesis. Int J Biol Markers 12:22–26
79. Paone G, De Angelis G, Munno R et al (1995) Discriminant analysis on small cell lung cancer and

non-small cell lung cancer by means of NSE and CYFRA-21.1. Eur Respir J 8:1136–1140
80. Paone G, De Angelis G, Portalone L et al (1997) Validation of an algorithm able to differentiate small-cell lung cancer (SCLC) from non-small-cell lung cancer (NSCLC) patients by means of a tumour marker panel: analysis of the errors. Br J Cancer 75:448–450
81. Jørgensen LG, Osterlind K, Genollá J et al (1996) Serum neuron-specific enolase (S-NSE) and the prognosis in small-cell lung cancer (SCLC): a combined multivariable analysis on data from nine centres. Br J Cancer 74:463–467
82. Esscher T, Steinholtz L, Bergh J et al (1985) Neurone specific enolase: a useful diagnostic serum marker for small cell carcinoma of the lung. Thorax 40:85–90
83. Takada M, Kusunoki Y, Masuda N et al (1996) Progastrin-releasing peptide (31–98) as a tumour marker of small-cell lung cancer: comparative evaluation with neuron-specific enolase. Br J Cancer 73:1227–1232
84. Giovanella L, Ceriani L, Bandera M et al (2001) Immunoradiometric assay of chromogranin A in the diagnosis of small cell lung cancer: comparative evaluation with neuron-specific enolase. Int J Biol Markers 16:50–55
85. Petrović M, Bukumirić Z, Zdravković V et al (2014) The prognostic significance of the circulating neuroendocrine markers chromogranin A, pro-gastrin-releasing peptide, and neuron-specific enolase in patients with small-cell lung cancer. Med Oncol 31:823
86. Broers JL, Carney DN, de Ley L et al (1985) Differential expression of intermediate filament proteins distinguishes classic from variant small-cell lung cancer cell lines. Proc Natl Acad Sci U S A 82:4409–4413
87. Kulpa J, Wójcik E, Reinfuss M et al (2002) Carcinoembryonic antigen, squamous cell carcinoma antigen, CYFRA 21-1, and neuron-specific enolase in squamous cell lung cancer patients. Clin Chem 48:1931–1937
88. Pujol JL, Boher JM, Grenier J et al (2001) Cyfra 21-1, neuron specific enolase and prognosis of non-small cell lung cancer: prospective study in 621 patients. Lung Cancer 31:221–231
89. Tiseo M, Ardizzoni A, Cafferata MA et al (2008) Predictive and prognostic significance of neuron-specific enolase (NSE) in non-small cell lung cancer. Anticancer Res 28:507–513
90. Andoh M, Gemma A, Takenaka K et al (1994) Serum neuron specific enolase level as a prognostic factor in non-small cell lung cancer. Intern Med 33:271–276
91. Diez M, Torres A, Ortega L et al (1993) Value of serum neuron-specific enolase in nonsmall cell lung cancer. Oncology 50:127–131
92. Yan HJ, Tan Y, Gu W (2014) Neuron specific enolase and prognosis of non-small cell lung cancer: a systematic review and meta-analysis. J BUON 19:153–156
93. Yao JC, Lombard-Bohas C, Baudin E et al (2010) Daily oral everolimus activity in patients with metastatic pancreatic neuroendocrine tumors after failure of cytotoxic chemotherapy: a phase II trial. J Clin Oncol 28:69–76
94. Cotterill SJ, Pearson AD, Pritchard J et al (2000) Clinical prognostic factors in 1277 patients with neuroblastoma: results of The European Neuroblastoma Study Group 'Survey' 1982–1992. Eur J Cancer 36:901–908
95. Zeltzer PM, Marangos PJ, Parma AM et al (1983) Raised neuron-specific enolase in serum of children with metastatic neuroblastoma. A report from the Children's Cancer Study Group. Lancet 2:361–363
96. Zeltzer PM, Marangos PJ, Evans AE et al (1986) Serum neuron-specific enolase in children with neuroblastoma. Relationship to stage and disease course. Cancer 57:1230–1234
97. Riley RD, Heney D, Jones DR et al (2004) A systematic review of molecular and biological tumor markers in neuroblastoma. Clin Cancer Res 10:4–12
98. Kintzel K, Sonntag J, Strauss E et al (1998) Neuron-specific enolase: reference values in cord blood. Clin Chem Lab Med 36:245–247
99. Missler U, Wiesmann M, Friedrich C et al (1997) S-100 protein and neuron-specific enolase concentrations in blood as indicators of infarction volume and prognosis in acute ischemic stroke. Stroke 28:1956–1960
100. Oh SH, Lee JG, Na SJ et al (2003) Prediction of early clinical severity and extent of neuronal damage in anterior-circulation infarction using the initial serum neuron-specific enolase level. Arch Neurol 60:37–41
101. Wunderlich MT, Lins H, Skalej M et al (2006) Neuron-specific enolase and tau protein as neurobiochemical markers of neuronal damage are related to early clinical course and long-term outcome in acute ischemic stroke. Clin Neurol Neurosurg 108:558–563
102. Brouns R, De Vil B, Cras P et al (2010) Neurobiochemical markers of brain damage in cerebrospinal fluid of acute ischemic stroke patients. Clin Chem 56:451–458
103. González-García S, González-Quevedo A, Fernández-Concepción O et al (2012) Short-term prognostic value of serum neuron specific enolase and S100B in acute stroke patients. Clin Biochem 45:1302–1307
104. Zaheer S, Beg M, Rizvi I et al (2013) Correlation between serum neuron specific enolase and functional neurological outcome in patients of acute ischemic stroke. Ann Indian Acad Neurol 16:504–508
105. Ahmad O, Wardlaw J, Whiteley WN (2012) Correlation of levels of neuronal and glial markers with radiological measures of infarct volume in

ischaemic stroke: a systematic review. Cerebrovasc Dis 33:47–54
106. Brea D, Sobrino T, Blanco M et al (2009) Temporal profile and clinical significance of serum neuron-specific enolase and S100 in ischemic and hemorrhagic stroke. Clin Chem Lab Med 47:1513–1518
107. Lee SY, Choi YC, Kim JH et al (2010) Serum neuron-specific enolase level as a biomarker in differential diagnosis of seizure and syncope. J Neurol 257:1708–1712
108. Wijdicks EF, Hijdra A, Young GB et al (2006) Practice parameter: prediction of outcome in comatose survivors after cardiopulmonary resuscitation (an evidence-based review): report of the Quality Standards Subcommittee of the American Academy of Neurology. Neurology 67:203–210
109. Meynaar IA, Oudemans-van Straaten HM, van der Wetering J et al (2003) Serum neuron-specific enolase predicts outcome in post-anoxic coma: a prospective cohort study. Intensive Care Med 29:189–195
110. Guzel A, Er U, Tatli M et al (2008) Serum neuron-specific enolase as a predictor of short-term outcome and its correlation with Glasgow Coma Scale in traumatic brain injury. Neurosurg Rev 31:439–444
111. Meric E, Gunduz A, Turedi S et al (2010) The prognostic value of neuron-specific enolase in head trauma patients. J Emerg Med 38:297–301
112. Vos PE, Jacobs B, Andriessen TM et al (2010) GFAP and S100B are biomarkers of traumatic brain injury: an observational cohort study. Neurology 75:1786–1793
113. Wibe E, Hannisdal E, Paus E et al (1992) Neuron-specific enolase as a prognostic factor in metastatic malignant melanoma. Eur J Cancer 28:1692–1695
114. Tofani A, Cioffi RP, Sciuto R et al (1997) S-100 and NSE as serum markers in melanoma. Acta Oncol 36:761–764
115. Shine BS, Hungerford J, Vaghela B et al (1990) Electrophoretic assessment of aqueous and serum neurone-specific enolase in retinoblastoma and ocular malignant melanoma. Br J Ophthalmol 74:427–430
116. Fosså SD, Klepp O, Paus E (1992) Neuron-specific enolase – a serum tumour marker in seminoma? Br J Cancer 65:297–299
117. Tandstad T, Klepp O (2003) Neuron-specific enolase in testicular cancer – clinical experiences with serum neuron-specific enolase in patients with testicular cancer at diagnosis and during follow-up. Acta Oncol 42:202–206
118. Takashi M, Haimoto H, Tanaka J et al (1989) Evaluation of gamma-enolase as a tumor marker for renal cell carcinoma. J Urol 141:830–834
119. Plowman PN (1989) Serum marker for Merkel cell tumour. Clin Radiol 40:542
120. Cunningham RT, Johnston CF, Irvine GB et al (1992) Serum neurone-specific enolase levels in patients with neuroendocrine and carcinoid tumours. Clin Chim Acta 212:123–131
121. Kawata M, Sekiya S, Hatakeyama R et al (1989) Neuron-specific enolase as a serum marker for immature teratoma and dysgerminoma. Gynecol Oncol 32:191–197
122. Grouzmann E, Gicquel C, Plouin PF et al (1990) Neuropeptide Y and neuron-specific enolase levels in benign and malignant pheochromocytomas. Cancer 66:1833–1835
123. O'Connor TP, Wade TP, Sunwoo YC et al (1992) Small cell undifferentiated carcinoma of the pancreas. Report of a patient with tumor marker studies. Cancer 70:1514–1519
124. Mokuno K, Kiyosawa K, Sugimura K et al (1994) Prognostic value of cerebrospinal fluid neuron-specific enolase and S-100b protein in Guillain-Barré syndrome. Acta Neurol Scand 89:27–30
125. Vermuyten K (1989) Determination of glial fibrillary acidic protein, S100, myelin basic protein and neuron specific enolase in cerebrospinal fluid from patients suffering from dementia. Acta Neurol Belg 89:318
126. Aksamit AJ Jr, Preissner CM, Homburger HA (2001) Quantitation of 14-3-3 and neuron-specific enolase proteins in CSF in Creutzfeldt-Jakob disease. Neurology 57:728–730
127. Egan MF, el-Mallakh RS, Suddath RL et al (1992) Cerebrospinal fluid and serum levels of neuron-specific enolase in patients with schizophrenia. Psychiatry Res 43:187–195

Components of the Plasminogen-Plasmin System as Biologic Markers for Cancer

10

Brandon J. McMahon and Hau C. Kwaan

Abstract

Members of the plasminogen-plasmin (PP) system participate in many physiologic functions. In particular, uPA, its receptor (uPAR) and its inhibitor PAI-1 play an important role in cell migration, cell proliferation and tissue remodeling. Through a number of interactions, these components of the PP system are also involved in the pathogenesis of many diseases. In cancer, they modulate the essential processes of tumor development, growth, invasion and metastasis as well as angiogenesis and fibrosis. Thus, quantification of uPA, uPAR and PAI-1 in tumors and, in some cases in the circulating blood, became of potential value in the prognostication of many types of cancer. These include cancer of the breast, stomach, colon and rectum, esophagus, pancreas, glioma, lung, kidney, prostate, uterine cervix, ovary, liver and bone. Published data are reviewed in this chapter. Clinical validation of the prognostic value has also been made, particularly in cancer of the breast. Inclusion of these biomarkers in the risk assessment of cancer patients is now considered in the risk-adapted management in carcinoma of the breast. Factors limiting its broader use are discussed with suggestions how these can be overcome. Hopefully the use of these biomarkers will be applied to other types of cancer in the near future.

Keywords

Biomarker • Cancer • PAI-1 • Thrombosis • uPA • uPA activity and lymph node involvement • uPA and PAI-1 expression • uPA/PAI-1 as biomarkers • uPA/PAI-1 in breast cancer • uPAR

B.J. McMahon, MD • H.C. Kwaan, MD, FRCP (✉)
Division of Hematology/Oncology, Feinberg School of Medicine, and the Robert H. Lurie Cancer, Northwestern University, Chicago, IL USA

Olson Pavilion, Room 8258, 710 N. Fairbanks Court, Chicago, IL 60611, USA
e-mail: h-kwaan@northwestern.edu

R. Scatena (ed.), *Advances in Cancer Biomarkers*, Advances in Experimental Medicine and Biology 867, DOI 10.1007/978-94-017-7215-0_10

10.1 Introduction

The Plasminogen-Plasmin System The proteolytic enzyme plasmin (Plm), derived from its precursor plasminogen (Plgn), was first believed to be responsible for dissolution of fibrin clot. Following this original discovery, more components were found to belong to this plasminogen-plasmin (PP) system [1–3]. The various components are shown in Fig. 10.1. Plgn is converted to Plm by the action of two plasminogen activators (PA), tissue-type PA (t-PA) and urokinase-type plasminogen activator (uPA). Their activities are controlled by a number of inhibitors, including plasminogen activator inhibitor type 1 (PAI-1) plasminogen activator inhibitor-1 [4], plasminogen activator inhibitor type 2 (PAI-2), thrombin activable fibrinolysis inhibitor (TAFI) [5] and protease nexin 1 (PN-1) [6]. They are also modulated by their respective receptors [7, 8].

Studies of the PP system have produced evidence that it is involved in many body functions, ranging from embryogenesis, cell migration, wound repair, angiogenesis, inflammation, apoptosis and fibrosis. The role of fibrinolysis belongs primarily to tPA, maintaining normal hemostasis and keeping circulating blood free from fibrin. However, the picture on the cell surface is different, with uPA being the prominent player. As shown in Fig. 10.2, several steps had been recognized. (1) uPA converts Plg bound to the Plg receptor on the cell surface to generate Plm. Plm then converts pro-metalloproteinase to metalloproteinase. (2) Both Plm and MMP can proteolyze the breakdown extracellular matrix. (3) Plm activates latent growth factors. (4) PAI-1 inactivates uPA and forms a complex with uPA and uPAR. This complex is internalized into the cell. (5) Following internalization, the uPA/uPAR/PAI-1 complex is broken down. While PAI-1 and uPA is removed, uPAR is externalized from the cell in a process of recycling. These steps enable cell migration, a process essential in tissue remodeling and in wound healing.

An additional step is cell signaling from uPAR [7, 9]. Through the GPI anchoring, uPAR can

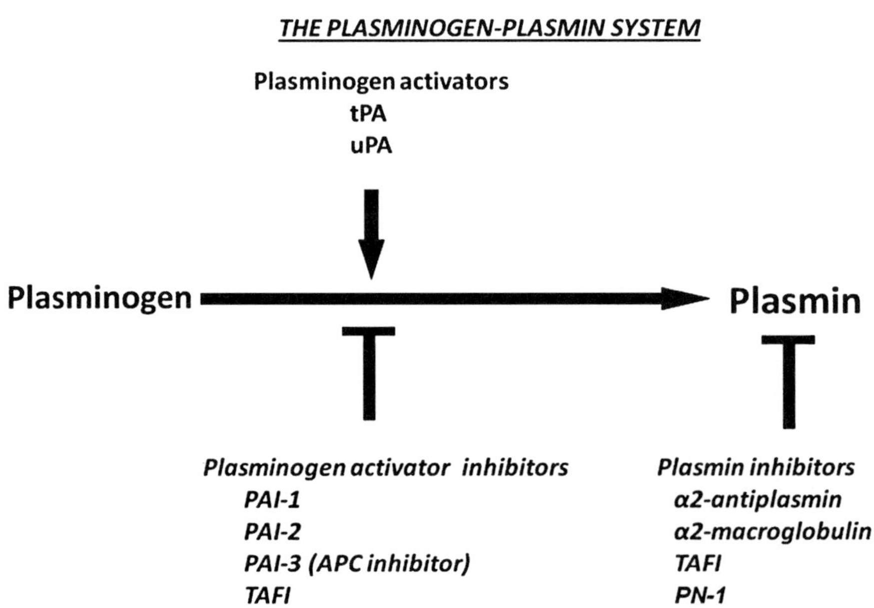

Fig. 10.1 Components of the plasminogen-plasmin system. *APC* activated protein C, *TAFI* thrombin activable fibrinolysis inhibitor

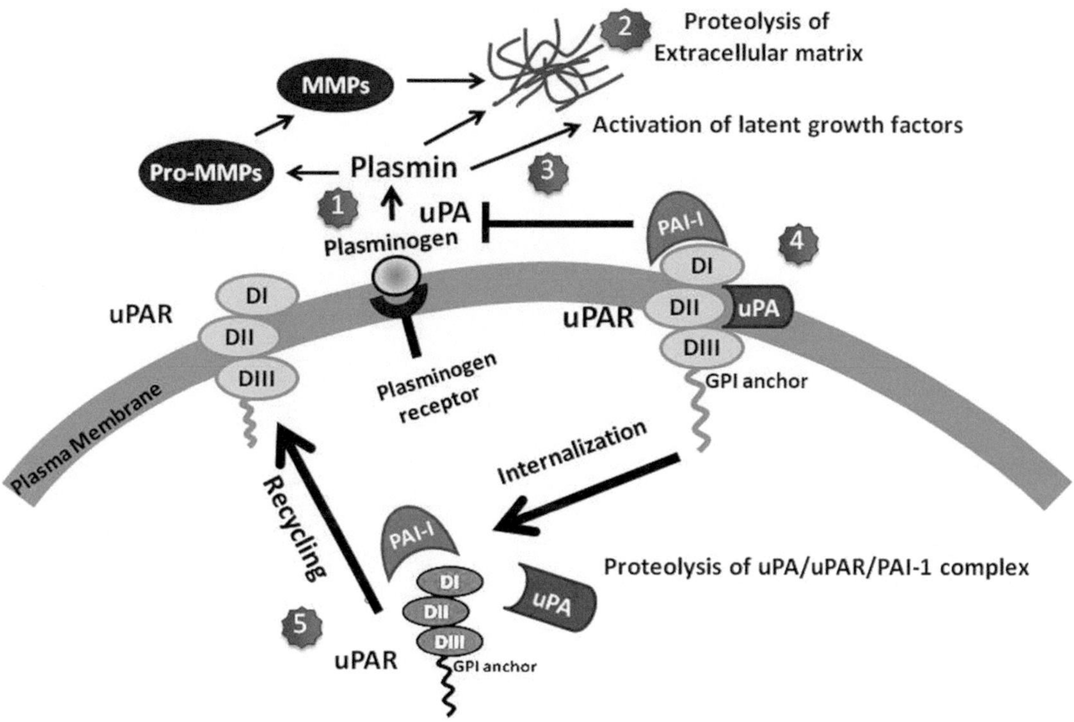

Fig. 10.2 Known steps in the activity of the plasminogen-plasmin system on the cell surface. (1) uPA converts Plg bound to the Plg receptor on the cell surface to generate Plm. Plm then converts pro-metalloproteinase to metalloproteinase (MMP). (2) Both plm and MMP can proteolyse the breakdown extracellular matrix.(3) Plm activates latent growth factors.(4) PAI-1 inactivates uPA and forms a complex with uPA and uPAR. This complex is internalized into the cell. (5) Following internalization, the uPA/uPAR/PAI-1 complex is broken down. While PAI-1 and uPA is proteolyzed, uPAR is exteriorized from the cell in the process of recycling

activate the G-protein kinases. These signals cell proliferation as well as apoptosis.

Role of the Plasminogen-Plasmin System in Diseases and in Cancer With such wide range of actions, it is now recognized that this system plays an important role in the pathogenesis of many diseases. In particular, it has been extensively studied in the various processes of tumor development, proliferation, invasion and tumor angiogenesis [10–16].

The relationship between fibrin and tumor was first noted by Billroth [17] who found tumor cells within a thrombus. Early in vitro observation was of liquefaction of growth media by malignant tumors was made by Carrel [18], while clinical record of fibrinolytic bleeding was made in patients with metastatic carcinoma of prostate [19]. Evidence of a possible causative role of plasminogen activator (PA) in malignancy was shown by the sharp increase in fibrinolytic activity in viral transformed fibroblasts [20]. This (PA) was later identified to be uPA [21]. Subsequently, abnormal levels of uPA have been found in most forms of cancer by tissue extraction, immunohistochemical staining and in situ hybridization. These include cancer of the breast, stomach, colon and rectum, esophagus, pancreas, glioma, lung, kidney, prostate, uterine cervix, ovary, liver and bone (Table 10.1). Of significance, uPA expression was found to be higher in the aggressive types of tumor, in metastatic more than in the primary tumor, and often in the invading front of the tumor [62–65]. One example was observed in adenocarcinoma of the prostate (Fig. 10.3) [66]. This association between

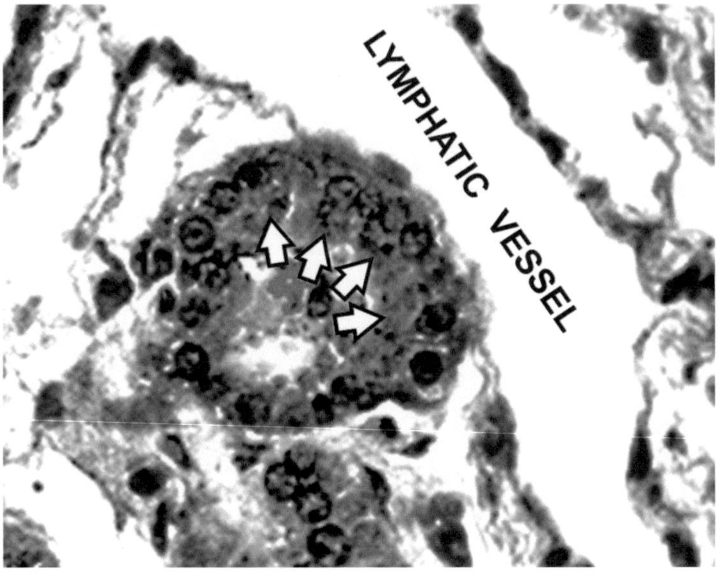

Fig. 10.3 Immunohistochemical staining of uPA of human adenocarcinoma of prostate showing the distribution of uPA at the invading front (*arrows*) of the tumor adjacent to a lymphatic channel (Reprinted with permission from Dano et al. [65], Kwaan et al. [66]

increased uPA expression and aggressive tumor behavior was also seen in carcinoma of breast [67], glioma [46] and many other tumors, both in vitro and in vivo. Experimental inhibition of uPA by various methods could impair tumor growth and metastasis, such as by anti-uPA antibodies [68, 69] or by transfection with uPA antisense genes [70, 71] or with PAI-1 gene [72]. Following the discovery of uPAR, it was also found to be expressed in many tumors [73–76] and to be associated with tumor aggressiveness [26, 33, 36, 50, 52, 53, 57, 77–79].

10.2 Clinical Validation of uPA, uPAR and PAI-1 as Biomarkers in Cancer

As has been outlined in detail above, key components of the fibrinolytic system may play a significant pathologic role in the growth and metastatic potential of many malignant processes. Inhibition of apoptosis, and increased levels of TGFB, FGF2, ILGF-1, and hepatocyte growth factor due to perturbations in the uPA system may add to tumor growth and progression. Metastatic spread can be enhanced through degradation of the extracellular matrix, and promotion of cellular adhesion. These in vitro adverse outcomes have indeed been demonstrated in clinical studies, with increased expression of uPA, uPAR, and/or PAI-1 being associated with poorer overall prognosis in multiple cancer types, including cancer of breast, stomach, colon and rectum, esophagus, pancreas, glioma, lung, kidney, prostate, uterine cervix, ovary, liver and bone (Table 10.1).

The impact of the uPA system on clinical outcomes in malignancies has been most extensively studied in breast cancer [23–28, 30, 31]. Indeed, expression of uPA has been demonstrated to be associated with more aggressive disease. Early studies demonstrated high uPA activity correlated with larger tumor size and lymph node involvement, in addition to a shorter disease-free survival [25]. Increased levels of uPA and PAI-1 were associated with a worse overall prognosis in a subsequent pooled analysis of over 8000 patients [23]. Interestingly, levels of uPA and PAI-1 were more predictive of both disease-free and overall survival than either estrogen receptor (ER) status or tumor size in this study, and findings were applicable to both lymph-node negative and positive disease. These and other studies have helped validate the utility of tumor uPA and PAI-1 expression in predicting disease course in breast cancer at the highest level of evidence (Level 1), and are the first novel biomarkers to achieve this [80].

Table 10.1 Components of the plasminogen-plasmin system as biomarkers in various types of cancer (Modified with permission from Kwaan et al. [22])

Clinical impact of uPA/PAI-1 biomarkers	
Disease site	Clinical findings
Breast	In lymph node negative disease, uPA & PAI-1 more predictive of RFS and OS than ER status [23]
	In node-negative disease, uPA & PAI-1 levels more informative than age, tumor size, and hormonal status; correlated with DFS; and predicted benefit from adjuvant chemotherapy [24]
	uPA stronger predictor of RFS than lymph node status, but not for OS. However, uPA predicts OS in node-negative disease, whereas ER status and tumor size do not [25]
	Lower OS with high uPAR and PAI-1 levels. High PAI-1 also corresponded to shorter RFS [26]
	High tumor PAI-1 mRNA results in shorter OS, but PAI-1 gene promoter polymorphism did not add prognostic information [27]
	In tumors with high uPA, high PAI-2 corresponds to favorable RFS and OS [28, 29]
	uPA and PAI-1 predict disease outcome and response to therapy, and statistically independent of tumor size, grade, ER/PR status [30–32]
Gastric	Higher uPA/uPAR expression associated with more advanced stage and higher mortality [33]
	High uPA corresponds to more aggressive disease, and prognostic in T1/T2, lymph node negative disease [34]
	High uPA/PAI-1 in resected tumors associated with decreased OS. PAI-1 is the only significant prognostic marker in multivariate analysis [35]
	uPA/uPAR/VEGF mRNA expression in resected gastric cancer tissue predicted poorer chance for survival [36]
	Higher uPA and PAI-1 expression seen in gastric cancer versus normal tissue, with decreased RFS seen with higher levels [37]
Colorectal cancer	Increased mortality risk with higher preoperative soluble uPAR levels [38]
	Same results as above [39]
	High uPA levels in carcinoma versus adenomatous polyp or normal mucosa. Higher uPA levels associated with lower OS, independent of tumor stage [40]
	Decreased OS associated with high uPAR levels, independent of age, stage, grade [41]
Esophageal	In both squamous and adenocarcinoma, high uPA expression is an independent predictor of disease outcome [42]
	Same results as above [43]
	uPA expression in squamous cell carcinoma associated with higher metastatic potential and shorter OS
	Higher PAI-2 expression associated with lower metastatic potential [44]
Glioma	Shorter OS associated with stronger cytoplasmic uPA staining. In higher grade glioma, poorer OS seen with uPA staining, age >50, tumor grade in multivariate analysis [45]
	uPA & PAI-1 expression seen in glioblastoma multiforme, but not in normal brain tissue or benign tumors [46]
Lung	Small cell lung cancer cells expressing uPA demonstrated chemotherapy resistance [47]
	TAFI levels higher in small cell versus adeno- or squamous cell carcinoma. Chemotherapy response higher seen in those with higher TAFI expression [48]
	Increased PAI-1 antigen associated with increased risk of death in non-small cell lung cancer [49]
Renal	Relapsed and/or metastatic disease corresponds with stronger tissue staining for uPA, uPAR, or PAI-1 [50]
	uPA, uPAR, and PAI-1 all overexpressed in kidney cancer compared to normal tissue [51]

(continued)

Table 10.1 (continued)

Clinical impact of uPA/PAI-1 biomarkers	
Disease site	Clinical findings
Prostate	uPA & uPAR levels higher in prostate than healthy controls, and levels correspond to more aggressive disease [52]
	uPA & uPAR levels higher in those with bone metastases versus organ confined disease [53]
	uPA & uPAR levels higher in those with bone metastases versus organ confined disease [54]
Cervical	Stronger uPA/PAI-1 staining correlates with more extensive disease and a lower OS rate [55].
Ovarian	Decreased OS with increased uPA & PAI-1 levels on univariate (but not multivariate) analysis [56]
Liver	Higher uPAR and tPA in malignant versus normal hepatocytes, with a lower OS in male patients with high uPA levels [57]
Chondrosarcoma	uPA overexpression associated with higher metastatic potential, and a lower 5-year survival rate [58]
Pancreatic	tPA, PAI-1, and PAI-2 were expressed in the majority of pancreatic cancer specimens. Strong PAI-2 expression associated with less peritoneal metastasis, as well as a better OS [59]
	Higher uPA and uPAR mRNA levels in pancreatic cancer specimens versus control tissue. Shorter OS in cancer patients with overexpression of both uPA and uPAR than in those without [60]
Oral	Oral squamous cell carcinoma tumors had higher uPA expression compared to dysplastic lesions [61]

RFS relapsed-free survival, *OS* overall survival, *ER* estrogen receptor, *PR* progesterone receptor, *DFS* disease-free survival

The ability of these markers to help aid in prognostication and predict response to therapy has resulted in their being included in the American Society of Clinical Oncology guidelines for use in treatment decisions [80]. In fact, there have been a number of clinical studies demonstrating that incorporating uPA/PAI-1 status into treatment decision algorithms can help predict which patients would most benefit from a more aggressive approach. An early, prospective multicenter study randomized lymph-node negative breast cancer patients based on tumor levels of uPA and PAI-1. Those patients with low levels of both markers were observed, while those high levels of one or both were randomized to either observation alone, or combination chemotherapy [24]. At 3 years of follow up, those patients considered high risk based on elevated uPA/PAI-1 levels gained significant benefit from chemotherapy, with a 43.8 % reduced probability of recurrent disease. A subsequent study, again in patients with lymph node negative disease, further supported the utility of using these markers in treatment decisions [23]. Patients with low levels of both uPA and PAI-1 had an excellent 5-year disease-free survival at over 90 %; however, those with high levels of one or both marker had 5-year disease free survival rates comparable to patients with lymph-node positive disease. The negative impact of uPA/PAI-1 was mitigated through use of systemic, adjuvant chemotherapy, with improvements in both disease-free and overall survival when cyclophosphamide-methotrexate-5FU (CMF) was used [23]. As CMF is no longer considered standard of care for adjuvant treatment, an updated prospective study using an anthracycline-docetaxel based regimen was recently completed with over 4000 patients enrolled [81, 82]. The Node Negative Breast Cancer-3 (NNBC-3) trial was conducted in the years 2002–2009, and compared uPA/PAI-1 tumor levels to more conventional clinic-pathologic features, and how use of adjuvant chemotherapy in both impacted the disease course.

Low risk patients did not receive adjuvant chemotherapy. High risk groups were randomized to treatment with either fluorouracil-epirubicin-cyclophosphamide (FEC) for six cycles, or three cycles of FEC followed by docetaxel for three cycles. Results are still pending, noting that the first interim analysis was recently presented at the San Antonio Breast Cancer Symposium in December 2012 [83]. This analysis only evaluated a different endpoint in the trial, which addressed whether addition of taxanes to adjuvant chemotherapy improved outcomes. The data on comparison of uPA/PAI-1 to other clinical features are not yet mature. Once available, they may further validate use of these biomarkers in clinical treatment decision making. It is noted that through review of prior studies, incorporating uPA/PAI-1 testing in patients with node-negative breast cancer as recommended by ASCO not only appears to have a positive effect on outcomes, but is also beneficial from an economic standpoint [84].

In addition to identifying those patients who would most benefit from adjuvant chemotherapy in node-negative breast cancer, uPA/PAI-1 biomarkers have also been helpful in predicting response to hormonal agents. Women with uPA and PAI-1 negative tumors were more likely to have a beneficial response to tamoxifen in one study, and this was independent of ER/PR status [29].

Although less robust compared to breast cancer, there are studies demonstrating the clinical implications of uPA/PAI-1 in other malignancies (Table 10.1). The majority of the investigations have focused on the prognostic impact of these biomarkers, with their increased expression being associated with a more aggressive disease, and therefore worse overall prognosis, across a wide range of malignancies. For example, one study in pancreatic cancer demonstrated that post-operative survival was half that in patients with overexpression of uPA and uPAR compared to those with only one or neither being overexpressed (9 versus 18 months) [60]. As has been shown in breast cancer, consideration for using these biomarkers in treatment decisions may be important, allowing health providers to reserve more aggressive treatment for those who are most likely to benefit. Indeed, one study demonstrated that those patients with small cell lung cancer expressing uPAR were more likely to be chemotherapy-resistant [47]. Conversely, high expression of thrombin activatable fibrinolysis inhibitor (TAFI) expression in lung cancer was associated with a better therapeutic response [48]. These studies show promise, but certainly more prospective investigations are needed in order to validate the use of fibrinolytic markers in treatment decisions in other cancers.

10.3 Drug Targets

A number of therapeutic agents have been developed targeting the components of the P-P system. Their current status is briefly reviewed here, since biomarkers are used in the clinical trials of these agents. They can be used in the characterization and risk classification of the respective tumors or as part of the outcome. The therapeutic agents cover a wide spectrum of monoclonal antibodies, targeted toxins, synthetic small molecules and peptides, or genetic knockdown such as antisense and siRNA. With the discovery of the active sites in the crystal structure of the P-P components, small molecules can be designed to block the respective active sites [85–90]. In the case of uPA, the S1 pocket at the active site requires a highly basic molecule for binding and inactivation. A pro-drug upamostat (WX-671) (Mesupron™) showed activity in carcinoma of head and neck [91], pancreatic cancer [92] and breast cancer [93]. The site of interaction between uPA and uPAR has also been targeted [94, 95]. Results of peptides and small molecules designed to block this site have been disappointing. In contrast, antisense or siRNA in knockdown of uPAR showed antitumor activity [96, 97]. Monoclonal antibodies against uPAR also demonstrated antitumor effect both in vitro and in vivo [98, 99]. Treatment with a monoclonal antibody to uPAR resulted in a decrease of primary tumor growth and reduced hepatic and retroperitoneal metastases in a mouse model of pancreatic cancer [100].

Similar benefit was seen in ovarian cancer [101]. PAI-1 as therapeutic target, on the other hand, has not been well studied in cancer, though a small molecule targeting PAI-1 XR5967, a diketopiperazine, had been shown to suppress tumor cell invasion and angiogenesis in vitro [102].

The demonstration that various inhibitors of the P-P system have antitumor effect is a proof of concept that several components of the P-P system discussed above are biomarkers of cancer with unfavorable prognosis. This would undoubtedly stimulate further developments in the near future with these markers.

10.4 Perspectives

Biomarkers in cancer are most often used as aid in diagnosis. However, they can also be useful to assess tumor aggressiveness and to classify the risks. The use of risk classification in an individual patient can allow intensive therapy given to those with high risks while the low risk patients can receive milder forms of treatment. The association of uPA and PAI-1 and the aggressiveness of tumors have been recognized for over 30 years. Yet, the use of uPA, its receptor uPAR and PAI-1 as biomarkers is limited. Even less utilized is the employment of these biomarkers in risk assessment to guide the management of a cancer patient. In order to improve the use of the biomarkers, one has to understand the causes of under-utilization. Several factors can be recognized. First, PAI-1 is an inhibitor of uPA. Yet, both uPA and PAI-1 are indicators of tumor aggressiveness. This apparent paradox, first pointed out by Binder, is due to the multiple and complex pathways in which uPA, uPAR and particularly PAI-1 affects tumor biology [22, 103]. As discussed in this article, the validity of these biomarkers has been verified in several clinical trials. As yet, these trials have not been able to alter clinical practice. Secondly, inhibition of uPA, uPAR or PAI-1 by various approaches has shown positive results in impairing the growth and metastasis in experimental tumors in animals but has not been able to have any impact on human cancers. Some of the agents used include the use monoclonal antibodies, gene manipulations such as the transfection of PAI-1 into experimental tumors, and synthetic small molecules designed to target uPA, uPAR or PAI-1. Without clinical trials showing significant effect of these agents in human tumors, there is less demand for the use of these biomarkers. At the time of this writing, there a few promising clinical trials, including the use of synthetic small molecules. Any successful outcome of these trials will add to the utility of the biomarkers discussed here.

References

1. Kwaan HC (1992) The biologic role of components of the plasminogen-plasmin system. Prog Cardiovasc Dis 34(5):309–316
2. Castellino FJ, Ploplis VA (2005) Structure and function of the plasminogen/plasmin system. Thromb Haemost 93(4):647–654
3. Rijken DC, Lijnen HR (2009) New insights into the molecular mechanisms of the fibrinolytic system. J Thromb Haemost 7(1):4–13
4. Declerck PJ, Gils A (2013) Three decades of research on plasminogen activator inhibitor-1: a multifaceted serpin. Semin Thromb Hemost 39(4):356–364, Mar 26, epub ahead of print
5. Vercauteren E, Gils A, Declerck PJ (2013) Thrombin activatable fibrinolysis inhibitor: a putative target to enhance fibrinolysis. Semin Thromb Hemost 39(4):365–372, Mar 26, epub ahead of print
6. Bouton MC, Boulaftali Y, Richard B, Arocas V, Michel JB, Jandrot-Perrus M (2012) Emerging role of serpinE2/protease nexin-1 in hemostasis and vascular biology. Blood 119(11):2452–2457
7. Ferraris GM, Sidenius N (2013) Urokinase plasminogen activator receptor: a functional integrator of extracellular proteolysis, cell adhesion, and signal transduction. Semin Thromb Hemost 39(4):347–355
8. Miles LA, Parmer RJ (2013) Plasminogen receptors: the first quarter century. Semin Thromb Hemost 39(4):329–337
9. Binder BR, Mihaly J, Prager GW (2007) uPAR-uPA-PAI-1 interactions and signaling: a vascular biologist's view. Thromb Haemost 97(3):336–342
10. Pepper MS (2001) Role of the matrix metalloproteinase and plasminogen activator-plasmin systems in angiogenesis. Arterioscler Thromb Vasc Biol 21(7):1104–1117
11. Andreasen PA, Egelund R, Petersen HH (2000) The plasminogen activation system in tumor growth, invasion, and metastasis. Cell Mol Life Sci 57(1):25–40

12. Kwaan HC (1992) The plasminogen-plasmin system in malignancy. Cancer Metastasis Rev 11(3–4):291–311
13. Dano K, Behrendt N, Hoyer-Hansen G et al (2005) Plasminogen activation and cancer. Thromb Haemost 93(4):676–681
14. Kwaan HC, McMahon B (2009) The role of plasminogen-plasmin system in cancer. Cancer Treat Res 148:43–66
15. Deryugina EI, Quigley JP (2012) Cell surface remodeling by plasmin: a new function for an old enzyme. J Biomed Biotechnol 2012:564259
16. Carroll VA, Binder BR (1999) The role of the plasminogen activation system in cancer. Semin Thromb Hemost 25(2):183–197
17. Billroth T (1878) Lectures on surgical pathology and therapeutics. A handbook for students and practitioners. The New Sydenham Society, London
18. Carrel A, Burrows MT (1911) Cultivation in vitro of malignant tumors. J Exp Med 13(5):571–575
19. Tagnon HJ, Whitmore WF Jr, Schulman P, Kravitz SC (1953) The significance of fibrinolysis occurring in patients with metastatic cancer of the prostate. Cancer 6(1):63–67
20. Ossowski L, Quigley JP, Kellerman GM, Reich E (1973) Fibrinolysis associated with oncogenic transformation. Requirement of plasminogen for correlated changes in cellular morphology, colony formation in agar, and cell migration. J Exp Med 138(5):1056–1064
21. Astedt B, Holmberg L (1976) Immunological identity of urokinase and ovarian carcinoma plasminogen activator released in tissue culture. Nature 261(5561):595–597
22. Kwaan HC, Mazar AP, McMahon BJ (2013) The apparent uPA/PAI-1 paradox in cancer: more than meets the eye. Semin Thromb Hemost 39(4):382–391, Mar 26, epub ahead of print
23. Look MP, van Putten WL, Duffy MJ et al (2002) Pooled analysis of prognostic impact of urokinase-type plasminogen activator and its inhibitor PAI-1 in 8377 breast cancer patients. J Natl Cancer Inst 94(2):116–128
24. Janicke F, Prechtl A, Thomssen C et al (2001) Randomized adjuvant chemotherapy trial in high-risk, lymph node-negative breast cancer patients identified by urokinase-type plasminogen activator and plasminogen activator inhibitor type 1. J Natl Cancer Inst 93(12):913–920
25. Duffy MJ, Duggan C, Mulcahy HE, McDermott EW, O'Higgins NJ (1998) Urokinase plasminogen activator: a prognostic marker in breast cancer including patients with axillary node-negative disease. Clin Chem 44(6 Pt 1):1177–1183
26. Grondahl-Hansen J, Peters HA, van Putten WL et al (1995) Prognostic significance of the receptor for urokinase plasminogen activator in breast cancer. Clin Cancer Res 1(10):1079–1087
27. Sternlicht MD, Dunning AM, Moore DH et al (2006) Prognostic value of PAI1 in invasive breast cancer: evidence that tumor-specific factors are more important than genetic variation in regulating PAI1 expression. Cancer Epidemiol Biomarkers Prev 15(11):2107–2114
28. Foekens JA, Buessecker F, Peters HA et al (1995) Plasminogen activator inhibitor-2: prognostic relevance in 1012 patients with primary breast cancer. Cancer Res 55(7):1423–1427
29. Foekens JA, Look MP, Peters HA, van Putten WL, Portengen H, Klijn JG (1995) Urokinase-type plasminogen activator and its inhibitor PAI-1: predictors of poor response to tamoxifen therapy in recurrent breast cancer. J Natl Cancer Inst 87(10):751–756
30. Harbeck N, Kates RE, Look MP et al (2002) Enhanced benefit from adjuvant chemotherapy in breast cancer patients classified high-risk according to urokinase-type plasminogen activator (uPA) and plasminogen activator inhibitor type 1 (n=3424). Cancer Res 62(16):4617–4622
31. Harbeck N, Kates RE, Schmitt M (2002) Clinical relevance of invasion factors urokinase-type plasminogen activator and plasminogen activator inhibitor type 1 for individualized therapy decisions in primary breast cancer is greatest when used in combination. J Clin Oncol 20(4):1000–1007
32. Harbeck N, Kates RE, Schmitt M et al (2004) Urokinase-type plasminogen activator and its inhibitor type 1 predict disease outcome and therapy response in primary breast cancer. Clin Breast Cancer 5(5):348–352
33. Ji F, Chen YL, Jin EY, Wang WL, Yang ZL, Li YM (2005) Relationship between matrix metalloproteinase-2 mRNA expression and clinicopathological and urokinase-type plasminogen activator system parameters and prognosis in human gastric cancer. World J Gastroenterol 11(21):3222–3226
34. Heiss MM, Babic R, Allgayer H et al (1995) Tumor-associated proteolysis and prognosis: new functional risk factors in gastric cancer defined by the urokinase-type plasminogen activator system. J Clin Oncol 13(8):2084–2093
35. Nekarda H, Schmitt M, Ulm K et al (1994) Prognostic impact of urokinase-type plasminogen activator and its inhibitor PAI-1 in completely resected gastric cancer. Cancer Res 54(11):2900–2907
36. Zhang L, Zhao ZS, Ru GQ, Ma J (2006) Correlative studies on uPA mRNA and uPAR mRNA expression with vascular endothelial growth factor, microvessel density, progression and survival time of patients with gastric cancer. World J Gastroenterol 12(25):3970–3976
37. Cho JY, Chung HC, Noh SH, Roh JK, Min JS, Kim BS (1997) High level of urokinase-type plasminogen activator is a new prognostic marker in patients with gastric carcinoma. Cancer 79(5):878–883
38. Stephens RW, Nielsen HJ, Christensen IJ et al (1999) Plasma urokinase receptor levels in patients with colorectal cancer: relationship to prognosis. J Natl Cancer Inst 91(10):869–874

39. Riisbro R, Christensen IJ, Nielsen HJ, Brunner N, Nilbert M, Fernebro E (2005) Preoperative plasma soluble urokinase plasminogen activator receptor as a prognostic marker in rectal cancer patients. An EORTC-receptor and biomarker group collaboration. Int J Biol Markers 20(2):93–102
40. Skelly MM, Troy A, Duffy MJ et al (1997) Urokinase-type plasminogen activator in colorectal cancer: relationship with clinicopathological features and patient outcome. Clin Cancer Res 3(10):1837–1840
41. Ganesh S, Sier CF, Heerding MM, Griffioen G, Lamers CB, Verspaget HW (1994) Urokinase receptor and colorectal cancer survival. Lancet 344(8919):401–402
42. Torzewski M, Sarbia M, Verreet P et al (1997) Prognostic significance of urokinase-type plasminogen activator expression in squamous cell carcinomas of the esophagus. Clin Cancer Res 3(12 Pt 1):2263–2268
43. Nekarda H, Schlegel P, Schmitt M et al (1998) Strong prognostic impact of tumor-associated urokinase-type plasminogen activator in completely resected adenocarcinoma of the esophagus. Clin Cancer Res 4(7):1755–1763
44. Shiomi H, Eguchi Y, Tani T, Kodama M, Hattori T (2000) Cellular distribution and clinical value of urokinase-type plasminogen activator, its receptor, and plasminogen activator inhibitor-2 in esophageal squamous cell carcinoma. Am J Pathol 156(2):567–575
45. Hsu DW, Efird JT, Hedley-Whyte ET (1995) Prognostic role of urokinase-type plasminogen activator in human gliomas. Am J Pathol 147(1):114–123
46. Landau BJ, Kwaan HC, Verrusio EN, Brem SS (1994) Elevated levels of urokinase-type plasminogen activator and plasminogen activator inhibitor type-1 in malignant human brain tumors. Cancer Res 54(4):1105–1108
47. Gutova M, Najbauer J, Gevorgyan A et al (2007) Identification of uPAR-positive chemoresistant cells in small cell lung cancer. PLoS One 2(2), e243
48. Hataji O, Taguchi O, Gabazza EC et al (2004) Increased circulating levels of thrombin-activatable fibrinolysis inhibitor in lung cancer patients. Am J Hematol 76(3):214–219
49. Pavey SJ, Hawson GA, Marsh NA (2001) Impact of the fibrinolytic enzyme system on prognosis and survival associated with non-small cell lung carcinoma. Blood Coagul Fibrinolysis 12(1):51–58
50. Hofmann R, Lehmer A, Buresch M, Hartung R, Ulm K (1996) Clinical relevance of urokinase plasminogen activator, its receptor, and its inhibitor in patients with renal cell carcinoma. Cancer 78(3):487–492
51. Swiercz R, Wolfe JD, Zaher A, Jankun J (1998) Expression of the plasminogen activation system in kidney cancer correlates with its aggressive phenotype. Clin Cancer Res 4(4):869–877
52. Shariat SF, Roehrborn CG, McConnell JD et al (2007) Association of the circulating levels of the urokinase system of plasminogen activation with the presence of prostate cancer and invasion, progression, and metastasis. J Clin Oncol 25(4):349–355
53. Miyake H, Hara I, Yamanaka K, Gohji K, Arakawa S, Kamidono S (1999) Elevation of serum levels of urokinase-type plasminogen activator and its receptor is associated with disease progression and prognosis in patients with prostate cancer. Prostate 39(2):123–129
54. Hienert G, Kirchheimer JC, Pfluger H, Binder BR (1988) Urokinase-type plasminogen activator as a marker for the formation of distant metastases in prostatic carcinomas. J Urol 140(6):1466–1469
55. Kobayashi H, Fujishiro S, Terao T (1994) Impact of urokinase-type plasminogen activator and its inhibitor type 1 on prognosis in cervical cancer of the uterus. Cancer Res 54(24):6539–6548
56. Kuhn W, Schmalfeldt B, Reuning U et al (1999) Prognostic significance of urokinase (uPA) and its inhibitor PAI-1 for survival in advanced ovarian carcinoma stage FIGO IIIc. Br J Cancer 79(11–12):1746–1751
57. De Petro G, Tavian D, Copeta A, Portolani N, Giulini SM, Barlati S (1998) Expression of urokinase-type plasminogen activator (u-PA), u-PA receptor, and tissue-type PA messenger RNAs in human hepatocellular carcinoma. Cancer Res 58(10):2234–2239
58. Hackel CG, Krueger S, Grote HJ et al (2000) Overexpression of cathepsin B and urokinase plasminogen activator is associated with increased risk of recurrence and metastasis in patients with chondrosarcoma. Cancer 89(5):995–1003
59. Takeuchi Y, Nakao A, Harada A, Nonami T, Fukatsu T, Takagi H (1993) Expression of plasminogen activators and their inhibitors in human pancreatic carcinoma: immunohistochemical study. Am J Gastroenterol 88(11):1928–1933
60. Cantero D, Friess H, Deflorin J et al (1997) Enhanced expression of urokinase plasminogen activator and its receptor in pancreatic carcinoma. Br J Cancer 75(3):388–395
61. Lescaille G, Menashi S, Cavelier-Balloy B et al (2012) EMMPRIN/CD147 up-regulates urokinase-type plasminogen activator: implications in oral tumor progression. BMC Cancer 12:115
62. Keer HN, Gaylis FD, Kozlowski JM, Bauer KD, Sinha AA, Wilson MJ, Kwaan HC (1991) Heterogeneity in plasminogen activator (PA) levels in human prostate cancer cell lines: increased PA activity correlates with biologically aggressive behavior. Prostate 18(3):201–214
63. Gaylis FD, Keer HN, Wilson MJ, Kwaan HC, Sinha AA, Kozlowski JM (1989) Plasminogen activators in human prostate cancer cell lines and tumors: correlation with the aggressive phenotype. J Urol 142(1):193–198

64. Kirchheimer JC, Pfluger H, Ritschl P, Hienert G, Binder BR (1985) Plasminogen activator activity in bone metastases of prostatic carcinomas as compared to primary tumors. Invasion Metastasis 5(6):344–355
65. Dano K, Romer J, Nielsen BS, Bjorn S, Pyke C, Rygaard J, Lund LR (1999) Cancer invasion and tissue remodeling–cooperation of protease systems and cell types. APMIS 107(1):120–127
66. Kwaan HC, Keer HN, Radosevich JA, Cajot JF, Ernst R (1991) Components of the plasminogen-plasmin system in human tumor cell lines. Semin Thromb Hemost 17(3):175–182
67. Duffy MJ, O'Grady P, Devaney D, O'Siorain L, Fennelly JJ, Lijnen HJ (1988) Urokinase-plasminogen activator, a marker for aggressive breast carcinomas. Preliminary report. Cancer 62(3):531–533
68. Ossowski L, Russo-Payne H, Wilson EL (1991) Inhibition of urokinase-type plasminogen activator by antibodies: the effect on dissemination of a human tumor in the nude mouse. Cancer Res 51(1):274–281
69. Kobayashi H, Gotoh J, Shinohara H, Moniwa N, Terao T (1994) Inhibition of the metastasis of Lewis lung carcinoma by antibody against urokinase-type plasminogen activator in the experimental and spontaneous metastasis model. Thromb Haemost 71(4):474–480
70. Yu HR, Schultz RM (1990) Relationship between secreted urokinase plasminogen activator activity and metastatic potential in murine B16 cells transfected with human urokinase sense and antisense genes. Cancer Res 50(23):7623–7633
71. Wilhelm O, Schmitt M, Hohl S, Senekowitsch R, Graeff H (1995) Antisense inhibition of urokinase reduces spread of human ovarian cancer in mice. Clin Exp Metastasis 13(4):296–302
72. Soff GA, Sanderowitz J, Gately S, Verrusio E, Weiss I, Brem S, Kwaan HC (1995) Expresion of plasminogen activator inhibitor type 1 by human prostate carcinoma cells inhibits primary tumor growth, tumor-associated angiogenesis, and metastasis to lung and liver in san athymic mouse model. J Clin Invest 96(6):2593–2600
73. Pyke C, Ralfkiaer E, Ronne E, Hoyer-Hansen G, Kirkeby L, Dano K (1994) Immunohistochemical detection of the receptor for urokinase plasminogen activator in human colon cancer. Histopathology 24(2):131–138
74. Bianchi E, Cohen RL, Thor AT, Todd RF 3rd, Mizukami IF, Lawrence DA, Ljung BM, Shuman MA, Smith HS (1994) The urokinase receptor is expressed in invasive breast cancer but not in normal breast tissue. Cancer Res 54(4):861–866
75. de Vries TJ, Quax PH, Denijn M, Verrijp KN, Verheijen JH, Verspaget HW, Weidle UH, Ruiter DJ, van Muijen GN (1994) Plasminogen activators, their inhibitors, and urokinase receptor emerge in late stages of melanocytic tumor progression. Am J Pathol 144(1):70–81
76. Weidle UH, Wollisch E, Ronne E, Ploug M, Behrendt N, de Vries TJ, Quax PH, Verheijen JH, van Muijen GN, Ruiter DJ (1994) Studies on functional and structural role of urokinase receptor and other components of the plasminogen activation system in malignancy. Ann Biol Clin 52(11):775–782
77. Pedersen H, Grondahl-Hansen J, Francis D et al (1994) Urokinase and plasminogen activator inhibitor type 1 in pulmonary adenocarcinoma. Cancer Res 54(1):120–123
78. Bruckner A, Filderman AE, Kirchheimer JC, Binder BR, Remold HG (1992) Endogenous receptor-bound urokinase mediates tissue invasion of the human lung carcinoma cell lines A549 and Calu-1. Cancer Res 52(11):3043–3047
79. Kariko K, Kuo A, Boyd D, Okada SS, Cines DB, Barnathan ES (1993) Overexpression of urokinase receptor increases matrix invasion without altering cell migration in a human osteosarcoma cell line. Cancer Res 53(13):3109–3117
80. Harris L, Fritsche H, Mennel R et al (2007) American Society of Clinical Oncology 2007 update of recommendations for the use of tumor markers in breast cancer. J Clin Oncol 25(33):5287–5312
81. Annecke K, Schmitt M, Euler U et al (2008) uPA and PAI-1 in breast cancer: review of their clinical utility and current validation in the prospective NNBC-3 trial. Adv Clin Chem 45:31–45
82. Schmitt M, Harbeck N, Brunner N et al (2011) Cancer therapy trials employing level-of-evidence-1 disease forecast cancer biomarkers uPA and its inhibitor PAI-1. Expert Rev Mol Diagn 11(6):617–634
83. Thomssen C (2012) First planned efficacy analysis of the NNBC 3-Europe trial: addition of docetaxel to anthracycline containing adjuvant chemotherapy in high risk node-negative breast cancer patients. In: San Antonio breast cancer symposium, pp 1–1313
84. Jacobs VR, Kates RE, Kantelhardt E et al (2013) Health economic impact of risk group selection according to ASCO-recommended biomarkers uPA/PAI-1 in node-negative primary breast cancer. Breast Cancer Res Treat 138(3):839–850
85. Nienaber V, Wang J, Davidson D, Henkin J (2000) Re-engineering of human urokinase provides a system for structure-based drug design at high resolution and reveals a novel structural subsite. J Biol Chem 275(10):7239–7248
86. Jensen JK, Thompson LC, Bucci JC et al (2011) Crystal structure of plasminogen activator inhibitor-1 in an active conformation with normal thermodynamic stability. J Biol Chem 286(34):29709–29717
87. Lin Z, Jiang L, Yuan C et al (2011) Structural basis for recognition of urokinase-type plasminogen activator by plasminogen activator inhibitor-1. J Biol Chem 286(9):7027–7032

88. Xu X, Gardsvoll H, Yuan C, Lin L, Ploug M, Huang M (2012) Crystal structure of the urokinase receptor in a ligand-free form. J Mol biol 416(5):629–641
89. Huai Q, Mazar AP, Kuo A et al (2006) Structure of human urokinase plasminogen activator in complex with its receptor. Science 311(5761):656–659
90. Law RH, Caradoc-Davies T, Cowieson N et al (2012) The X-ray crystal structure of full-length human plasminogen. Cell Rep 1(3):185–190
91. Meyer JE, Brocks C, Graefe H et al (2008) The oral serine protease inhibitor WX-671 – first experience in patients with advanced head and neck carcinoma. Breast Care (Basel) 3(s2):20–24
92. Heinemann V, Ebert MP, Laubender RP, Bevan P, Mala C, Boeck S (2013) Phase II randomised proof-of-concept study of the urokinase inhibitor upamostat (WX-671) in combination with gemcitabine compared with gemcitabine alone in patients with non-resectable, locally advanced pancreatic cancer. Br J Cancer 108(4):766–770
93. Goldstein LJ, Oliveria CT, Heinrich B et al (2012) A randomized double-blindphase II study of the combination of WX-671 plus capecitabine vs. capecitabine monothrapry in first-line HER-2 negaive metastatic breast cancer (MBC). In: CTRC-AACR San Antonio breast cancer symposium, 5-20-01
94. Kriegbaum MC, Persson M, Haldager L et al (2011) Rational targeting of the urokinase receptor (uPAR): development of antagonists and non-invasive imaging probes. Curr Drug Targets 12(12):1711–1728
95. Wang F, Eric Knabe W, Li L et al (2012) Design, synthesis, biochemical studies, cellular characterization, and structure-based computational studies of small molecules targeting the urokinase receptor. Bioorg Med Chem 20(15):4760–4773
96. Gorantla B, Asuthkar S, Rao JS, Patel J, Gondi CS (2011) Suppression of the uPAR-uPA system retards angiogenesis, invasion, and in vivo tumor development in pancreatic cancer cells. Mol Cancer Res 9(4):377–389
97. Gondi CS, Rao JS (2009) Therapeutic potential of siRNA-mediated targeting of urokinase plasminogen activator, its receptor, and matrix metalloproteinases. Methods Mol Biol 487: 267–281
98. Van Buren G 2nd, Gray MJ, Dallas NA et al (2009) Targeting the urokinase plasminogen activator receptor with a monoclonal antibody impairs the growth of human colorectal cancer in the liver. Cancer 115(14):3360–3368
99. Rabbani SA, Ateeq B, Arakelian A et al (2010) An anti-urokinase plasminogen activator receptor antibody (ATN-658) blocks prostate cancer invasion, migration, growth, and experimental skeletal metastasis in vitro and in vivo. Neoplasia 12(10):778–788
100. Bauer TW, Liu W, Fan F et al (2005) Targeting of urokinase plasminogen activator receptor in human pancreatic carcinoma cells inhibits c-Met- and insulin-like growth factor-I receptor-mediated migration and invasion and orthotopic tumor growth in mice. Cancer Res 65(17):7775–7781
101. Kenny HA, Leonhardt P, Ladanyi A et al (2011) Targeting the urokinase plasminogen activator receptor inhibits ovarian cancer metastasis. Clin Cancer Res 17(3):459–471
102. Brooks TD, Wang SW, Brunner N, Charlton PA (2004) XR5967, a novel modulator of plasminogen activator inhibitor-1 activity, suppresses tumor cell invasion and angiogenesis in vitro. Anticancer Drugs 15(1):37–44
103. Binder BR, Mihaly J (2008) The plasminogen activator inhibitor "paradox" in cancer. Immunol Lett 118(2):116–124

Part III

Tumor Markers – A Critical Revision: Hormones

The Role of Human Chorionic Gonadotropin as Tumor Marker: Biochemical and Clinical Aspects

11

Lorenza Sisinni and Matteo Landriscina

Abstract

Tumor markers are biological substances that are produced/released mainly by malignant tumor cells, enter the circulation in detectable amounts and are potential indicators of the presence of a tumor. The most useful biochemical markers are the tumor-specific molecules, i.e., receptors, enzymes, hormones, growth factors or biological response modifiers that are specifically produced by tumor cells and not, or minimally, by the normal counterpart (Richard et al. Principles and practice of gynecologic oncology. Wolters Kluwer Health, Philadelphia, 2009). Based on their specificity and sensitivity in each malignancy, biomarkers are used for screening, diagnosis, disease monitoring and therapeutic response assessment in clinical management of cancer patients.

This chapter is focused on human chorionic gonadotropin (hCG), a hormone with a variety of functions and widely used as a tumor biomarker in selected tumors. Indeed, hCG is expressed by both trophoblastic and non-trophoblastic human malignancies and plays a role in cell transformation, angiogenesis, metastatization, and immune escape, all process central to cancer progression. Of note, hCG testing is crucial for the clinical management of placental trophoblastic malignancies and germ cell tumors of the testis and the ovary. Furthermore, the production of hCG by tumor cells is accompanied by varying degrees of release of the free subunits into the circulation, and this is relevant for the management of cancer patients (Triozzi PL, Stevens VC, Oncol Rep 6(1):7–17, 1999).

The name chorionic gonadotropin was conceived: chorion derives from the latin *chordate* meaning afterbirth, gonadotropin indicates that the hormone is a gonadotropic molecule, acting on the ovaries and promoting steroid production (Cole LA, Int J Endocrinol Metab 9(2):335–352, 2011).

L. Sisinni
Laboratory of Pre-Clinical and Translational Research, IRCCS, Referral Cancer Center of Basilicata, Rionero in Vulture, PZ, Italy

M. Landriscina (✉)
Clinical Oncology Unit, Department of Medical and Surgical Sciences, University of Foggia, Viale Pinto, 1, 71100 Foggia, Italy
e-mail: matteo.landriscina@unifg.it

R. Scatena (ed.), *Advances in Cancer Biomarkers*, Advances in Experimental Medicine and Biology 867, DOI 10.1007/978-94-017-7215-0_11

The function, the mechanism of action and the interaction between hCG and its receptor continue to be the subject of intensive investigation, even though many issues about hCG have been well documented (Tegoni M et al., J Mol Biol 289(5):1375–1385, 1999).

Keywords
Core fragment of hCGβ • Germ cell tumors • Gestational trophoblastic disease • HCG antibodies specificity • hCG biochemical structure • hCG biological functions • hCG determination • hCG in clinical practice • HCG in other non-trophoblastic cancer • hCG α-subunit • hCG β-subunit • hCGβcf

Abbreviation

hCGβcf Core fragment of hCGβ

11.1 Biochemical Structure

As we know today, hCG is a hormone with a molecular weight of approximately 36,000 Da, comprising a 92 amino acid α-subunit and a 145 amino acid β-subunit which are held together by non-covalent hydrophobic and ionic interactions (Fig. 11.1) [1, 2]. The α-subunit is common to all members of the glycoprotein hormone family, such as follicle stimulating hormone (FSH), thyroid stimulating hormone (TSH) and luteinizing hormone (LH). While both α and β-subunits are necessary for the binding to the receptor, the β-subunit is responsible for the specific activity of the hormone [3]. The hCG receptor, belonging to the same family as the G-protein receptors with seven transmembrane helices, plays a role in the specificity of the response: it is distinct from FSH, TSH, and LH receptors, and it is modulated by different physiological stimuli [4, 5]. Both α and β-subunits of hCG have two N-linked glycosylation sites (Asn-52 and -78 on the α-subunit and Asn-13 and -30 on the β-subunit) (Fig. 11.1a, b); in addition, four O-linked glycosylation sites are present at the Ser-rich C terminus of the β-subunit (Ser121, -127, -132, -138) (Fig. 11.1b). Thus, the β-subunit is responsible for the structural and the functional specific properties of the biologically active glycoprotein heterodimer of hCG.

Over the past decade, researches established that the trophoblast uses two independent pathways, involving villous and extravillous trophoblast cells, in order to produce three different hCG variants, all of them sharing the β-subunit, but characterized by different physiological functions and distinct roles in evolution: the native hCG, the hyperglycosylated form of hCG (hyp-hCG) and the free β-subunit (hCGβ) [6, 7]. The syncytyotrophoblast, that is generated from the villous trophoblast cells, produces regular hCG, while the extravillous invasive trophoblast produces hyp-hCG [8]. As above mentioned, 20–30 % of the total molecular weight of hCG is due to oligosaccharide side chains, this contributing to the structural difference between the different forms of hCG, for instance increasing the molecular weight of hyp-hCG to 41,000 Da as compared to 36,000 Da for native hCG [9, 10]. While native hCG has monoantennary (8 sugar residues) and biantennary (11 sugar residues) N-linked oligosaccharides, as well as trisaccharide O-linked oligosaccharides (3 sugar residues), hyp-hCG has larger fucosylated triantennary (15 sugars) N-linked oligosaccharides and double-size O-linked hexasaccharides (6 sugar residues) [11]. The free β-subunit of hCG represents the alternatively glycosylated monomeric variant of

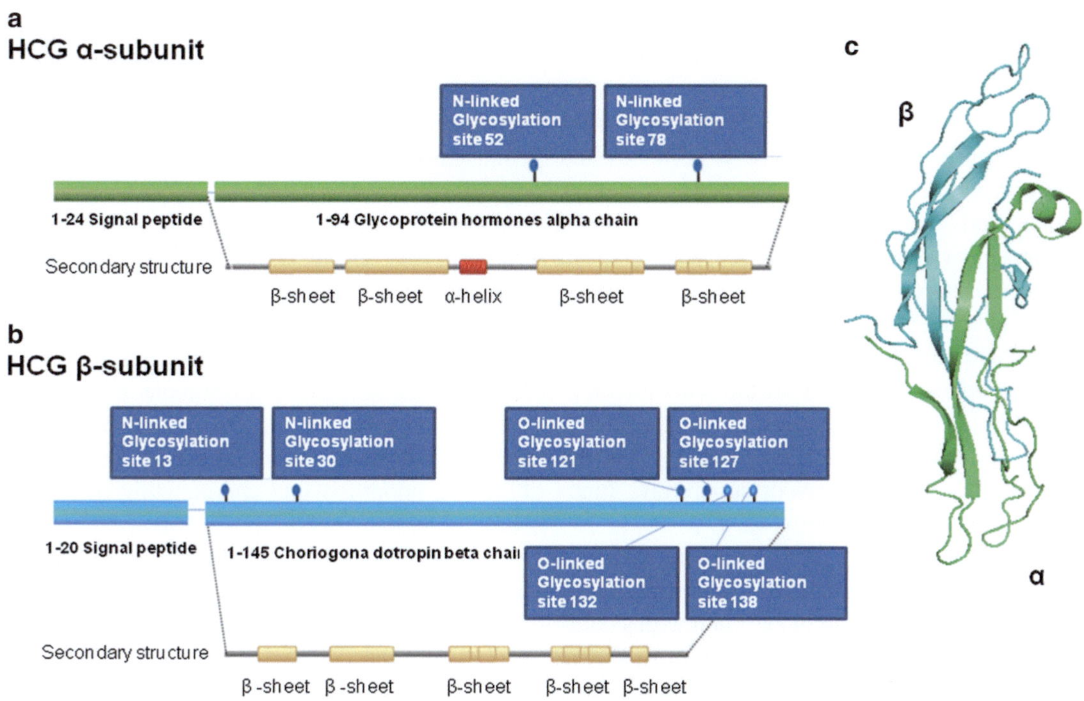

Fig. 11.1 Structural representation of hCG. (**a**). hCG α-subunit. The protein is subdivided in two parts: the signal peptide, that comprises amino acids 1–24, and the glycoprotein hormone (amino acids 1–94), corresponding at the mature protein. The N-linked glycosilation sites (52, 78) are indicated. The secondary structure includes 4 β-sheets and 1 α-helix. (**b**). hCG β-subunit. The protein is subdivided in two parts: the signal peptide, that comprises amino acids 1–20, and the chorionic gonadotropin (amino acids1-145), corresponding at the mature protein. The N-linked glycosilation sites (13, 30) and the O-linked glycosilation sites (121, 127, 132, 138) are indicated. The secondary structure shows that this subunit includes 5 β-sheets. (**c**). Ribbon diagram of hCG using the pdb code 1HCN. The α-subunit is indicated in green and the β-subunit in *light blue*. The secondary structural elements are labeled

hCG, generated by several non-trophoblastic malignancies [2, 8].

11.2 Biological Functions

The biological activity of hCG was first described at the beginning of the last century and further studied in the following decades [12–15]. Indeed, hCG is produced by trophoblast cells during the first weeks of pregnancy to take over from LH in promoting progesterone production by ovarian corpus luteal cells, preventing menstrual bleeding. The science of hCG has advanced in the last 10 years and we know today that hCG promotes progesterone production for only 3–4 weeks following pregnancy implantation and that this function is active for approximately 10 % of the length of pregnancy. Indeed, hCG reaches a peak after 10 weeks from gestation start, or almost 1 month after progesterone promotion is complete, then continues to be produced through the length of pregnancy [16].

Even though the most established function of hCG is progesterone promotion, we now know that hCG has also uterine, fetal and placental functions in pregnancy. From the time of implantation, for the subsequent 3 weeks, hCGs are produced by trophoblast cells to take over corpus luteal progesterone. Then, there are sufficient syncytiotrophoblast cells in the placenta to take over progesterone production from corpus luteal cells [16]. Several research groups have shown that hCG is also active in promoting angiogenesis and vasculogenesis in the uterus during pregnancy [15, 17, 18] and this insures maximal blood supply to the invading placenta and optimal nutrition to the fetus [19]. HCG treatment was shown to promote growth of pericytes and vascular endothelial cell *in vitro* [18], as well as retinal perivascular and endothelial cells [20], suggesting a role of hGC and its receptor in angiogenesis. In addition, hCG secreted by glial cell may influence the perivascular structure in normal and pathological conditions [20, 21].

HCG appears to be one of the numerous factors acting to prevent rejection of the fetoplacental tissue: several observations suggest that the hormone has an inhibitory or suppressive function on macrophage activity [22, 23].

As previously described, there are different variants of hCG with specific biological functions, produced by different cells and with a common hCG β-subunit. These variants includes hyp-hCG and free β-subunit, besides native hCG. Hyp-hCG is the principal variant of hCG produced in early pregnancy and comprises an average of 87 % of the total hCG produced in serum during the third week, 51 % during the fourth week and 43 % during the fifth week of gestation. Hyp-hCG levels then dwindle to <1 % of total hCG during the 2nd and 3rd trimesters of pregnancy. These data are consistent with hyp-hCG having a function in promoting implantation in early pregnancy [24, 25]. However, several authors reported additional functions specific for hyp-hCG. The evidence that hyp-hCG is involved in blocking apoptosis and likely metalloproteinase promoting activity suggests that hyp-hCG may be an antagonist of TGFβ receptor, thus controlling functions in cytotrophoblast cells. Other studies showed that hyp-hCG acts on choriocarcinoma cells (cancer of cytotrophoblast cells) promoting invasion [7, 24]. Indeed, hyp-hCG is the principal variant of hCG made by choriocarcinoma cells [7, 26], and its role in choriocarcinoma invasion has been demonstrated by independent groups, each showing that this molecules promotes migration and invasion of cancer cells in Matrigel chamber [24, 27, 28].

On the another hand, there is the free β-subunit of hCG that has a major role in non-gestational neoplasm carcinogenesis, as a promoter of either malignant transformation and poor patient's outcome. In such a context, the regulation of TGFβ receptor function is a key mechanism responsible for the role of the free β-subunit in tumor progression [29–32]: hCGβ is, indeed, produced by bladder cancer cells and inhibits TGFβ activity in bladder tumor cells [33], this leading to cancer growth and malignancy [22, 33]. Thus, both hyp-hCG and free β-subunit promote cancer cell growth and invasion [24, 26, 29, 31, 34–36], as well as both hCG variants function similarly by blocking apoptosis and antagonizing the TGFβ receptor signaling [28, 31, 35–38].

Major efforts are ongoing in order to use different hCG β-subunit derivatives as vaccines in the treatment of non-gestational malignancies. In such a perspective, preliminary achievements have been reported with anti-hCGβ immune responses improving cancer patient's outcome [39–43]. Indeed, the association of free β-subunit detection and poor prognosis, in combination with site specific hCG β-subunit vaccine technology, suggests a plausible route for the development of adjuvant cancer therapies specifically targeting patients with free β-subunit producing non-gestational tumors [16].

11.3 Clinical Use of hCG Determination in Clinical Practice

Understanding the complexity of the biology of these molecules, as well as the nuances of hCG testing are challenging, yet critical to practice management in oncology. As reported in the following paragraphs, hCG is a good marker of gestational trophoblastic malignancies and it is a key diagnostic and prognostic tool during the diagnosis and the follow-up of germ cell tumors. Indeed, the clinical use of hCG in gestational trophoblastic and germ cell diseases is strongly linked to the understanding of the respective role of hCG molecules in invasion and metastases formation. In addition, serum from many patients with non-trophoblastic tumors contains hCG-immunoreactivity, which, with few exceptions, consists of hCGβ, even though expression of native hCG occasionally occurs in various tumors. Elevated expression of hCGβ in serum, urine, or tumor tissues is a strong indicator of adverse prognosis in many non-trophoblastic tumors [44]. However, hCG and hCGβ are also expressed at low levels by many normal tissues. In such a scenario, sensitive and specific assays showed that both hCG and hCGβ can be detected at low concentrations in serum and urine from most men and non-pregnant women. Thus, the development of novel technologies to measure specific hCG variants (i.e., native hCG, hyp-hCG, hCGβ) in blood and urine has led to a better understanding of the changing spectrum of hCG clinical value in human trophoblastic and non-trophoblastic malignancies.

11.3.1 Gestational Trophoblastic Diseases

hCG is elevated in all cases of gestational trophoblastic disease (GTD) and serves as ideal tumor marker. GTDs are disorders of the pregnancy and include a spectrum of diseases from the potentially premalignant hydatidiform mole to the highly aggressive choriocarcinoma. All trophoblastic tumors produce hCG, and monitoring of therapy is largely based on the determination of hCG in serum [45]. Indeed, in these malignancies there is a close correlation between hCG levels and tumor burden, and hCG levels are used in staging and daily clinical management.

Hydatidiform moles are divided into two cytogenetically, morphologically, and clinically well characterized syndromes: i.e., complete and partial moles [46]. Indeed, both complete and partial hydatidiform mole is a pregnancy comprising solely placental tissue. In particular, in a complete hydatidiform mole there is the product of an empty ovum with no female haploid set, a diandrogenous fertilization leading to a diploid gestation composed entirely of hygromatous cysts of villous placental tissue. By contrast, a partial hydatidiform mole originates in an ovum with an inactive haploid set, a diandrogenous fertilization leading to a triploid gestation composed of villous trophoblastic and fetal elements [47]. Persistent trophoblastic disease may develop from both partial and complete moles. Choriocarcinoma is a malignancy of transformed cytotrophoblast cells, that occasionally can be associated with a complete mole. The cell transformation inhibits cytotrophoblast differentiation to syncytiotrophoblast cells, so the majority of cases are characterized by a predominance of malignant cytotrophoblast cells. Cytotrophoblast cells produce hCG β-subunit and/or hyp-hCG which drive tumor cell growth and invasion [24, 48, 49].

There is no better example of a tumor marker than total hCG in gestational trophoblastic diseases, being both the sensitivity and the specificity for trophoblast malignant tissues close to 100 %. The amount of hydatidiform mole or tumor tissue is directly proportional to the circulating concentration of total hCG. Hyp-hCG is also an absolute tumor marker of invasion and malignancy in invasive mole and choriocarcinoma.

Pharmacological therapy of choriocarcinoma is monitored by serial assays of hCG in serum until the levels are undetectable (or within the reference interval) and thereafter at regular time intervals for up to 2 years. During the follow-up, assay of hCG alone is mostly sufficient, but simultaneous determination of hCGβ can sometimes reveal a relapse earlier than hCG [50]. The half-life of hCGβ is longer than that of hCG [51], and therefore the hCGβ/hCG ratio will increase when the levels of hCG decrease after successful therapy.

Patients with molar disease are monitored with hCG determinations after evacuation of the mole to detect persistent trophoblastic disease. Serum hCG should be determined 48 h after tumor evacuation and every 1–2 weeks until the levels are undetectable. Follow-up determinations should be continued at 1- to 2-month intervals for 6–12 months. Deviation from the normal regression corridor indicates risk of persistent disease requiring chemotherapy [52]. In such a perspective, hCG represents an ideal marker for disease management and treatment decision. Indeed, chemotherapy is recommended if plateauing or rising hCG levels are observed in 3–4 consecutive samples taken during 2–3 weeks, but according to other recommendations, chemotherapy should be considered only if the hCG level is higher than 10,000 IU/l at 5 weeks, 1000 IU/l at 8 weeks, or detectable at 24 weeks [53].

Placental site trophoblastic tumor is a slowly growing and often treatment-resistant form of trophoblastic cancer that develops after pregnancy or molar disease, sometimes with a delay of years. The hCG levels are usually low in relation to tumor burden, but hCG determinations are essential for monitoring of this disease [54, 55].

11.3.2 Germ Cell Tumors

Serum hCG can also be detected in patients with non-trophoblastic cancers, being gynecologic cancers prominent in this group. In non-trophoblastic malignancies, the sensitivity of hCG is lower than for other markers in current clinical use, except in germ-cell tumors with a chorionic component.

Germ cell tumors, despite their rarity, constitute the most common cancer in males between the age of 15 and 35. This disease is highly curable, with long-term remissions being observed in more than 90 % of patients following treatment, whether by surgery, radiation therapy, chemotherapy, or a combination of them. Germ cell tumors comprise more than 90 % of the tumors arising in the testis and 20 % of those in the ovary. While 99 % of testicular germ cell tumors are malignant, more than 90 % of the ovarian ones are benign teratomas. Thus, malignant germ cell tumors are 6–10 times more common in the testis than in the ovary and gonadal tumors are also much more common than extragonadal ones [56, 57].

Testicular cancers are of two main types, seminomas and non-seminomatous germ cell tumors (NSGCT), which differ with respect to marker expression. More than 90 % of NSGCTs contain a mixture of various histological types, i.e., embryonal carcinoma, choriocarcinoma, teratoma, and yolk sac tumor, also-called endodermal sinus tumor [58, 59]. NSGCTs have a shorter survival compared to seminomatous cancers, due to the more aggressive behavior and the more complex therapeutic approach. In case of uncertain diagnosis, treatment imposed is generally that of nonseminomatous tumors that is based, depending on the stage, on systemic chemotherapy followed by retroperitoneal radiotherapy (or retroperitoneal linfectomy), in addition to the removal of the testis and the surrounding tissue.

Tissue expression of hCG is detected in syncytiotrophoblast cells of NSGCTs and in syncytiotrophoblastic components found in about 20 % of seminomas [59]. While hCG may be expressed by both seminomas and NSGCTs, high serum concentrations (>300–1000 IU/l) occur nearly exclusively in NSGCTs [60]. Indeed, elevated serum concentrations of hCG occur in 40–50 % of patients with NSGCT and 15–20 % of those with seminomas [61]. In addition, 20–40 % of seminoma patients have elevated serum levels of hCGβ alone [61, 62]. It is likely that the increase of hCG or hCGβ levels in seminomas is due to the presence of rare nonseminomatous elements.

Because of the higher reference limit for hCG respect to hCGβ (16 pmol/l for hCG vs. 2 pmol/l for hCGβ), tumors producing only hCGβ will be detected later by an assay measuring hCG and hCGβ together than by a specific hCGβ assay [62]. Thus, the independent evaluation of hCG and hCGβ may facilitate an earlier detection of a relapse of disease in monitoring testicular cancers. Furthermore, it is important to note that in the course of therapy hCG can give indications on the proliferation rate of the tumor, since a precise correlation between the value of the markers and tumor mass was not always observed, as chemotherapy may induce the block of synthesis and secretion of hCG, but not major effects on the growth of the tumor [63].

Among female germ cell tumors, dysgerminomas are more frequent, followed by endodermal sinus tumors, immature teratomas, mixed germ cell tumors, and embryonal carcinomas [64].

Immature teratomas and yolk sac tumors are common during early childhood, while dysgerminomas and mixed tumors are common in girls and young adults [57, 65]. Dysgerminomas often express hCG, this likely being the mechanism of precocious puberty in young girls bearing these malignancies [66, 67]. Other germ cell tumors, especially embryonal carcinomas, may also express hCG. Yolk sac tumors regularly produce α-fetoprotein (αFP) and only rarely hCG [58, 68].

11.3.2.1 Prognosis and Therapy

According to the TNM classification of germ cell tumors, strongly elevated concentrations of hCG, αFP, or lactic dehydrogenase (LDH) in serum are associated with adverse prognosis. Thus, these serum markers are used for staging and prognostic evaluation of testicular germ cell tumors [58, 69, 70]. A serum hCG concentration over 1000–10,000 IU/l is a strong negative prognostic factor, with a close correlation between risk of recurrence and marker serum levels [71, 72].

The levels of hCG (or αFP) are relevant in the daily clinical management of germ cell tumors. The curves of marker decline after surgery and/or during chemotherapy reflect the efficacy of the treatment [73, 74]. Indeed, upon removal of the primary tumor, a slow hCG decline is an indicator of residual disease and, thus, a criteria to start adjuvant chemotherapy [75]. Furthermore, in patients with metastatic disease and elevated marker levels, the serial evaluation of hCG is a critical decision tool. Indeed, the normal half-life of hCG is about 1.5 days and a half-life exceeding 3.5 days during chemotherapy is associated with increased probability of drug resistance and adverse prognosis. The half-time should be estimated during two cycles of chemotherapy using regression analysis of weekly determinations between days 7 and 56 [76]. Persisting marker elevation after chemotherapy indicates residual disease and the need for further therapy [58, 77, 78]. Furthermore, it is important to note that therapy may selectively destroy certain histological components of the tumor, and this may cause a shift in marker expression [79]. Therefore, multiple markers are used during follow-up even if only one (or no) marker is elevated before therapy. Indeed, about 70 % of the patients have elevated tumor markers at relapse [44, 68].

11.3.3 HCG in Other Non-trophoblastic Cancer

High concentrations of hCG have been observed in human tumors that do not derive from the trophoblastic tissue. In particular, carcinomas of the pancreas, ovary and breast may have hormone increases, this suggesting that the protein is produced by (i) the whole tumor cell population, or, more likely, (ii) a subclone of poorly-differentiated tumor cells. For this reason, it has been suggested that the stretch of DNA for the synthesis of hCG has phylogenetically very ancient origins [80].

Expression of hCG is observed in a variable proportion of many non-trophoblastic tumors. This immunoreactivity mainly consists of hCGβ, while hCG expression is rare [81–83]. In the past, most studies analyzed non-trophoblastic tumors by evaluating both hCG and hCGβ with the aim of measuring total hCGβ increase, even though some patients also have slightly elevated hCG levels [81]. Expression of hCG at the tissue level has been demonstrated by both radioimmunoassay on tissue extracts and immunohistochemistry on histological specimens [66, 84]. Expression of hCGβ has been demonstrated at the mRNA level by RT-PCR and sequencing both in normal and malignant tissues [44, 85].

11.3.3.1 Bladder Cancer

Among non-trophoblastic cancers, transitional cell carcinoma (TCC) of the bladder and urinary tract is the tumor in which hCG immunoreactivity has been more extensively evaluated. Studies in bladder cancer have shown that hCG production, while not diagnostic, is a very good indicator of poor prognosis through correlations with resistance to radiotherapy and rapid metastatic behavior. These clinical findings led to *in vitro* studies that have shown a direct proliferative activity of hCG on bladder carcinoma cell lines, this leading to inhibition of apoptosis and a parallel increase in cell population.

The frequency of elevated levels of hCG in TCCs ranges from 10 % to 75 %, depending on the type of patients, the laboratory assay, and the cut-off limit. Studies with specific assays showed that the immunoreactivity in serum consists of hCGβ, but moderate elevation of hCG has also been observed [83, 86, 87], and there are also rare cases of trophoblastic cancer in the bladder. Bladder cancer cell lines often express hCGβ, but expression has been observed both in malignant and "normal" urothelial cells [88].

11.3.3.2 Renal Cancer

Much evidence suggest that renal cell cancer is linked to increased hCG levels: data on high expression of hCG in renal cancer were first obtained by radioimmunoassay in concentrated urine [89] and by immunohistochemistry in tumor tissues [90]. A large study used a highly sensitive assay to demonstrate elevated serum levels of hCGβ in 23 % of patients with renal cell carcinoma. However, these authors failed in demonstrating a correlation between hormone expression and tumor stage and grade. Elevated serum levels have been proposed as an independent prognostic factor [91], even though the association between hCGβ expression and patient outcome was not confirmed by studies that evaluated hormone levels in tumor tissues by immunohistochemistry and/or RT-PCR [92].

11.3.3.3 Prostate Cancer

An early study reported hCG in the serum of one of 16 prostate cancer patients and the expression of hCG by immunohistochemistry in less than 10 % of prostatic adenocarcinomas. However, by using more sensitive methods, such as RT-PCR assay, hCGβ was detected both in normal and malignant prostatic tissues [93, 94]. Furthermore, increased hCG immunoreactivity was observed in the urine of few prostate cancer patients and the immunoreactive material in urine was found to consist of a low molecular form of hCG (i.e., hCGβ core fragment, hCGβcf,) [44, 95], comprising amino acids 6–40 and 55–92 linked together by disulfide bridges [96].

11.3.3.4 Gastrointestinal Cancers

Some patients with gastrointestinal cancer have been reported to have high serum concentrations of hCG, this finding suggesting that, within the context of these epithelial malignancies, there may be sporadic tumor cells expressing this hormone. The frequency of elevated hCG levels is highest in biliary (60 %), pancreatic (46 %), and gastric (40 %) carcinomas [81, 97], and less frequent in liver (20 %) [84, 97, 98] and colorectal (15 %) cancers [99, 100]. Furthermore, tissue expression of hCGβ has been detected in all gastrointestinal cancers and this finding is in agreement with the detection of hCGβ expression in many normal tissues of the gastrointestinal tract, and it may explain why slightly elevated circulating levels of hCG and hCGβ are occasionally observed in patients with benign diseases [82, 97].

Tissue expression or elevated serum levels of hCGβ have been found to be associated with adverse prognosis in most [98–100], but not all studies [101]. However, the correlation between tissue and serum expression is often weak, and in some studies, tissue expression has not been found to predict prognosis [101]. In such a scenario, several reports have shown that the production of hCG by tumor cells is associated with a more aggressive behavior in gastric cancers, and serum hCGβ appears to be an independent prognostic factor in this malignancy [44, 102]. The presence of hCG in cancer tissues has been demonstrated in some patients with colorectal cancers by immunohistochemistry. Indeed, the detection of a minority of hCG-positive cells in this cancer was associated with greater local invasion and the presence of lymph node and liver metastases [103]. Expression of hCG in hepatocellular cancer is rare [104, 105], but elevated serum levels may occur in advanced disease [83, 98].

11.3.3.5 Neuroendocrine Tumors

Since the majority of neuroendocrine tumors (NET) secretes peptides and amines, these are used as markers both for diagnosis and monitoring of therapy. In this context, an important marker is hCG α-subunit, which is particularly useful to determine the malignant potential of a NET, even though many NETs also express hCG β-subunit [106–108]. Non-functioning pituitary tumors and somatotroph adenomas often cause elevated serum levels of hCGα, as well as tissue expression of the α-subunit has been demonstrated in craniopharyngiomas [109–111]. However, comparative studies showed that chromogranin A and B are more useful markers respect to the hCG subunits [109, 110].

11.3.3.6 Lung Cancer

Evidence of hCG immunoreactivity has been frequently observed in cell lines from non-small cell lung carcinoma (NSCLC) and less often from small cell lung carcinoma (SCLC) [112]. HCG or its subunits are present in 72 % of NSCLCs, 10 % of SCLCs, one extrapulmonary small cell carcinoma, and carcinoid tumors, whereas related glycoprotein hormones are undetectable [112]. Interestingly, elevated urine levels of hCGβcf have been found in 49 % of the cases of NSCLCs, and studies on serum indicated that this was derived from hCGβ [113].

Tissue expression of hCG was observed in 30–80 % of lung tumors by immunohistochemistry [90, 114, 115]. In serum, hCGβ levels above 5 IU/l were detected in 12–14 % of small cell lung cancers and these were associated with short survival [116, 117]. Taken together, these results suggest that when measured by a sensitive assay, hCGβ serum levels might be clinically useful in the management of lung cancer [44].

11.3.3.7 Breast Cancer

The relationship between breast cancer and hCGβ expression has been widely investigated. Indeed, expression of hCGβ mRNA can be detected both in normal and malignant breast tissue by RT-PCR [118, 119]. Furthermore, between 10 % and 50 % of patients with breast cancer have been found to have slightly increased hCG-immunoreactivity in serum [84, 120–122]. However, clearly elevated levels are rare, and this finding has been ascribed to menopausal status and cross-reaction with LH in early radioimmunoassays. Thus, serum determinations have not been considered clinically useful [123, 124].

Several reports described very aggressive phenotypes where hCGβ has been detected, and lower response rates to radiotherapy and chemotherapy in breast cancer patients where hCGβ was elevated. However, when determined by sensitive and specific assays, hCGβ was found to be elevated in half of the patients with advanced disease but, like other tumor markers, changes in hCGβ levels did not reliably reflect the response to chemotherapy [125].

11.3.3.8 Gynecological Cancers

HCG-positive sera were found in 26.7 % of patients with benign and 67 % of patients with malignant ovarian tumors. Ovarian cancer tissue was positive for hCG expression in 68 % of cases and different studies identified significant differences in hCG tissue expression respect to tumor grade, but no differences with regard to the histological subtypes. However, immunoassays measuring hCG and hCGβ together have not been found to be useful in monitoring nontrophoblastic gynecological cancers.

The recent introduction of assays specific for hCGβcf in urine showed that expression of hCG-like molecules is common in nontrophoblastic gynecological tumors [126, 127]. Indeed, elevated urine levels of hCGβcf have been observed in preoperative samples from 20 % to 75 % of patients with various gynecological cancers with similar frequencies in ovarian, endometrial, cervical, and vulvovaginal carcinomas [96, 127–129]. Furthermore, elevated levels of hCGβcf in urine have also been reported to be predictive of adverse prognosis in vulvovaginal and cervical cancer. Finally, the combined use of hCGβcf in urine and CA125 in serum has been found to improve the diagnostic accuracy in ovarian cancer [130]. In spite of this, hCGβcf testing has not become a routine method apparently because variations in urinary flow rate adversely affect assay reliability [44].

11.3.3.9 Head and Neck Cancer

Head and neck cancer is the sixth most common type of cancer in the world. Histopathologically, squamous-cell carcinoma (SCC) is by far the most frequent variant of this disease. After curative treatment, about 50 % of the patients develop a recurrence, and 80 % of the relapses occur within the first 2 years of follow-up, this suggesting that a reliable tumor marker may be extremely useful in patients monitoring. hCGβ expression has been identified in 29 of 45 (64 %) of SCC from the oral cavity, indicating that hCGβ is produced by the majority of these tumors [131]. HCGβ was also investigated as a prognostic marker in patients with cancers of the oral cavity and oropharynx. Among different forms of SCC of the head and neck region, tumors of the oral cavity and oropharynx were particularly associated with poor prognosis and hCGβ was demonstrated to be an independent prognostic marker [132]. Thus, elevated hCGβ in serum may identify a high-risk subgroup of patients in these malignancies.

11.3.3.10 Retinoblastoma

Retinoblastoma account for 11 % of cancer cases in the first 4 years of life [133] and a link between retinoblastoma incidence and in vitro fertilization upon treatment with the gonadotropin hormone has been pointed out by several authors [21, 134–136]. In such a perspective, several preclinical observations support this hypothesis. Indeed, human retina produces this gonadotropin that acts as a neuroactive molecule [21], as well as Müller glial and retinal pigmented epithelial cells secrete hCG that affects neighbor cells expressing its receptor, namely cone photoreceptors. Furthermore, much evidence suggests that hCG receptor is expressed within the human retina. Using a rabbit antibody raised against the common receptor for luteinizing and gonadotropin hormones (LHR), researchers observed a diffused staining throughout the retina with an increased specific signal in cells located in the first rows of the photoreceptor layer and in structures of the outer plexiform layer, corresponding to the synaptic connection of the photoreceptors with the inner retina [21]. Furthermore, by using an anti-synaptophysin antibody to reveal synapses in the plexiform layer, Dukic-Stefanovic et al. observed the co-localization of the LHR and synaptophysin in large synaptic structures corresponding morphologically to cone [21]. Thus, altogether these observations suggest that cone photoreceptors strongly express LHR at their membrane. Finally, recent evidence suggests that Y79 retinoblastoma cells line, a cone precursor tumor, expresses the LHR and authors observed the hCG receptor concentrated at the cancer cell membrane [21]. When treated with hCG, Y79 cells showed an increase in proliferation rate, this suggesting a potential activity of hCG on retinoblastoma cells and a potential risk on the incidence of retinoblastoma due to gonadotropin use in women infertility treatment [21, 133]. However, other studies failed in establishing a clear link between hCG therapy and this specific type of cancer, even though an increased risk of pediatric cancers after infertility treatment have been globally demonstrated [134–136]. The discrepancy between these studies may be due to the low incidence of retinoblastoma (1 out of 15–20,000 children), leading to only few cases after infertility treatment [21].

11.4 Measurement of hCG

The expressions "β-hCG assay" or "hCG-beta assay" are misleadingly used to describe assays that measure both hCG and hCGβ. The International Federation of Clinical Chemistry and Laboratory Medicine (IFCC) recommends that assays should be exactly defined according to what they measure, for example, hCG and hCGβ separately or hCG + hCGβ together [137]. This issue in extremely relevant in the clinical setting, since the diagnostic value of hCG depends on the specificity and sensitivity of the method used for its detection. Based on the methodology, these assays can be distinguished in:

(a) Competitive, where there is a competition between molecules of hCG present in the sample to be evaluated and molecules of hCG added to the system in defined quantity.

The molecules may be labeled with radioactive iodine (isotope 125) or linked to solid particles (latex or erythrocytes).

(b) Non-competitive (sandwich), in which the assay is based on a secondary labeled antibody. This secondary antibody, linked to iodine 125 (IRMA), enzymes (IEMA, CLIA), or fluorescent molecules (IFMA) forms a sandwich with the first antibody, generally linked to a solid support (polystyrene of the tube, wells or beads), and the antigen (hCG) [138]. A particular application of the sandwich method was exploited for test strips with solid support for rapid diagnosis on urine. The various methods used can be both quantitative and qualitative. If the method is quantitatively, the results are expressed in international units respect to the volume, while if it is qualitatively, the result is considered positive whether it is above a threshold value. For diagnosis of pregnancy, qualitative detection methods on urine with rather small sensitivity and subsequent confirmation by quantitative methods are accepted. By contrast, the evaluation of hCG as tumor marker requires the use of quantitative methods on serum with high specificity and sensitivity [139].

11.4.1 HCG Antibodies Specificity

The antibodies to the hCG products can be divided into polyclonals and monoclonals. The polyclonal antibodies can be directed to: (a) the full length hCG, antibodies that cross-react with LH and often used for the measurement of LH, (b) the β subunit of hCG, and (c) the carboxyterminal peptide of hCG. Vaitukaitis et al. in [140] obtained antisera directed towards the β-subunit, with low cross-reactivity with the LH [140], using the subunit isolated and purified by Morgan [141]. By contrast, the carboxyterminal domain of hCG acts as an antigen only if joined to a large molecule, with the formation of antibodies recognizing the peptide bound to thyroglobulin.

The development of monoclonal antibodies to hCG has facilitated the design of assays specific for the various forms of hCG [81, 142–145]. The monoclonal antibodies, obtained from hybridomas of immunocompetent cells of mouse and human myeloma origin, have surely some advantages: (i) recognition of a single antigen with a specific constant affinity, (ii) conserved characteristics of the produced immunoglobulin, and (iii) disappearance of cross-reactivity with LH. There are numerous groups that have obtained preparations of monoclonal antibodies to the hCG. Indeed, 16 distinct antigenic regions have been defined: 5 epitopes are located on hCGα (α1–α5) and 7 on hCGβ (β1–β5, β7–β9).

Nearly all monoclonal antibodies recognize peptide epitopes and do not differentiate between hCG variants differing with respect to glycosylation [146]. The expression "hyp-hCG" is ambiguous, it was initially used to denote hCG containing complex carbohydrates [10], but it is also used to denote hCG measured by assays using antibody B152 [147]. Presently, virtually all commercial assays are based on the sandwich principle and use monoclonal or a combination of monoclonal and polyclonal antibodies [148].

Serum or plasma samples are used for quantitative hCG determination, while urine is mainly used for detection of hCG in pregnancy tests. The immunoreactivity measured by these assays in urine reflects those of hCG and hCGβ in plasma, and they have been widely used as cancer markers [82, 149, 150]. If pregnancy can be ruled out, an elevated serum level of hCG may be an indicator of cancer, even though unrecognized false positive results may lead to inappropriate therapy and serious complications. Low concentrations of hCG and its subunits can be detected in serum and plasma from healthy men and nonpregnant women. Pituitary secretion of hCG can be induced by gonadotropin releasing hormone, while estrogen treatment of postmenopausal women causes suppression of hCG production [151]. Thus, most of hCG detectable in normal serum is derived from the pituitary. Furthermore, the genes for both hCG subunits are expressed at low levels in the testis, breast, prostate, and skeletal muscle, but it is not known whether hCG expression in these tissues affects its serum levels. The serum concentrations of hCGβ are lower than those of hCG, and they do not increase with age [82]. In women, the postmenopausal levels of hCG (up to 5 IU/l corresponding to 16 pmol/l) are 5–10 times higher than those of hCGβ (<2 pmol/l). Therefore, assays measuring both forms together will not detect moderately elevated levels of hCGβ.

Low-level expression of hCGβ occurs in many tissues that do not express hCGα, i.e., bladder, adrenal, colon, thyroid, and uterus, but the mRNA levels are about 10,000-fold lower than those in the placenta. These tissues are potential sources of hCGβ in plasma of men and non-pregnant women, but their relative contribution is still unknown [152].

The concentrations for hCGβ are expressed in IU/l based on its own standard (3rd IS) [137], and, when measured by assays detecting hCGβ and hCG together, the values are based on the units for hCG. Different is the situation for hCG, because its concentration increases with the age in both women and men, being lower in men than in women. Depending on age, there are different reference values: the upper reference limit of hCG is 3–5 IU/l in women and 0.7–3 IU/l in men. However, several commercially available assays are poorly sensitive and there is notable variation in assay calibration. Therefore, an upper reference limit of 5–10 IU/l for hCG is used by many laboratories for both men and women.

Chemotherapy often causes suppression of gonadal function causing a "postmenopausal" condition with hCG levels up to 5–10 IU/l both in men and women. When necessary, testosterone therapy can be used to obtain suppression of the hCG level and, thus, identify this iatrogenic hCG elevation. HCG and hCGβ are excreted into urine, and the hCG concentrations are on average 50 % of those in plasma [153]. A major part of the hCG immunoreactivity in urine consists of hCGβcf [95, 126, 149, 154]. Reference values for various forms of hCG in urine have been published [81], but these depend on the specific method used. Because the protein concentrations in urine are highly dependent on urinary flow rate, urine measurements of hCG, hCGβ, and hCGβcf are not used for monitoring of cancer patients.

11.5 Conclusions

A complete understanding the complexity of the biology of hCG hormone is a prerequisite for its use as a tumor marker in practice management of cancer patients. As reported in this review, hCG is a good marker of gestational and non-gestational malignancies. Indeed, hCG testing plays a crucial role in the management of placental trophoblastic disease as well as in germ cell tumors of the testis and the ovary. Expression of hCGβ is also common in non-trophoblastic cancers, hCGβ in serum and hCGβcf in urine can be used to improve the diagnostic and prognostic accuracy for some tumors, even though its clinical use in non-trophoblastic diseases is far to be standardized. In this direction, several authors suggested a prognostic/predictive value for hCG or its variants in several non-trophoblastic tumors. Thus, new clinical studies need to be designed to evaluate the relevance of hCGβ in the stratification of patients for clinical trials and in the identification of tumors who might benefit from more aggressive therapy based on its prognostic value.

Acknowledgements This work was supported by grants from the Associazione Italiana per la Ricerca sul Cancro (AIRC, IG13128) and from the Italian Ministry of Health (GR-2010-2310057) to ML.

References

1. Bahl OP, Carlsen RB, Bellisario R, Swaminathan N (1972) Human chorionic gonadotropin: amino acid sequence of the alpha and beta subunits. Biochem Biophys Res Commun 48(2):416–422
2. Banerjee P, Fazleabas AT (2011) Extragonadal actions of chorionic gonadotropin. Rev Endocr Metab Disord 12(4):323–332
3. Pierce JG, Parsons TF (1981) Glycoprotein hormones: structure and function. Annu Rev Biochem 50:465–495
4. McFarland KC, Sprengel R, Phillips HS, Köhler M, Rosemblit N, Nikolics K, Segaloff DL, Seeburg PH (1989) Lutropin-horiogonadotropin receptor: an

unusual member of the G protein-coupled receptor family. Science 245(4917):494–499
5. Minegishi T, Nakamura K, Takakura Y, Miyamoto K, Hasegawa Y, Ibuki Y, Igarashi M, Minegish T (1990) Cloning and sequencing of human LH/hCG receptor cDNA corrected to Minegishi T. Biochem Biophys Res Commun 172(3):1049–1054
6. Handschuh K, Guibourdenche J, Tsatsaris V, Guesnon M, Laurendeau I, Evain-Brion D et al (2007) Human chorionic gonadotropin expression in human trophoblasts from early placenta: comparative study between villous and extravillous trophoblastic cells. Placenta 28(2–3):175–184
7. Cole LA (2010) Structures of free a-subunit and free b-subunit. In: Cole LA (ed) Human chorionic gonadotropin (hCG). Elsevier, Oxford
8. Handschuh K, Guibourdenche J, Tsatsaris V, Guesnon M, Laurendeau I, Evain-Brion D, Fournier T (2007) Human chorionic gonadotropin produced by the invasive trophoblast but not the villous trophoblast promotes cell invasion and is down-regulated by peroxisome proliferator-activated receptor-a. Endocrinology 148:5011–5019
9. Morgan FJ, Birken S, Canfield RE (1975) The amino acid sequence of human chorionic gonadotropin. The alpha subunit and beta subunit. J Biol Chem 250(13):5247–5258
10. Elliott MM, Kardana A, Lustbader JW, Cole LA (1997) Carbohydrate and peptide structure of the alphaand beta-subunits of human chorionic gonadotropin from normal and aberrant pregnancy and choriocarcinoma. Endocrine 7(1):15–32
11. Wu H, Lustbader JW, Liu Y, Canfield RE, Hendrickson WA (1994) Structure of human chorionic gonadotropin at 2.6 å resolution from MAD analysis of the selenomethionyl protein. Structure 2:545–558
12. Aschner B (1912) Ueber die function der hypophyse. Pflugers Arch Gesamte Physiol 146:1–147
13. Aschheim S, Zondek B (1927) Das Hormon des hypophysenvorderlappens: testobjekt zum Nachweis des hormons. Klin Wochenschr 6:248–252
14. Rao CV, Griffin LP, Carman FR Jr (1977) Prostaglandin F2 alpha binding sites in human corpora lutea. J Clin Endocrinol Metab 44:1032–1037
15. Rao CV (1979) Differential properties of human chorionic gonadotropin and human luteinizing hormone binding to plasma membranes of bovine corpora luteal. Acta Endocrinol 90:696–710
16. Cole LA (2010) Biological functions of hCG and hCG-related molecules. Reprod Biol Endocrinol 8:102
17. Toth P, Lukacs H, Gimes G, Sebestyen A, Pasztor N, Paulin F, Rao CV (2001) Clinical importance of vascular hCG/LH receptors – a review. Reprod Biol 1:5–11
18. Berndt S, Blacher S, d'Hauterive PS, Thiry M, Tsampalas M, Cruz A, Pequeux C, Lorquet S, Munaut C, Noel A, Foidart JM (2009) Chorionic gonadotropin stimulation of angiogenesis and pericyte recruitment. J Clin Endocrinol Metab 94:4567–4574
19. Licht P, Russu V, Wildt L (2001) On the role of human chorionic gonadotropin (hCG) in the embryo-endometrial microenvironment: implications for differentiation and implantation. Semin Reprod Med 19:37–47
20. Carmichael DN, Morgan NG, Scarpello JHB (1994) Human chorionic-gonadotropin stimulates the growth of retinal vascular cells. Diabetologia 38:A275
21. Dukic-Stefanovic S, Walther J, Wosch S, Zimmermann G, Wiedemann P, Alexander H, Claudepierre T (2012) Chorionic gonadotropin and its receptor are both expressed in human retina, possible implications in normal and pathological conditions. PLoS One 7(12), e52567
22. Akoum A, Metz CN, Morin M (2005) Marked increase in macrophage migration inhibitory factor synthesis and secretion in human endometrial cells in response to human chorionic gonadotropin hormone. J Clin Endocrinol Metab 90:2904–2910
23. Wan H, Marjan A, Cheung VW, Leenen PJM, Khan NA, Benner R, Kiekens RCM (2007) Chorionic gonadotropin can enhance innate immunity by stimulating macrophage function. J Leukoc Biol 82:926–933
24. Cole LA, Dai D, Butler SA, Leslie KK, Kohorn EI (2006) Gestational trophoblastic diseases: 1. Pathophysiology of hyperglycosylated hCG-regulated neoplasia. Gynecol Oncol 102:144–149
25. Sasaki Y, Ladner DG, Cole LA (2008) Hyperglycosylated hCG the source of pregnancy failures. Fertil Steril 89:1781–1786
26. Cole LA, Butler SA, Khanlian SA, Giddings A, Muller CY, Seckl MJ et al (2006) Gestational trophoblastic diseases: 2.Hyperglycosylated hCG as a reliable marker of active neoplasia. Gynecol Oncol 102:150–158
27. Lei ZM, Taylor DD, Gercel-Taylor C, Rao CV (1999) Human chorionic gonadotropin promotes tumorigenesis of choriocarcinoma JAR cells. Troph Res 13:147–159
28. Hamade AL, Nakabayashi K, Sato A, Kiyoshi K, Takamatsu Y, Laoag-Fernandez JB, Ohara N, Maruo T (2005) Transfection of antisense chorionic gonadotropin β gene into choriocarcinoma cells suppresses the cell proliferation and induces apoptosis. J Clin Endocrinol Metab 90:4873–4879
29. Cole LA, Perini F, Birken S, Ruddon RW (1984) An oligosaccharide of the O-linked type distinguishes the free from the combined form of hCG alpha-subunit. Biochem Biophys Res Commun 122:1260–1267
30. Khoo NK, Bechberger JF, Shepherd T, Bond SL, McCrae KR, Hamilton GS, Lala PK (1998) SV40 Tag transformation of the normal invasive trophoblast results in a premalignant phenotype I Mechanisms responsible for hyperinvasiveness and resistance to anti-invasive action of TGFβ. Intl J Cancer 77:429–439

31. Butler SA, Ikram MS, Mathieu S, Iles RK (2000) The increase in bladder carcinoma cell population induced by the free beta subunit of hCG is a result of an anti-apoptosis effect and not cell proliferation. Br J Cancer 82:1553–1556
32. Staun-Ram E, Shaleu E (2005) Human trophoblast function during implantation process. Reprod Biol Endocrinol 3:56
33. Butler SA, Staite EM, Iles RK (2003) Reduction of bladder cancer cell growth in response to hCG beta CTP37 vaccinated mouse serum. Oncol Res 14:93–100
34. Hoshina M, Boime I, Mochizuki M (1984) Cytological localization of hPL, hCG, and mRNA in chorionic tissue using in situ hybridization. Acta Obstet Gynaecol Jpn 36:397–404
35. Butler SA, Iles RK (2003) Ectopic human chorionic gonadotrophin β secretion by epithelial tumors and human chorionic gonadotrophin β-induced apoptosis in Karposi's sarcoma is there a connection? Clin Cancer Res 9:4666–4673
36. Iles RK (2007) Ectopic hCGβ expression by epithelial cancer: malignant behavior metastasis and inhibition of tumor cell apoptosis. Mol Cell Endocrinol 260:264–270
37. Carter WB, Sekharem M, Coppola D (2006) Human chorionic gonadotropin induces apoptosis in breast cancer. Breast Cancer Res Treat 100:S243–S244
38. Li D, Wen X, Ghali L, Al-Shalabi FM, Docherty SM, Purkis P, Iles RK (2008) hCGβ expression by cervical squamous carcinoma – in vivo histological association with tumor invasion and apoptosis. Histopathology 53:147–155
39. Moulton HM, Yoshihara PH, Mason DH, Iversen PL, Triozzi PL (2002) Active specific immunotherapy with b-human chorionic gonadotropin peptide vaccine in patients with metastatic colorectal cancer: antibody response is associated with improved survival. Clin Cancer Res 8:2044–2051
40. Iversen PL, Mourich DV, Moulton HM (2003) Monoclonal antibodies to two epitopes of b-human chorionic gonadotropin for the treatment of cancer. Curr Opin Mol Ther 5:156–160
41. Delves PJ, Roitt IM (2005) Vaccines for the control of reproduction–status in mammals and aspects of comparative interest. Dev Biol 121:265–273
42. Delves PJ, Iles RK, Roitt IM, Lund T (2007) Designing a new generation of antihCG vaccines for cancer therapy. Mol Cell Endocrinol 260:276–281
43. Guan QD, Wang Y, Chu YW, Wang LX, Ni J, Guo Q, Xiong SD (2007) The distinct effects of three tandem repeats of C3d in the immune responses against tumor-associated antigen hCGbeta by DNA immunization. Cancer Immunol Immunother 56: 875–884
44. Stenman U-H, Alfthan H, Hotakainen K (2004) Human chorionic gonadotropin in cancer. Clin Biochem 37:549–561
45. Bagshawe KD (1992) Choriocarcinoma. A model for tumor markers. Acta Oncol 31:99–106
46. Fisher RA (1993) Newlands ES. Rapid diagnosis and classification of hydatidiform moles with polymerase chain reaction. Am J Obstet Gynecol 168:563–569
47. Szulman AE, Surti U (1982) The syndromes of hydatidiform mole: I. Cytogenetic and morphologic correlations. Am J Obstet Gynecol 131:665
48. Cole LA, Khanlian SA, Riley JM, Butler SA (2006) Hyperglycosylated hCG (hCG-H) in gestational implantation, and in choriocarcinoma and testicular germ cell malignancy tumorigenesis. J Reprod Med 51:919–929
49. Cole LA, Butler SA (2008) Hyperglycosylated hCG and its free β-subunit, tumor markers and tumor promoters: a review. J Reprod Med 53:499–510
50. Vartiainen J, Alfthan H, Lehtovirta P, Stenman U-H (1998) Identification of choriocarcinoma by the hCG beta-to-hCG proportion in patients with delayed diagnosis caused by contraceptive use. Contraception 57:257–260
51. Korhonen J, Alfthan H, Ylostalo P, Veldhuis J, Stenman U-H (1997) Disappearance of human chorionic gonadotropin and its alpha- and beta-subunits after term pregnancy. Clin Chem 43:2155–2163
52. Yedema KA, Verheijen RH, Kenemans P, Schijf CP, Borm GF, Segers MF et al (1993) Identification of patients with persistent trophoblastic disease by means of a normal human chorionic gonadotropin regression curve. Am J Obstet Gynecol 168: 787–792
53. Matsui H, Iitsuka Y, Yamazawa K, Tanaka N, Mitsuhashi A, Seki K et al (2003) Criteria for initiating chemotherapy in patients after evacuation of hydatidiform mole. Tumour Biol 24:140–146
54. Feltmate CM, Genest DR, Goldstein DP, Berkowitz RS (2002) Advances in the understanding of placental site trophoblastic tumor. J Reprod Med 47:337–341
55. Papadopoulos AJ, Foskett M, Seckl MJ, McNeish I, Paradinas FJ, Rees H et al (2002) Twenty-five years' clinical experience with placental site trophoblastic tumors. J Reprod Med 47:460–464
56. Talerman A (1985) Germ cell tumours. Ann Pathol 5:145–157
57. Mayordomo JI, Paz-Ares L, Rivera F, Lopez-Brea M, Lopez Martin E, Mendiola C et al (1994) Ovarian and extragonadal malignant germ-cell tumors in females: a single-institution experience with 43 patients. Ann Oncol 5:225–231
58. Bosl GJ, Motzer RJ (1997) Testicular germ-cell cancer. N Engl J Med 337:242–253
59. Mostofi FK, Sesterhenn IA, Davis CJ Jr (1988) Developments in histopathology of testicular germ cell tumors. Semin Urol 6:171–188
60. Ruther U, Rothe B, Grunert K, Bader H, Sessler R, Nunnensiek C et al (1994) Role of human chorionic gonadotropin in patients with pure seminoma. Eur Urol 26:129–133

61. Mann K, Saller B, Hoermann R (1993) Clinical use of HCG and hCG beta determinations. Scand J Clin Lab Invest Suppl 216:97–104
62. Saller B, Clara R, Spottl G, Siddle K, Mann K (1990) Testicular cancer secretes intact human choriogonadotropin (hCG) and its free betasubunit: evidence that hCG (+hCG-beta) assays are the most reliable in diagnosis and follow-up. Clin Chem 36:234–239
63. Braunstein GD (1979) Use of chorionic gonadotropin as a tumor marker in cancer. In: Herberman RB, McIntire KR (eds) Immunodiagnosis of cancer. Marcel Dekker Inc, New York, pp 383–409
64. Zalel Y, Piura B, Elchalal U, Czernobilsky B, Antebi S, Dgani R (1996) Diagnosis and management of malignant germ cell ovarian tumors in young females. Int J Gynaecol Obstet 55:1–10
65. Harms D, Janig U (1986) Germ cell tumours of childhood. Report of 170 cases including 59 pure and partial yolk-sac tumours. Virchows Arch A Pathol Anat Histopathol 409:223–239
66. Kurman RJ, Norris HJ (1976) Embryonal carcinoma of the ovary: a clinicopathologic entity distinct from endodermal sinus tumor resembling embryonal carcinoma of the adult testis. Cancer 38:2420–2433
67. Roger M, Chaussain JL, Blacker C, Feinstein MC (1984) Tumors secreting choriogonadotropin in children. Ann Med Intern (Paris) 135:381–384
68. Stenman U-H, Alfthan H (2002) Markers for testicular cancer. In: Diamandis E, Fritsche H, Lilja H, Chan D, Schwartz M (eds) Tumor markers. Physiology, pathobiology, technology, and clinical applications. AACC Press, Washington, DC, pp 351–359
69. Sobin L, Wittekind C (1997) TNM classification of malignant tumors, 5th edn. Wiley-Liss, New York
70. Sturgeon CM, Duffy MJ, Stenman UH et al (2008) National academy of clinical biochemistry laboratory medicine practice guidelines for use of tumor markers in testicular, prostate, colorectal, breast, and ovarian cancers. Clin Chem 54(12):e11–e79
71. Vogelzang NJ (1987) Prognostic factors in metastatic testicular cancer. Int J Androl 10:225–237
72. Mead GM, Stenning SP (1993) Prognostic factors in metastatic non-seminomatous germ cell tumours: the medical research council studies. Eur Urol 23:196–200
73. Kohn J (1978) The dynamics of serum alphafetoprotein in the course of testicular teratoma. Scand J Immunol 8(Suppl 8):103
74. Lange PH, Vogelzang NJ, Goldman A, Kennedy BJ, Fraley EE (1982) Marker half-life analysis as a prognostic tool in testicular cancer. J Urol 128:708–711
75. Pierotti MA, van Harten W, Licitra L, Lombardo C (2011) European options and recommendations for cancer diagnosis and therapy, 1st edn. Organisation of European Cancer Institutes European Economic Interest Grouping Publisher, OECI-EEIG Reg. , Brussels
76. Mazumdar M, Bajorin DF, Bacik J, Higgins G, Motzer RJ, Bosl GJ (2001) Predicting outcome to chemotherapy in patients with germ cell tumors: the value of the rate of decline of human chorionic gonadotrophin and alpha-fetoprotein during therapy. J Clin Oncol 19:2534–2541
77. Coogan CL, Foster RS, Rowland RG, Bihrle R, Smith ER Jr, Einhorn LH et al (1997) Postchemotherapy retroperitoneal lymph node dissection is effective therapy in selected patients with elevated tumor markers after primary chemotherapy alone. Urology 50:957–962
78. Toner G (1990) Serum tumor-marker half-life during chemotherapy allows early prediction of complete response and survival in nonseminomatous germ cell tumors. Cancer Res 50:5904–5910
79. Czaja JT, Ulbright TM (1992) Evidence for the transformation of seminoma to yolk sac tumor, with histogenetic considerations. Am J Clin Pathol 97:468–477
80. Banfi G, Casari E, Murone M, Bonini P (1990) La coriogonadotropina umana. Medical systems S.P.A
81. Alfthan H, Haglund C, Dabek J, Stenman U-H (1992) Concentrations of human chorionic gonadotropin, its h-subunit and the core fragment of the h-subunit in serum and urine of men and nonpregnant women. Clin Chem 38:1981–1987
82. Alfthan H, Haglund C, Roberts P, Stenman U-H (1992) Elevation of free h-subunit of human choriogonadotropin and core h fragment of human choriogonadotropin in the serum and urine of patients with malignant pancreatic and biliary disease. Cancer Res 52:4628–4633
83. Marcillac I, Troalen F, Bidart JM, Ghillani P, Ribrag V, Escudier B et al (1992) Free human chorionic gonadotropin beta subunit in gonadal and nongonadal neoplasms. Cancer Res 52:3901–3907
84. Braunstein GD, Vaitukaitis JL, Carbone PP, Ross GT (1973) Ectopic production of human chorionic gonadotrophin by neoplasms. Ann Intern Med 78:39–45
85. Lazar V, Diez SG, Laurent A, Giovangrandi Y, Radvanyi F, Chopin D et al (1995) Expression of human chorionic gonadotropin beta subunit genes in superficial and invasive bladder carcinomas. Cancer Res 55:3735–3738
86. Crawford RA, Iles RK, Carter PG, Caldwell CJ, Shepherd JH, Chard T (1998) The prognostic significance of beta human chorionic gonadotrophin and its metabolites in women with cervical carcinoma. J Clin Pathol 51:685–688
87. Hotakainen K, Ljungberg B, Paju A, Rasmuson T, Alfthan H, Stenman UH (2002) The free betasubunit of human chorionic gonadotropin as a prognostic factor in renal cell carcinoma. Br J Cancer 86:185–189
88. Iles RK, Chard T (1989) Immunochemical analysis of the human chorionic gonadotrophin-like material secreted by 'normal' and neoplastic urothelial cells. J Mol Endocrinol 2:107–112
89. Fukutani K, Libby JM, Panko WB, Scardino PT (1983) Human chorionic gonadotropin detected in

urinary concentrates from patients with malignant tumors of the testis, prostate, bladder, ureter and kidney. J Urol 129:74–77
90. Kuida CA, Braunstein GD, Shintaku P, Said JW (1988) Human chorionic gonadotropin expression in lung, breast, and renal carcinomas. Arch Pathol Lab Med 112:282–285
91. Hotakainen K, Haglund C, Paju A, Nordling S, Alfthan H, Rintala E et al (2002) Chorionic gonadotropin beta-subunit and core fragment in bladder cancer: mRNA and protein expression in urine, serum and tissue. Eur Urol 41:677–685
92. Hotakainen K, Ljungberg B, Haglund C, Nordling S, Paju A, Stenman UH (2003) Expression of the free beta-subunit of human chorionic gonadotropin in renal cell carcinoma: prognostic study on tissue and serum. Int J Cancer 104:631–635
93. Purnell DM, Heatfield BM, Trump BF (1984) Immunocytochemical evaluation of human prostatic carcinomas for carcinoembryonic antigen, nonspecific cross-reacting antigen, beta- chorionic gonadotrophin, and prostate-specific antigen. Cancer Res 44:285–292
94. Span PN, Thomas CM, Heuvel JJ, Bosch RR, Schalken JA, vd Locht L et al (2002) Analysis of expression of chorionic gonadotrophin transcripts in prostate cancer by quantitative Taqman and a modified molecular beacon RT-PCR. J Endocrinol 172:489–495
95. Papapetrou PD, Sakarelou NP, Braouzi H, Fessas P (1980) Ectopic production of human chorionic gonadotropin (hCG) by neoplasms: the value of measurements of immunoreactive hCG in the urine as a screening procedure. Cancer 45:2583–2592
96. Birken S, Agosto G, Amr S, Nisula B, Cole L, Lewis J et al (1988) Characterization of antisera distinguishing carbohydrate structures in the beta-carboxyl-terminal region of human chorionic gonadotropin. Endocrinology 122:2054–2063
97. Louhimo J, Carpelan-Holmstrom M, Alfthan H, Stenman U-H, Jarvinen HJ, Haglund C (2002) Serum HCG beta, CA 72-4 and CEA are independent prognostic factors in colorectal cancer. Int J Cancer 101:545–548
98. Louhimo J, Finne P, Alfthan H, Stenman U-H, Haglund C (2002) Combination of hCGb, CA 19-9 and CEA with logistic regression improves accuracy in gastrointestinal malignancies. Anticancer Res 22:1759–1764
99. Carpelan-Holmström M, Haglund C, Lundin J, Alfthan H, Stenman U-H, Roberts P (1996) Independent prognostic value of preoperative serum markers CA 242, specific tissue polypeptide antigen and human chorionic gonadotrophin beta, but not of carcinoembryonic antigen or tissue polypeptide antigen in colorectal cancer. Br J Cancer 74:925–929
100. Lundin M, Nordling S, Lundin J, Alfthan H, Stenman UH, Haglund C (2001) Tissue expression of human chorionic gonadotropin beta predicts outcome in colorectal cancer: a comparison with serum expression. Int J Cancer 95:18–22
101. Webb A, Scott-Mackie P, Cunningham D, Norman A, Andreyev J, O'Brien M et al (1995) The prognostic value of CEA, beta HCG, AFP, CA125, CA19-9 and C-erb B-2, beta HCG immunohistochemistry in advanced colorectal cancer. Ann Oncol 6:581–587
102. Louhimo J, Kokkola A, Alfthan H, Stenman UH, Haglund C (2004) Preoperative hCGbeta and CA 72-4 are independent prognostic factors in gastric cancer. Int J Cancer 111(6):929–933
103. Yamaguchi A, Ishida T, Nishimura G, Kumaki T, Katoh M, Kosaka T, Yonemura Y, Miyazaki I (1989) Human chorionic gonadotropin in colorectal cancer and its relationship to prognosis. Br J Cancer 60(3):382–384
104. Zseli J, Csillag J, Tulassay Z, Tarjan G, Moksony I (1984) Gonadotropinsecreting liver cancer in ulcerative colitis. Wien Klin Wochenschr 96:5–8
105. Louhimo J, Nordling S, Alfthan H, von Boguslawski K, Stenman U-H, Haglund C (2001) Specific staining of hCGh in benign and malignant gastrointestinal tissue with monoclonal antibodies. Histopathology 38:418–424
106. Kahn CR, Rosen SW, Weintraub BD, Fajans SS, Gorden P (1977) Ectopic production of chorionic gonadotropin and its subunits by islet-cell tumors. A specific marker for malignancy. N Engl J Med 297:565–569
107. Oberg K, Wide L (1981) hCG and hCG subunits as tumour markers in patients with endocrine pancreatic tumours and carcinoids. Acta Endocrinol (Copenh) 98:256–260
108. Grossmann M, Trautmann ME, Poertl S, Hoermann R, Berger P, Arnold R et al (1994) Alpha-subunit and human chorionic gonadotropinbeta immunoreactivity in patients with malignant endocrine gastroenteropancreatic tumours. Eur J Clin Invest 24:131–136
109. Ridgway EC, Klibanski A, Ladenson PW, Clemmons D, Beitins IZ, McArthur JW et al (1981) Pure alpha-secreting pituitary adenomas. N Engl J Med 304:1254–1259
110. Oppenheim DS, Kana AR, Sangha JS, Klibanski A (1990) Prevalence of alpha-subunit hypersecretion in patients with pituitary tumors: clinically nonfunctioning and somatotroph adenomas. J Clin Endocrinol Metab 70:859–864
111. Tachibana O, Yamashima T, Yamashita J, Takabatake Y (1994) Immunohistochemical expression of human chorionic gonadotropin and pglycoprotein in human pituitary glands and craniopharyngiomas. J Neurosurg 80:79–84
112. Bepler G, Jaques G, Oie HK, Gazdar AF (1991) Human chorionic gonadotropin and related glycoprotein hormones in lung cancer cell lines. Cancer Lett 58(1-2):145–150
113. Yoshimura M, Nishimura R, Murotani A, Miyamoto Y, Nakagawa T, Hasegawa K et al (1994) Assessment

of urinary beta-core fragment of human chorionic gonadotropin as a new tumor marker of lung cancer. Cancer 73:2745–2752
114. Wilson TS, McDowell EM, McIntire KR, Trump BF (1981) Elaboration of human chorionic gonadotropin by lung tumors: an immunocytochemical study. Arch Pathol Lab Med 105:169–173
115. Slodkowska J, Szturmowicz M, Rudzinski P, Giedronowicz D, Sakowicz A, Androsiuk W et al (1998) Expression of CEA and trophoblastic cell markers by lung carcinoma in association with histological characteristics and serum marker levels. Eur J Cancer Prev 7:51–60
116. Szturmowicz M, Wiatr E, Sakowicz A, Slodkowska J, Roszkowski K, Filipecki S et al (1995) The role of human chorionic gonadotropin beta subunit elevation in small-cell lung cancer patients. J Cancer Res Clin Oncol 121:309–312
117. Szturmowicz M, Slodkowska J, Zych J, Rudzinski P, Sakowicz A, Rowinska-Zakrzewska E (1999) Frequency and clinical significance of beta- subunit human chorionic gonadotropin expression in non-small cell lung cancer patients. Tumour Biol 20:99–104
118. Bieche I, Lazar V, Nogues C, Poynard T, Giovangrandi Y, Bellet D et al (1998) Prognostic value of chorionic gonadotropin beta gene transcripts in human breast carcinoma. Clin Cancer Res 4:671–676
119. Span PN, Manders P, Heuvel JJ, Thomas CM, Bosch RR, Beex LV et al (2003) Molecular beacon reverse transcription-PCR of human chorionic gonadotropin-beta-3,-5, and-8 mRNAs has prognostic value in breast cancer. Clin Chem 49:1074–1080
120. Tormey DC, Waalkes TP, Simon RM (1977) Biological markers in breast carcinoma: II. Clinical correlations with human chorionic gonadotrophin. Cancer 39:2391–2396
121. Castro A, Buschbaum P, Nadji M, Voigt W, Tabei S, Morales A (1979) Ectopic human chorionic gonadotropin in breast carcinoma. Experientia 35:1392–1393
122. Caffier H, Brandau H (1983) Serum tumor markers in metastatic breast cancer and course of disease. Cancer Detect Prev 6:451–457
123. Borkowski A, Puttaert V, Gyling M, Muquardt C, Body JJ (1984) Human chorionic gonadotropin-like substance in plasma of normal nonpregnant subjects and women with breast cancer. J Clin Endocrinol Metab 58:1171–1178
124. Monteiro JC, Ferguson KM, McKinna JA, Greening WP, Neville AM (1984) Ectopic production of human chorionic gonadotrophin-like material by breast cancer. Cancer 53:957–962
125. Sjöström J, Alfthan H, Joensuu H, Stenman UH, Lundin J, Blomqvist C (2001) Serum tumour markers CA 15-3, TPA, TPS, hCGbeta and TATI in the monitoring of chemotherapy response in metastatic breast cancer. Scand J Clin Lab Invest 61:431–441
126. Birken S, Armstrong EG, Kolks MA, Cole LA, Agosto GM, Krichevsky A et al (1988) Structure of the human chorionic gonadotropin beta-subunit fragment from pregnancy urine. Endocrinology 123:572–583
127. Carter PG, Iles RK, Neven P, Ind TE, Shepherd JH, Chard T (1994) The prognostic significance of urinary beta core fragment in premenopausal women with carcinoma of the cervix. Gynecol Oncol 55:271–276
128. Alberti C, Sacchini P, Coltellini P (1990) Occult carcinoma in urology. Nosografy and diagnosis. Minerva Urol Nefrol 42:85–93
129. Schwartz BF, Auman R, Peretsman SJ, Moul JW, Deshon GE, Hernandez J et al (1996) Prognostic value of BHCG and local tumorinvasion in stage I seminoma of the testis. J Surg Oncol 61:131–133
130. Kinugasa M, Nishimura R, Koizumi T, Morisue K, Higashida T, Natazuka T et al (1995) Combination assay of urinary beta-core fragment of human chorionic gonadotropin with serum tumor markers in gynecologic cancers. Jpn J Cancer Res 86:783–789
131. Bhalang K, Kafrawy AH, Miles DA (1999) Immunohistochemical study of the expression of human chorionic gonadotropin-beta in oral squamous cell carcinoma. Cancer 85:757–762
132. Hedstrom J, Grenman R, Ramsay H, Finne P, Lundin J, Haglund C et al (1999) Concentration of free hCGbeta subunit in serum as a prognostic marker for squamous-cell carcinoma of the oral cavity and oropharynx. Int J Cancer 84:525–528
133. Abramson DH, Schefler AC (2004) Update on retinoblastoma. Retina 24:828–848
134. Anteby I, Cohen E, Anteby E, BenEzra D (2001) Ocular manifestations in children born after in vitro fertilization. Arch Ophthalmol 119:1525–1529
135. Marees T, Dommering CJ, Imhof SM, Kors WA, Ringens PJ et al (2009) Incidence of retinoblastoma in Dutch children conceived by IVF: an expanded study. Hum Reprod 24:3220–3224
136. Moll AC, Imhof SM, Cruysberg JR, Schouten-van Meeteren AY, Boers M (2003) Incidence of retinoblastoma in children born after in-vitro fertilisation. Lancet 361:309—310
137. Stenman U-H, Bidart JM, Birken S, Mann K, Nisula B, O'Connor J (1993) Standardization of protein immunoprocedures. Choriogonadotropin (CG). Scand J Clin Lab Invest 216(Suppl):42–78
138. Vaitukaitis JL (1977) Human chorionic gonadotropin. In: Fuchs F, Klopper A (eds) Endocrinology of pregnancy. Harper and Row, New York
139. Hussa RO, Rinke ML, Schweitzer PG (1985) Discordant human chorionic gonadotropin results, causes and solutions. Obstet Gynecol 65:211
140. Vaitukaitis JL, Braunstein GD, Ross GT (1972) A radioimmunoassay which specifically measures

human chorionic gonadotropin in the presence of human luteinizing hormone. Am J Obstet Gynecol 113:751–758

141. Morgan FJ, Canfield RE (1971) Nature of the subunits of human chorionic gonadotropin. Endocrinology 88:1045
142. Bidart JM, Ozturk M, Bellet DH, Jolivet M, Gras-Masse H, Troalen F et al (1985) Identification of epitopes associated with hCG and the beta hCG carboxyl terminus by monoclonal antibodies produced against a synthetic peptide. J Immunol 134:457–464
143. Ehrlich PH, Moustafa ZA, Krichevsky A, Birken S, Armstrong EG, Canfield RE (1985) Characterization and relative orientation of epitopes for monoclonal antibodies and antisera to human chorionic gonadotropin. Am J Reprod Immunol Microbiol 8:48–54
144. Norman RJ, Poulton T, Gard T, Chard T (1985) Monoclonal antibodies to human chorionic gonadotropin: implications for antigenic mapping, immunoradiometric assays, and clinical applications. J Clin Endocrinol Metab 61:1031–1038
145. Schwarz S, Berger P, Wick G (1985) Epitope-selective, monoclonal-antibody-based immunoradiometric assays of predictable specificity for differential measurement of choriogonadotropin and its subunits. Clin Chem 31:1322–1328
146. Schwarz S, Krude H, Klieber R, Dirnhofer S, Lottersberger C, Merz WE et al (1991) Number and topography of epitopes of human chorionic gonadotropin (hCG) are shared by desialylated and deglycosylated hCG. Mol Cell Endocrinol 80:33–40
147. Birken S, Krichevsky A, O'Connor J, Schlatterer J, Cole L, Kardana A et al (1999) Development and characterization of antibodies to a nicked and hyperglycosylated form of hCG from a choriocarcinoma patient: generation of antibodies that differentiate between pregnancy hCG and choriocarcinoma hCG. Endocrine 10:137–144
148. Cole LA (1997) Immunoassay of human chorionic gonadotropin, its free subunits, and metabolites. [see comments]. Clin Chem 43:2233–2243
149. Cole LA, Wang YX, Elliott M, Latif M, Chambers JT, Chambers SK et al (1988) Urinary human chorionic gonadotropin free beta-subunit and beta-core fragment: a new marker of gynecological cancers. Cancer Res 48:1356–1360
150. Iles RK, Persad R, Trivedi M, Sharma KB, Dickinson A, Smith P et al (1996) Urinary concentration of human chorionic gonadotrophin and its fragments as a prognostic marker in bladder cancer. Br J Urol 77:61–69
151. Stenman UH, Alfthan H, Ranta T, Vartiainen E, Jalkanen J, Seppälä M (1987) Serum levels of human chorionic gonadotropin in nonpregnant women and men are modulated by gonadotropin-releasing hormone and sex steroids. J Clin Endocrinol Metab 64:730–736
152. Bellet D, Lazar V, Bieche I, Paradis V, Giovangrandi Y, Paterlini P et al (1997) Malignant transformation of nontrophoblastic cells is associated with the expression of chorionic gonadotropin beta genes normally transcribed in trophoblastic cells. Cancer Res 57:516–523
153. Norman RJ, Menabawey M, Lowings C, Buck RH, Chard T (1987) Relationship between blood and urine concentrations of intact human chorionic gonadotropin and its free subunits in early pregnancy. Obstet Gynecol 69:590–593
154. Papapetrou PD, Nicopoulou SC (1986) The origin of a human chorionic gonadotropin beta-subunit-core fragment excreted in the urine of patients with cancer. Acta Endocrinol (Copenh) 112: 415–422
155. Cole LA (2011) hCG, the centerpiece of life and death. Int J Endocrinol Metab 9(2):335–352
156. Barakat RR, Markman M, Randall ME (2009) Principles and practice of gynecologic oncology. Wolters Kluwer Health, Philadelphia
157. Tegoni M, Spinelli S, Verhoeyen M, Davis P, Cambillau C (1999) Crystal structure of a ternary complex between human chorionic gonadotropin (hCG) and two Fv fragments specific for the alpha and beta-subunits. J Mol Biol 289(5):1375–1385
158. Triozzi PL, Stevens VC (1999) Human chorionic gonadotropin as a target for cancer vaccines. Oncol Rep 6(1):7–17

Part IV

Tumor Markers – A Critical Revision: Oncofetal Proteins

Biomarkers for Hepatocellular Carcinoma (HCC): An Update

12

Dave Li and Shinji Satomura

Abstract

The past decades have witnessed increased use of biomarkers in disease management. A biomarker is any characteristic that can be objectively measured and evaluated as an indicator of normal biological process, pathogenic process, or pharmacological response to a therapeutic intervention. The clinical measurements of biomarkers can be carried out in vivo using imaging modalities like ultrasound (US), computed tomography (CT), and magnetic resonance imaging (MRI), as well as in vitro utilizing serum or plasma or other body fluids as specimens. In contrast to the imaging modalities, a prominent value of serum biomarkers is that they could be biologically relevant and disease-specific to pathophysiologic or pathologic process of disease development. This article provides an update of serum biomarkers for hepatocellular carcinoma (HCC) in risk assessment for early detection through surveillance.

Keywords

AFP-L3 • AFP-L3 clinical performance • Alpha-fetoprotein isoforms • Chip-based microfluidic assay • Chronic hepatitis • Cirrhosis • DCP clinical performance • Des-gamma-carboxy prothrombin (DCP) • HCC • HCC biomarkers • HCC risk factors • Level of evidence • Liver fibrosis

12.1 Introduction: Some Important Issues Associated with HCC Early Detection Through Risk Assessment in Surveillance

The past decades have witnessed increased use of biomarkers in disease management. A biomarker is any characteristic that can be objectively measured and evaluated as an indicator of normal biological process, pathogenic process, or pharmacological response to a therapeutic intervention

I am grateful to Julia Li of University of Maryland College Park in Washington, DC for her review of the manuscript and comments.

D. Li, M.D., Ph.D. (✉) • S. Satomura, Ph.D.
Wako Life Sciences, Inc.,
Mountain View, CA 94043, USA
e-mail: daijunli@verizon.net

R. Scatena (ed.), *Advances in Cancer Biomarkers*, Advances in Experimental Medicine and Biology 867, DOI 10.1007/978-94-017-7215-0_12

[1]. The clinical measurements of biomarkers can be carried out in vivo using imaging modalities like ultrasound (US), computed tomography (CT), and magnetic resonance imaging (MRI) as well as in vitro utilizing serum or plasma or other body fluids as specimens. In contrast to the imaging modalities, a prominent value of serum biomarkers is they could be biologically relevant and disease-specific to pathophysiologic or pathologic process of disease development.

Alpha-fetoprotein (AFP) has been widely used although it has not been formally approved or cleared by the U.S. Food and Drug Administration (FDA) as a cancer biomarker for hepatocellular carcinoma (HCC). Recently the regulatory agency has cleared two novel and specific HCC serum biomarkers for risk assessment for HCC, Alpha-fetoprotein-L3 (AFP-L3) and Des-γ-decarboxyprothrombin (DCP). AFP-L3 is a glycosylation variant of the AFP [2]. DCP is abnormal coagulation protein produced in liver and a precursor of thrombin in the coagulation cascade [3]. This review article will focus on analytical and clinical validity of the AFP-L3 and DCP as serum biomarkers and provide an overview of their potential clinical utilities in HCC management especially for early detection through risk assessment. I critically review some recent clinical research data up to 2012. The discussions are mainly from clinical laboratory perspectives with focus on the new microfluidic chip-based assay system, *μTASWako™i30*. This article discusses some important investigator-initiated studies and reports reflecting user experiences which have enriched the knowledge base of the novel oncology biomarkers and their potentials in medical practice.

12.1.1 Natural History: Disease Spectrum and Cellular Heterogeneity

Natural history of malignant disease and its relation to disease development is increasingly delineated and defined at the molecular levels [4], which offer ample opportunities and rich sources for biomarker assay developments. The disease development of HCC, like many other human malignancies, is not an event but a process which spans from physiological changes such as quantitative variations of biomolecules to pathological modifications of qualitative natures such somatic mutations [5].

Major risk factors in natural history of HCC have been understood thanks to intensive medical research on the viral etiology and mechanisms of the hepatitis B and C virus. Primary liver cancer is mostly HCC, the malignant disease of the hepatocytes [6]. Chronic hepatitis infections including hepatitis B in the Southeast Asia countries and hepatitis C in the West have been attributed to the rise in incidence of HCC over the past decades. In fact, the HCC has the fastest rising cancer incidence in the US [7]. Chronic hepatitis C infection will become cirrhotic within 20–30 years, however, as many as 40 % of chronic hepatitis B patients may not have clinical evidence of liver cirrhosis as a precursor to HCC [8].

HCC, also similar to most other human cancers, is heterogeneous [9, 10] which may be non-heritable in the sources of cellular diversity such as arising from different cancer stem cells [11] or heritable such as from driver mutations in different signal transduction pathways within the HCC cancer cell population [12]. Therefore depending on the driver mutation, HCC is probably not a single disease entity, instead is a collective term for many subgroups of the liver malignancies.

The early HCC is clinically manageable or curable [8]. The diagnosis for early intervention decision has shifted to relying more on non-invasive clinical diagnosis based on dynamic imaging modalities instead of histology in recent years [13]. In order to treat HCC more effectively, the size of the tumor nodule(s) when they are found by screening ideally should be single and less than 2–3 cm in diameter [14]. Given the background liver disease of cirrhosis, a liver nodule of <1 cm in diameter is rarely diagnosed as liver cancer [15]. A liver nodule, when detected, the size of <1–2 cm is considered to be in the early stages for the purpose of the discussion.

Serum biomarkers are useful assisting in the characterization of a liver nodule for evaluating likelihood of HCC occurrence, or its downstream risk of evolving into HCC within a specific time-frame. Surveillance can improve survival by reducing deaths using US and serum biomarker [16–18]. In Japan, surveillance has been embedded into medical practice [19, 20]. Although clinical conditions limiting successful management of HCC exist, such as the residual liver functions among others in patients with the HCC, early detection of HCC do offer additional treatment options. It has been observed that patients with end stage liver diseases could have excellent long term survival if pre-matured deaths from HCC can be prevented through surveillance and liver transplantation [21, 22].

12.1.2 Serum Biomarkers: Specificity Versus Sensitivity

American Association for the Study of Liver Diseases (AASLD) has recommended that HCC surveillance should be based on US every 3–6 months for patients at high risk for HCC [15]. These patients are mainly chronic HBV carriers of Asian males over 40 years and female over 50 years old and cirrhotic HCV infection [15]. It is concluded that US is effective as the first line HCC surveillance [15]. However, some medical experts are quick to point out that US is limited by its relatively low sensitivity and therefore the high false negative rate for use in the HCC surveillance. US demonstrated marginal performance in clinical sensitivity for HCC surveillance with sensitivity of 60 % on average [23]. Furthermore, US is also operator-dependent with significant performance variations among hospitals and medical centers around the country. The US images are subject to human interpretations and are vulnerable to human errors. The effective use of US in surveillance has been hampered by poor reproducibility [24]. Other limiting factors for diagnostic grade of US results are physiological or pathological in nature such as fatty liver disease associated with metabolic syndrome, interference from the anatomical barriers adjacent to the liver such as lung or stomach that could sometime obscure the imaging producing less granular pictures. The background cirrhotic liver could also have potential cripple effect on US quality.

There should be no doubt that serum biomarkers could provide additional diagnostic or prognostic information. More information would likely change the clinical impression on likelihood of HCC especially in some challenging clinical diagnostic situations which more often than not is the rule rather than the exception in HCC management because of the background or underlying liver cirrhosis leading to the HCC development.

Serum biomarkers can signal the early development of HCC. In general, HCC is derived from liver cirrhosis presenting as background liver disease of high grade dysplastic nodules due to the chronic viral hepatitis infection [25]. Liver nodule(s) can be detected by US as mass(es) of sufficiently large size, say, for example when it reaches 2 cm in diameter or greater. Serum biomarkers can be an early warning alerting the development of HCC. Early diagnosis by surveillance is associated with lower mortality risk [18]. The HCC with seropositive AFP-L3 is reported to be correlated to short doubling time in tumor volume, and increased arterial supplies of tumor nodule, thereby clinically aggressive with poorer prognosis [26, 27]. Newer generation of the AFP-L3 assay is highly sensitive for pathologically advanced HCC [28]. It is worth noting that the pathologically advanced HCC may be more clinically aggressive even they are small in size for example <2 cm [26].

Clinically useful Serum biomarkers should have several key characteristics. They must be cancer specific, non-invasive and safe to use, convenient and easy to apply in different clinical settings, and acceptable to patients. They are expected being sensitive to the underlying disease. However, clinical sensitivity could be affected by a variety of analytical and biological reasons. Undesirable detection limit of assay technology could affect the clinical sensitivity. Improvement in assay's detection limit can increase the true sensitivity but also the false positive rate by decreasing the assay specificity simultaneously. Biologically, tumor heterogeneity could also curtail the sensitivity of a laboratory assay because some cancer may not produce certain biomolecules as serum biomarkers especially in early stage. It was suggested this is also the case in HCC [29, 30]. There are different subgroups of HCC. For instance, approximately 20–80 % of the HCC do not have elevated AFP depending on tumor size at diagnosis [31]. This has been a significant issue when clinicians use AFP for referral of patients suspicious of HCC for imaging confirmation.

The clinical sensitivity can be significantly improved by advanced assay technology with drastic improvement in lower detection limit thereby higher analytical sensitivity. For example, the *i30* AFP-L3 and DCP assay platform based on microfluidic chip has greatly improved the analytical sensitivity [32]. But physicians are compelled to address the issue of "false positivity" of the test results. It is expected that the surveillance strategy for HCC management with multiple periodic sampling could in some degrees provide practical solution to the issue with respect to whether these seropositive AFP-L3 and DCP cases are authentic HCC in patients at high risk for the malignant liver disease.

The other reason for the low clinical sensitivity of some cancer biomarkers must be biological due largely to cancer is heterogeneous with many subgroups as demonstrated by recent studies in breast cancer [4]. It is clear also from molecular studies that HCC is likely not a single disease entity according to the underlying molecular alterations [33]. Clinical presentations show HCC is seropositive with AFP, or AFP-L3 or DCP with only some degrees of overlapping patterns although some HCCs are seropositive with all the current available HCC biomarkers [29, 30]. How the phenotypic variation patterns related to biologic behavior can be interpreted for directing treatments remains to be determined. This also suggests that some serum biomarkers complementary to the existing ones remain to be discovered. But it should be clear that usefulness of any single biomarker in HCC surveillance is limited.

Combined use of serum biomarkers can maximize the clinical sensitivity (or specificity depending decision rule). Overall test results can be registered as positive using algorithm of "OR" or "AND" rule depending on the clinical context [34]. This offers a rationale and testable hypothesis for using multiple serum biomarkers simultaneously in hoping for achieving higher clinical sensitivity and/or specificity. As a matter of fact, recent studies did have provided "prove of concept" of such approach [35, 36].

12.1.3 Assay Calibration: From Data to Information

Information must be extracted from the data in order for the data become useful or actionable to clinicians. In this sense, the information is the data which are interpretable for further clinical actions [5]. Structured data from quantitative measurements have intrinsic values such as measurement concentrations of cancer biomarkers CA125 or CA19-9. These clinical data may not have any information simply because we do not know what they are actually meant. For serum biomarkers, one approach for extracting meaningful information from measurement data are through comparison to a Gold Standard which could be histology from biopsied or surgical specimens, or in the case of early diagnosis of HCC, clinical diagnosis based on dynamic imaging modalities such as four phase contrast CT or MRI. Tissue morphology by staining have provided disease diagnostic standard for human diseases. Medical sciences have evolved in recent years for HCC diagnosis. Clinical diagnosis and decision for early intervention can be made based on clinical diagnosis which relied on dynamic CT or MRI. It is worth noting that tumor size has been integrated in the HCC definition in the AASLD clinical practice guideline for HCC management.

Until now, the cancer biomarker assays have not been calibrated based on tumor size as a clinical parameter as a gold standard. This has led to spectrum bias in many studies reported of performance characteristics using the serum biomarkers. The possibility of the use of cancer biomarkers calibrated based on smaller tumor size from imaging would represent a paradigm shift in medical diagnosis which can set the diagnostic threshold lower for detecting earlier stage of HCC. How effective these serum biomarkers are for early detection remains to be determined by clinical studies in relevant clinical contexts.

12.1.4 Level of Evidences: From Clinical Validity to Utility

Safety and effectiveness are the basis of the FDA clearance and approval of the serum biomarkers for marketing in the U.S. which constitute the regulatory framework for medical devices. The evidences can be obtained from observational study or clinical experiment. For regulatory clearance or approval, observational study with clear intended use and indication for use in retrospective or prospective designs can be used to collect the validation data for demonstrating the safety and effectiveness. The most commonly used clinical parameters are sensitivity and specificity for effectiveness and false positive and false negative for safety which should be evaluated in light of a specific clinical context i.e. the intended use and indication for use as proposed for the serum biomarkers.

Pepes et al. have proposed five phases of biomarker development for early detection of cancer: (a) preclinical exploratory studies (phase 1); (b) clinical assay and validation (phase 2); (c) retrospective longitudinal (phase 3); (d) prospective screening (phase 4); and (e) cancer control (phase 5) [37]. These ordered phases of biomarker development have provided a framework for rational development and clinical adoption of serum biomarkers for cancer early detection.

The data from different phases of the evaluation stage present different levels of evidences. National Comprehensive Cancer Network (NCCN) Task Force on Evaluating Clinical Utility of Tumor Markers in Oncology has affirmed the level of evidence in their newly released practice guideline on cancer serum biomarker evaluation [38]. A system of the levels of evidence has been outlined as in Table 12.1.

Table 12.1 Tumor marker utility grading system level of evidence

Level	Interpretation
I	Prospective, marker primary objective, well-powered or meta-analysis
II	Prospective, marker the secondary objective
III	Retrospective, outcomes, multivariate analysis (most currently published marker studies are level of evidence III)
IV	Retrospective, outcomes, univariate analysis
V	Retrospective, correlation with other marker, no outcomes

Most clinical studies leading to FDA clearance or approval likely remain in phase 3 developmental stage providing relatively low levels of evidence for clinical utility. It would be challenging in convincing clinicians that the tumor markers with regulatory clearance or approval have clinical utilities satisfying their unmet medical needs. Clinically, the only reason for diagnostic testing is treatment decision [39]. A biomarker would have clinical utilities if it can direct treatment based on high level of evidences from well-designed clinical studies. However, clinical utility can be suggested by observational study with robust designs [40].

12.2 HCC: Risk Factors and Clinical Measurements

12.2.1 Chronic Hepatitis, Liver Fibrosis and Cirrhosis

Chronic liver diseases in forms of liver fibrosis or cirrhosis are precursor of liver failure and HCC, the end stages of the liver disease. Worldwide the most common causes of chronic liver disease are chronic hepatitis B and C virus infection. After decades of the initial HBV or HCV infection, a pathological process in liver characterized by stepwise progressions of chronic liver disease could lead to fibrosis and cirrhosis, eventually to liver failure or primary liver cancer. The hepatitis B virus B and C virus infection are the major risk factors for HCC. Relative risk (RR) for HCC with HBV infection is approximately 100 compared to non-carriers; in cirrhotic HBV carrier, the RR was 961 compared to uninfected controls [8]. HCC risk was also drastically increased to 20–200 times in HCV-infected patients compared to HCV-negative controls [41]. The conversion rate of HCC is 1–6 % per year among the chronic hepatitis patients with cirrhosis [6]. It has been reported that obesity and diabetes from metabolic syndrome are associated with HCC as the emerging risk factor of HCC [42, 43].

There are multiple clinical staging systems for liver cancer for predicting the prognosis of HCC. The major ones include American Joint Commission on Cancer (AJCC) Tumor-Node-Metastasis (TNM) system, the Barcelona Clinic Liver Cancer (BCLC) System, Cancer of the Liver Italian Program (CLIP), and the Okuda System, etc. [14]. Although none of these scoring systems have been universally accepted, they invariably incorporate some most important considerations for survival of HCC, namely (a) severity of the underlying liver disease; (b) tumor size; (c) intrahepatic micro-invasion; and (d) metastasis [44]. In a retrospective cohort study published in 2009, Nathan et al. compared six major staging systems for HCC with an early HCC prognostic score [45], and concluded that an early HCC prognostic score is superior to the AJCC TNM system for predicting survival of patients with early HCC after liver resection or liver transplantation. The investigators found that all the major HCC staging systems performed poorly in patients with early HCC. This is likely due to the fact that liver functions are not accounted for in the staging schemes [14].

AASLD Clinical Practice Guideline on HCC Management recommends use of US every 3–6 months for HCC surveillance for patients at risk for HCC. NCCN Clinical Practice Guideline in Oncology on Hepatocellular Carcinoma recommends utilizing both US and serum biomarker AFP for screening patients in an interval of every 6 months. Overseas the J-HCC/Japan Society of Hepatology (JSH) recommends use of serum biomarkers AFP, AFP-L3 and DCP every 3–4 months for the patients at high risk for HCC in addition to US [20].

Other imaging modalities such as dynamic contrast CT and MRI have been used for annual surveillance of patients at risk for HCC although they tend to be utilized more in confirmative diagnosis, especially in tertiary health care settings. The imaging modalities are technically demanding and not as convenient as testing of patient specimens being drawn and sent to reference laboratories. Similar to serum biomarkers, the imaging modalities are, in general, of relatively low sensitivity but of high specificity. In recent years, the treatments of HCC can be initiated according to the clinical diagnosis provided by the vascular characteristics on imaging of the liver malignancies, thereby representing a new framework of clinical utility of biomarkers.

12.2.2 Clinical Measurements: Enzyme Aberration in Glycosylation and Carboxylation

Clinical measurements of serum biomarkers have focused on changes of protein concentration in circulation. However, variations in protein concentration such as hormones and growth factors are thought to be mostly physiological phenomenon reflecting feedback regulations instead of pathological presentation [5]. The operating ranges of most of the cancer biomarker assays are probably well above the concentration gradients of many biologically important molecules in cancer early development [46]. Furthermore, although in biology, information flows from DNA to RNA, to proteins, it is post-translational modifications such as protein phosphorylation and glycosylation that empowers protein molecules with functional significance.

At the molecular levels, AFP-L3 is a glycosylation variant of AFP with α-1,6 core fucosylation on reducing terminus of N-acetylglucosamine of AFP molecule which is the AFP fraction reactive to lectin Lens culinaris agglutinin [2]. The elevation of AFP-L3 in HCC results from over-expression of fucosyltransferase Fut 8 which is responsible for core-fucosylation of proteins in the liver and other enzymes facilitating synthesis of GDP-glucose, the substrate of the fucosyltransferase [47]. Fucosylation is one of the most common post-translational modifications of

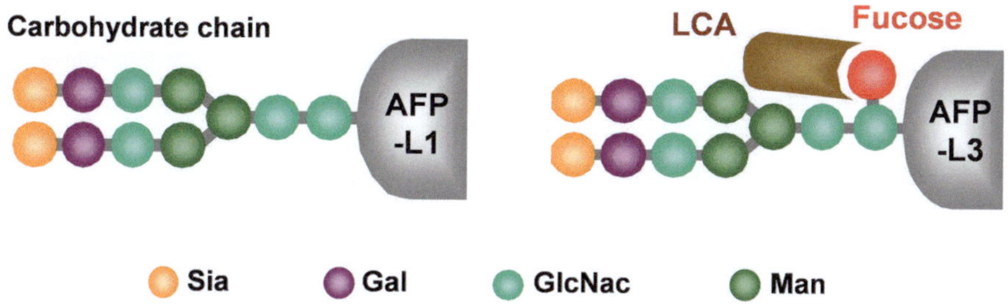

Fig. 12.1 Alpha-fetoprotein (AFP) isoforms: AFP-L1 (*left*), and AFP-L3 (*right*). Note: Sialic acid (*Sia*); Galatose (*Gal*); N-Acetylglucosamine (*GlcNac*); Mannose (*Man*) (http://www.wakodiagnostics.com/afpl3test.html)

proteins in physiology. Increase in fucosylation has also been reported in inflammation and cancer. Fucosylated glycoproteins are involved in biological functions of adhesion molecules and growth factor receptors through Notch signaling [48]. Core fucosylation is reported crucial for cytokine receptor activation [49]. The increased concentration of AFP-L3 is also due to increased release of the AFP-L3 from hepatocytes in HCC into plasma which is normally secreted into the bile duct (Fig. 12.1) [50].

Patients with primary malignant hepatic tumors seropositive for AFP-L3 and low AFP concentrations appear of unique clinicopathologic features. It is reported these cancers have a higher incidence of non-HCC primary liver cancer derived from cholangiocytes. They also had a high frequency of poorly differentiated tumors and sarcomatous changes, and showed a poor prognosis [51]. HCC patients who were positive for AFP-L3 and negative for DCP demonstrated histopathologic features of more advanced HCC compared with those who were seropositive for DCP alone such as infiltrative growth with an irregular margin and showing poorly differentiation of the HCC [52]. In fact, Okuda et al. found that a subgroup of intrahepatic cholangiocarcinoma (ICC) are seropositive for AFP-L3 and those with combined hepatocellular and cholangiocarcinoma have features close to HCC. The investigators thought that these liver cancers may be different from the ICC which is seropositive with CA19-9 [53]. This suggests that AFP-L3 seropositive HCC is a subtype of primary liver cancer with more aggressive behaviors.

DCP or proteins induced by vitamin K absence or antagonist-II (PIVKA II) is an abnormal form of the coagulation protein produced by the liver in HCC. Prothrombin is also known as the Coagulation Factor II of the blood coagulation cascade. In normal liver, the prothrombin undergoes post-translational carboxylation before release into the peripheral blood. The carboxylation converts specific amino-terminal glutamic acid residues to γ-carboxyglutamic acid [54]. The vitamin K dependent carboxylase responsible for the carboxylation is absent in malignant cells, and an abnormal prothrombin with all or some of unconverted glutamic acid is released into the circulation instead. The non-carboxylated form i.e. DCP is a biomarker for HCC (Fig. 12.2). Some subgroups of HCC, probably due to malfunction of carboxylase, secrete the unmodified precursor, DCP. In a study comparing hypervascular and hypovacular HCC, Matsubara et al. found that DCP production is associated with tumor angiogenesis of HCC [55]. Yuan et al. reported that the DCP levels in HCC tissue with portal vein invasion were significantly greater than in HCC tissues without portal vein invasion

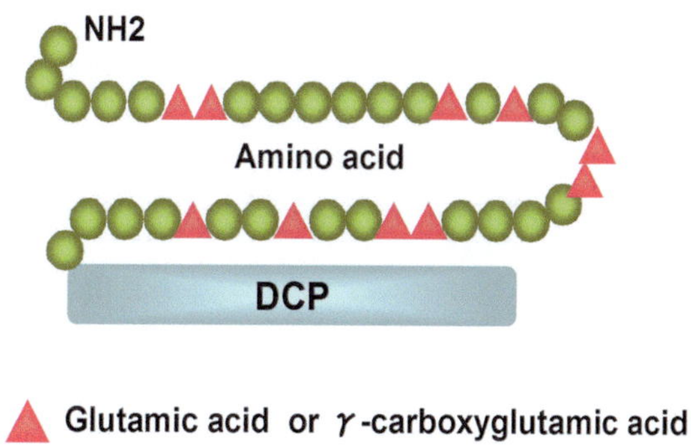

Fig. 12.2 Des-gamma-carboxy prothrombin (DCP) (http://www.wakodiagnostics.com/pivka_dcptest.html)

[56]. In addition, recent studies have revealed that DCP functions as a growth factor and might play significant roles in cancer progression [57]. Durazo et al. showed that DCP has a direct correlation to tumor size in patients with single lesion [58].

It has been suggested that the both AFP-L3 and DCP are associated with tumor aggressiveness of HCC [59]. In particular, AFP-L3 is related to progression from moderately differentiated to poorly differentiated HCC, whereas DCP is more specific to vascular invasion and is therefore likely to be a useful indicator of vascular invasion [60].

12.2.3 History of AFP-L3 Developments and Technical Features

AFP-L3 is a glycoform with core fucose glycosylation. Based on its affinity to lectin Len culinaris agglutinin, AFP can be sub-fractionated into three distinctive species i.e. L1, L2 and L3 according to their reactivity to Lens culinaris of migration pattern of affinity electrophoresis. Investigations found that the L1 was elevated in inflammation of liver. The L3 is tumor-specific for HCC. The micro-heterogeneity of the glycan structural variation between AFP-L1 and AFP-L3 is due to presence of an α-1,6, core fucose at the reducing end of the N-acetylglucosamine of AFP [2].

The first clinical laboratory assay on AFP-L3 was developed with a lectin-affinity electrophoresis method. The lectin lens culinaris was used to separate the three fractions of the AFP based on its reactivity to the agglutinin. Detection of the L3 ratio in percentage to L1 was achieved by dye-labeled antibodies and quantification by densitometry. An automated assay was developed for clinical use in 1997 in Japan on a liquid phase binding immunoassay platform, (LiBASys). The AFP-L3% reading was generated when AFP is >10 ng/mL with a minimal detectable limit of AFP-L3 at 0.8 ng/mL [61]. The LiBASys AFP/AFP-L3 assays were cleared by the FDA for risk assessment of HCC in the U.S. in April of 2005. Subsequently, the DCP assay was also cleared by the regulatory agency for the same indication for use, and was added to the test menu. Since then the assay technologies have continued to evolve. Since 2009, the assays have migrated to a state-of-the-art immunoassay platform based on microfluidic chip as an electrokinectic analyte transport assay (EATA). With deployment of the second generation of the assay instrument, the analytical sensitivity has increased with further diminishing the minimal detection limit to 0.3 ng/mL of AFP-L3. The assay range of AFPL3% has been extended from 0.6 to 1000 ng/mL of AFP [62]. The assay system can provide accurate and precise percent ratio AFP-L3 reading over the entire assay range of AFP from 0.6 to 1000 ng/mL. This has rendered significant improvement in assay sensitivity while maintaining the clinical specificity facilitating clinical applications for early detection of smaller HCC. Furthermore, the fully automated features in designs of the analyzer have greatly shortened the assay turnaround time to less than 10 min [62].

12.2.4 Technical Features of Chip-based Microfluidic Assay and Analytical Performance

The EATA immunoassay on the microfluidic chip immunoassay platform can carry out reagent and sample mixing, concentration, reaction, and also can integrate all other assay steps on chip. The microfluidic chip was made with precision injection modeled from poly(methyl methacrylate-PMMA) plastic resin, and the channels were formed by bonding of plastic film to the modeled chip. PMMA has no ionizable group. Using a non-charged substrate has minimized electrostatic interactions between the analytes and the micro-channel's surface; and helped to reduce the electroosmotic flow (EOF) which can assists in clean and clinical assay grade quality separation of the immunocomplexes in the capillary electrophoresis on chip [63].

The EATA immunoassay is highly sensitive using <10 nL of actual serum size of specimen per measurement. The underpinning technology of high analytical therefore the high clinical sensitivity is isotachophoresis (ITP) which allows target analyte to be highly concentrated prior to detection using laser-activated immunophorescence dyes. ITP has been demonstrated to enhance analyte concentration by as much as three orders of magnitude enhancing the analytical sensitivity of the assays [63].

DNA-conjugated antibody has been employed for precisely control, adjustment and fine-tuning the electrophorectic mobility of immunocomplexes by varying the length of the conjugated oligonucleotides. The immunocomplex is also bound to another fluorescent-labeled antibody specific for the analyte which is under controlled for unidirectional migration together with the specimen and reagents from beginning to end of the assaying process on chip [63].

The advanced technical features of the microfluidic assay platform are attributed to the exceptional performance characteristics in analytical validations. The reproducibility of the assays is demonstrated that the coefficient variation (CV) is within 2 % for AFP and 3 % for AFP-L3. The assays' imprecision is reduced to minimum. The proportional bias has been shown within 2–3 % in comparison to the electrophoresis and LiBASys methods. The systemic bias of the assays in general is less than 5–6 %. In serial dilution experiments, the AFP-L3% has been shown held in a constant level over the entire assay range with changes in AFP concentrations in a reportable range from 0.6 to 1000 ng/mL [62].

12.3 Clinical Performance: Parameters and Interpretations

12.3.1 Clinical Validity: Parameters

The clinical parameters most commonly used in evaluating and demonstrating the clinical validity are sensitivity and specificity which are relatively unaffected by prevalence of the disease in population. Since the clinical sensitivity and specificity of a test are trade-offs depending on the assay cut-off value which should be determined and chosen according to the indication for use of the assay. It is unreasonable to expect an assay to have both very high sensitivity and specificity since human disease is a spectrum in development, especially the degenerative disease such as cardiovascular, metabolic, and malignant disorders. The purpose of diagnosis is to treat patients. The threshold of making definitive diagnosis is a balance between costs and benefits [64]. The benefit is therefore also depending on effective treatments available. Of importance in assessing the clinical validity and utility of the assays is the indication for use and the clinical context the assay is applied. For example, diagnosis tools such as serum biomarkers could be used for rule-in or a rule-out diagnosis. The selection of a clinically valid cut-off for assay requires a clinical context. For the rule-in diagnosis, a positive testing would be more valuable with high specificity to avoid unacceptable level of false positive results, whereas for rule-out diagnosis, negative testing result is more important with high sensitivity and low false negative rate.

In general, the microfluidic chip-based AFP-L3 and DCP assays are highly specific for early HCC although the clinical sensitivity and specificity vary by the cut-off threshold chosen and by tumor size which the assays designed to detect. These HCC usually featured by low AFP concentration <20 ng/mL. For assay with high clinical sensitivity, negative test results are more informative. The assay with high NPV from high sensitivity is used for screening or surveillance in clinics. The seronegative result can rule out suspicious HCC. In contrast, seropositive data of AFP-L3 and DCP should be cautious in interpretation since the potential false positive results need to be teased out. The performance of the AFP, AFP-L3 and DCP assay on microfluidic assay platform of *μTASWako i30* are summarized in Table 12.2 [65–67].

The clinical performance characteristics as shown in the Table are clearly influenced by the cut-off selected according to the proposed indication for use of the medical devices. They could be affected as well by tumor characteristics such as tumor size which the medical devices are expected to detect, and the staging system used for categorizing the malignant disease. Since

Table 12.2 Clinical performance of AFP-L3, and DCP assays on *μTASWako i30*[a]

HCC serum marker	Sensitivity	Specificity
AFP-L3 (%)		
>1 %	68 %	81 %
>5 %	40–53 %	54–87 %
>7 %	24–41 %	92 %
>10 %	12–21 %	97–98 %
>15 %	9 %	97 %
AFP-L3 (5 %)		
≤2 cm	37 %	
>2 and ≤3 cm	46 %	
>2 and ≤3 cm	44 %	
>5 cm	47 %	
DCP (mAU/mL)		
>40	56 %	95 %
DCP (40 mAU/mL)		
≤2 cm	24 %	
>2 and ≤3 cm	52 %	
>2 and ≤3 cm	64 %	
>5 cm	78 %	

[a]All study subjects had AFP<20 ng/mL

dynamic imaging has been widely accepted for clinical diagnosis of HCC, the disease definition of HCC should be specified including information of imaging modality and the contrast reagents used. Also because of the background liver cirrhosis, size of the tumor nodule for definitive HCC diagnosis is also important for the performance characterization.

The serum biomarkers, when used individually especially at the lower cutoff, have demonstrated comparable performance to ultrasonography. Recent research data have indicated that serum biomarkers when used in parallel or simultaneously, can maximize the clinical sensitivity while maintaining clinically acceptable specificity to meet the operating requirement of performance for HCC surveillance [36, 66]. Feng reported that combined AFP and DCP with cut-off threshold set at >6 ng/mL and >100 mAU/mL, respectively, can significantly improve the clinical sensitivity of the overall testing to 94.5 % [34]. Separately, Volk et al. also demonstrated the similar results for early stage HCC [35].

Recent study data further indicated that the combined use of all three current available HCC serum biomarkers can improve performance of the overall test result for early HCC. Hanaoka [36] showed that the overall sensitivity of AFPL3 plus DCP can be boosted to 78 % while maintaining the specificity basically the same as the respective serum biomarker at 86 %. For early HCC i.e. those with tumor nodule <2 cm in diameter, the sensitivity of the biomarkers were 24 % for DCP (using 40 mAU/mL as a cut-off) and 37 % for AFP-L3 (using 5 % as a cut-off) (Table 12.2), respectively. The relatively low sensitivities are not unexpected which may be due to tumor biology of the early HCC since the HCC is highly heterogeneous [68] as being reflective of discernible and yet non-overlapping expression patterns of the HCC biomarkers. This is echoed by Sherman M. who reported that 20–80 % of the HCC did not produce AFP depending on the tumor size at diagnosis [31]. Of note is that breast cancer has multiple subgroups with distinct clinical outcomes which may also be represented in HCC as well [14]. This further implies that the expectation of any single laboratory testing can achieve extremely high sensitivity while maintaining high clinical specificity may be unrealistic. Therefore although high clinical sensitivity is desirable for cancer screening and surveillance, it is a complex issue involving not only assay performance but also related to the gold standard employed for the performance comparison, as well as to intrinsic tumor biology.

Many serum HCC biomarkers of potential clinical usefulness have been found such as Glypican-3, Golgi protein 73 (GP73), and osteopontin [69, 70]. Due largely to the intrinsic biological heterogeneity, some HCC were not detected by every serum HCC biomarker. Thereby the performance characteristics especially the sensitivity would vary significantly among different serum biomarkers. It is expected that this performance gap would be narrowed with additional new discoveries of HCC serum biomarkers followed by parallel applications of multiple serum biomarkers in the testing algorithm. Recently, Shen et al. reported that a new serum biomarker of Dickkopf-1 (DKK1) could complement AFP in detecting HCC subtypes in patients of sero-negative AFP [71].

AFP-L3 and DCP are highly specific cancer biomarkers. AFP is a tissue specific embryonic antigen. It is re-expressed in some human cancers distinctively such as in testicular and primary liver cancer. It is clear that the elevation of AFP is more related to tissue necroinflamamtory reaction of hepatocytes of the underlying chronic viral infections [3]. Empirical data demonstrated AFP is consists of different glycoforms with reactivity to Lens culinaris. AFP-L1 is the major AFP fraction presenting in the necroinflammatory reaction that would likely elevated at liver tissue regeneration after necrosis. AFP-L3 is cancer-specific [3]. The practical implications for the finding of AFP-L3 is HCC-specific would be far-reaching in risk assessment, screening or surveillance, and diagnosis. Other potential clinical utilities of the serum biomarkers could include predicting prognosis and monitoring recurrence after treatments in surgical resection, radiofrequency ablation (RFA), and liver transplantation. It has been reported that the AFP-L3 concentration has fallen significantly beyond half-life of the serum protein in circulation in patients treated successfully by surgery and RFA in those patients presumably had not intrahepatic invasion or metastasis [72, 73]. Retrospective data analysis also suggested the patient cohort with low AFP-L3 < 5 % who had undergone successful surgical resection showed better long term survival compared to those with AFP-L3 > 5 % [68]. In comparison, AFP and DCP have been utilized as prognostic biomarkers in liver transplant for predicting recurrence and outcomes in the same study, but they were not associated with favorable outcome in survival [66]. Therefore, it appears AFP-L3 could be used for directing treatment and predicting prognosis of the treatments.

12.3.2 Test Interpretation: The Caveats

When interpreting test results of AFP-L3 and DCP, keep in mind that the sensitivity and specificity are conditional probabilities. The clinical parameters of sensitivity and specificity are useful but limited for at least by two reasons. The first is these are population level statistics. They cannot be easily applied in individual patient because one has to assume that the clinical truth about the disease status is already known. This is not true in clinical decision making using the biomarkers [74]. In addition, verification bias could affect the performance characteristics of a diagnostic device if gold standard is not applied across the entire study population for assessing the assay performance characterizations. This could happen when the test negative patients in a study have no imaging data to confirm the lack of HCC. This is not unusual in many oncology device investigations. For instance, due to ethical consideration, some patients in a study with negative lab testing results may not be subject to the same rigorous verification of disease status by tissue biopsy as the positive cases were. This is not trivial in clinical validation of oncology study.

In contrast, positive and negative predictive value (PPV and NPV) of testing could offer useful information for the assessment of risk or probability of HCC at individual level. However, PPV and NPV could be affected by pre-test probability i.e. the prevalence of the disease. For HCC, disease prevalence is relatively low in population, approximately 5 % among the patients at risk for HCC at least in North America. Under such circumstance, a diagnostic test may be unproductive in terms of the information yield from the testing procedure.

This brings us to another aspect of the testing utilization of the AFP-L3 and DCP in surveillance of HCC risk. Surveillance is repeat use of screening for patients at risk for HCC which is a targeted screening using AFP-L3 and DCP assay in patients of chronic hepatitis and cirrhosis [15]. Outside the United States, surveillance is established in medical protocol for HCC management in some countries. For example, Japanese government has sponsored and endorsed the practice guideline of HCC surveillance employing US and the novel HCC serum biomarkers [20]. Periodic and serial sampling is imperative for accurate assessment of the HCC risk in clinical decision making using the serum biomarkers in surveillance. In this case, changes of the serum biomarkers in value compared to baseline may make more clinical senses than simply look at an individual test result at any random time point. The assay interpretation in surveillance should rely on trending of the measurement values of the serum biomarker variation overtime. Multiple readings of AFP-L3 and DCP may mitigate the risk of false negative testing result or can even help to address the concern of false positive result of the tests which may be a more efficient way to identify the patients of early HCC.

In evaluating of performance of a diagnostic test, a test is informative if sensitivity plus specificity is >1.0 or if PPV is greater than prevalence [75]. But its acceptance in medical practice in HCC management will depend on understanding of what is the actionable information derived from the testing procedure to answer the question of whether a patient should be treated. For most diagnostic testing, such information could be only feasible from post-market or phase 4 clinical study design, or from user experiences since the HCC nodules have to be found in order to be treated.

HCC is a future event in the context of risk assessment. The clinical parameters appropriate for this purpose are relative risk (RR) and odds ratio (OR). The value of RR and OR > 1.0 with 95 % confidence interval not bracketing 1.0 is considered statistically significant. For risk assessment, it is meaningful if these values are much greater than 1.0 [76]. Furthermore, a timeframe associated with the risk implied should also be specified for RR. The RR of HCC for positive AFP-L3 and DCP is 10.6 and 4.8, respectively when the cut-off of AFP-L3 is set at10 % and DCP at 7.5 ng/mL (product package inserts, Wako Life Sciences, Inc., Mountain View, CA) indicating that the risk of HCC of seropositive AFP-L3 and DCP is 10 and 5 times higher, respectively, in next 2 years compared to those with the assay results remain negative.

12.4 Summary: Potential Clinical Utilities

AFP-L3 and DCP are the serum biomarkers with FDA clearance for marketing in the United States for the indication for use of risk assessment of HCC development in conjunction with other clinical information. The criteria of the regulatory clearance are safety and effectiveness of the device for the stated indication for use. The safety of the device for use in risk assessment is further ensured by the statement that the devices should be used in conjunction with other clinical diagnostic modalities for decision making. Fundamentally, the patient safety is driven by the biological nature of the serum biomarkers i.e. their disease-specificities in general and tissue specificities in particular. High specificity implies that elevation of AFP-L3 and DCP in circulation is pathognomonic for HCC irrespective of the gold standard in use for performance comparison. High specificity is also indicative of the devices are of low false positive rate. A positive assay alerts of early HCC development in the patients with excessive risks for HCC because the high PPV of such testing is revealing, and the patients should be followed-up closely for confirmation. The dilemma facing clinicians in interpreting the assay results is that they will have to find the tumor nodule in order to initiate medical or surgical interventions in a timely manner. Technology advances in clinical measurements sometime indeed pose unintended challenges instead of immediate answers to clinicians.

While the high specificity of the HCC biomarkers could be indicative of high risk of HCC, the high clinical sensitivity is desirable but it should be secondary to clinical specificity. The improvement in clinical sensitivity was largely limited by the assay technology in the past, but also by the gold standard used for performance comparison now. With advancement in technologies for clinical measurements, as demonstrated in the cases of AFP-L3 and DCP, it has become apparent that value of the clinical laboratory tests will depend on understanding of the clinical significance of the testing results with clear clinical utilities. User experience should be important in delineating the clinical usefulness of the HCC biomarkers. It should also be pointed out that the clinical sensitivity and specificity can be improved significantly by serial sampling and the combined use of the cancer biomarkers in parallel or in tandem in algorithms or by adding newer or more sensitive biomarkers in the future.

The complexities of human biology in disease developments unraveled by the improvements in measurement technologies suggest further collaborative efforts for determining the potential clinical utilities of the novel cancer biomarkers are necessary. Perhaps biomedical informatics can come to our helps in the near future in this regard with integrative data modeling tools for clinical algorithms in clinical decision making.

References

1. Biomarkers Definitions Working Group (2001) Biomarkers and surrogate endpoints: preferred definitions and conceptual framework. Clin Pharmacol Ther 69:89–95
2. Li D, Mallory T, Satomura S (2001) AFP-L3: a new generation of tumor marker for hepatocellular carcinoma. Clin Chim Acta 313:15–19
3. Weitz IC, Liebman HA (1993) Des-gamma-carboxy (abnormal) prothrombin and hepatocellular carcinoma: a critical review. Hepatology 18:990–997
4. Chen R, Mias GI, Li-Pook-Than J, Jiang L, Lam HY, Chen R et al (2012) Personal omics profiling reveals dynamic molecular and medical phenotypes. Cell 148(6):1293–1307
5. Li DJ, Chan DW (2010) Decoding the protein folding pattern of serum biomarkers: alternative strategy for cancer biomarker validation? Clin Proteom 6:53–55
6. Institute of Medicine of National Academies (2010) Hepatitis and liver cancer a national strategy for prevention and control hepatitis B and C. The National Academies Press, Washington, DC
7. Everhart JE, Ruhl CE (2009) Burden of digestive diseases in the United States Part III: overall and upper gastrointestinal diseases. Gasteroenterology 136:1134–1144
8. Sherman M (2010) Hepatocellular carcinoma: epidemiology, surveillance, and diagnosis. Semin Liver Dis 30:3–16
9. Heppner GH (1984) Tumor heterogeneity. Cancer Res 44:2259–2265
10. Altschuler SJ, Wu LF (2010) Cellular heterogeneity: do differences make a difference? Cell 141:559–563
11. Marusky A, Polyak K (2010) Tumor heterogeneity: cause and consequence. Biochim Biophys Acta 1805:105–117
12. McClenllan J, King M-C (2010) Genetic heterogeneity in human disease. Cell 141:210–217
13. El-Serag H (2011) Hepatocellular carcinoma. N Engl J Med 365:1118–1127
14. Sherman M (2011) Hepatocellular carcinoma: screening and staging. Clin Liver Dis 15:323–334
15. Bruix JG, Sherman M (2005) Management of hepatocellular carcinoma. Hepatology 42:1208–1236
16. Chen JG, Parkin DM, Chen QG, Lu JH, Shen QJ, Zhang BC, Zhu YR (2003) Screening for liver cancer: results of randomized controlled trial in Qidong, China. J Med Screen 10:204–209
17. Zhang BH, Yang BH, Tang ZY (2004) Randomized controlled trial of screening for hepatocellular carcinoma. J Cancer Res Clin Oncol 130:417–422
18. El-Serag HB, Kramer JR, Chen GH, Duan Z, Richardson PA, Davila JA (2011) Effectiveness of AFP and ultrasound tests on hepatocellular carcinoma mortality in HCV-infected patients in the USA. Gut 60:992–997
19. Izumi N (2010) Diagnostic and treatment algorithm of the Japanese Society of Hepatology: a consensus-based practice guideline. Oncology 78(suppl 1):78–86
20. Song P, Tobe RG, Inagaki Y, Kokudo N, Hasegawa K, Sugawara Y, Tang W (2012) The management of hepatocellular carcinoma around the world: a comparison of guidelines from 2001 to 2011. Liver Int 32(7):1053–1063. doi:10.1111/j.1478-3231.2012.02792.x
21. Stravitz RT, Heuman DM, Chand N, Sterling RK, Shiffman ML, Luketic VA, Sanyal AJ, Habib A, Mihas AA, Giles HC, Maluf DG, Cotterell AH, Posner MP, Fisher RA (2008) Surveillance for hepatocellular carcinoma in patients with cirrhosis improves outcome. Am J Med 121:119–126
22. Doyle MB, Vachharajani N, Maynard E, Shenoy S, Anderson C, Wellen JR, Lowell JA, Chapman WC (2012) Liver transplantation for hepatocellular carcinoma: long-term results suggest excellent Outcomes. J Am Coll Surg 215(1):19–28
23. Colli A, Fraquelli M, Casazza G, Massironi S, Colucci A, Conte D, Duca P (2006) Accuracy of ultrasonography, spiral CT, magnetic resonance, and alpha-fetoprotein in diagnosing hepatocellular carcinoma: a systematic review. Am J Gastroenterol 10:513–523
24. Marrero JA (2011) The role of serum biomarkers in hepatocellular carcinoma surveillance. Gastroenterol Hepatol 7:821–823
25. Matsui O, Kobayashi S, Sanada J, Kouda W, Ryu Y, Kozaka K, Kitao A, Nakamura K, Gabata T (2011) Hepatocelluar nodules in liver cirrhosis: hemodynamic evaluation (angiography-assisted CT) with special reference to multi-step hepatocarcinogenesis. Abdom Imaging 36:264–272
26. Kumada T, Nakano S, Takeda I, Kiriyama S, Sone Y, Hayashi K, Katoh H, Endoh T, Sassa T, Satomura S (1999) Clinical utility of Lens culinaris agglutinin-reactive alpha-fetoprotein in small hepatocellular carcinoma: special reference to imaging diagnosis. J Hepatol 30:125–130
27. Tada T, Kumada T, Toyoda H, Kiriyama S, Sone Y, Tanikawa M, Hisanaga Y, Kitabatake S, Kuzuya T, Nonogaki K, Shimizu J, Yamaguchi A, Isogai M, Kaneoka Y, Washizu J, Satomura S (2005) Relationship between Lens culinaris agglutinin-reactive alpha-fetoprotein and pathologic features of hepatocellular carcinoma. Liver Int 25:848–853

28. Kudo M (2011) Hepatocellular carcinoma in 2011 and beyond: from the pathogenesis to molecular targeted therapy. Oncology 81(suppl 1):1–10
29. Sterling RK, Jeffers L, Gordon F, Venook AP, Reddy KR, Satomura S, Kanke F, Schwartz ME, Sherman M (2009) Utility of Lens culinaris agglutinin-reactive fraction of alpha-fetoprotein and des-gamma-carboxy prothrombin, alone or in combination, as biomarkers for hepatocellular carcinoma. Clin Gastroenterol Hepatol 7:104–113
30. Toyoda H, Kumada T, Kiriyama S, Sone Y, Tanikawa M, Hisanaga Y, Yamaguchi A, Isogai M, Kaneoka Y, Washizu J (2006) Prognostic significance of simultaneous measurement of three tumor markers in patients with hepatocellular carcinoma. Clin Gastroenterol Hepatol 4:111–117
31. Sherman M (2010) The resurrection of alphafetoprotein. J Hepatol 52:939–940
32. Kagebayashi C, Yamaguchi I, Akinaga A, Kitano H, Yokoyama K, Satomura M, Kurosawa T, Watanabe M, Kawabata T, Chang W, Li C, Bousse L, Wada HG, Satomura S (2009) Automated immunoassay system for AFP-L3% using on-chip electrokinetic reaction and separation by affinity electrophoresis. Anal Biochem 388:306–311
33. Frenette C, Gish RG (2011) Hepatocellular carcinoma: molecular and genomic guideline for the clinician. Clin Liver Dis 15:307–321
34. Feng Z (2010) Classification versus association models: should the same methods apply? Scand J Clin Lab Invest Suppl 242:53–58
35. Volk ML, Hernandez JC, Su GL, Lok AS, Marrero JA (2007) Risk factors for hepatocellular carcinoma may impair the performance of biomarkers: a comparison of AFP, DCP, and AFP-L3. Cancer Biomark 3:79–87
36. Hanaoka T, Sato S, Tobita H, Miyake T, Ishihara S, Akagi S, Amano Y, Kinoshita Y (2011) Clinical significance of the highly sensitive fucosylated fraction of α-fetoprotein in patients with chronic liver disease. J Gastroenterol Hepatol 26:739–744
37. Pepe MS, Etzioni R, Feng Z, Potter JD, Thompson ML, Thornquist M, Winget M, Yasui Y (2001) Phases of biomarker development for early detection of cancer. J Natl Cancer Inst 93:1054–1061
38. Febbo PG, Ladanyi M, Aldape KD, De Marzo AM, Hammond ME, Hayes DF, Iafrate AJ, Kelley RK, Marcucci G, Ogino S, Pao W, Sgroi DC, Birkeland ML (2011) NCCN Task Force report: evaluating the clinical utility of tumor markers in oncology. J Natl Compr Canc Netw 9(Suppl 5):S1–S32
39. Newman TB, Kohn MA (eds) (2009) Evidence-based diagnosis. Cambridge University Press, New York
40. Pepe MS, Feng Z, Janes H, Bossuyt PM, Potter JD (2008) Pivotal evaluation of the accuracy of a biomarker used for classification or prediction: standards for study design. J Natl Cancer Inst 100(20): 1432–1438
41. Sherman M (2010) Epidemiology of hepatocellular carcinoma. Oncology 78(Suppl 1):7–10
42. Nordenstedt H, White DL, El-Serag HB (2010) The changing pattern of epidemiology in hepatocellular carcinoma. Dig Liver Dis 42(Suppl 3):S206–S214
43. Welzel TM, Graubard BI, Zeuzem S, El-Serag HB, Davila JA, McGlynn KA (2011) Metabolic syndrome increases the risk of primary liver cancer in the United States: a study in the SEER-Medicare database. Hepatology 54:463–471
44. Curley SA, Barnett CC Jr, Abdalla EK (2010) Staging and prognostic factors in hepatocellular carcinoma. UpToDate (Version 18.3: September 2010). http://www.uptodate.com/online/content/topic.do?topicKey+gicancer/12573&view=print. Accessed Jan 2011
45. Nathan H, Mentha G, Marques HP, Capussotti L, Majno P, Aldrighetti L, Pulitano C, Rubbia-Brandt L, Russolillo N, Philosophe B, Barroso E, Ferrero A, Schulick RD, Choti MA, Pawlik TM (2009) Comparative performances of staging systems for early hepatocellular carcinoma. HPB (Oxford) 11:382–390
46. Anderson NL, Anderson NG (2002) The human plasma proteome: history, character, and diagnostic prospects. Mol Cell Proteomics 1:845–867
47. Meany DL, Chan DW (2011) Aberrant glycosylation associated with enzymes as cancer biomarkers. Clin Proteomics 8:7–14
48. Miyoshi E, Moriwaki K, Nakagawa T (2008) Biological function of fucosylation in cancer biology. J Biochem 143:725–729
49. Schachter H (2005) The search for glycan function: fucosylation of the TGF-beta1 receptor is required for receptor activation. Proc Natl Acad Sci U S A 102:15721–15722
50. Nakagawa T, Takeishi S, Kameyama A, Yagi H, Yoshioka T, Moriwaki K, Masuda T, Matsumoto H, Kato K, Narimatsu H, Taniguchi N, Miyoshi E (2010) Glycomic analyses of glycoproteins in bile and serum during rat hepatocarcinogenesis. J Proteome Res 9:4888–4896
51. Okuda H, Saito A, Shiratori K, Yamamoto M, Takasaki K, Nakano M (2005) Clinicopathologic features of patients with primary malignant hepatic tumors seropositive for alpha-fetoprotein-L3 alone in comparison with other patients seropositive for alpha-fetoprotein-L3. J Gastroenterol Hepatol 20:759–764
52. Okuda H, Nakanishi T, Takatsu K, Saito A, Hayashi N, Yamamoto M, Takasaki K, Nakano M (2002) Clinicopathologic features of patients with hepatocellular carcinoma seropositive for alpha-fetoprotein-L3 and seronegative for des-gamma-carboxy prothrombin in comparison with those seropositive for des-gamma-carboxy prothrombin alone. J Gastroenterol Hepatol 17:772–778
53. Okuda H, Shiratori K, Yamamoto M, Takasaki K, Nakano M (2006) Clinicopathologic features of patients with intrahepatic cholangiocarcinoma who are seropositive for alpha-fetoprotein-L3 and those with combined hepatocellular and cholangiocarcinoma. J Gastroenterol Hepatol 21:869–873

54. Liebman HA, Furie BC, Tong MJ, Blanchard RA, Lo KJ, Lee SD, Coleman MS, Furie B (1984) Des-gamma-carboxy (abnormal) prothrombin as a serum marker of primary hepatocellular carcinoma. N Engl J Med 310:1427–1431
55. Matsubara M, Shiraha H, Kataoka J, Iwamuro M, Horiguchi S, Nishina SI, Takaoka N, Uemura M, Takaki A, Nakamura S, Kobayashi Y, Nouso K, Yamamoto K (2012) Des-γ-carboxyl prothrombin is associated with tumor angiogenesis in hepatocellular carcinoma. J Gastroenterol Hepatol 27(10):1602–1608. doi:10.1111/j.1440-1746.2012.07173.x
56. Yuan LW, Tang W, Kokudo N, Sugawara Y, Karako H, Hasegawa K, Aoki T, Kyoden Y, Deli G, Li YG, Makuuchi M (2004) Measurement of des-gamma-carboxy prothrombin levels in cancer and non-cancer tissue in patients with hepatocellular carcinoma. Oncol Rep 12:269–273
57. Inagaki Y, Tang W, Makuuchi M, Hasegawa K, Sugawara Y, Kokudo N (2011) Clinical and molecular insights into the hepatocellular carcinoma tumour marker des-γ-carboxyprothrombin. Liver Int 31:22–35
58. Durazo FA, Blatt LM, Corey WG, Lin JH, Han S, Saab S, Busuttil RW, Tong MJ (2008) Des-gamma-carboxyprothrombin, alpha-fetoprotein and AFP-L3 in patients with chronic hepatitis, cirrhosis and hepatocellular carcinoma. J Gastroenterol Hepatol 23:1541–1548
59. Yuen MF, Lai CL (2005) Serological markers of liver cancer. Best Pract Res Clin Gastroenterol 19(1):91–99
60. Miyaaki H, Nakashima O, Kurogi M, Eguchi K, Kojiro M (2007) Lens culinaris agglutinin-reactive alpha-fetoprotein and protein induced by vitamin K absence II are potential indicators of a poor prognosis: a histopathological study of surgically resected hepatocellular carcinoma. J Gastroenterol 42:962–968
61. Yamagata Y, Shimizu K, Nakamura K, Henmi F, Satomura S, Matsuura S, Tanaka M (2003) Simultaneous determination of percentage of Lens culinaris agglutinin-reactive alpha-fetoprotein and alpha-fetoprotein concentration using the LiBASys clinical auto-analyzer. Clin Chim Acta 327:59–67
62. Kagebayashi C, Yamaguchi I, Akinaga A, Kitano H, Yokoyama K, Satomura M, Kurosawa T, Watanabe M, Kawabata T, Chang W, Li C, Bousse L, Wada HG, Satomura S (2009) Automated immunoassay system for AFP-L3% using on-chip electrokinetic reaction and separation by affinity electrophoresisAnal. Biomolecules 388:306–311
63. Kawabata T, Wada HG, Watanabe M, Satomura S (2008) Electrokinetic analyte transport assay for alpha-fetoprotein immunoassay integrates mixing, reaction and separation on-chip. Electrophoresis 29:1399–1406
64. Pauker SG, Kassirer JP (1980) The threshold approach to clinical decision making. N Engl J Med 302:1109–1117
65. Tamura Y, Igarashi M, Kawai H, Suda T, Satomura S, Aoyagi Y (2010) Clinical advantage of highly sensitive on-chip immunoassay for fucosylated fraction of alpha-fetoprotein in patients with hepatocellular carcinoma. Dig Dis Sci 55:3576–3583
66. Toyoda H, Kumada T, Tada T, Kaneoka Y, Maeda A, Kanke F, Satomura S (2011) Clinical utility of highly sensitive Lens culinaris agglutinin-reactive alpha-fetoprotein in hepatocellular carcinoma patients with alpha-fetoprotein <20 ng/mL. Cancer Sci 102:1025–1031
67. Toyoda H, Kumada T, Tada T (2011) Highly sensitive Lens culinaris agglutinin-reactive α-fetoprotein: a new tool for the management of hepatocellular carcinoma. Oncology 81(Suppl 1):61–65
68. Thomas MB, Jaffe D, Choti MM, Belghiti J, Curley S, Fong Y, Gores G, Kerlan R, Merle P, O'Neil B, Poon R, Schwartz L, Tepper J, Yao F, Haller D, Mooney M, Venook A (2010) Hepatocellular carcinoma: consensus recommendations of the National Cancer Institute Clinical Trials Planning Meeting. J Clin Oncol 28:3994–4005
69. Malaguarnera G, Giordano M, Paladina I, Berretta M, Cappellani A, Malaguarnera M (2010) Serum markers of hepatocellular carcinoma. Dig Dis Sci 55:2744–2755
70. Shang S, Plymoth A, Ge S, Feng Z, Rosen HR, Sangrajrang S, Hainaut P, Marrero JA, Beretta L (2012) Identification of osteopontin as a novel marker for early hepatocellular carcinoma. Hepatology 55:483–490
71. Shen Q, Fan J, Yang XR, Tan Y, Zhao W, Xu Y, Wang N, Niu Y, Wu Z, Zhou J, Qiu SJ, Shi YH, Yu B, Tang N, Chu W, Wang M, Wu J, Zhang Z, Yang S, Gu J, Wang H, Qin W (2012) Serum DKK1 as a protein biomarker for the diagnosis of hepatocellular carcinoma: a large-scale, multicentre study. Lancet Oncol 13:817–826
72. Kobayashi M, Hosaka T, Ikeda K, Seko Y, Kawamura Y, Sezaki H, Akuta N, Suzuki F, Suzuki Y, Saitoh S, Arase Y, Kumada H (2011) Highly sensitive AFP-L3% assay is useful for predicting recurrence of hepatocellular carcinoma after curative treatment pre- and postoperatively. Hepatol Res 41:1036–1045
73. Tateishi R, Shiina S, Yoshida H, Teratani T, Obi S, Yamashiki N, Yoshida H, Akamatsu M, Kawabe T, Omata M (2006) Prediction of recurrence of hepatocellular carcinoma after curative ablation using three tumor markers. Hepatology 44:1518–1527
74. Moons KG, Harrell FE (2003) Sensitivity and specificity should be de-emphasized in diagnostic accuracy studies. Acad Radiol 10:670–672
75. Kondratovich MV (2008) Comparing two medical tests when results of reference standard are unavailable for those negative via both tests. J Biopharm Stat 18:145–166
76. Pepe MS, Janes H, Longton G, Leisenring W, Newcomb P (2004) Limitations of the odds ratio in gauging the performance of a diagnostic, prognostic, or screening marker. Am J Epidemiol 159:882–890

Part V

Tumor Markers – A Critical Revision: Cytokeratins

Mucins and Cytokeratins as Serum Tumor Markers in Breast Cancer

13

Andrea Nicolini, Paola Ferrari, and Giuseppe Rossi

Abstract

Structural and functional characteristics of mucins and cytokeratins are shortly described. Thereafter, those commonly used in breast cancer as serum tumor markers are considered. First CA15.3, MCA, CA549, CA27.29 mucins and CYFRA21.1, TPA, TPS cytokeratins alone or in association have been examined in different stages and conditions. Then their usefulness in monitoring disease-free breast cancer patients is evaluated. The central role of the established cut-off and critical change, the "early" treatment of recurrent disease and the potential benefit in survival are other issues that have been highlighted and discussed. The successive sections and subsections deal with the monitoring of advanced disease. In them, the current recommendations and the principal findings on using the above mentioned mucins and cytokeratins have been reported. A computer program for interpreting consecutive measurements of serum tumor markers also has been illustrated. The final part of the chapter is devoted to mucins and cytokeratins as markers of circulating and disseminated tumor cells and their usefulness for prognosis.

Keywords

Breast cancer • Breast cancer follow-up • CA15.3 • CA27.29 • CA549 • CTCs • CTCs detection • CYFRA21.1 • Cytokeratins • Cytokeratins structure • DTCs • DTCs detection • MCA • Mucins • Mucins and cytokeratins • Mucins structure • Serum TMs • TPA • TPS

A. Nicolini (✉) • P. Ferrari
Department of Oncology, Transplantations and New Technologies in Medicine, University of Pisa, Italy
e-mail: andrea.nicolini@med.unipi.it

G. Rossi
Unit of Epidemiology and Biostatistics, National Council of Research, Pisa, Italy

R. Scatena (ed.), *Advances in Cancer Biomarkers*, Advances in Experimental Medicine and Biology 867, DOI 10.1007/978-94-017-7215-0_13

13.1 Introduction

Mucins (MUCs) are normally expressed by epithelial cells and contribute to the lubrication of hollow tubular surfaces such as ducts and the passages in the respiratory and gastrointestinal systems. They also serve as a mechanical barrier to extrinsic physical and biological attacks. Mucins play an important role in the development of breast cancer, and an altered expression of mucins is associated with cancer progression. Recent studies have identified a differential expression of both membrane bound (MUC1, 4 and 16) and secreted mucins (MUC2, 5 AC, 5B and 6) in breast cancer tissues when compared with the non-neoplastic breast tissues. Functional studies have also uncovered many roles of mucins during the progression of breast cancer, which include modulation in proliferative, invasive and metastatic potential of tumor cells [1].

Cytokeratins are involved in the stability of epithelial cells and in many intracellular signal cascades [2, 3]. Breast ducts contain two types of epithelial cells, inner luminal cells and outer basal/myoepithelial cells. These cells can be distinguished by their immunophenotype [4]. Most investigators have addressed breast carcinoma precursors by analyzing expression of cytokeratins (CKs) as differentiation markers, since their expression is thought to remain stable throughout carcinogenesis [5]. Breast cancers are thought to arise from luminally differentiated epithelial cells, as evidenced by strong expression of CK8, CK18 and CK19, similar to the situation in the cells lining the lumen of normal breast ducts [5–7]. A small fraction of breast cancers express CK5 together with its major partners CK14 and CK17 [6, 8, 9] which are normally found in the basal cell layer of the mammary duct [5–7, 10]. Tumors expressing these CKs have been named 'basal-type' breast cancer. Breast cancers are generally thought to express either luminal (CK8/18/19þ) or basal (CK5/14þ) cytokeratins [11–13]. However, some CK5/14- and CK8/18-coexpressing tumors have also been found [6, 8, 10, 14]. It has been proposed that tumors positive for CK5 originate from multipotent CK5-expressing progenitor cells [6, 10, 15, 16] located between the basal/suprabasal and luminal cell layers in normal ducts [10]. CK5-positive progenitor epithelial cells can gradually differentiate towards glandular and myoepithelial lineages [6, 10, 15, 16].

13.2 Biochemistry of Mucin-Like Breast Cancer Antigens and Cytokeratins

MUCs include a family of high molecular weight, heavily O-glycosylated proteins that are differentially expressed in several epithelial malignancies. MUCs are broadly classified structurally into two main classes: membrane-bound mucins (1, 3A-B, 4, 12-13, 15-17, and 20) and secreted or gel-forming mucins (2, 5 AC, 5B, 6-8 and 19). MUCs are distinct in the sequence, domain organization, length, and number of their respective tandem repeat sequences [1].

Various monoclonal antibodies react with high molecular weight mucin-like proteins which are located in neoplastic mammary cells, i.e. carbohydrate antigen 15.3 (CA15.3), mucin-like carcinoma-associated antigen (MCA), carbohydrate antigen 549 (CA549), breast cancer mucin (BCM) [17, 18]. CA15.3 is a serum mucin-like tumor associated glycoprotein corresponding to an immuno-dominant epitope in the extracellular portion of the membrane bound mucin MUC1. It has a molecular weight of 300 Kda and is recognized by two monoclonal antibodies: 115 D8 against milk fat membrane and DF 3 against breast carcinoma cell line. CA15.3 is the most widely used mucin-like antigen in breast cancer. MCA is a serum mucin-like glycoprotein (molecular weight 350–500 KDa). The monoclonal antibody that tests for it recognizes a repetitive epitope in the peptide part of the MCA molecule. CA549 is a high-molecular weight mucin (molecular weight 400–500 Kda) which is recognized by two different monoclonal antibodies; the first (BCAE549) is directed against a human breast cancer line and the second (BCAN154) against the membranes of milk fat globules.

Cytokeratins (CKs) belong to a family of proteins which co-polymerise generating heterodimers, then tetramers, which combine forming intermediate filaments. At this moment 54 genes coding for human keratin are known, and they can be divided in two broad groups: 28 of type I and 26 of type II. Type I citokeratins are made up of relatively small acidic subunits (40–56 KDa) which are encoded on chromosome 17q21.2. They include 17 keratins from squamous epithelium and 11 from simple columnar epithelium (K9-10, K12-28 and K31-40). Type II citokeratins are made up of slightly larger basic subunits (53 and 67 KDa) which are encoded on chromosome 12q23.3. They include 20 keratins from squamous epithelium and six from simple columnar epithelium (K1-8, and K71-86) [2, 3]. Each epithelial tissue has a characteristic combination of cytokeratins that is maintained even after malignant transformation [19]. CKs 1-6 and 9-17 are found in the squamous epithelium, CKs 7-8 and 18-19 in the simple columnar epithelium.

Cytokeratin fragments are soluble in serum with a half-life of 10–15 h, and can be detected as aggregates by monoclonal antibodies. Tissue polypeptide antigen (TPA) is formed by a simple chain with a molecular weight between 22 and 23 Kda and probably consists of proteolytic fragments of CKs 8, 18 and 19. TPA is produced during late S and G2 phases of cell cycle and its positivity is linked to a rapid cellular proliferation [20, 21]. Tissue polypeptide-specific antigen (TPS) test is believed to detect CKs 18 and 19; TPS is recognized by a monoclonal antibody against the M3 epitope [22]. Cytokeratin fragment 21.1 (CYFRA 21.1) is a fragment of CK 19 with low molecular weight (3 KDa) recognized by two monoclonal antibodies: KS19.1 and BM12.21.

Figures 13.1 and 13.2 show the structure of mucins and cytokeratins.

The principal mucins and cytokeratins, their structure, molecular weight and monoclonal antibodies commonly used to recognize them are shown in Table 13.1.

13.3 Mucins and Cytokeratins as Serum Tumor Markers in Different Stages of Breast Cancer and in Other Conditions

Some mucins and cytokeratins are commonly used as serum tumor markers in breast cancer. However, high levels of them has been found also in other cancers or in benign conditions.

13.3.1 Mucins (CA15.3, MCA, CA549, CA27.29)

CA15.3 is the most used mucin-like antigen in breast cancer. High CA15.3 values may be observed also in ovarian cancer, endometrial carcinoma and non small cell lung cancer [23, 24]. Megaloblastic anemia, renal failure, liver, infectious pulmonary and autoimmune diseases, ovarian cysts, endometriosis, benign breast lesions, oral contraceptive use, pregnancy and treatment with G-CSF are common benign reasons of CA15.3 increase [25–32].

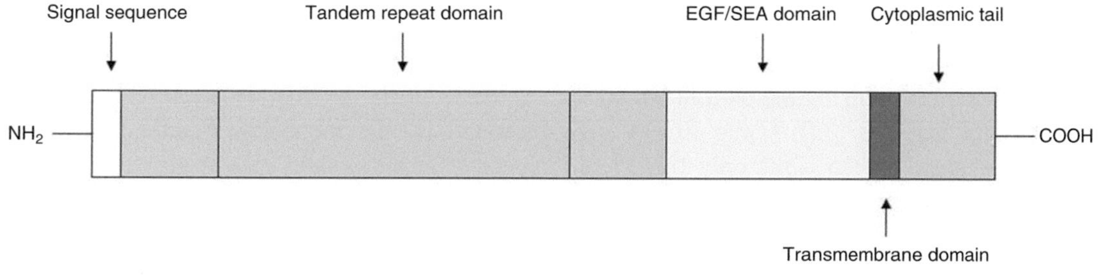

Fig. 13.1 Structure of MUC-1. The extracellular region contains sites of O- and N-linked glycosilation and is predominantly composed of variable number of tandem repeats

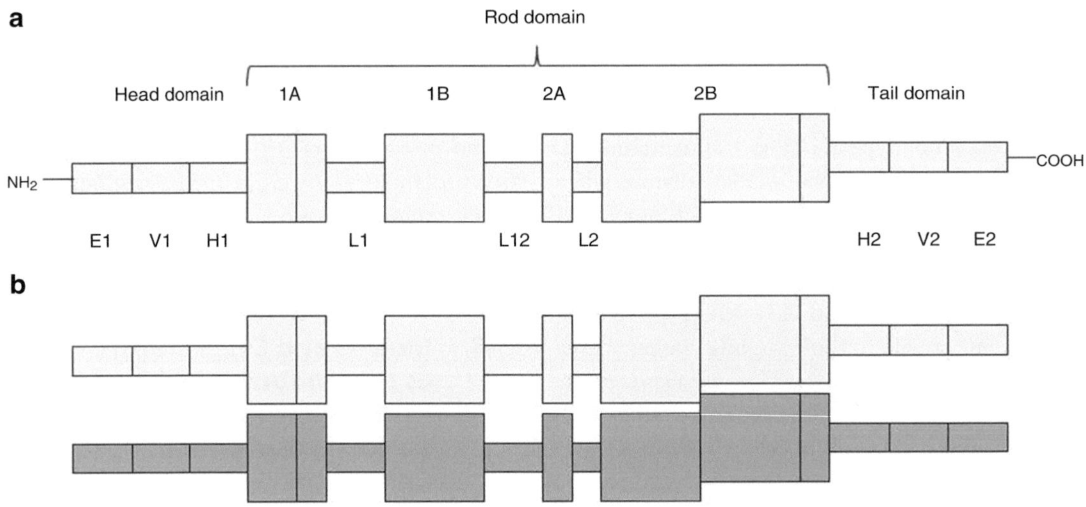

Fig. 13.2 Structure of keratin molecule. A: keratin protein molecules with domains and subdomains. B: heterodimer: type I/II keratin protein molecules in parallel alignment

Table 13.1 Principal characteristics of some mucins and cytokeratins commonly used as serum tumor markers in breast cancer

Tumor marker	Structure	Molecular weight (KDa)	mAb for detection
CA15.3	Glycoprotein	300	115D8, DF3
MCA	Glycoprotein	350–500	b-12
CA549	Glycoprotein	400–500	BCAE549, BCAN154
CYFRA21.1	CK 19 fragment	3	KS19.1, BM12.21
TPA	CKs 8, 18 and 19 fragments	22–23	KS
TPS	CKs 18 and 19	14	M3

mAb monoclonal antibody

CA15.3 levels appear to correlate with stage of BC. In a study, 6/108 (6 %) stage 1, 5/52 (10 %) stage 2 and 9/39 stage 3 (18 %) BC patients had elevated serum CA15.3 levels (≥30 U/ml) at diagnosis. In a 12-month follow-up during which serum CA15.3 levels were measured once every 3 months, CA15.3 declined to normal value in all but three patients who were then diagnosed with metastatic disease [33]. CA15.3 levels in serum are elevated in 50–80 % of metastatic patients [34]. Using ELISA and normality defined as <25 U/ml, only 1/14 (7 %) patients with local recurrence of BC had elevated CA15.3 levels. Twenty-two from twenty-three (96 %) patients with both local recurrence and distant metastasis had elevated circulating CA15.3 levels [34].

MCA is a MUC-1 associated antigen; elevated levels are observed in breast, ovary, gastrointestinal cancers, and in pregnancy, endometriosis, ovarian cysts, benign lesions of breast, kidney and liver [31].

CA549 has been found elevated in other types of tumors, like ovarian, prostate and lung cancer, in pregnancy and in benign conditions of the breast [31].

CA27.29 is a MUC-1 associated antigen detected by the monoclonal antibody B27.29, specific for the protein core of the MUC1 product; it has comparable results to CA15.3, although it seems more sensitive to limited variations in tumor extension [35]. Elevated levels of this marker are observed also in ovary, gastrointestinal, kidney, endometrium, liver, lung and thyroid cancer, and in pregnancy, endometriosis, benign lesions of breast, kidney and liver [31].

To compare the two breast tumour markers, CA15-3 and MCA using Receiver Operating Characteristic (ROC) curve analysis, 196 patients "presenting" with breast carcinoma had serum CA15-3 and MCA concentrations measured. Using these markers as indicators of stage IV disease at the recommended laboratory level, true positive rates (TPR) and false positive rates (FPR) were obtained as follows: CA15-3 TPR=75 %, FPR=7.4 %, MCA TPR=80 %, FPR=59.1 %. By increasing the CA15-3 cutoff level to 45 U/ml, a TPR and FPR of 75 % and 0.6 %, respectively were obtained. By increasing the MCA cutoff level to 23 U/ml, a TPR and FPR of 65 % and 2.3 %, respectively, were obtained. These findings show that CA15-3 is a superior indicator of metastatic breast disease than MCA at recommended laboratory levels, and by altering the cutoff points, the specificity and sensitivity for both these markers can be improved [36].

13.3.2 Cytokeratins (CYFRA 21.1, TPA, TPS)

13.3.2.1 CYFRA21.1

Breast carcinoma has been demonstrated to express CK19 fragments in the primary and metastatic lesions and CK19 mRNA is detectable in peripheral blood from patients affected by breast cancer. In a study, serum CYFRA 21.1, CEA and CA 15.3 were measured in the sera from 212 BC patients, including 96 with untreated primary disease (54 stage I-II, 18 stage III and 24 stage IV), 30 regional (chest-wall and/or lymph-nodes) and 68 metastatic (haematogenous metastases) relapsing disease. One hundred healthy age-matched females and 65 patients affected by benign mammary gland disease (including 38 patients with mastopathy and 27 with fibroadenoma) were enrolled as controls. Serum levels of all markers increased from controls to patients affected by breast cancer, from stage I-II to stage IV of the breast cancer and from local to advanced recurrence [37]. In another paper, the authors studied serum CYFRA 21-1 in breast carcinoma based on evidence that breast carcinoma expresses cytokeratin 19 fragments and that CYFRA 21-1 is a specific antigen for cytokeratin 19 fragments. The serum samples of 86 patients with primary breast carcinoma, 14 patients with recurrent breast carcinoma, 22 patients with benign mammary disease, and 25 healthy controls were provided for measurements of CYFRA 21-1, carcinoembryonic antigen (CEA), and CA 15-3. The relation between clinicopathologic features, prognosis, and disease free survival with serum CYFRA 21-1 was studied. There was no difference between the serum CYFRA 21-1 levels from patients with benign mammary disease and those from healthy controls. The sensitivities of CYFRA 21-1 for patients with International Union Against Cancer Stage IV and recurrent tumors were 60 % and 64.2 %, respectively, which were as high as those for CA 15-3 and superior to those for CEA. The hematogenous recurrence showed a very high sensitivity of 89 %. According to the increments of T, N, and M factor numbers, the serum CYFRA 21-1 levels were elevated. No correlation between CYFRA 21-1 and CEA was observed and the correlation between CYFRA 21-1 and CA 15-3 was weak. The univariate and multivariate analyses for survival revealed that serum CYFRA 21-1 levels were an independent indicator of prognosis [38]. In another study from the same author, the sera from 173 patients with primary breast cancer or recurrent disease were measured for CYFRA 21-1, carcinoembryonic antigen (CEA), and carbohydrate antigen 15-3 (CA 15-3) levels. The positive rates of serum CYFRA 21-1 for stage IV (n=12) or recurrent disease (n=26) were 83.3 and 84.6 %, respectively, while those of serum CEA were 41.7 and 26.9 %, and those of serum CA 15-3 were 83.3 and 34.6 %. The elevated preoperative levels of serum CYFRA 21-1 decreased to normal levels after curative operation, whereas they remained abnormally high after noncurative operation. There was a significantly high frequency of recurrence in patients with elevated levels of serum CYFRA 21-1 preoperatively compared to those with normal levels of the marker preoperatively. The positive rate of serum CYFRA 21-1 alone was higher than that of an assay combining CEA with CA 15-3, in both primary and recurrent cases (28.8 vs. 18.8 and 84.6 vs. 46.2 %, respectively) [39].

13.3.2.2 TPA, TPS, TPA(cyk), CYFRA 21.1

In a study, the different behaviour of TPA, TPS, TPA(cyk) and CYFRA 21.1 were investigated in serum samples, mainly of metastasized cancer patients. The TPA (cyk) test determines cytokeratin 8 and 18 fragments. By selecting individual samples with a high and a low TPA/TPS ratio, it could be proven that no correlation existed in these samples between TPS and CYFRA 21.1. A good correlation was established between the TPA test and the CYFRA 21.1 test, and intermediate correlations were present between these tests and TPA (cyk) [40].

Many other studies report that serum CKs have low specificity and a raise can be observed in a wide range of cancers [19, 40–45]. Acute and chronic infections, acute and chronic inflammation, liver chirrosis, cholestasis, renal failure, and also pregnancy are the most common non malignant causes of serum cytokeratins high levels [31, 46–50].

TPA Compared with CEA and CA15.3

Specificity and sensitivity of CA15.3 have been evaluated in another study and they were compared with those of CEA and TPA. Serum concentrations of all three TMs were determined in 618 individuals: 80 healthy controls, 421 patients with local breast cancer who became free of disease following locoregional treatment, and 117 patients with disseminated disease. Radioimmunoassay (RIA) was the method employed, and the cut-off values obtained were 30 U/ml for CA 15.3, 5 ng/ml for CEA, and 120 U/l for TPA. The results showed CA 15.3 and CEA specificities to be analogous (95.7 % and 95.5 %, respectively), while TPA specificity (81.9 %) was lower ($p<0.001$). During adjuvant therapy, CA 15.3 serum levels were seen to increase, followed by a normalization of concentration after terminating therapy. On the other hand, CA 15.3 and TPA sensitivities (64.1 % and 67.5 %, respectively) were greater than for CEA (44.4 %, $p<0.01$). It was concluded that (a) CA 15.3 is a useful TM for breast cancer, as it offers a greater sensitivity than CEA and a higher specificity than TPA; (b) combining CA 15.3 and CEA fails to increase CA 15.3 sensitivity; (c) combining CA 15.3 with TPA increases false-positives therefore likely it does offer no additional benefit [51].

TPA, a Proliferation Tumor Marker

Unlike CEA and CA15.3, that are usually considered tumor burden markers, as their values tend to correlate with the stage of disease, there are data suggesting that TPA is a tumor proliferation marker.

Particularly, a study evaluated TPA in serum and tumor cell cytosol of breast cancer patients, for which proliferative activity, determined by the thymidine labelling index (TLI) technique, was also available. High serum TPA levels were associated with unfavourable clinicopathological characteristics whereas a higher tumor cell cytosol TPA level was associated with better cytohistological tumor differentiation. When analyzing cases in which serum and tumor cell cytosol TPA values were higher than 100 U/L and 500 U/mg cytosol protein, respectively, serum TPA was positively associated with TLI, while cytosolic TPA resulted negatively associated with TLI. A strong inverse relationship between cytosolic and serum TPA was evident [52]. In another study, TPA and CA 15.3 concentrations were routinely determined in serum of patients treated for breast cancer during a 15-month period. ROC curves did not show differences in the ability to differentiate between NED and PD on the basis of matching tumor marker values. During monitoring of patients with NED, TPA levels showed fluctuations of more than 25 % that were not disease related. It was concluded that CA 15.3 is a more slowly reacting marker of tumor burden than TPA, which is an immediate indicator of cell turnover [53].

13.4 Post-operative Follow-Up of Breast Cancer Using Serum TMs for an "Early" Detection of Relapse

Mainly basing upon two prospective randomized trials conducted in early nineties, it is commonly thought that in the post-operative monitoring of asymptomatic patients routine use of serum TMs with conventional instrumental examinations provide no advantage in survival or ability to palliate recurrent disease [54–59]. Therefore, in post-therapy surveillance and follow-up of primary breast cancer, current guidelines recommend clinical exam and routine breast imaging, and do not support the use of TMs such as CEA and CA15.3 and radiological examinations unless investigationally [60]. In spite of this, in clinical practice, many patients are submitted also to serial serum TMs measurement and an instrumental follow up, with repeated US and bone scans. The European Group on Tumor Markers (EGTM) and the National Academy of Clinical Biochemistry (NSCB) recommend the use of TMs for the diagnosis of early recurrences, mainly because the use of TMs may decrease the frequency of using imaging techniques, thereby reducing costs [61, 62]. In fact, diagnostic imaging are carried out only in patients suspected by clinical symptoms or by a TM increase. However, it must be highlighted that the most common guidelines, specifically those issued by Clinical Societies, are sometimes based on "old" trials, therefore new clinical evidences are needed.

13.4.1 Cut-off Value and Critical Change (CC)

Interpretation of serum TMs value is a central issue. In fact, it is well known that an "ideal" marker, with 100 % specificity and sensitivity, does not exist. Intra- (CVP) and inter- (CVG) individual biological variation, analytical imprecision (CVA), and indices of individuality affect serum TMs values. In a study, the average CVP and CVG obtained from 22 healthy women were, respectively, 6.2 % and 62.9 % (CA 15.3), 9.3 % and 86.8 % (CEA), and 28.3 % and 133 % (TPA). The indices of individuality were all <0.6: 0.2 (CA 15.3), 0.15 (CEA), and 0.2 (TPA). CVA depended on the concentration of the analytes. CVP and CVA determine what constitutes a significant difference between sequential results. Assuming a CVA of 11.2 % (CA 15.3), 9.5 % (CEA), or 11.9 % (TPA), results must differ by 30 %, 31 %, or 72 %, respectively, for $P \leq 0.05$. Therefore, they all should be considered to define at the best cut-off and critical change (CC). In fact, conventional cut-off limits are inappropriate for follow-up of breast cancer [63] and for having a cost-effective TMs accuracy with early detection of recurrences [64–67]. The addition of more markers, particularly CA15.3 and TPA to CEA proved to be useful for increasing sensitivity approximately up to 90 % with a lower decrease in specificity (Table 13.2). An appropriate cut-off and CC are necessary to get high sensitivity and specificity. A CC is a significant variation between two serum TM values determined in two consecutive blood samples withdrawn at relative short interval (few weeks).

Table 13.2 Specificity and sensitivity of serum TMs for early detection of recurrences according to the number of the evaluated markers: a meta-analysis of 22 studies

	Specificity %			Sensitivity %		
Tm (n)	Range	Median	Difference % between medians	Range	Median	Difference % between medians
1	90–98	96	–	33–69	54	–
2	82.5–95	88	−8 (1 vs. 2)	61–88	78.5	+24 (1 vs. 2)
3	79–91	84	−12 (1 vs. 3)	85–95	90	+36 (1 vs. 3)

There are discrepancies in the criteria to define a critical change [40, 62, 63, 68–71]. The EGTM considers a significant change to be an increase in previous levels of at least 25 %, which must be confirmed by a second measurement obtained within 1 month and at least one of them above the normal level. If the TMs continue to increase, this indicates disease progression [40, 72–74].

Also in our Center, since a long time a dynamic evaluation was considered to define CC. In particular, in the event of a high value, if the tumour marker(s) re-measured within 2–4 weeks had decreased to the normal level, the initial elevated value was considered to be an isolated elevated value (IEV). The elevated tumour marker was considered to be progressive (progressive increase, PI) when it was 30 %, or more, higher in the sample withdrawn 2–4 weeks following the initial elevated value. Otherwise, two equally high values were regarded to be a constant elevation (CE). In disease-free patients CE and/or PI in one or more markers, unexplained by a clear concomitant benign pathology, was considered the predictive increase, that is the kind of increase to predict relapse with an established tumour marker panel [75, 76]. In 2008, to rule out any interpretation of serum TMs, we proposed a CC according to a formula based on an individual reference limit (IRL) as cut-off value. Five consecutive blood samples are regularly withdrawn within 6 months at the beginning of the follow-up and the five serum values are considered for each marker;

IRL (cut off value) is : mean + 2SD (+3SD for TPA) when SD is ‡ 20% of mean; otherwise, SD is taken as 20% of mean.

This cut-off value is adjusted every 2.5 years and two serum TMs values higher than IRL is considered a CC. So, the CC has been defined considering both mathematical criteria (within-subject biological and statistical variability) and observational findings (rising levels at the relapse) [77].

13.4.2 Mucins

The most widely used serum TMs for post-operative breast cancer surveillance are antigens associated with the MUC-1 gene family and CEA, which are recommended by the EGTM [62].

13.4.2.1 CEA

Carcinoembryonic antigen (CEA) is a high molecular weight (180 Kda) glycoprotein which is synthesized in the developing embryo. Its natural function is unknown, although it is believed that it could be related to cell recognition or adhesion mechanisms because of its resemblance with immunoglobulins. Other molecules with a great similarity with CEA, known as CEA family, are encoded by about ten genes located on chromosome 19 [78]. Several benign conditions can cause increased serum CEA levels, like smoking, thyroiditis, hypothyroidism, inflammatory bowel disease, liver chirrosis, biliary obstruction, pancreatitis, renal failure, chronic obstructive lung disease, pneumonia, tuberculosis, ovarian cyst [31, 61, 79–82]. Elevated serum values of CEA can be detected in patients with breast, gastrointestinal, ovary and lung cancer. In breast cancer, its specificity and sensitivity as single marker are reported to be ranging from 92 % to 98 % and from 30.5 % to 50.5 % respectively depending on criteria of positivity. The reported interval between increase and diagnosis of recurrence ranges from 2 to 18 months (mean, 5.2 months) [50, 64, 66, 76, 83].

13.4.2.2 CA15.3

In a large study of 3953 patients with breast cancer followed for detection of disease recurrence, 274 of the 784 patients (35 %) who had recurrence of the disease had at least one abnormally elevated CA15.3 measurement (>30 U/ml) [84]. Another study examined the value of CA15-3 as an alternative to conventional bone scintigraphy for diagnosing breast cancer metastases. A total of 218 patients with breast cancer was evaluated over a 4-year period. Serum CA15-3 levels were obtained at 3-monthly intervals and bone scintigraphy annually or if the patient developed locomotor symptoms or exhibited elevated CA15-3 levels. Of these patients, 33 with metastatic breast carcinoma had an elevated tumour marker level at the time of diagnosis of their metastases; bone metastases alone = 15/17 (88 %), soft tissue metastases alone = 2/6 (33 %), simultaneous bony and soft tissue metastases = 7/10 (70 %). The preponderance of an elevated CA15-3 in metastatic bone disease, be it in isolation or in combination with non-bone metastases, yields a sensitivity, specificity and positive predictive value of 81.5 %, 66 % and 92 %, respectively. Although 22 of the 27 patients had an elevated CA15-3 at the time of diagnosis of their bone metastases, the remaining five patients (with tumour marker levels in the normal range) showed a similar, albeit a delayed, increase (median = 3 months). Thus, all metastatic bone disease patients demonstrated elevated marker levels [33]. Two hundred and forty three female breast cancer patients with localised disease were followed prospectively with CA15.3 after primary treatment until the first relapse. In the follow-up period, the CA15-3 was analysed every 6 months. During the 5 years of follow-up, 59 (24 %) relapses were discovered. CA15-3 was elevated in 21/59 (36 %) of the relapsed cases at least once. The 59 patients were subjected to 199 tests, of which 25 (13 %) were positive. Among the 184 patients without recurrence, there were 6 (3 %) with a positive CA15-3 level. The test failed to detect locoregional relapse or contralateral breast cancer. It was elevated in approximately half of bone-only metastases and in all of the liver-only metastases. In the pulmonary-only recurrences, the marker value was not elevated. Authors conclude that the CA15-3 is not sensitive enough to indicate the first relapse earlier than other methods [85].

13.4.2.3 CEA-CA15.3 Association

Many studies have shown that serial determination of CA15.3 and CEA is useful for the early detection of recurrences [50, 64, 85, 86].

Sixty-two women who had undergone curative surgery for pT1-2 pN0-1 M0 breast cancer developed local recurrences, distant metastases or contralateral BC during a median relapse time of 53 months (range 25–149 months). Sensitivity of CEA, CA 15-3, and CEA + CA 15-3 together was 40.3 %, 41.9 % and 59.7 %, respectively. No correlation (p = NS) was found between tumor markers sensitivity and type of recurrence, surgical procedure, histologic subtypes and hormone receptors rate. CEA significantly ($p < 0.01$) correlated with the size of the tumor and axillary node status and CA 15-3 with the age of the patients [87]. In a prospective study, serial serum determinations of CEA and CA15.3 every 3–6 months were performed in 1023 patients (mean follow-up 6.2 years) with no evidence of residual disease (NED) after radical surgery; 246 patients developed metastases during the follow-up. CEA and CA 15.3 were elevated (>10 ng/ml or >60 U/ml, respectively) prior to diagnosis of metastases in 40 % (98/246) and 41 % (37/91) of the patients with recurrence, with a lead time of 4.9 ± 2.2 and 4.2 ± 2.3 months, respectively. When patients with locoregional recurrences were excluded, sensitivity improved to 46 % (CEA) and 54 % (CA 15.3), and to 64 % with both TMs. Specificity of the tumor markers was 99 % for both TMs [66]. In a study conducted in 8000 breast cancer patients, CEA and CA15.3 were in the normal range (CEA < 6 microg/L and CA15.3 < 40 U/L) before surgery, and increased only before the development of distant metaseases. Twenty four patients participated in a prospective study in which they were monitored every 3 months after an increase of CEA and/or CA15.3 until the metastases were detected clinically. Half of these patients developed metastases within 5 months after CA15.3 or CEA increase, while in the remaining 12 patients the time interval between increase and detection of metastases was much longer [88].

In another study, 103 women with pT1-2, pN0-1, M0 operated for breast cancer were followed up for at least 5 years and CEA and CA 15-3 serum levels were measured every 6 months. During the follow-up, 21 (20.4 %) patients showed recurrence and overall CEA and CA 15-3 sensitivity was 38.1 % and 61.1 %, with 98.8 %

and 91.2 % specificity, respectively [64]. More recently, a prospective Iranian study assessed the value of CEA and CA15-3 in 159 patients with primary breast cancer. CEA and CA15-3 assays (mean 14 per patient) were performed at diagnosis, end of surgery and chemotherapy and every 3 months in the first 2 years and every 6 months in second 2 years of the follow-up period. During the follow-up, 33 patients (20.8 %) presented symptomatic metastasis. A significant relationship was seen between metastasis status and positive CEA and CA15-3 levels. The sensitivity and specificity were 66.7 % and 98.4 % for CEA and 84.8 % and 91.3 % for CA15-3 respectively. Optimum cut-offs were 4.95 ng/mL and 30.5 U/mL for CEA and CA15-3 [89].

13.4.2.4 Lead Time and Diagnostic Accuracy of CEA and CA15.3

The lead time is the time interval between the first TM increase and the instrumental diagnosis of recurrence. The majority of authors report a led time ranging between 2 and 18 months (mean 5.2 months) [50, 64, 65, 76, 85]. Sensitivity in early diagnosis of recurrence is low in locoregional recurrences and high in distant metastases [66, 85]. Published papers show that CA15.3 is the TM of choice in the early diagnosis of recurrence, but EGTM guidelines advise the inclusion of CEA to increase sensitivity by 5–20 %. Using the commercial kit cut-off values, the proportion of high TM values due to reasons other than recurrence was 6.6 % for CA15.3 and 5 % for CEA. Other studies have reported a specificity ranging from 92 % to 99 % for these two TMs. The use of a dynamic criterion, at least two successive increases in each of them of more than 15 % compared to the previous measurement, increased specificity to over 99 % [90].

13.4.2.5 CEA-CA15.3-MCA Association

A prospective study comparing the abilities of CA15.3, mucin-like carcinoma associated antigen (MCA), and CEA to predict the onset of metastasis in BC patients observed that CA15.3, at a cut-off of >27 U/ml, could predict metastasis in 36 % of BC patients compared to 64 % for MCA and 33 % for CEA. CA15.3 elevation in the serum appeared to be more sensitive (78–96 % sensitive with a range of 56–140 U/ml) to detect patients with mixed metastasis (both bony and soft tissue metastasis) than those with either an isolated bony or soft tissue metastasis (32–75 % sensitivity for bone metastasis, range: 21–40 U/ml and 47–83 % sensitivity for soft tissue metastasis, range: 22–67 U/ml). While MCA was a better marker of early metastasis than either CA15.3 or CEA, neither marker was very good at predicting disease relapse [91].

13.4.3 Cytokeratins in Addition to Mucins

Various studies have suggested the inclusion of cytokeratins with or without CEA, in breast cancer follow-up.

13.4.3.1 CA15.3-CEA-TPA

A study investigated the ability of CA 15.3, CEA, and TPA to predict or exclude metastases in bone/viscera during adjuvant treatment and follow-up of high-risk breast cancer patients. Ninety of them were followed up with TMs, clinical examination, and imaging techniques. During the marker monitoring period, four patients developed a recurrence confined to skin or lymph nodes, 21 developed metastases to bone or viscera, and 65 females had no evidence of metastases. CA 15.3, CEA, and TPA correctly classified 48 %, 10 %, and 19 % of the patients with metastases in bone/viscera, and 100 %, 94 %, and 98 % without. The NPV (86 %) indicated that when CA 15.3 did not signal recurrence, metastases to bone or viscera were not likely [92]. The same TM panel was evaluated by Nicolini et al. in 285 breast cancer patients. In particular, the CA15-3 sensitivity for an "early" diagnosis was compared with those of the two other markers in order to define the most suitable association. Moreover, in a subset of 169 non relapsed patients with a prolonged follow-up (40±8 months) CA15-3 specificity was investigated. During post-operative follow-up, in 27 (10 %) patients, distant metastases occurred. CA15-3, CEA and TPA sensitivity were 46 %, 7 % and 63 % respectively. When each tumour marker was considered in combination, CA15-3-CEA-TPA association showed a higher sensitivity (87 %) than both CA15-3-TPA (83 %) and the CEA-TPA (70 %). Serum CA15-3 increase preceded the certain sign of metastases 2.7±2.6 months. Shortly before appearance of distant metastases, CE and/or PI in serum CA15-3 values occurred in all evaluated patients except three in whom IEVs were found as well. In 24 (14 %) of the 169 non relapsed patients, high serum CA15-3 values occurred. In 16 of these 24 patients, an IEV was found, while four (2.3 %) or the eight remaining ones with CE and/or PI were falsely suspected of metastases. In this group of non relapsed patients, chronic liver failure, diabetes and/or hepatic steatosis were the reasons more commonly responsible for the CA15-3 increase. These data indicate that in the post-operative follow-up of breast cancer patients, TPA is the most useful tumour marker and TPA-CA15-3 the most suitable association. Contemporaneous measurement of serum CEA levels only slightly increases sensitivity and PPV of TPA-CA15-3 combination [50]. More recently, after we have adopted the previously mentioned IRL and CC in 186 disease free breast cancer patients, those falsely suspected have been evaluated. Every 100 person/years, 1.8 %, 6 %, 0.8 % and 8.4 % were patients falsely suspected for relapse with CEA, TPA, CA15.3 and CEA-TPA-CA15.3 association respectively.

13.4.3.2 CA15.3-CEA-TPS

The efficacy of CEA and CA15.3 tumor markers in monitoring breast cancer was evaluated in 831 patients. Three hundred and forty-nine patients were monitored for either a minimum of 5 years or until time of recurrence. CA 15.3 and TPS sensitivities were 71.9 % and 66.3 % in metastatic patients, respectively and in them the addition of TPS to CA 15.3 increased the sensitivity to 87.6 %. During post-surgical follow-up CA 15.3 was elevated in 65.7 % and TPS in 61.3 % of patients with recurrence. The combination of TPS and CA 15.3 increased the overall sensitivity by 12.7 % [44]. Given et al. examined TPS, CA15.3 and CEA in 1082 breast cancer patients, 277 of whom had a recurrence. The mean follow-up was 4.4 years. Sensitivity, specificity, PPV and NPV of CA 15-3, TPS and CEA for visceral, bony and locoregional recurrence were calculated. CA 15.3 was the most sensitive marker, 68 % for visceral and 69 % for bony recurrence. TPS showed 64 % and 51 % specificity, and CEA 27 % and 46 % for visceral and bony recurrence respectively. The PPV of CA 15.3 was 47 % for visceral and 54 % for bony recurrence, and was greater than that for TPS (visceral 25 %, bony 21 %) or CEA (visceral 18 %, bony 26 %). The sensitivity of CA 15.3 and TPS for locoregional recurrence was low at 23 % and 17 % respectively. A combination of CA 15.3, TPS and CEA failed to increase the sensitivity of CA 15.3 for visceral recurrence. However, a marginally increased sensitivity was recorded for combined CA 15.3 and TPS (70 %) and for combined CA 15.3, TPS and CEA (71 %) in bony recurrence. The mean lead time in visceral recurrence for TPS and CA 15.3 were 8 and 10 months respectively. In patients with bony recurrence the mean lead time for TPS and CA 15.3 were 7.5 and 8.25 months. Mean lead time increased to 9 and 11 months for bony and visceral recurrence respectively when CA 153 and TPS were combined. Sensitivity in the early diagnosis of distant metastases was 21–25 % for TPS, 47–54 % for CA15.3 and 18–26 % for CEA. Specificity was over 90 % for CA15.3 and CEA, while TPS showed more than 12 % false positive results [86].

13.4.3.3 CEA-CA15.3-CYFRA21.1

In the study previously mentioned by Giovanella et al., 48 patients previously treated by surgery and without any evidence of disease were enrolled to evaluate the role of serum TMs in the monitoring for recurrence of the disease. The comparison of diagnostic accuracy in the detection of primary and relapsing breast cancer showed no significant differences between markers. CEA and CYFRA 21.1 detected less recurrences than CA 15.3. Authors concluded that these data showed no significant improvement in the diagnosis and follow-up of breast cancer by CYFRA 21.1 and CEA assays compared to CA 15.3 assay and recommended that the CYFRA 21.1 assay should not be employed in clinical practice [37].

13.4.3.4 CA15.3-MCA-CEA-TPA

A study prospectively monitored 209 post-operative breast cancer patients with simultaneous serum level estimations of CA15.3, MCA, TPA and CEA; 141 (67.5 %) were free of recurrence and 68 (32.5 %) developed metastases during the follow-up. The sensitivity of tumor markers were 68.2 % for CA15.3, 34.1 % for CEA, 72.7 % for MCA and TPA. The combination of CA15.3 with TPA or MCA with TPA showed a trend for improved sensitivity of both markers ($p=0.06$), with no specific loss of specificity ($p=0.11$). The addition of CEA to CA15.3 or MCA did not provide additional information for clinical evaluation. Patients with elevated tumor marker determinations had significantly shorter survival than those with values within the normal range. Two serial, progressively increasing values of tumor markers during the follow-up strongly predicted recurrence. Authors concluded that the co-measurement of CA15.3 with TPA or MCA with TPA is justifiable in monitoring breast cancer patients postoperatively [93]. In this study, and in the study by Vizcarra et al. already mentioned, adding a cytokeratin resulted in an increase in sensitivity, but it resulted in a decrease in specificity as well (over 15 % false positive results for TPA) [93, 94].

13.4.4 Usefulness of Serum TMs in Addition to Conventional Instrumental Examinations During an Instrumental-Biochemical Follow-Up

A few studies have addressed the usefulness of serum TMs in addition to conventional instrumental examinations for diagnosis of distant metastases.

13.4.4.1 Bony Skeleton

A study was conducted in order to specify the precise role of bone scintigraphy and serum CEA and CA 15-3 assays in the monitoring of breast cancers in order to optimize their use. In patients with bone metastasis, serum CEA levels were abnormal in 23/49 cases and CA 15-3 serum concentrations were elevated above the cut-off in 33/49 cases. Among patients without bone metastasis, CEA and CA 15-3 serum concentrations were normal in 50/74 and 55/74 cases respectively. The combination of the two markers improved the diagnostic sensitivity. Authors conclude that although serial tumor marker measurements are an efficient and cost effective method of monitoring disease progression, it does not allow prediction of the bone scan results; so it is not justifiable to reject a bone scintigraphy on the basis of these markers [95]. A study was performed in 25 patients with breast cancer, previously surgically treated to correlate serum levels of CA15-3, CEA and bone scintigraphy. All patients underwent whole body scintigraphy. CA15.3 and CEA were measured by radioimmunoassay. Bone scintigraphy revealed bone metastases in 16 (64 %) patients. Significant differences in CA15.3 level was found in patients with metastases compared to patients without metastases [96]. Another study retrospectively evaluated 120 bone scans of patients with breast carcinoma Results of the bone scans were grouped as normal, equivocal and metastatic. Cutoff levels of 4.8 U/mL for CEA and 38 U/mL for CA 15-3 were accepted. Bone scintigraphy revealed metastases in 16 patients. Sixty-one patients had normal scans and in 47 patients metastases could not be ruled out. In patients with metastases, CA 15-3 was elevated in 8 and CEA was higher than the upper limit in 6 [97]. Eighty-nine women with BC who had undergone bone scintigraphy as part of their follow-up were retrospectively evaluated in order to establish the diagnostic value of bone scan in association with measurements of serum CEA, CA 15-3 and TPA levels. Serum tumor markers levels were compared with the results of bone scintigraphy. Serum CEA, CA 15-3 and TPA levels of 7 ng/ml, 35 U/ml and 90 U/l, respectively, were adopted as the upper limit of normal. Serum CA 15-3 was significantly higher in patients with a positive bone scan ($p=0.017$). For CEA and TPA, no significant difference was found between patients with and without bone metastases. Twenty-five of seventy patients (36 %) with normal CEA had bone metastases. Four of 50 (8 %) patients with normal

CA 15-3 and 15 of 51 (29 %) patients with normal TPA had a positive bone scan. The combination of CA 15-3 with TPA showed 100 % sensitivity in detecting bone metastases. In all 42 patients without bone metastases, CA 15-3 and/or TPA levels were normal [98]. In another study bone scan (99 mTc-MDP) and CA15-3 were evaluated in 35 patients with breast cancer. The serum CA15-3 was measured by electrochemoluminescence (ECLIA) method with 30 U/mL as cutoff value. According to bone scan results, 24 (68.8 %) patients revealed bone metastasis. The mean level of serum CA15-3 was significantly higher in patients with bone metastasis than in those without metastasis (26.37 ± 4.74 U/mL vs. 19.09 ± 1.99 U/mL; $p < 0.001$). There was not significant relation between the serum level of CA15-3 and the extent of bone metastasis. Coordinates of the curve study yielded a cut-off point >21.8 U/mL for the serum level of CA15-3, with a sensitivity and specificity of 91.7 % and 91 %, respectively [99]. A retrospective study assessed the value of a serum tumour marker panel in selecting among the patients with equivocal BS those with bone metastases. Two hundred and ninety seven breast cancer patients were followed-up after mastectomy with serial determinations of a CEA-TPA-CA15.3 tumour marker panel, BS and liver echography. The tumour marker panel was used to select patients with equivocal BS for examination of suspicious bone areas by further imaging techniques. Up to December 1995, 158 (53 %) patients showed an equivocal BS and 47 patients developed bone metastases. In the 158 patients with equivocal BS, prolonged clinical and imaging follow-up over 45 months (mean; range 12–120) was used to ascertain the presence or absence of bone metastases. In these 158 patients the negative predictive value and positive predictive value of the tumour marker panel to predict bone metastases was 97 % and 75 % respectively. This study shows that in breast cancer patients the CEA-TPA-CA15.3 tumour marker panel has a high value in selecting those patients with bone metastases, or at high risk of developing clinically-evident bone metastases, among the large number of subjects with equivocal BS [75].

13.4.4.2 Liver

CEA, carbohydrate antigen CA19-9 (CA19-9), thymidine kinase (TK), TPA, TPS and CYFRA 21-1 were evaluated in differential diagnosis between benign liver lesions and liver metastases of breast cancer. Serum levels of CYFRA 21-1, TPA, TPS and CEA were significantly higher in patients with liver metastases of breast cancer in contrast to healthy controls and patients with benign liver lesions (p-value < 0.05) [100].

13.4.4.3 Multiorgans (Bony Skeleton, Thorax and Abdomen)

The relationship between serum serial CA15.3 values and 18 F-fluorodeoxyglucose (FDG) positron emission tomography (PET)/computed tomography (CT) findings in BC follow-up was assessed in a further study. Authors retrospectively selected 60 patients with previous history of BC, already submitted to surgery and other treatments. Three serial measures of Ca15.3 were collected within 1 year before PET/CT examination, respectively, at 12–9 months, 9–3 months and 3–0 months. Clinical outcome or imaging follow-up data were used to define disease relapse. The increase in tumor marker value was compared with PET/CT results and disease relapse. PET/CT was negative in 36 (60 %) and positive in 24 (40 %) patients. Coefficient of variation of the Ca15.3 serial determinations was significantly higher in patients with positive than negative PET/CT (39 % vs. 24 %, $p < 0.05$). Disease relapse was found in 25 (42 %) patients, of these 21 (88 %) had positive PET/CT. ROC analyses showed that an increase of Ca15.3 between the 2nd and 3rd measures have better individuated positive PET/CT and disease relapse (AUC 0.65 and 0.64, respectively; p < 0.05) [101]. A retrospective Japanese study analyzed the lead time by periodic measurements of serum CEA and CA15-3 in 233 patients who underwent breast cancer surgery. Both tumor marker levels were measured every 3 months for the first 5 years, every 6 months for the next 5 years, then annually. Physical examination and chest X-ray were routinely done at the same time, and bone or computed tomographic scans were done if the tumor marker levels were elevated or clinical symptoms appeared. In patients with recurrent disease, the mean lead times were −333.9 days for CEA and −210.6 days for CA15-3, respectively. Elevated tumor marker levels were found much later than recurrence [102]. Another retrospective study by our group assessed the value of a serum tumour marker panel in selecting from among the patients with equivocal chest X-ray (CXR) or liver echography (LE) those with thoracic or liver metastases respectively. We focused on a series of 377 patients including 341 non-relapsed plus 36 with liver or thoracic metastases. The patients were followed-up after mastectomy with serial determinations of a panel of CEA-TPA-CA15.3 tumour markers, bone scintigraphy, CXR and LE. Up to December 1999, equivocal CXR occurred in 23 (6.1 %) patients of whom 11 (47.8 %) developed thoracic metastases; 14 (3.7 %) patients showed an equivocal LE of whom five developed liver metastases. In the 37 patients with equivocal CXR or equivocal LE prolonged clinical and imaging follow-up over 41 ± 36 months (mean ± SD, range 3–163) was used to ascertain the presence or absence of thoracic or liver metastases. In the 23 patients with equivocal CXR the negative and positive predictive values of the tumour marker panel to predict thoracic metastases were 92 % and 100 % respectively. In the 14 patients with equivocal LE the negative and positive predictive values of the tumour marker panel for prediction of liver metastases were 90 % and 100 % respectively. So in breast cancer patients the CEA-TPA-CA15.3 tumour marker panel showed a high value for selecting those patients at high risk of developing clinically evident pulmonary or liver metastases from amongst those subjects with equivocal CXR or equivocal LE [76]. In a similar study, data of 427 breast cancer patients submitted to an intensive follow-up after mastectomy were retrospectively reviewed by the same authors. Among the 427 patients operated on for breast cancer, 221 patients with a total of 332 equivocal instrumental examinations (bone scintigraphy, $n = 286$; chest X-ray, $n = 29$; liver echography, $n = 17$) were reviewed. All 221 patients were followed up clinically, biochemically and instrumentally until there was a clear definition of their condition, metastatic or not, for an average time of 35 months. Concomitant clinical symptoms were also taken into consideration. Among the 221 patients with equivocal bone scintigraphy, chest X-ray and liver echography, tumour markers showed a positive predictive value of 69 %, 93 % and 83 % and a negative predictive value of 98 %, 86 % and 91 %, respectively, for the indication of the metastatic or benign origin of the equivocal instrumental imaging. Clinical symptoms were not helpful in predicting metastatic disease (sensitivity, specificity and accuracy of 60 %, 53 % and 54 %, respectively). Basing upon these data, a short monitoring with the CEA-TPA-CA15.3 tumour marker panel is suggested to confirm or exclude metastatic disease in those patients who are suspected to have metastases following common instrumental investigations. This monitoring can avoid false positive diagnoses [103].

13.4.5 "Early" Treatment of Recurrent Disease

This is a very controversial issue. In spite the two above mentioned prospective randomized trials do not support the usefulness of an early detection of relapse, few pilot studies have reported on survival benefit from an "early" treatment of recurrent disease using serum TMs.

13.4.5.1 Pilot Studies Supporting Survival Benefit

Nicolini et al. studied 50 patients with an increase in TMs but no clinical or radiological evidence of disease. Twenty-eight patients were treated 13.5 ± 10 months (mean ± s.d.) before the clinical and/or radiological occurrence of distant metastases that were suspected because of an increase in the tumour markers (patients treated 'early'). Their outcome was compared with that of 22 similar patients who were treated only after a definite radiological diagnosis was achieved (patients treated 'not early'). The groups were similar for all the major prognostic factors (menopause, staging, hormone dependency). The time to progression and the overall survival were significantly greater in the treated group. In particular, for patients treated 'early', the survival curves up to 30 months after salvage treatment and up to 72 months after mastectomy showed greater survival than those for the patients treated later (42.9 % vs. 13.6 % and 42.9 % vs. 22.7 % respectively; $P=0.04$ in both instances). These data suggest that treatment triggered by rising tumour markers before clinical and/or radiological appearance of distant metastases can be useful in prolonging both the asymptomatic interval and the duration of response of some relapsed patients [104]. These findings at least in part also have been observed by Jaeger et al. [88]. We successively confirmed our data in 68 metastatic patients. Thirty-six (53 %) received salvage treatment at the time of significant increase in one or more components of CEA-TPA-CA15.3 tumour marker panel and negative instrumental examinations ("tumour marker guided" treatment) and 32 (47 %) were treated only after radiological confirmation of metastases (conventional treatment). The prognostic factors of the two groups did not show any statistically significant difference. The time from one or more tumour marker increase to clear clinical and/or radiological signs of distant metastases (lead time) was significantly prolonged in the 36 patients with "tumour marker guided" treatment (17.3 ± 13.1 vs. 2.9 ± 2.9 months, $P<0.001$, Wilcoxon test) as well as the survival curves from salvage therapy and from mastectomy (the proportion of survivors was: at 36 months from salvage therapy 28 % vs. 9 %, $P=0.0094$; at 84 months from mastectomy 42 % vs. 19 %, $P=0.0017$). The multivariate Cox analysis showed that time from mastectomy to tumour marker increase and "tumour marker guided" salvage treatment were the only significantly different variables ($P=0.00001$ and 0.005, respectively). These data confirmed that "tumour marker guided" salvage treatment significantly prolongs disease-free and overall survivals of relapsing responsive patients [105]. These interesting data have not yet received confirmation by randomized, multicenter, prospective trials. Such trials cannot be easily planned. In fact, they arise some ethical reasons on patients treated without certain signs of metastatic disease, due to the potential toxicity of the administered drugs.

13.5 Monitoring of Advanced Disease According to Current Guidelines

In advanced or metastatic disease, current guidelines recommend a response to treatment evaluation every 2–4 cycles of chemotherapy by history, physical-clinical examination, routine blood tests and radiological examinations. The interval between assessments may be prolonged in case of indolent disease and long lasting responses. Serum TMs, such as CA15.3 and/or CEA, if initially elevated, are considered helpful in monitoring response. However, a change in TM alone is not recommended as the only determinant for treatment decisions. In fact, a flare of TM can occur in the first 6 weeks of an efficacious therapy and this must be considered when interpreting serial values [57, 58, 60, 106] It has been reported that the use of serum TMs in therapy monitoring may reduce the follow-up expenses by up 50 % as compared to the use of imaging techniques [107] and EGTM guidelines advise the measurement of CA15.3 and CEA in the metastatic breast cancer follow-up, especially in patients with non measurable disease [61, 62]. Other clinical societies, such as the British Association of Surgical Oncology, recommend the use of TMs in monitoring the efficacy of treatment [108].

13.5.1 Serum TMs for Monitoring of Metastatic Disease

Monitoring response to treatment using TMs may provide earlier information than that obtained with imaging methods. In addition, with some new "biological" drugs, RECIST criteria are often inadequate [39, 40, 68–71, 109–112]. A decrease of at least 50 % indicates a response. It is important to carry out the measurement at the pre-therapy check in order to avoid wrongly evaluating transient increases during chemotherapy or radiotherapy, possibly related to cell destruction [40, 71–73]. EGTM guidelines recommend pre-cycle measurement of CEA and CA15.3 in patients receiving chemotherapy and at least every 3 months in patients receiving hormone therapy. In metastatic disease, the reported sensitivity of CA15.3 varies from 42 % to 82 % and that of CEA from 35.5 % to 50.5 % [51, 57, 61, 62, 93, 113–116]. Various authors have suggested to add a cytokeratin (TPA, TPS or Cyfra 21.1) in order to improve sensitivity [37, 40, 50, 68, 69, 117, 118].

13.5.2 Mucins

13.5.2.1 CA15.3

A study included 122 patients in whom the CA15-3 level showed either a decline (92 patients) or an acute surge followed by a decline (30 patients) after chemotherapy. The clinical characteristics between the two groups and the CA 15-3 kinetics using ROC curves were analyzed. Patients with a surge had a significantly higher risk of disease progression than patients without a surge (P=0.004; odds ratio 2.62; 95 % CI 1.45–4.72). The clinicopathologic characteristics were significantly different between the two groups with respect to the distribution of ER, PR, and HER2 status, relapse-free survival, and the severity and extent of the involved organs. For patients with a surge, a CA 15-3 slope threshold >≥0.0038 was chosen with a sensitivity of 80.0 % and a specificity of 80.4 %. The area under the curve was 0.847 (95 % CI 0.771–0.906; P=0.0001). A significant correlation between PFS and CA 15-3 slope was shown with Cox-regression modeling (P=0.036; hazard ratio [HR], 2.1; 95 % CI 1.01–4.14). These kinetics might serve as a good predictive marker of treatment response and response duration [119]. In mestatatic disease, serial measurement of serum CA15.3 levels with a cut-off of 33 U/ml (prior to start of therapy and then at 2, 4, and 6 months after starting therapy) significantly correlated with progression of the disease (non-progression being defined as having either a complete/partial response or stable disease). The sensitivity and specificity of CA15.3 in detecting progressive disease were 85 % and 91 % at 2 months, 96 % and 96 % at 4 months, and 92 % and 100 % at 6 months respectively [120, 121].

13.5.2.2 CA549

A study investigated whether the serum tumour marker CA549 gave early and reliable information about disease activity among metastatic breast cancer patients during cytostatic treatment and follow-up. Fifty females were monitored clinically and with the tumour marker CA549. Response evaluation was based upon clinical (World Health Organization) and elaborated CA549 criteria, respectively. In 113 blindly and matched evaluations, concordance appeared in 73/113 and discordance in 40/113 evaluations. In 27, discordance concerned degree of response, in two clinical progression followed marker progression after the end of the study, and in 11 progressive disease was established by clinical investigation alone. CA 549 response excluded clinical progression in bone or viscera and reversed. Clinical progression within 2 months in viscera and bone was predicted among 91 % by marker progression. Clinical progression was excluded among 93 % without marker progression [122].

13.5.2.3 CEA-CA15.3 Association

An established biochemical index for monitoring therapy in patients with metastatic breast cancer was tested prospectively in a multicentre study. The index uses two serum tumour markers – carcinoembryonic antigen (CEA) and carbohydrate antigen 15-3 (CA15-3) along with erythrocyte sedimentation rate (ESR). Sixty-seven patients treated by either endocrine or chemotherapy had CA15-3, CEA and ESR measured at diagnosis of metastases and sequentially during therapy. Two markers, CA15-3 and CEA, were measured on a further 16 patients giving a total of 83 patients who were assessable for CA15-3 and CEA. Of the patients with CA15-3, CEA and ESR measured at diagnosis of metastases 84 % (56/67) had elevation of one or more markers. During therapy the number with elevated marker(s) rose to 96 % (64/67). Changes in the markers were in line with and often pre-dated therapeutic outcome as assessed by the International Union Against Cancer (UICC) criteria both for remission and progression. Patients without elevation of markers on diagnosis subsequently showed a rise in the marker(s) at or before documented disease progression by UICC. The three women in whom markers were at no time significantly elevated remained in remission. The results using CA15-3 and CEA were similar but 12 % less patients were assessable. It was concluded that CA15-3 and CEA (with and without ESR) provide an objective method to guide therapy in patients with metastatic breast cancer [69].

The utility of computer simulation models for performance comparisons of different tumor marker assessment criteria to define progression or nonprogression of metastatic breast cancer was investigated. Clinically relevant values for progressive CA15.3 and CEA concentrations were combined with representative values for background variations in a computer simulation model. Fifteen criteria for assessment of longitudinal tumor marker data were obtained from the literature and computerized. Modulation of the background variation, the starting concentrations, and the cutoffs enabled identification of criteria that were robust against false-positive signals of progression. The computer simulation model showed to be a fast, effective, and inexpensive approach for comparing the diagnostic potential of assessment criteria during clinically relevant conditions of steady-state and progressive disease. Authors concluded that the proposed model can be used to generate tumor marker assessment criteria for a variety of malignancies and to compare and optimize their diagnostic performance [71].

When CA15.3, CEA and ESR were used as a panel of serum markers in monitoring therapeutic response, over 90 % of patients are biochemically assessable. A biochemical index score comprising these three markers has been devised retrospectively, validated prospectively, in a single centre and in a multicentre study. Biochemical assessment by serum markers correlated with clinical/radiological (UICC) assessment and often pre-dated remission and progression shown by UICC criteria. Authors stated that it is also the only validated method in monitoring metastatic breast cancer with disease unassessable by UICC criteria (e.g. sclerotic bone metastases, irradiated lesions) [123].

To clarify the significance of CEA and CA 15-3 in monitoring advanced breast cancer, the Tumor Marker Study Group of the Japanese Breast Cancer Society conducted a large-scale retrospective study. The findings of 528 patients from four clinical trials and seven institutes with advanced breast cancer were collected. Three hundred and forty-eight patients, in whom both serum CEA and CA 15-3 were measured during therapy, were selected for analysis. The pretreatment positivity rate of CA 15-3 was significantly higher than that of CEA ($p<0.0001$). Time-to-progression (TTP) in CEA- and CA 15-3-positive patients was significantly shorter than TTP in negative patients. The changes in either marker level correlated well with response to therapy in marker-positive patients but not in negative patients. TTP in the marker-positive patients with a greater than 20 %-reduction in either marker level during therapy was significantly longer than that in positive patients without such a reduction ($p<0.01$ for CEA and CA 15-3) [124].

The Tumor Marker Study Group of the Japanese Breast Cancer Society conducted also a prospective study. Patients with advanced breast cancer who were treated with systemic therapy between January and December 2002 were recruited from five collaborative institutes in Japan. The patients were monitored every 4 weeks using three serum tumor markers, CEA, CA 15-3 and NCC-ST-439 during the therapy. Findings from 108 eligible patients were analyzed. The pretreatment positivity rates were 51.9 % for CEA, 50 % for CA 15-3, and 34.3 % for NCC-ST-439. The changes in each marker level at 8 and 12 weeks but not at 4 weeks after the start of therapy seemed to correlate with the response to therapy in pretreatment marker-positive patients but not in negative patients. The Cox proportional hazard model revealed a greater than 20 % reduction in CEA, CA 15-3 or NCC-ST-439 levels at 4, 8 and/or 12 weeks after the start of therapy to be an independent predictive factor for longer time-to-progression (TTP) in pretreatment marker-positive patients. This prospective study supported the findings obtained from the previous retrospective study that in pretreatment marker-positive patients (1) the changes in serum tumor marker levels after the start of therapy correlate with the response to therapy; and (2) a greater than 20 % reduction in the tumor marker levels is a favorable predictive factor for TTP during systemic therapy. When the pretreatment serum level of these markers is over the respective cut-off value, sequential measurement of them may be useful for evaluating the efficacy of treatment as well as monitoring the outcome of patients with advanced breast cancer [125]

To predict the response to chemotherapy of patients with metastatic or recurrent breast cancer using serum TMs, a study retrospectively analyzed a training set of 105 patients with metastatic or recurrent breast cancer. Their chemotherapeutic response had been evaluated according to the World Health Organization (WHO)'s response criteria. The model for predicting response using CEA, CA15-3, and NCC-ST-439 was determined using the area under the ROC (ROC-AUC) and the overall misclassification rate (OMR) in a random cross-validation. The prediction model was then verified in a consecutive set of 64 patients. Their response had been evaluated using the response evaluation criteria in solid tumors (RECIST). The best prediction model consisted of the serum CEA, CA15-3, and NCC-ST-439 levels, but the prediction formula varied according to the baseline CA15-3 level (elevated or normal). The overall ROC-AUC and OMR in the training set were 0.83 and 0.19, respectively. The overall ROC-AUC and OMR in the verification set were 0.72 and 0.28, respectively. When the verification set was stratified according to either the objective response or the predicted response, the time-to-progression, but not the overall survival, was significantly different. This model for predicting the response to first-line chemotherapy of patients with metastatic or recurrent breast cancer predicted the outcome of more than 70 % of the patients in an independent verification set [126].

13.5.3 Cytokeratins

During therapy, monitoring of metastasized patients with TPA, TPS, TPA (cyk) and CYFRA21.1 could show a different pattern of reactivity and the different test results during therapy monitoring are not always easy to interpretate [40].

13.5.3.1 CYFRA21.1

In both previously mentioned studies by Nakata et al. [38, 39], the measurement of the serum CYFRA 21-1 titer in patients with breast carcinoma was useful in monitoring for recurrence and well correlated with response to chemotherapy.

13.5.4 Mucins and Cytokeratins

13.5.4.1 CA15.3, CEA, TPA

To clarify the usefulness of the serial combination assay of serum CEA, CA 15-3 and TPA in monitoring the clinical course of patients during therapy, the relationship between the initial changes and the kinetic patterns of the markers after therapy and the objective responses was investigated. When an increase or decrease of over 20 % in these markers was taken as significant, then the initial changes in all three markers significantly correlated with the therapeutic responses ($P<0.01$). Five distinct kinetic patterns in the marker levels were observed. A paradoxical kinetic pattern of CEA and CA 15-3 levels – that is, an "initial surge and subsequent drop" – was seen in one-third of the responders. The TPA levels tended to exhibit a "steady decline" pattern in those responders. The sensitivity and specificity of the kinetic patterns to predict the clinical courses were significantly higher than those obtained from the analysis of initial changes. These findings thus suggest that adequate knowledge of the unique kinetics of each marker may help to make a more accurate prediction of the therapeutic responses [127].

In an above mentioned study by A Nicolini et al., in metastatic patients serum TPA values showed the highest sensitivity and paralleled clinical and/or instrumental signs better than the CA15-3 and even more than CEA values. The reported data indicated that in the post-operative follow-up of breast cancer patients, TPA is the most useful tumour marker and TPA-CA15-3 the most suitable association. Contemporaneous measurement of serum CEA levels only slightly increases sensitivity and positive predictive value of TPA-CA15-3 combination [50].

In another study, authors investigated whether model systems integrating stochastic variation into criteria for marker assessment could be used for monitoring metastatic breast cancer. A total of 3989 serum samples was obtained from 204 patients receiving first-line chemotherapy. Each sample was analyzed for CA 15.3, CEA, and TPA. The efficiency for identifying progression and nonprogression was 94 % during therapy, with no false-positive marker results for progressive disease. At clinical progressive disease, the median positive lead time was 35 days during therapy. Tumor marker assessment may document that a therapy is effective and ought to be continued in spite of adverse toxic effects, and that a treatment is ineffective and should be stopped to prevent unnecessary toxicity [68].

In a further study of the same author, 192 patients were monitored during first-line chemotherapy for metastatic breast cancer and during follow-up. Blood specimens were sampled approximately every 4 weeks. Steady state concentrations were registered for 77 (CA 15.3), 96 (CEA), and 127 (TPA) patients with below cutoff level values and for 28 (CA 15.3), 25 (CEA), and 11 (TPA) patients with above cutoff level values. Clinical and marker progression was registered for 75 (CA 15.3), 62 (CEA), and 57 (TPA) patients. The coefficients of total variation of steady state concentrations (comprising the intra- and interassay analytical imprecision and the within subject biological variation) were higher below (14.9 % CA 15.3, 15.4 % CEA, 25.9 % TPA) than above cutoffs (9.6 % CA 15.3,6.0 % CEA, 19.9 % TPA). The variability was similar for CA 15.3 and CEA but higher for TPA. During progression the rates of increase in concentrations were similar for CA 15.3 (0.0257) and CEA (0.0214) and lower than for TPA (0.0346). These data indicated that criteria for assessment of sequential tumor marker concentrations should consider the marker in question, the steady state variability, the cutoff value, and the rate of increase during disease progression [74].

13.5.4.2 CA15.3, TPS, TPA

The clinical utility of CA 15-3, TPS, TPA, human chorionic gonadotropin (hCGbeta) and tumour-associated trypsin inhibitor (TATI) as indicators of chemotherapy response was assessed in advanced breast cancer. Serum was prospectively collected in one center before treatment (after the first course of chemotherapy) and at response evaluation from 57 patients taking part in a multicentre randomized trial comparing docetaxel with sequential methotrexate and 5-fluorouracil in the treatment of advanced breast cancer. The pretreatment levels of the serum markers were not predictors of the later response to treatment. Changes in the TPS level showed the strongest association with clinical response after the first course of chemotherapy and CA 15.3 at the best response evaluation. However, distinct mismatches occurred with every marker. The most problematic error was an increase in marker levels in patients with clinical responses, which might have caused interruption of therapy. This occurred in 8 % and 17 % of patients after the first course of chemotherapy and in 4 % and 17 % of patients at the best response evaluation with CA 15.3 and TPS, respectively. Moreover, after the first course of chemotherapy only 39 % and 33 % of the patients with progressive disease could be identified on the basis of increasing levels of CA 15.3 and TPS respectively. Later, TPA and TPS were found to be better indicators of clinical disease progression than CA 15.3. In conclusion, in this study changes in CA 15.3 or TPS levels usually correlated with clinical response, but owing to distinct discordances, authors did not recommend them to be used as sole indicators of response to chemotherapy in advanced breast cancer [128].

Recently, the EGTM has convened a multidisciplinary panel of scientists to plan a trial aimed at defining guidelines on tumor biomarker evaluation in cancer patients monitoring. The panel proposed a four-phase model for biomarker-monitoring trial analogous to that in use for the investigation of new drugs. In phase I, biomarker kinetics and correlation with tumor burden will be assessed. Phase II will evaluate the ability of the biomarker to identify, exclude, and/or predict a change in disease status. In phase III, the effectiveness of tumor biomarker-guided intervention will be assessed by measuring patient outcome in randomized trials. Phase IV will consist of an audit of the long-term effects after biomarker monitoring has been included into standard patient care [129].

13.6 A Computer Program for Interpreting Consecutive Measurements of Serum TMs

It is time-consuming to process and compare the clinical and marker information registered during monitoring of breast cancer patients. To facilitate the assessment, a computer program for interpreting consecutive measurements also was developed. The intraindividual biological variation, the analytical precision profile, the cutoff limit, and the detection limit for each marker are entered and stored in the program. The assessment procedure for marker signals considers the analytical and biological variation of the applied markers. The software package contains a database that can store the interpretation of the measurements as evaluation codes together with patient demographics, information about treatment type, dates for treatment periods, control periods, and evaluation codes for clinical activity of disease. The consecutive concentrations for a patient are imported temporarily into the program from outside sources and presented graphically. Marker concentrations to be compared are selected with the computer mouse and the significance of the difference is calculated by the program. The program has an option for calculating the lead time of marker signals versus clinical information. The program facilitates the monitoring of individual breast cancer patients with tumor marker measurements. It may also be implemented in trials investigating the utility of potential new markers in breast cancer as well as in other malignancies [130].

13.7 Mucins and Cytokeratins as Markers of Circulating Tumor Cells/Disseminated Tumor Cells

13.7.1 Circulating Tumor Cells (CTCs)

Recently, technological advances permitted to detect and enumerate CTCs in peripheral blood of cancer patients. Because of the rarity of CTCs in the blood, the majority of these technologies use some kind of enrichment step, followed by a detection step.

13.7.1.1 Assays for CTCs Detection

The most commonly enrichment method is immunomagnetic separation with antibody-based magnetic capture, in which magnetically bound antibodies are directed against the epithelial cell adhesion molecule (EpCAM), so that EpCAM-positive cells are selected or against clusters of differentiation 45 (CD45) so that CD45-positive cells are not selected. There are various techniques for the detection of CTCs, including direct antibody-based methods in which antibodies are directed against CKs, such as immunocytochemistry, immunofluorescence, or flow cytometry, and indirect nucleic acid-based methods that measure messenger RNA (mRNA) transcript expression levels by reverse transcriptase polymerase chain reaction (RT-PCR) [131]. CellSearch (Veridex LLC, Raritan, NJ), a semi-automated, fluorescence-based microscopic assay, is the only standardized, objective test approved by the US Food and Drug Administration for the detection of CTCs in patients with metastatic breast, prostate, and colorectal cancer. This assay is a combined enrichment and detection system that uses EpCAM antibodies for enrichment. The enriched cells are subsequently subjected to immunofluorescent staining using CD45 and CK antibodies (CK8, CK18, CK19) for detection. The cells are recognized as CTCs if they are CK-positive and CD45-negative and have the signatures of malignant cells, including large size and large nuclei with or without nucleoli. Cells are analyzed using an automated microscope and counted using a cell spotter analyzer [132]. Another CTC detection test is the AdnaTest Breast Cancer Select/Detect (AdnaGen, Langenhagen, Germany), which is based on the analysis of tumor-associated mRNA isolated from CTCs after immunomagnetic separation that uses EpCAM and mucin 1 (MUC1) as the targets. For detection of CTCs, multiplex RT-PCR is performed to analyze the relative expression levels for three tumor-associated transcripts: human epidermal growth factor 2 (HER2), MUC1, and GA733-2. This test is scored positive if at least one of the PCR transcript products for the three markers is detected at a concentration of >0.15 ng/microL [133]. Technologies based on morphologic evaluation are very specific but they are generally less sensitive. Molecular methods, which allow for the concomitant evaluation of multiple markers, such as CK19, MUC1, and mammaglobin, are generally more sensitive, but they may generate false positive results due to low expression of the tested marker in noncancerous cells [131].

13.7.1.2 CTCs for Prognosis and Monitoring of Breast Cancer

In breast cancer, CTCs detection has been evaluated as prognostic value in both metastatic and disease-free patients and as tool to monitor advanced disease. The majority of clinical trials used the CellSearch for CTCs enumeration. In the DETECT study, the CellSearch assay with cut-off level of five or more cells/7.5 microL was used to evaluate 221 metastatic breast cancer patients; 116 (50 %) of them had positive CTCs. Median overall survival (OS) was 18.1 months for CTC positive patients and 27 months for CTC negative patients ($p<0.001$). In multivariate analysis, the presence of CTCs was an independent predictor for OS [134]. In another study, in a cohort of 302 disease-free breast cancer patients, CTCs were measured by the CellSearch assay. Authors identified one or more CTCs in 73 (24 %) patients who showed both decreased progression free survival (PFS) and OS. Patients with two or more CTCs had decreased PFS and OS than patients with less than two CTCs. Similarly, patients with three or more CTCs had decreased PFS and OS than patients with less than three CTCs [135]. As regard to disease monitoring, in 2009 Liu et al. evaluated CTC levels and imaging in 68 metastatic breast cancer patients receiving chemotherapy or endocrine therapy during a median follow-up of 13.3 months. They demonstrated a statistically significant correlation between CTC levels and radiographic disease progression [136]. In the United States, a phase III clinical trial (Southwest Oncology Group, SWOG S0500) is ongoing in metastatic breast cancer patients to determine: (a) whether CTC monitoring can be used to predict the response to treatment at an early time, and thereby promptly discontinue ineffective anticancer drugs and switch to another therapy if a response is unlikely; (b) whether outcomes can be improved by adhering to this procedure. Moreover the potential of CTCs is not restricted to simple enumeration of tumor cells. Since the phenotype of CTCs may differ from that of the primary tumor, clinical trials have been initiated to establish targeted treatment strategies based on expression profiles of CTCs [137].

13.7.2 Disseminated Tumor Cells (DTCs)

The detection of disseminated tumor cells (DTCs) in the bone marrow have been used to identify micro-metastasis, and therefore, predict prognosis in breast cancer patients [138].

13.7.2.1 Assays for DTCs Detection

DTCs are rare with only 10–20 cells among millions of bone marrow cells. Therefore, procedures have been developed for their enrichment prior to detection and further characterization [139, 140]. There are 2 different methods to screen bone marrow aspirates for DTCs, namely cytologic/cytometric (antibody-based) and molecular approaches [141]. Among the cytologic methods, immunocytochemistry is the most widely used approach [140, 142].

Antibodies against various epithelium-specific antigens such as cytoskeleton-associated cytokeratins, surface adhesion molecules or growth factor receptors are applied [140, 143]. The main advantage of cytologic methods is the opportunity to combine immunostaining with the morphology of the cells so that both cell size and shape as well as the nucleus/plasma relation might be estimated and illegitimate expression of the protein of interest in bone marrow cells can be excluded as far as possible. The pan-anti-cytokeratin antibodies A45-B/B3 or AE1/AE3 against a wide spectrum of cytokeratins are recommended as standard application, thereby ensuring detection of DTCs also in cells that have downregulated the expression of individual cytokeratins in the course of EMT [144].

Nucleic acid-based techniques enable the detection of DTCs also at the single cell level. Measurement of epithelium-specific or more organ-specific mRNA species such as cytokeratin 19 or mammaglobin mRNA by RT-PCR has been proven as promising approach to detect DTCs in bone marrow samples [145–148]. Multimarker real-time RT-PCRs have the potential to improve the method even in case of downregulation of the expression of a single gene [149, 150]. A new technique, designated EPISPOT (epithelial immunospot) detects proteins secreted/released/shed from single epithelial cancer cells. In breast cancer, the release of cytokeratin-19 (CK19) and mucin-1 (MUC1) were measured and it was demonstrated that many patients with apparently localized tumors harbored viable DTCs. Preliminary clinical data showed that patients with DTC-releasing CK19 have an unfavorable outcome [151].

Sensitivity, Specificity and Clinical Relevance of DTCs

A study aimed at examining the mucin expression profile of DTCs in the bone marrow of preoperative BC patients showed that MUC2, MUC3, MUC5B, MUC6, and MUC7 were detectable in at least one bone marrow specimen [152]. MUC5B was the most discriminating mucin marker, distinguishing between healthy and cancer patients with a sensitivity of 47 % and specificity of 100 %. Based on the results in the bone marrow, a nested RT-PCR assay was designed to detect MUC5B transcripts in the peripheral blood of BC patients. This test was moderately sensitive (52 %) but highly specific (100 %), suggesting it could be used clinically to identify the appearance of DTCs in BC patients. When applied to the bone marrow samples of BC patients collected at the time of surgery, however, nested PCR for MUC5B was as sensitive (19.5 %) as that for carcino-embryonic antigen (CEA, 17 %) and inferior to PCR for CK19 (41 % sensitivity) in identifying DTCs. While the diagnostic potential of MUC5B remains to be examined further, the study uncovered that MUC5B expression in the bone marrow positively correlates with the size of the tumor and stage (but not the nodal status). These results suggest a role for the mucin in the metastasis of BC cells. Immunomagnetic separation using one or more anti-MUC1 antibodies is now commonly used to isolate DTCs from the peripheral blood of BC patients. Further, the percentage of MUC1-positive DTCs increased progressively with increasing stage of the disease (0 %, 6 %, and 33 % positive cases in stage 1, 2, and 3, respectively), nodal involvement (7 %, 16 %, and 33 % positivity in patients without nodal involvement, or with N1 and N2 disease, respectively) and metastasis [1, 153].

Several studies have demonstrated worse prognosis following detection of DTCs in bone marrow of breast cancer patients [154, 155]. In a pooled analysis evaluating the results from 9 different European centers, including a total of 4703 patients, Braun et al. [156] have reported that approximately 30 % of women with primary breast cancer have DTCs in bone marrow, and in a multivariate analysis, the 10-year follow-up of these patients revealed a significantly decreased overall survival, when compared to patients without DTCs. The presence of DTCs in bone marrow was significantly associated with higher tumor stage, worse differentiation, lymph node metastasis and negativity in hormone receptor expression. Prognostic relevance was shown for all subgroups, even among those patients with small tumors and without lymph node metastasis.

Although using different antibodies and detection methods, almost all investigators participating in this pooled analysis used anti-cytokeratin antibodies to screen for DTCs in the BM [156]. Moreover, the persistence of DTCs in BM from breast cancer patients after adjuvant therapy was predictive for a subsequent disease recurrence [157, 158].

References

1. Mukhopadhyay P, Chakraborty S, Ponnusamy MP, Lakshmanan I, Jain M, Batra SK (2011) Mucins in the pathogenesis of breast cancer: implications in diagnosis, prognosis and therapy. Biochim Biophys Acta 1815(2):224–240
2. Hatzfeld M, Franke WW (1985) Pair formation and promiscuity of cytokeratins: formation in vitro of heterotypic complexes and intermediate-sized filaments by homologous and heterologous recombinations of purified polypeptides. J Cell Biol 101(5 Pt 1):1826–1841
3. Schweizer J, Bowden PE, Coulombe PA, Langbein L, Lane EB, Magin TM, Maltais L, Omary MB, Parry DA, Rogers MA, Wright MW (2006) New consensus nomenclature for mammalian keratins. J Cell Biol 174(2):169–174
4. Laakso M, Loman N, Borg A, Isola J (2005) Cytokeratin 5/14-positive breast cancer: true basal phenotype confined to BRCA1 tumors. Mod Pathol 18(10):1321–1328
5. Moll R, Franke WW, Schiller DL, Geiger B, Krepler R (1982) The catalog of human cytokeratins: patterns of expression in normal epithelia, tumors and cultured cells. Cell 31(1):11–24
6. Boecker W, Buerger H, Schmitz K, Ellis IA, van Diest PJ, Sinn HP, Geradts J, Diallo R, Poremba C, Herbst H (2001) Ductal epithelial proliferations of the breast: a biological continuum? Comparative genomic hybridization and high-molecular-weight cytokeratin expression patterns. J Pathol 195(4):415–421
7. Chu PG, Weiss LM (2002) Keratin expression in human tissues and neoplasms. Histopathology 40(5):403–439
8. Malzahn K, Mitze M, Thoenes M, Moll R (1998) Biological and prognostic significance of stratified epithelial cytokeratins in infiltrating ductal breast carcinomas. Virchows Arch 433(2):119–129
9. Korsching E, Packeisen J, Agelopoulos K, Eisenacher M, Voss R, Isola J, van Diest PJ, Brandt B, Boecker W, Buerger H (2002) Cytogenetic alterations and cytokeratin expression patterns in breast cancer: integrating a new model of breast differentiation into cytogenetic pathways of breast carcinogenesis. Lab Invest 82(11):1525–1533
10. Boecker W, Buerger H (2003) Evidence of progenitor cells of glandular and myoepithelial cell lineages in the human adult female breast epithelium: a new progenitor (adult stem) cell concept. Cell Prolif 36(Suppl 1):73–84
11. Wetzels RH, Kuijpers HJ, Lane EB, Leigh IM, Troyanovsky SM, Holland R, van Haelst UJ, Ramaekers FC (1991) Basal cell-specific and hyperproliferation-related keratins in human breast cancer. Am J Pathol 138(3):751–763
12. Birnbaum D, Bertucci F, Ginestier C, Tagett R, Jacquemier J, Charafe-Jauffret E (2004) Basal and luminal breast cancers: basic or luminous? (review). Int J Oncol 25(2):249–258
13. Perou CM, Sørlie T, Eisen MB, van de Rijn M, Jeffrey SS, Rees CA, Pollack JR, Ross DT, Johnsen H, Akslen LA, Fluge O, Pergamenschikov A, Williams C, Zhu SX, Lønning PE, Børresen-Dale AL, Brown PO, Botstein D (2000) Molecular portraits of human breast tumours. Nature 406(6797):747–752
14. Abd El-Rehim DM, Pinder SE, Paish CE, Bell J, Blamey RW, Robertson JF, Nicholson RI, Ellis IO (2004) Expression of luminal and basal cytokeratins in human breast carcinoma. J Pathol 203(2):661–671
15. Bánkfalvi A, Ludwig A, De-Hesselle B, Buerger H, Buchwalow IB, Boecker W (2004) Different proliferative activity of the glandular and myoepithelial lineages in benign proliferative and early malignant breast diseases. Mod Pathol 17(9):1051–1061
16. Boecker W, Moll R, Dervan P, Buerger H, Poremba C, Diallo RI, Herbst H, Schmidt A, Lerch MM, Buchwalow IB (2002) Usual ductal hyperplasia of the breast is a committed stem (progenitor) cell lesion distinct from atypical ductal hyperplasia and ductal carcinoma in situ. J Pathol 198(4):458–467
17. Tobias R, Rothwell C, Wagner J, Green A, Liu YS (1985) Development and evaluation of a radioimmunoassay for the detection of a monoclonal antibody defined breast tumor-associated antigen 115D8/DF3. Clin Chem 31:986
18. Bray KR, Koda JE, Gaur PK (1987) Serum levels and biochemical characteristics of cancer-associated antigen CA-549, a circulating breast cancer marker. Cancer Res 47(22):5853–5860
19. Sawant SS, Zingde SM, Vaidya MM (2008) Cytokeratin fragments in the serum: their utility for the management of oral cancer. Oral Oncol 44(8):722–732
20. Bjorklund B, Bjorklund V (1957) Antigenicity of pooled human malignant and normal tissues by cytoimmunological technique; presence of an insoluble, heat-labile tumor antigen. Int Arch Allergy Appl Immunol 10(3):153–184
21. Sundström BE, Stigbrand TI (1994) Cytokeratins and tissue polypeptide antigen. Int J Biol Markers 9(2):102–108
22. Bonfrer JM, Groeneveld EM, Korse CM, van Dalen A, Oomen LC, Ivanyi D (1994) Monoclonal anti-

body M3 used in tissue polypeptide-specific antigen assay for the quantification of tissue polypeptide antigen recognizes keratin 18. Tumour Biol 15(4): 210–222

23. Moore RG, Brown AK, Miller MC, Skates S, Allard WJ, Verch T, Steinhoff M, Messerlian G, DiSilvestro P, Granai CO, Bast RC Jr (2008) The use of multiple novel tumor biomarkers for the detection of ovarian carcinoma in patients with a pelvic mass. Gynecol Oncol 108(2):402–408
24. Molina R, Auge JM, Escudero JM, Marrades R, Viñolas N, Carcereny E, Ramirez J, Filella X (2008) Mucins CA 125, CA 19.9, CA 15.3 and TAG-72.3 as tumor markers in patients with lung cancer: comparison with CYFRA 21-1, CEA, SCC and NSE. Tumour Biol 29(6):371–380
25. Filella X, Cases A, Molina R, Jo J, Bedini JL, Revert L, Ballesta AM (1990) Tumor markers in patients with chronic renal failure. Int J Biol Markers 5(2):85–88
26. Szekanecz E, Szucs G, Szekanecz Z, Tarr T, Antal-Szalmás P, Szamosi S, Szántó J, Kiss E (2008) Tumor-associated antigens in systemic sclerosis and systemic lupus erythematosus: associations with organ manifestations, immunolaboratory markers and disease activity indices. J Autoimmun 31(4): 372–376
27. Wong RC, Klingberg S, Wilson R (2002) CA15-3 and cancer associated serum antigenassays are alternatives to the KL-6 assay for measuring serum MUC-1 levels in patients with interstitial lung disease associated with polymyositis/dermatomyositis. J Rheumatol 29(9):2021–2022
28. Okada M, Suzuki K, Nakanishi T, Nakashima M (2006) Serum levels of KL-6 are positively correlated with those of CA15-3 in patients with interstitial pneumonia associated with collagen diseases. Respirology 11(4):509–510
29. Symeonidis A, Kouraklis-Symeonidis A, Apostolopoulos D, Arvanitopoulou E, Giannakoulas N, Vassilakos P, Zoumbos N (2004) Increased serum CA-15.3 levels in patients with megaloblastic anemia due to vitamin B12 deficiency. Oncology 67(5–6):359–367
30. Dehaghani AS, Ghiam AF, Hosseini M, Mansouri S, Ghaderi A (2007) Factors influencing serum concentration of CA125 and CA15-3 in Iranian healthy postmenopausal women. Pathol Oncol Res 13(4):360–364
31. Zervoudis S, Peitsidis P, Iatrakis G, Panourgias E, Koureas A, Navrozoglou I, Dubois JB (2007) Increased levels of tumor markers in the follow-up of 400 patients with breast cancer without recurrence or metastasis: interpretation of false-positive results. J BUON 12(4):487–492
32. Pentheroudakis G, Malamou-Mitsi V, Briasoulis E, Damala K, Vassou A, Vartholomatos G, Kolaitis N, Pavlidis N (2004) The neutrophil, not the tumor: serum CA 15-3 elevation as a result of granulocyte–colony-stimulating factor-induced neutrophil MU1C overexpression and neutrophilia in patients with breast carcinoma receiving adjuvant chemotherapy. Cancer 101(8):1767–1775
33. O'Brien DP, Horgan PG, Gough DB, Skehill R, Grimes H, Given HF (1992) CA15-3: a reliable indicator of metastatic bone disease in breast cancer patients. Ann R Coll Surg Engl 74(1):9–11
34. Geraghty JG, Coveney EC, Sherry F, O'Higgins NJ, Duffy MJ (1992) CA 15-3 in patients with locoregional and metastatic breast carcinoma. Cancer 70(12):2831–2834
35. Gion M, Mione R, Leon AE, Lüftner D, Molina R, Possinger K, Robertson JF (2001) CA27.29: a valuable marker for breast cancer management. A confirmatory multicentric study on 603 cases. Eur J Cancer 37(3):355–363
36. O'Brien DP, Gough DB, Skehill R, Grimes H, Given HF (1994) Simple method for comparing reliability of two serum tumour markers in breast carcinoma. J Clin Pathol 47(2):134–137
37. Giovanella L, Ceriani L, Giardina G, Bardelli D, Tanzi F, Garancini S (2002) Serum cytokeratin fragment 21.1 (CYFRA 21.1) as tumour marker for breast cancer: comparison with carbohydrate antigen 15.3 (CA 15.3) and carcinoembryonic antigen (CEA). Clin Chem Lab Med 40(3):298–303
38. Nakata B, Ogawa Y, Ishikawa T, Ikeda K, Kato Y, Nishino H, Hirakawa K (2000) SerumCYFRA 21-1 is one of the most reliable tumor markers for breast carcinoma. Cancer 89(6):1285–1290
39. Nakata B, Takashima T, Ogawa Y, Ishikawa T, Hirakawa K (2004) Serum CYFRA 21-1 (cytokeratin-19 fragments) is a useful tumour marker for detecting disease relapse and assessing treatment efficacy in breast cancer. Br J Cancer 91(5): 873–878
40. van Dalen A (1996) Significance of cytokeratin markers TPA, TPA (cyk), TPS and CYFRA 21.1 in metastatic disease. Anticancer Res 16(4B): 2345–2349
41. Kawaguchi H, Ohno S, Miyazaki M, Hashimoto K, Egashira A, Saeki H, Watanabe M, Sugimachi K (2000) CYFRA 21-1 determination in patients with esophageal squamous cell carcinoma: clinical utility for detection of recurrences. Cancer 89(7): 1413–1417
42. Berglund A, Molin D, Larsson A, Einarsson R, Glimelius B (2002) Tumour markers as early predictors of response to chemotherapy in advanced colorectal carcinoma. Ann Oncol 13(9):1430–1437
43. Ecke TH, Schlechte HH, Schulze G, Lenk SV, Loening SA (2005) Four tumour markers for urinary bladder cancer–tissue polypeptide antigen (TPA), HER-2/neu (ERB B2), urokinase-type plasminogen activator receptor (uPAR) and TP53 mutation. Anticancer Res 25(1B):635–641
44. D'Alessandro R, Roselli M, Ferroni P, Mariotti S, Spila A, Aloe S, Carone MD, Abbolito MR,

Carlini S, Perri P, Ricciotti A, Botti C, Conti F, Vici P, Chiappetta NR, Cognetti F, Buonomo O, Guadagni F (2001) Serum tissue polypeptide specific antigen (TPS): a complementary tumor marker to CA 15-3 in the management of breast cancer. Breast Cancer Res Treat 68(1):9–19

45. Barak V, Goike H, Panaretakis KW, Einarsson R (2004) Clinical utility of cytokeratins as tumor markers. Clin Biochem 37(7):529–540
46. Nakayama M, Satoh H, Ishikawa H, Fujiwara M, Kamma H, Ohtsuka M, Sekizawa K (2003) Cytokeratin 19 fragment in patients with nonmalignant respiratory diseases. Chest 123(6):2001–2006
47. Nakahama H, Tanaka Y, Fujita Y, Fujii M, Sugita M (1998) CYFRA 21-1 and ProGRP, tumor markers of lung cancer, are elevated in chronic renal failure patients. Respirology 3(3):207–210
48. Sarandakou A, Protonotariou E, Rizos D (2007) Tumor markers in biological fluids associated with pregnancy. Crit Rev Clin Lab Sci 44(2):151–178
49. Gonzalez-Quintela A, Mallo N, Mella C, Campos J, Perez LF, Lopez-Rodriguez R, Tome S, Otero E (2006) Serum levels of cytokeratin-18 (tissue polypeptide-specific antigen) in liver diseases. Liver Int 26(10):1217–1224
50. Nicolini A, Colombini C, Luciani L, Carpi A, Giuliani L (1991) Evaluation of serum CA15-3 determination with CEA and TPA in the post-operative follow-up of breast cancer patients. Br J Cancer 64(1):154–158
51. Vizcarra E, Lluch A, Cibrián R, Jarque F, Alberola V, Belloch V, García-Conde J (1996) Value of CA 15.3 in breast cancer and comparison with CEA and TPA: a study of specificity in disease-free follow-up patients and sensitivity in patients at diagnosis of the first metastasis. Breast Cancer Res Treat 37(3):209–216
52. Correale M, Reshkin S, Tedone T, Abbate I, Mangia A, Schittulli F, Paradiso A (1996) Cytokeratins and proliferation in breast cancer patients. Int J Oncol 9(5):1007–1012
53. Bonfrer JM, Korse CM (1999) TPA and CA 15.3 measurements for breast cancer monitoring in a routine setting. Int J Biol Markers 14(1):40–44
54. Rosselli Del Turco M, Palli D, Cariddi A, Ciatto S, Pacini P, Distante V (1994) Intensive diagnostic follow-up after treatment of primary breast cancer. A randomized trial. National Research Council Project on Breast Cancer follow-up. JAMA 271(20): 1593–1597
55. Smith TJ, Davidson NE, Schapira DV, Grunfeld E, Muss HB, Vogel VG 3rd, Somerfield MR (1999) American Society of Clinical Oncology 1998 update of recommended breast cancer surveillance guidelines. J Clin Oncol 17(3):1080–1082
56. Bast RC Jr, Ravdin P, Hayes DF, Bates S, Fritsche H Jr, Jessup JM, Kemeny N, Locker GY, Mennel RG, Somerfield MR, American Society of Clinical Oncology Tumor Markers Expert Panel (2001) 2000 update of recommendations for the use of tumor markers in breast and colorectal cancer: clinical practice guidelines of the American Society of Clinical Oncology. J Clin Oncol 19(6):1865–1878. Erratum in: J Clin Oncol 2001 Nov 1;19(21):4185–4188, J Clin Oncol 2002 Apr 15;20(8):2213
57. Harris L, Fritsche H, Mennel R, Norton L, Ravdin P, Taube S, Somerfield MR, Hayes DF, Bast RC Jr, American Society of Clinical Oncology (2007) American Society of Clinical Oncology 2007 update of recommendations for the use of tumor markers in breast cancer. J Clin Oncol 25(33):5287–5312
58. Pestolazzi BC, Lupoeai-Gely E, Jost LM, Bergh J (2005) ESMO minimum clinical recommendations for diagnosis, adjuvant treatment and follow-up of primary breast cancer. Ann Oncol 16:157–159
59. Goldhirsch A, Wood WC, Gelber RD, Coates AS, Thürlimann B, Senn HJ, 10th St. Gallen conference. (2007) Progress and promise: highlights of the international expert consensus on the primary therapy of early breast cancer 2007. Ann Oncol 18(7):1133–1144. Erratum in: Ann Oncol 2007 Nov;18(11):1917
60. http://www.nccn.org/professionals/physician_gls/f_guidelines.asp
61. Sturgeon CM, Duffy MJ, Stenman UH, Lilja H, Brünner N, Chan DW, Babaian R, Bast RC Jr, Dowell B, Esteva FJ, Haglund C, Harbeck N, Hayes DF, Holten-Andersen M, Klee GG, Lamerz R, Looijenga LH, Molina R, Nielsen HJ, Rittenhouse H, Semjonow A, Shih IM, Sibley P, Sölétormos G, Stephan C, Sokoll L, Hoffman BR, Diamandis EP, National Academy of Clinical Biochemistry (2008) National Academy of Clinical Biochemistry laboratory medicine practice guidelines for use of tumor markers in testicular, prostate, colorectal, breast, and ovarian cancers. Clin Chem 54(12):e11–e79
62. Molina R, Barak V, van Dalen A, Duffy MJ, Einarsson R, Gion M, Goike H, Lamerz R, Nap M, Sölétormos G, Stieber P (2005) Tumor markers in breast cancer – European Group on Tumor Markers recommendations. Tumour Biol 26(6):281–293
63. Sölétormos G, Schiøler V, Nielsen D, Skovsgaard T, Dombernowsky P (1993) Interpretation of results for tumor markers on the basis of analytical imprecision and biological variation. Clin Chem 39(10): 2077–2083
64. Lumachi F, Brandes AA, Boccagni P, Polistina F, Favia G, D'Amico DF (1999) Long-term follow-up study in breast cancer patients using serum tumor markers CEA and CA 15-3. Anticancer Res 19(5C):4485–4489
65. Jäger W, Kissing A, Cilaci S, Melsheimer R, Lang N (1994) Is an increase in CA 125 in breast cancer patients an indicator of pleural metastases? Br J Cancer 70(3):493–495
66. Molina R, Zanón G, Filella X, Moreno F, Jo J, Daniels M, Latre ML, Giménez N, Pahisa J, Velasco M et al (1995) Use of serial carcinoembryonic antigen and CA 15.3 assays in detecting relapses in

breast cancer patients. Breast Cancer Res Treat 36(1):41–48
67. Nicolini A, Carpi A (2000) Postoperative follow-up of breast cancer patients: overview and progress in the use of tumor markers. Tumour Biol 21(4):235–248
68. Sölétormos G, Nielsen D, Schiøler V, Skovsgaard T, Dombernowsky P (1996) Tumor markers cancer antigen 15.3, carcinoembryonic antigen, and tissue polypeptide antigen for monitoring metastatic breast cancer during first-line chemotherapy and follow-up. Clin Chem 42(4):564–575
69. Robertson JF, Jaeger W, Syzmendera JJ, Selby C, Coleman R, Howell A, Winstanley J, Jonssen PE, Bombardieri E, Sainsbury JR, Gronberg H, Kumpulainen E, Blamey RW (1999) The objective measurement of remission and progression in metastatic breast cancer by use of serum tumour markers. European Group for Serum Tumour Markers in Breast Cancer. Eur J Cancer 35(1):47–53
70. Williams MR, Turkes A, Pearson D, Twining P, Griffiths K, Blamey RW (1999) The use of serum carcinoembryonic antigen to assess therapeutic response in locally advanced and metastatic breast cancer. A prospective study with external review. Eur J Surg Oncol 14:417–422
71. Sölétormos G, Hyltoft Petersen P, Dombernowsky P (2000) Progression criteria for cancer antigen 15.3 and carcinoembryonic antigen in metastatic breast cancer compared by computer simulation of marker data. Clin Chem 46(7):939–949
72. Quayle JB (1982) Tumour lysis as a factor affecting blood levels of CEA. Br J Cancer 46(2):213–219
73. Yasasever V, Dinçer M, Camlica H, Karaloğlu D, Dalay N (1997) Utility of CA 15-3 and CEA in monitoring breast cancer patients with bone metastases: special emphasis on "spiking" phenomena. Clin Biochem 30(1):53–56
74. Sölétormos G, Petersen PH, Dombernowsky P (2000) Assessment of CA 15.3, CEA and TPA concentrations during monitoring of breast cancer. Clin Chem Lab Med 38(5):453–463
75. Nicolini A, Ferrari P, Sagripanti A, Carpi A (1999) The role of tumour markers in predicting skeletal metastases in breast cancer patients with equivocal bone scintigraphy. Br J Cancer 79(9–10): 1443–1447
76. Nicolini A, Carpi A, Ferrari P, Anselmi L, Spinelli C, Conte M, Miccoli P (2000) The role of tumour markers in improving the accuracy of conventional chest X-ray and liver echography in the post-operative detection of thoracic and liver metastases from breast cancer. Br J Cancer 83(11):1412–1417
77. Nicolini A, Fancelli S, Ferrari P, Anselmi L (2012) Reducing radiological imaging during post-operative monitoring of breast cancer patients with serum CEA-TPA-CA15.3 tumor marker (TM) panel and an individual reference limit (IRL). In: Proceedings of the 26th international congress and exhibition of Computer Assisted Radiology and Surgery (CARS), vol 7, Suppl 1:S243
78. Thompson JA, Pande H, Paxton RJ, Shively L, Padma A, Simmer RL, Todd CW, Riggs AD, Shively JE (1987) Molecular cloning of a gene belonging to the carcinoembryonic antigen gene family and discussion of a domain model. Proc Natl Acad Sci U S A 84(9):2965–2969
79. Cases A, Filella X, Molina R, Ballesta AM, Lopez-Pedret J, Revert L (1991) Tumor markers in chronic renal failure and hemodialysis patients. Nephron 57(2):183–186
80. Collazos J, Genollà J, Ruibal A (1992) Evaluation of the behavior of carcinoembryonic antigen in cirrhotic patients. Int J Biol Markers 7(4):244–248
81. Amino N, Kuro R, Yabu Y, Takai SI, Kawashima M, Morimoto S, Ichihara K, Miyai K, Kumahara Y (1981) Elevated levels of circulating carcinoembryonic antigen in hypothyroidism. J Clin Endocrinol Metab 52(3):457–462
82. Shapiro M, Scapa E (2000) Elevated carcinoembryonic antigen (CEA) levels in a patient with no malignancy. Hepatogastroenterology 47(31):163–164
83. Uehara M, Kinoshita T, Hojo T, Akashi-Tanaka S, Iwamoto E, Fukutomi T (2008) Long-term prognostic study of carcinoembryonic antigen (CEA) and carbohydrate antigen 15-3 (CA 15-3) in breast cancer. Int J Clin Oncol 13(5):447–451
84. Keshaviah A, Dellapasqua S, Rotmensz N, Lindtner J, Crivellari D, Collins J, Colleoni M, Thürlimann B, Mendiola C, Aebi S, Price KN, Pagani O, Simoncini E, Castiglione Gertsch M, Gelber RD, Coates AS, Goldhirsch A (2007) CA15-3 and alkaline phosphatase as predictors for breast cancer recurrence: a combined analysis of seven International Breast Cancer Study Group trials. Ann Oncol 18(4):701–708
85. Kokko R, Holli K, Hakama M (2002) Ca 15-3 in the follow-up of localised breast cancer: a prospective study. Eur J Cancer 38(9):1189–1193
86. Given M, Scott M, Mc Grath JP, Given HF (2000) The predictive of tumour markers CA 15-3, TPS and CEA in breast cancer recurrence. Breast 9(5): 277–280
87. Lumachi F, Brandes AA, Ermani M, Bruno G, Boccagni P (2000) Sensitivity of serum tumor markers CEA and CA 15-3 in breast cancer recurrences and correlation with different prognostic factors. Anticancer Res 20(6C):4751–4755
88. Jäger W, Krämer S, Palapelas V, Norbert L (1995) Breast cancer and clinical utility of CA 15-3 and CEA. Scand J Clin Lab Invest Suppl 221:87–92
89. Bahrami A, Mortazavizadeh MR, Yazdi MF, Chamani M (2012) Serial tumour markers serum carcinoembryonic antigen and cancer antigen 15-3 assays in detecting symptomatic metastasis in breast cancer patients. East Mediterr Health J 18(10): 1055–1059
90. Briasoulis E, Andreopoulou E, Tolis CF, Bairaktari E, Katsaraki A, Dimopoulos MA, Fountzilas G,

Seferiadis C, Pavlidis N (2001) G-CSF induces elevation of circulating CA 15-3 in breast carcinoma patients treated in an adjuvant setting. Cancer 91(5):909–917
91. Bieglmayer C, Szepesi T, Neunteufel W (1988) Follow-up of metastatic breast cancer patients with a mucin-like carcinoma-associated antigen: comparison to CA 15.3 and carcinoembryonic antigen. Cancer Lett 42(3):199–206
92. Sölétormos G, Nielsen D, Schiøler V, Skovsgaard T, Winkel P, Mouridsen HT, Dombernowsky P (1993) A novel method for monitoring high-risk breast cancer with tumor markers: CA 15.3 compared to CEA and TPA. Ann Oncol 4(10):861–869
93. Pectasides D, Pavlidis N, Gogou L, Antoniou F, Nicolaides C, Tsikalakis D (1996) Clinical value of CA 15-3, mucin-like carcinoma-associated antigen, tumor polypeptide antigen, and carcinoembryonic antigen in monitoring early breast cancer patients. Am J Clin Oncol 19(5):459–464
94. Vizcarra E, Lluch A, Cibrián R, Jarque F, García-Conde J (1994) CA 15.3, CEA and TPA tumor markers in the early diagnosis of breast cancer relapse. Oncology 51(6):491–496
95. Yildiz M, Oral B, Bozkurt M, Cobaner A (2004) Relationship between bone scintigraphy and tumor markers in patients with breast cancer. Ann Nucl Med 18(6):501–505
96. Begić A, Kucukalić-Selimović E, Obralić N, Durić O, Lacević N, Skopljak A (2006) Correlation between bone scintigraphy and tumor markers in patients with breast carcinoma. Bosn J Basic Med Sci 6(1):75–77
97. Gedik GK, Kiratli PO, Tascioglu B, Aras T (2006) Comparison of bone scintigraphy with serum tumor markers of CA 15-3 and carcinoembryonic antigen in patients with breast carcinoma. Saudi Med J 27(3):317–322
98. Zissimopoulos A, Matthaios D, Matthaiou E, Mantadakis E, Karaitianos I (2007) Association between bone scintigraphy and serum levels of tumor markers in the detection of bone disease in breast cancer patients. J BUON 12(4):505–511
99. Mohammadzadeh M, Alikhah H, Zareh AG (2010) Comparison of bone scan with carbohydrate antigen 15-3 for evaluation of bone metastasis of breast cancer. Pak J Biol Sci 13(4):175–179
100. Liska V, Holubec L Jr, Treska V, Vrzalova J, Skalicky T, Sutnar A, Kormunda S, Bruha J, Vycital O, Finek J, Pesta M, Pecen L, Topolcan O (2011) Evaluation of tumour markers as differential diagnostic tool in patients with suspicion of liver metastases from breast cancer. Anticancer Res 31(4):1447–1451
101. Evangelista L, Baretta Z, Vinante L, Cervino AR, Gregianin M, Ghiotto C, Bozza F, Saladini G (2011) Could the serial determination of Ca15.3 serum improve the diagnostic accuracy of PET/CT?: results from small population with previous breast cancer. Ann Nucl Med 25(7):469–477
102. Nakamura T, Kimura T, Umehara Y, Suzuki K, Okamoto K, Okumura T, Morizumi S, Kawabata T (2005) Periodic measurement of serum carcinoembryonic antigen and carbohydrate antigen 15-3 levels as postoperative surveillance after breast cancer surgery. Surg Today 35(1):19–21
103. Nicolini A, Carpi A, Ferrari P, Pieri L (2003) Utility of a serum tumour marker panel in the post-operative follow-up of breast cancer patients with equivocal conventional radiological examinations. Tumour Biol 24(6):275–280
104. Nicolini A, Anselmi L, Michelassi C, Carpi A (1997) Prolonged survival by 'early' salvage treatment of breast cancer patients: a retrospective 6-year study. Br J Cancer 76(8):1106–1111
105. Nicolini A, Carpi A, Michelassi C, Spinelli C, Conte M, Miccoli P, Fini M, Giardino R (2003) "Tumour marker guided" salvage treatment prolongs survival of breast cancer patients: final report of a 7-year study. Biomed Pharmacother 57(10):452–459
106. Cardoso F, Harbeck N, Fallowfield L, Kyriakides S, Senkus E, ESMO Guidelines Working Group (2012) Locally recurrent or metastatic breast cancer: ESMO Clinical Practice Guidelines for diagnosis, treatment and follow-up. Ann Oncol 23(Suppl 7):vii11–vii19
107. Schöndorf T, Hoopmann M, Warm M, Neumann R, Thomas A, Göhring UJ, Eisberg C, Mallmann P (2002) Serologic concentrations of HER-2/neu in breast cancer patients with visceral metastases receiving trastuzumab therapy predict the clinical course. Clin Chem 48(8):1360–1362
108. British Association of Surgical Oncology Guidelines (1999) The management of metastatic bone disease in the United Kingdom. The Breast Specialty Group of the British Association of Surgical Oncology. Eur J Surg Oncol 25(1):3–23
109. Tondini C, Hayes DF, Gelman R, Henderson IC, Kufe DW (1988) Comparison of CA15-3 and carcinoembryonic antigen in monitoring the clinical course of patients with metastatic breast cancer. Cancer Res 48(14):4107–4112
110. Robertson JF, Whynes DK, Dixon A, Blamey RW (1995) Potential for cost economies in guiding therapy in patients with metastatic breast cancer. Br J Cancer 72(1):174–177
111. Iwase H, Kobayashi S, Itoh Y, Fukuoka H, Kuzushima T, Iwata H, Yamashita T, Naitoh A, Itoh K, Masaoka A (1995) Evaluation of serum tumor markers in patients with advanced or recurrent breast cancer. Breast Cancer Res Treat 33(1):83–88
112. http://www.eortc.be/recist/
113. Lumachi F, Ermani M, Brandes AA, Basso S, Basso U, Boccagni P (2001) Predictive value of different prognostic factors in breast cancer recurrences: multivariate analysis using a logistic regression model. Anticancer Res 21(6A):4105–4108
114. Duffy MJ (2006) Serum tumor markers in breast cancer: are they of clinical value? Clin Chem 52(3):345–351

115. Guadagni F, Ferroni P, Carlini S, Mariotti S, Spila A, Aloe S, D'Alessandro R, Carone MD, Cicchetti A, Ricciotti A, Venturo I, Perri P, Di Filippo F, Cognetti F, Botti C, Roselli M (2001) A re-evaluation of carcinoembryonic antigen (CEA) as a serum marker for breast cancer: a prospective longitudinal study. Clin Cancer Res 7(8):2357–2362
116. De La Lande B, Hacene K, Floiras JL, Alatrakchi N, Pichon MF (2002) Prognostic value of CA 15.3 kinetics for metastatic breast cancer. Int J Biol Markers 17(4):231–238
117. Schuurman JJ, Bong SB, Einarsson R (1996) Determination of serum tumor markers TPS and CA 15-3 during monitoring of treatment in metastatic breast cancer patients. Anticancer Res 16(4B): 2169–2172
118. Willsher PC, Beaver J, Blamey RW, Robertson JF (1995) Serum tissue polypeptide specific antigen (TPS) in breast cancer patients: comparison with CA 15.3 and CEA. Anticancer Res 15(4):1609–1611
119. Kim HS, Park YH, Park MJ, Chang MH, Jun HJ, Kim KH, Ahn JS, Kang WK, Park K, Im YH (2009) Clinical significance of a serum CA15-3 surge and the usefulness of CA15-3 kinetics in monitoring chemotherapy response in patients with metastatic breast cancer. Breast Cancer Res Treat 118(1):89–97
120. Dixon AR, Price MR, Hand CW, Sibley PE, Selby C, Blamey RW (1993) Epithelial mucin core antigen (EMCA) in assessing therapeutic response in advanced breast cancer – a comparison with CA15.3. Br J Cancer 68(5):947–949
121. Laessig D, Nagel D, Heinemann V, Untch M, Kahlert S, Bauerfeind I, Stieber P (2007) Importance of CEA and CA 15-3 during disease progression in metastatic breast cancer patients. Anticancer Res 27(4A):1963–1968
122. Sölétormos G, Nielsen D, Schiøler V, Skovsgaard T, Dombernowsky P (1992) Carbohydrate antigen 549 in metastatic breast cancer during cytostatic treatment and follow-up. Eur J Cancer 28A(4–5):845–850
123. Cheung KL, Robertson FR (2003) Objective measurement of remission and progression in metastatic breast cancer by the use of serum tumour markers. Minerva Chir 58(3):297–303
124. Kurebayashi J, Yamamoto Y, Tanaka K, Kohno N, Kurosumi M, Moriya T, Nishimura R, Ogawa Y, Taguchi T, Tumor Marker Study Group of the Japanese Breast Cancer Society, Japan (2003) Significance of serum carcinoembryonic antigen and CA 15-3 in monitoring advanced breast cancer patients treated with systemic therapy: a large-scale retrospective study. Breast Cancer 10(1):38–44
125. Kurebayashi J, Nishimura R, Tanaka K, Kohno N, Kurosumi M, Moriya T, Ogawa Y, Taguchi T (2004) Significance of serum tumor markers in monitoring advanced breast cancer patients treated with systemic therapy: a prospective study. Breast Cancer 11(4):389–395
126. Yonemori K, Katsumata N, Noda A, Uno H, Yunokawa M, Nakano E, Kouno T, Shimizu C, Ando M, Tamura K, Takeuchi M, Fujiwara Y (2008) Development and verification of a prediction model using serum tumor markers to predict the response to chemotherapy of patients with metastatic or recurrent breast cancer. J Cancer Res Clin Oncol 134(11):1199–1206
127. Sonoo H, Kurebayashi J (1996) Serum tumor marker kinetics and the clinical course of patients with advanced breast cancer. Surg Today 26(4):250–257
128. Sjöström J, Alfthan H, Joensuu H, Stenman UH, Lundin J, Blomqvist C (2001) Serum tumour markers CA 15-3, TPA, TPS, hCGbeta and TATI in the monitoring of chemotherapy response in metastatic breast cancer. Scand J Clin Lab Invest 61(6):431–441
129. Sölétormos G, Duffy MJ, Hayes DF, Sturgeon CM, Barak V, Bossuyt PM, Diamandis EP, Gion M, Hyltoft-Petersen P, Lamerz RM, Nielsen DL, Sibley P, Tholander B, Tuxen MK, Bonfrer JM (2013) Design of tumor biomarker-monitoring trials: a proposal by the European Group on Tumor Markers. Clin Chem 59(1):52–59
130. Sölétormos G, Schiøler V (2000) Description of a computer program to assess cancer antigen 15.3, carcinoembryonic antigen, and tissue polypeptide antigen information during monitoring of metastatic breast cancer. Clin Chem 46(8 Pt 1):1106–1113
131. Krishnamurthy S (2012) The emerging role of circulating tumor cells in breast cancer. Cancer Cytopathol 120(3):161–166
132. Cristofanilli M, Budd GT, Ellis MJ, Stopeck A, Matera J, Miller MC, Reuben JM, Doyle GV, Allard WJ, Terstappen LW, Hayes DF (2004) Circulating tumor cells, disease progression, and survival in metastatic breast cancer. N Engl J Med 351(8): 781–791
133. Andreopoulou E, Yang LY, Rangel KM, Reuben JM, Hsu L, Krishnamurthy S, Valero V, Fritsche HA, Cristofanilli M (2012) Comparison of assay methods for detection of circulating tumor cells in metastatic breast cancer: AdnaGen AdnaTest BreastCancer Select/Detect™ versus Veridex CellSearch™ system. Int J Cancer 130(7):1590–1597
134. Müller V, Riethdorf S, Rack B, Janni W, Fasching PA, Solomayer E, Aktas B, Kasimir-Bauer S, Pantel K, Fehm T, DETECT Study Group (2012) Prognostic impact of circulating tumor cells assessed with the CellSearch System™ and AdnaTest Breast™ in metastatic breast cancer patients: the DETECT study. Cancer Res 14(4):R118
135. Lucci A, Hall CS, Lodhi AK, Bhattacharyya A, Anderson AE, Xiao L, Bedrosian I, Kuerer HM, Krishnamurthy S (2012) Circulating tumour cells in non-metastatic breast cancer: a prospective study. Lancet Oncol 13(7):688–695
136. Liu MC, Shields PG, Warren RD, Cohen P, Wilkinson M, Ottaviano YL, Rao SB, Eng-Wong J, Seillier-Moiseiwitsch F, Noone AM, Isaacs C (2009)

Circulating tumor cells: a useful predictor of treatment efficacy in metastatic breast cancer. J Clin Oncol 27(31):5153–5159

137. Banys M, Müller V, Melcher C, Aktas B, Kasimir-Bauer S, Hagenbeck C, Hartkopf A, Fehm T (2013) Circulating tumor cells in breast cancer. Clin Chim Acta 423:39–45
138. Ross JS, Slodkowska EA (2009) Circulating and disseminated tumor cells in the management of breast cancer. Am J Clin Pathol 132(2):237–245
139. Alix-Panabières C, Müller V, Pantel K (2007) Current status in human breast cancer micrometastasis. Curr Opin Oncol 19(6):558–563
140. Lacroix M (2006) Significance, detection and markers of disseminated breast cancer cells. Endocr Relat Cancer 13(4):1033–1067
141. Riethdorf S, Pantel K (2008) Disseminated tumor cells in bone marrow and circulating tumor cells in blood of breast cancer patients: current state of detection and characterization. Pathobiology 75(2):140–148
142. Pantel K, Brakenhoff RH (2004) Dissecting the metastatic cascade. Nat Rev Cancer 4(6):448–456
143. Wölfle U, Müller V, Pantel K (2006) Disseminated tumor cells in breast cancer: detection, characterization and clinical relevance. Future Oncol 2(4): 553–561
144. Fehm T, Braun S, Muller V, Janni W, Gebauer G, Marth C, Schindlbeck C, Wallwiener D, Borgen E, Naume B, Pantel K, Solomayer E (2006) A concept for the standardized detection of disseminated tumor cells in bone marrow from patients with primary breast cancer and its clinical implementation. Cancer 107(5):885–892
145. Schoenfeld A, Kruger KH, Gomm J, Sinnett HD, Gazet JC, Sacks N, Bender HG, Luqmani Y, Coombes RC (1997) The detection of micrometastases in the peripheral blood and bone marrow of patients with breast cancer using immunohistochemistry and reverse transcriptase polymerase chain reaction for keratin 19. Eur J Cancer 33(6):854–861
146. Smith BM, Slade MJ, English J, Graham H, Lüchtenborg M, Sinnett HD, Cross NC, Coombes RC (2000) Response of circulating tumor cells to systemic therapy in patients with metastatic breast cancer: comparison of quantitative polymerase chain reaction and immunocytochemical techniques. J Clin Oncol 18(7):1432–1439
147. Zhong XY, Kaul S, Lin YS, Eichler A, Bastert G (2000) Sensitive detection of micrometastases in bone marrow from patients with breast cancer using immunomagnetic isolation of tumor cells in combination with reverse transcriptase/polymerase chain reaction for cytokeratin-19. J Cancer Res Clin Oncol 126(4):212–218
148. Bossolasco P, Ricci C, Farina G, Soligo D, Pedretti D, Scanni A, Deliliers GL (2002) Detection of micrometastatic cells in breast cancer by RT-pCR for the mammaglobin gene. Cancer Detect Prev 26(1):60–63
149. Ring AE, Zabaglo L, Ormerod MG, Smith IE, Dowsett M (2005) Detection of circulating epithelial cells in the blood of patients with breast cancer: comparison of three techniques. Br J Cancer 92(5):906–912
150. Benoy IH, Elst H, Philips M, Wuyts H, Van Dam P, Scharpé S, Van Marck E, Vermeulen PB, Dirix LY (2006) Prognostic significance of disseminated tumor cells as detected by quantitative real-time reverse-transcriptase polymerase chain reaction in patients with breast cancer. Clin Breast Cancer 7(2):146–152
151. Alix-Panabières C (2012) EPISPOT assay: detection of viable DTCs/CTCs in solid tumor patients. Recent Results Cancer Res 195:69–76
152. Berois N, Varangot M, Sóñora C, Zarantonelli L, Pressa C, Laviña R, Rodríguez JL, Delgado F, Porchet N, Aubert JP, Osinaga E (2003) Detection of bone marrow-disseminated breast cancer cells using an RT-PCR assay of MUC5B mRNA. Int J Cancer 103(4):550–555
153. Bölke E, Orth K, Gerber PA, Lammering G, Mota R, Peiper M, Matuschek C, Budach W, Rusnak E, Shaikh S, Dogan B, Prisack HB, Bojar H (2009) Gene expression of circulating tumour cells and its correlation with tumour stage in breast cancer patients. Eur J Med Res 14(8):359–363
154. Braun S, Pantel K, Müller P, Janni W, Hepp F, Kentenich CR, Gastroph S, Wischnik A, Dimpfl T, Kindermann G, Riethmüller G, Schlimok G (2000) Cytokeratin-positive cells in the bone marrow and survival of patients with stage I, II, or III breast cancer. N Engl J Med 342(8):525–533
155. Gebauer G, Fehm T, Merkle E, Beck EP, Lang N, Jäger W (2001) Epithelial cells in bone marrow of breast cancer patients at time of primary surgery: clinical outcome during long-term follow-up. J Clin Oncol 19(16):3669–3674
156. Braun S, Vogl FD, Naume B, Janni W, Osborne MP, Coombes RC, Schlimok G, Diel IJ, Gerber B, Gebauer G, Pierga JY, Marth C, Oruzio D, Wiedswang G, Solomayer EF, Kundt G, Strobl B, Fehm T, Wong GY, Bliss J, Vincent-Salomon A, Pantel K (2005) A pooled analysis of bone marrow micrometastasis in breast cancer. N Engl J Med 353(8):793–802
157. Janni W, Rack B, Schindlbeck C, Strobl B, Rjosk D, Braun S, Sommer H, Pantel K, Gerber B, Friese K (2005) The persistence of isolated tumor cells in bone marrow from patients with breast carcinoma predicts an increased risk for recurrence. Cancer 103(5):884–891
158. Wiedswang G, Borgen E, Kåresen R, Qvist H, Janbu J, Kvalheim G, Nesland JM, Naume B (2004) Isolated tumor cells in bone marrow three years after diagnosis in disease-free breast cancer patients predict unfavorable clinical outcome. Clin Cancer Res 10(16):5342–5348

Part VI

Tumor Markers – A Critical Revision: Carbohydrate Markers

The Role of CA 125 as Tumor Marker: Biochemical and Clinical Aspects

14

Patrizia Bottoni and Roberto Scatena

Abstract

CA 125 also known as mucin 16 or MUC16 is a large membrane glycoprotein belonging to the wide mucin family, encoded by the homonymous *MUC16* gene. Following its discovery in the blood of some patients with specific types of cancers or other benign conditions, CA125 has found application as a tumor marker of ovarian cancer. Thirty years after its discovery, use of CA 125 is still FDA-recommended to monitor response to therapy in patients with epithelial ovarian cancer and to detect residual or recurrent disease in patients who have undergone first-line therapy and would be considered for second-look procedures. However, due to its limited specificity and sensitivity, CA 125 alone cannot still be an ideal biomarker. Increased clinical performance, in terms of better sensitivity and specificity in identifying epithelial ovarian cancer relapse, has been obtained by combined use of CA 125 with HE4, another ovarian cancer marker recently introduced in clinical use. Significant advancements have been achieved more recently, due to the introduction of FDA-approved ROMA and OVA1 algorithms to evaluate the risk of ovarian cancer for patients with a pelvic mass.

Keywords

CA 125 • CA 125 clinical use • CA 125 measurement • CA 125 nadir • HE4 • Membrane-associated mucins • MUC16 • MUC16 biochemical structure • Mucins biological functions • OVA1 algorithm • Ovarian cancer • Ovarian cancer monitoring • ROMA algorithm • Secreted mucins

P. Bottoni (✉) • R. Scatena
Institute of Biochemistry and Clinical Biochemistry,
School of Medicine, Catholic University,
Largo Gemelli 8, 00168 Rome, Italy
e-mail: patrizia.bottoni@rm.unicatt.it

R. Scatena (ed.), *Advances in Cancer Biomarkers*, Advances in Experimental Medicine and Biology 867, DOI 10.1007/978-94-017-7215-0_14

14.1 Introduction: Biochemical Structure

CA125 is a large transmembrane glycoprotein, the largest of the class of membrane-associated mucins (MAMs) to which it belongs.

For long debated whether the mucin family members were secreted or associated with the cell membrane, it is now known that both two classes of mucins exist, the secreted mucins and the cell-surface associated mucins, including different members that have common structural features. Mucin consists typically of a protein backbone, termed apomucin, covered with many O-linked oligosaccharides and a number of N-glycan chains [1]. The range and chemical composition of structures that are created by branched O-linked oligosaccharides are immense. In addition, many post-translational modifications, including glycosylation, sialylation and sulfation may then occur on mature mucin glycoproteins often in a cell-type specific manner. Structural feature that is common to all mucins and differentiate them from other membrane-bound glycoproteins, the exceptions being MUC14, MUC15, and MUC18 [2], is the centrally located tandem-repeat (TR) domain [3–5], which comprises TRs of identical or highly similar sequences particularly rich in proline, threonine, and serine and for this also known as a PTS domain [6]. The TR regions, whose number and specific sequence is highly variable among different mucins, provides a scaffold on which cells build complex oligosaccharide structures. The TR repeats typically consist from 5 to 100 potential glycosylation sites per repeat, and this peculiar TR arrays contribute increased 'stoichiometric power' to a confined area, thereby creating a locally high concentration of specific molecular structures. Also regions surrounding the TRs can contain carbohydrate structures which can be potential binding sites for interacting partners. The non-glycosylated regions of mucins consist of many structural motifs and domains [7] that might play a pathophysiological role [1].

In addition to glycosylated TR regions, common to all the mucin family members, additional structural motifs are present in the amino and carboxy termini of mucin protein backbones. Based on their biochemical features and physiological fate, mucin class are grouped into two structurally distinct categories: the secreted and the membrane-associated mucins.

14.1.1 Secreted Mucins

Next to the centrally located variable number TR sequences, which are unique to each MUC gene, the secreted mucins contain characteristic cysteine rich, cysteine knot and von Willebrand C and D domains (named D because of its homology with dimerisation domain of von Willebrand factor) at the N- or C-termini of the monomers, which are linked through disulphide bridges.

These domains are deemed to be responsible for oligomerization of the very large core-proteins.

Secretory mucins are further subdivided into those gel-forming and non-gel-forming. The first include the large secretory mucins with cysteine-rich motifs, MUC2, MUC5AC, MUC5B, MUC6, encoded by a cluster of genes at the chromosomal locus 11p15 and evolved from a common ancestor with von Willebrand factor (VWF). More recently has been identified and characterized MUC 19, another cysteine-rich secretory mucin, encoded by a gene showing 12q12 chromosomal location [8]. MUC7 and MUC9, instead, are smaller secreted mucins that do not oligomerize and do not form gels [9]. Also MUC18 do not form gels, and lacks the VWF D4 or C1, C2 domains typically present in the carboxy end of large secretory mucins. For a more detailed description we refer to some exhaustive review [9, 10].

14.1.2 Membrane-Associated Mucins

Cell-surface-associated mucins, which form the largest group of mucins, are bound to cells by an integral transmembrane domain and have relatively short cytoplasmic tails (CT) domain, often containing sites of phosphorilation that interact with mediators of signal transduction and other cytoskeleton-associated proteins [11]. On the extracellular side of the membrane-associated unit most MAMs have one, but also two or three domains which show significant homology to the epidermal-growth-factor (EGF) family members. The precise functions of EGF-like domains remains to be established, however, experimental evidence support their role in mediating interactions between cell-surface-associated mucins and members of EGF receptors (ERBB) family, which are involved in regulation of cellular growth, differentiation, motility and inflammation [12]. Another important functional module widely distributed among cell surface associated proteins is the SEA domain, so named after the first three proteins in which it was identified (Sperm protein, Enterokinase and Agrin). It is an extracellular domain of ~120 amino acids, of which an about 80-residue conserved region and an about 40-residue segment that separates the conserved region from the subsequent C-terminal domains. Characteristically located between the *O*-glycosylated PTS repeats and the transmembrane domain, SEA module contains autocatalytic proteolytic cleavage site that leads to the release of the large extracellular mucin into the mucus gel layer. This involvement of SEA domain in the cleavage of proteins has been well investigated in MUC1 [13]. Generally present in only one unit in the mucins, SEA domains can also to be present in more modules, such as in MUC16, which contains multiple SEA domains. The presence of multiple SEA domains, but no EGF-like domains, in MUC16 emphasizes the diversity in the evolution and potential function of the different MAMs [10]. Common feature of the ectodomains of MAMs is the heavy O-glycosylation, for which up to 80 % of the mass of the mucin is O-glycans, with galactose, N-acetylgalactosamine, N-acetylglucosamine and sialic acids as the main sugars with minor amounts of fucose, mannose and glucose.

14.1.2.1 MUC16: Biochemical Structure

In the genome, MUC16 is localized in 19p13.2 chromosome and is coded by sequences present within approximatively 179 kb of genomic DNA. MUC16 protein, also known as CA125 antigen, is a MAM, the largest of the class. With a core peptide of 22,152 amino acids and a molecular weight of 2,353,428 Da, MUC 16 is more than twice as long as MUC1 and MUC4.

MUC16 is composed of three different domains: an N-terminal domain, a central tandem repeat region, and a carboxy terminal domain. The N-terminal and tandem repeat domains are entirely extracellular and highly O-glycosylated. In particular, the N-terminal domain consists of 12,070 amino acids rich in serine/threonine residues and has been reported to contain the major O-glycosylation known to be present in CA125. The MUC16 protein back bone is composed of tandem repeat region, which has more than 60 repeat domains of 156 amino acids each. Though not all individually similar, most of the repeat units, which, such as any mucins, are rich in serine, threonine and proline residues, recur more than once inside the sequence. In the tandem-repeat domain of MUC16 there is also a small cysteine ring region on which are thought to be present the epitopes for known anti-CA125 antibodies (OC125 and M11).

The carboxy-terminal domain has 284 amino-acids and consists in an extra cellular region, a transmembrane and a cytoplasmic tail. The extracellular part of the carboxy-terminal domain contains multiple SEA modules, many N-glycosylation sites and some O-glycosylation sites. It has been reported to harbor also a putative cleavage site. The MUC16 cytoplasmic tail is 31 amino acids long and contains several potential phosphorylation sites, in particular a putative tyrosine phosphorylation site (RRKKEGY), which was first recognized in Src family protein. Recently, it has been shown that MUC16 cytoplasmic tail, which contains a polybasic amino-acid sequence, can interact with cytoskeleton through ERM (ezrin/radixin/moesin) actin-binding proteins.

14.2 Biological Functions

14.2.1 Physiology

All mucins are highly O-glycosylated in tissue-specific manner and in function of specific roles that they play at these locations. The properties and the wide variety of types of mucins expressed by epithelia, reflecting their different structural organization, the nature of their post-translational modifications, the degree of intramolecular and intermolecular crosslinking, has raised interest for further investigation into the biochemical properties and biological implications of mucins and their functional roles in normal and malignant cells.

Mucins produced by secretory epithelial cells of the gastrointestinal, respiratory, and urinogenital tracts contribute to confer normal physiological lubrification and protection to epithelial surfaces ducts and lumens within the human body. Keeping epithelial surfaces hydrated, needed for the lubrication and normal functioning of ducts and passageways, may guarantee to the epithelial cells also an effective protection from infections and injuries [7, 14]. The continuous need for maintaining mucosal protection against all external aggressive forces requires a normal turnover of the barrier. From this it results a dynamic and balanced process of mucin biosynthesis, secretion and degradation at mucosal surfaces that relies on the availability of specific proteases and glycosidases secreted by other mucosal cells or present in the extracellular microflora [9]. In addition, mucins play an important role in renewal and differentiation of the epithelium, in modulation of cell adhesion and cell signalling and immuno suppression [15].

Secreted mucins show patterns of expression that are restricted to specialized organs and cell types that secreted them into the extracellular space. They are key components in most mucus gels that protects underlying epithelia from adverse conditions by forming a chemical barrier that limits exposure to various injuries, including bacteria, virus, pH, ingested toxins, reactive oxygen species (ROS) and proteolytic enzymes in the gastrointestinal tract, and suppresses the inflammatory response. Mucin 2 (MUC2), the major secreted mucin lining the gastrointestinal mucosa, functions by suppressing inflammation in the intestinal tract and inhibiting the development of intestinal tumours [10]. Near the cell surface, the secreted mucin layer might interact with MAMs or other cell-surface molecules, thus contributing also in this way to physicochemical protection of the epithelial cell surfaces by maintaining the local molecular environment with respect to hydration, ionic composition and concentration, and accessibility of macromolecules [7].

Unlike the secreted mucins, MAMs are released from the apical cell membrane by enzymatic cleavage of the N-terminal subunit into the mucous gel; alternative splicing can also produce secreted variants [1]. From an evolutionist point of view, the inclusion of a transmembrane component provides many advantages to the epithelial cell. Informations about the condition of the external environment can be transmitted to the interior of the cell, to indicate that a normal status exists at the cell surface or that inflammation processes and other forms of stress are present. In such way, MAMs behaves as cell-surface receptors and sensors, and conduct signals in response to changes in conformation or ligand status of their extracellular domains. All that leads to coordinated cellular responses that include proliferation, differentiation, apoptosis and secretion of specialized cellular products [7], thus providing an additional level of defence to promote the growth, repair and survival of epithelial cells. In fact, among the multiple biological functions of MAMs, of particular importance is their role in signal transduction. The presence in many MAMs (specifically in MUC3A, MUC3B, MUC4, MUC12, MUC13, and MUC17) of two or three EGF-like domains might allow these membrane mucins to interact with the ErbB receptors and regulate EGF-receptor-mediated cell signalling, whose excessive signalling is well-known to be associated with the development of a wide variety of tumours.

14.2.2 Pathophysiology

Alterations in mucin forms and amounts can occur in numerous pathologic processes, including lung diseases such as asthma, bronchitis, cystic fibrosis and chronic obstructive pulmonary disease.

Mucus and mucins play in fact a fundamental role in disease mechanisms leading to the characteristic mucus hypersecretion, pulmonary obstruction, reduced mucociliary clearance and subsequent infection.

More importantly, mucins have multiple implications in cancer development. It is well known that mucins are overexpressed and aberrantly glycosylated in many adenocarcinomas, including in the breast, lung, gastric, colorectal, pancreatic, cervical and ovarian cancers. These aberrant forms can derive from deregulation of expression of mucin core proteins and alteration of enzymatic glycosylation events, which may be by incomplete synthesis or neosynthesis, with subsequent expression of novel, pathological combinations of different mucins. This results in an enormous selective advantage for tumor cell, which, by acquiring a widest range of potential ligands for interaction with other receptors at the cell surface, modifies its behaviour and enhances its survival ability during invasion and metastatic events. The changes in mucin expression lead in general to a loss of normal epithelial function, with decreased mucosal protection. In addition, the control of local environment by mucins and the capture of growth factors and cytochines can contribute not only to cell proliferation, invasion and metastasis, but also to affect the ability of immune, inflammatory and stromal cells to interact with the tumour, with subsequent impact, more or less direct, on the development and maintenance of immune responses, which are frequently suppressed in malignancies that overexpressed mucins [16].

Also the interactions between transmembrane mucins and several protein partners seems to be very important to regulate different molecular and cellular events, including cell-cell/protein-protein binding, signal transduction and protein stabilization. In fact, carbohydrate structures present in the highly glycosylated TR region or outside the TR region of mucins make them potential candidates to interact with several carbohydrate binding proteins, including the galectin family. Among the 14 known galectins, it has been observed an interaction of galectin-3 with both MUC16 (also called CA125) and MUC1, and of galectin-1 with MUC16 [17, 18]. In particular, following the observation that MUC16 is also a potent inhibitor of natural killer (NK) cell responses in vitro [19], it has been hypothesized that the interaction of the galectin-1 with MUC16 may be important in the attachment of the mucin to the NK cell surface, thus promoting metastasis and evading immune responses [20]. The association of cell surface mucins with galectin-3 has been reported to contribute to the ocular surface epithelial barrier, which is critical to preventing damage to and infection of wet-surfaced epithelia [17]. Furthermore, of particular importance is the direct interaction occurs between mesothelin, a glycosylphosphatidylinositol-linked cell surface protein present on mesothelial/ovarian cancer cells, and MUC16 [21, 22]. This interaction, which relies on MUC16-N-glycosylation, seems to involve the MUC16 TR region and mesothelin residues 296–359 [23, 24]. The biological importance of MUC16-mesothelin interaction in facilitating cell-cell adhesion, thus promoting the metastasis of ovarian cancer cells has aroused lively interest in its potential therapeutic implication. Additionally, the identification of the MUC16-interacting region in mesothelin has favoured the design of antibodies against MUC16 that can be used as potential agents to inhibit the MUC16-mesothelin interaction, thus inhibiting ovarian cancer cell metastasis. Furthermore, the characterization of the interacting domains in both the two partner proteins is opening new ways for the development of specific pharmacological tools against these interactions [23]. Further studies are needed, however, to determine the in vivo effectiveness of all these novel potential therapeutic agents.

14.3 Measurement of CA 125

CA 125 was discovered by Bast et al. in [25], with the development of a murine monoclonal antibody (OC 125) produced by immunizing a mouse with OVCA 433 cell line, derived from a patient with ovarian serous carcinoma. The first immunoassay for CA 125 developed and commercialized in [26] used the OC 125 antibody for both capture and detection [27].

A second-generation assay (CA125 II) typically uses the monoclonal antibody, M11, as the capture antibody and OC 125 as the conjugate antibody. Other FDA-cleared assays for CA 125, which employ antibodies other than the OC 125 and M11 antibodies, are available on automated immunoassay platforms. Notably, although the majority of manufacturers reports similar reference intervals, the concentrations of CA125 can vary because of differences in calibration, assay design, and reagent specificities [28]. It follows that, at present, results obtained with different assay methods cannot be used interchangeably. As recommended on National Academy of Clinical Biochemistry Laboratory Medicine Practice Guidelines for Use of Tumor Markers, in the absence of an International Standard for CA125, it is then suitable that manufacturers specify all features of the used method and laboratories indicate them on their clinical reports. For all that, patients should be monitored with a single assay or rebaselined if there is a change in adopted methodology [29].

14.3.1 Sensitivity, Specificity

In a healthy population, CA 125 serum levels are <35 U/mL. This cutoff was determined from the distribution of values in healthy individuals so as to include 99 % of normals [30]. Values tend to decline with menopause and aging. Elevations of CA 125 assay values may be found in approximately 1–2 % of healthy individuals [26] and in 5 % of individuals with nonmalignant conditions such as in women in the follicular phase of the menstrual cycle [31] and in individuals with cirrhosis [32, 33], hepatitis [34], endometriosis [35, 36], first trimester pregnancy [37, 38], ovarian cysts [39], and pelvic inflammatory disease [38, 40]. Increased CA 125 values have been reported in 28 % of subjects with non-ovarian malignancies which include breast, lung liver pancreatic, colon, stomach, biliary tract [34, 41] cervical [34, 40] uterine [33] fallopian tube [40] and endometrial carcinomas [42]. Therefore, CA-125 has poor specificity as biomarker for ovarian cancer because of many inflammatory conditions in the abdominal area that cause fluctuations in CA-125 levels, and other non-ovarian malignancies which result often in false positives. CA 125 has limited sensitivity in detecting ovarian cancer. Elevated levels of CA 125 have be found in about 50 % of patients with early stage ovarian cancer, meaning that CA 125 has particularly poor sensitivity for ovarian cancer before the onset of symptoms. Furthermore, CA 125 is elevated in 90 % of patients with stage II disease, and more than 90 % with stage III and IV, whereas the remainder do not express this antigen. The concentration of CA 125 correlates with tumor size and staging. The use of CA 125 to detect ovarian cancer, especially in early stages of disease, can frequently lead to false negatives with important clinical implications. It follow in fact that patients that receive false negatives could not receive required cares and an appropriate treatment for their disease. CA 125 determination may be then useful in the evaluation of the disease status in patients with advanced endometriosis, but is not useful in screening for ovarian cancer in asymptomatic populations.

Another issue that should be consider in measuring CA 125 is the possible interference which may be observed in presence of heterophilic antibodies in the serum, similarly to other immunoassays [43, 44]. In particular, individuals who follow a therapeutic protocol with monoclonal antibodies by parenteral routes may produce anti-mouse antibodies. Serum specimens from these patients may produce erroneous results in such assay.

14.4 CA 125 Determination in Clinical Practice

14.4.1 Ovarian Cancer Statistics

Ovarian cancer is the seventh most common cancer in women worldwide (18 most common cancer overall) and the second most common gynaecological cancer after uterus. Worldwide, nearly 239,000 women were estimated to have been diagnosed with ovarian cancer, with incidence rates varying across the world. The highest incidence of ovarian cancer was in Central and Eastern Europe and Northern America, and the lowest in Western Africa and Asia, but this partly reflects varying data quality worldwide. The most striking international difference occurs in Japan, which has lower rates of ovarian cancer than in Europe. In Europe, ovarian cancer is the 13th most common cancer overall and the fifth most common cancer for females with around 65,600 new cases diagnosed in 2012. Some of this variation may be explained by different prevalence of risk factors, use of screening, and diagnostic methods. Morphologically, ovarian cancer is composed of different tumor categories including surface epithelial tumors, sex-cord stromal tumors, and germ cell tumors [45]. Of these, epithelial tumors (carcinomas) are the most common, representing the 80–90 % of overall ovarian malignancies, and are divided into the following histologic types: serous, mucinous, endometrioid, clear cell, and transitional [46]. Data on prevalence and mortality clearly indicate that serous ovarian carcinoma represents the most important of all primary ovarian carcinomas [47]. Importantly, this distinct histological features result in different clinical behavior, tumorigenesis and pattern of gene expression, with subsequent and considerable clinical implications.

The latest statistics available on mortality for ovarian cancer are of 2012 and indicate that, worldwide, around 152,000 women were estimated to have died from ovarian cancer in 2012, with mortality rates varying across the world. Data related to the same year 2012 estimate that in Europe around 42,700 women have died from ovarian cancer [48]. Since ovarian cancer often has no symptoms at the early stages, its diagnosis happens generally when the disease is in advanced stage. That implies that, even though 10-year survival from ovarian cancer has almost doubled over the last 40 years, it remains however still poor, ranging from approximately 30–50% at 5 years after diagnosis (which compares the 5-year survival of people with the cancer to the survival of others at the same age who do not have cancer). As often happens for other types of cancer, early detection is often crucial for a better outcome of the disease. Statistical data recently reported show, in fact, that ovarian cancer survival is highest in younger women, who are more often diagnosed with early cancer.

14.4.2 CA 125 as a Screening and Diagnostic Biomarker for Ovarian Cancer

Due to its limited specificity and sensitivity, CA 125 alone is not useful as a screening assay for ovarian cancer detection in asymptomatic population. A single measurement of CA 125 cannot be interpreted, without use of other diagnostic techniques, as absolute evidence of the presence or absence of disease. Screening is however recommended by the NACB Panel or by other authoritative organizations in at-risk women with a family history of hereditary ovarian cancer, in conjunction with pelvic examination and ultrasound testing [49–51]. To improve the clinical usefulness of CA 125 for screening/early detection, several strategies has been suggested, including approaches combining CA125 with ultrasound, longitudinal measurements of CA125, and measurement of CA125 in combination with other recently proposed multimarker panels [27, 52–55].

The recognition that early detection of ovarian cancer may have the potential to considerably improve prognosis prompted the development, in the last few years, of a number of large prospective trials to evaluate the potential role for CA125 in screening for ovarian cancer in asymptomatic populations. A total of 82,487 low-risk postmenopausal women were screened using an annual ultrasound and CA125 determination in a Japanese Shizuoka Cohort Study of Ovarian Cancer Screening. The trial showed encouraging sensitivity (77.1 %) and specificity (99.9 %) with a more effectiveness in detecting cancer at an early stage (63 %) compared to the control arm (38 %) [56].

The Prostate, Lung, Colorectal and Ovarian (PLCO) Cancer Screening Trial was designed to determine the effect of specific cancer screening tests on cause-specific mortality. Enrollment for this randomized controlled trial began in November 1993 and concluded in July 2001. Planned follow-up was for up to 13 years from randomization. A total of 68,616 women aged 55–74 were enrolled, of whom 30,630 underwent screening, between 1993 and 2007, for serum CA125 and transvaginal ultrasound for 4 years followed by CA125 alone for a further 2 years. Data from this study indicate that annual screening for ovarian cancer as performed in the PLCO trial with simultaneous CA-125 and transvaginal ultrasound does not reduce disease-specific mortality in women at average risk for ovarian cancer but does increase invasive medical procedures and complications in women undergoing surgery for false positive results [57].

If the PLCO trial has reported no mortality benefit of ovarian cancer screening, also the largest prospective randomized trial realized so far, the United Kingdom Collaborative Trial of Ovarian Cancer Screening (UKCTOCS), has been designed to assess the effect of screening with serial CA125 measurements and transvaginal sonography on cause-specific mortality. Between 2001 and 2005, a total of 202,638 postmenopausal women aged 50–74 years were randomly assigned to no treatment (control; $n = 101{,}359$); annual CA125 screening (interpreted by a 'Risk of Ovarian Cancer' algorithm, ROCA) with transvaginal ultrasound as a second-line test (multimodal screening [MMS]; $n = 50{,}640$); or annual screening with transvaginal ultrasound (USS; $n = 50{,}639$) alone. The use of longitudinal algorithm ROCA, that compares the CA125 profile of cases to that of healthy women and incorporates age-specific incidence of ovarian cancer in estimating risk, seems to shown encouraging performance characteristics both on prevalence and incidence screening [58]. Data from the UKCTOCS suggest that CA125 rise within normal range can be detected by the ROCA well before any abnormalities are detected on transvaginal imaging. Whether this converts into a mortality impact will be known as soon as the results will be available [59].

If not recommended by NACB for use in screening asymptomatic women, CA 125 is however considered useful in distinguishing benign from malignant disease in women, particularly in postmenopausal women with suspicious ovarian masses, thus facilitating orientation for a more o less extensive surgical intervention. If in premenopausal women several benign conditions that cause increased values of CA 125 may be a confounding factors, thus rendering more difficult the discrimination of benign from malignant disease, in postmenopausal women elevated concentrations of CA125>95 kU/L can discriminate malignant from benign pelvic masses with a positive predictive value of 95 % [27].

14.4.3 CA 125 as Biomarker for Ovarian Cancer Prognosis and Monitoring of Therapeutic Effect

Measuring CA 125 is actually considered standard of care by many for ovarian cancer patient surveillance. Monitoring response to therapeutic treatment is in fact the primary FDA-indicated use for CA 125 in patients with epithelial ovarian cancer. The second FDA-indicated use is to detect residual or recurrent disease during the follow up of patients who have undergone first-line therapy and would be considered for second-look procedures.

Generally, in monitoring studies, elevations of CA 125>35 U/mL after debulking surgery and chemotherapy indicate that residual disease is likely (>95 % accuracy). A persistently rising CA 125 value after three cycles of chemotherapy suggests progressive malignant disease and poor therapeutic response. However, CA-125 levels below 35 U/mL do not rule-out recurrence, because patients with histopathologic evidence of ovarian carcinoma may have CA-125 test concentrations within the range of healthy individuals. Then clinical decisions for these patients should not be based on a CA-125 test concentration below 35 U/mL.

Currently, there is general consensus about the recommendation of CA 125 measurement for monitoring response to treatment and detecting disease recurrence. However, which may be the best evaluation criteria of CA 125-based response remains still debated [60–62]. In 2011, the Gynecologic Cancer Intergroup (GCIG), in evaluating the criteria of CA 125 use to define progression-free survival after first-line therapy as well as the criteria to define response to treatment in recurrent disease, suggested that CA 125 alone can be used to evaluate the effectiveness of treatment [63]. The commonly accepted response criterion is a 50 % decrease in CA 125 as compared to the pretreated sample, which should be taken 2 weeks before treatment. According to NACB ovarian cancer panel recommendation, subsequent samples should be taken at 2–4 weeks during treatment and at intervals of 2–3 weeks during follow-up [28]. Then, if CA 125 monitoring is actually considered a relatively sensitive and cost-effective test to follow up of ovarian cancer patients, however other methods such as physical examination, CT scan, and ultrasound are also important for detecting residual disease. Of note, the retrospective study of Gadducci et al. [64] assessed the pattern of failures of 412 patients with recurrent ovarian cancer followed up with different surveillance protocols. Follow-up by using clinical examination, imaging technique and serum CA 125 raised the suspect of recurrent disease in the 80 % of patients, while only 23 % of them were detected by CA 125 measurement alone [64]. It is likely that the GCIG progression or recurrence criteria, based on CA 125 monitoring, might be so strict as they do not allow to detect disease progression in those patients whose CA 125 levels are less than two times the upper limit of the reference range or nadir value [62].

The possible advantages related to use of CA 125 nadir have been recently evaluated in several retrospective studies, suggesting that the nadir serum CA-125 level, in women achieving a clinically-defined complete response to primary chemotherapy, accurately defined the risk of relapse [65, 66]. According to these reports, the retrospective analysis of Markman et al. [67] demonstrated that the baseline CA-125 level before initiation of maintenance chemotherapy may be of strong prognostic value. In particular, baseline CA-125 levels distributed into subgroups for values of (A) <or=10 U/mL, (B) 11–20 U/mL, and (C) 21–35 U/mL, was highly statistically significant in strongly predicting the risk of subsequent relapse. At premaintenance baseline CA-125 values <or=10 U/mL corresponds to a superior progression-free survival compared with higher levels in the normal CA-125 range. Given findings of different prognostic groupings existing within the commonly regarded normal CA-125 range, Liu et al. [68] evaluated another criterion to detect early signal of progressive disease, by predicting progression if CA $125 \geq 20$ U/mL on two consecutive occasions for patients with CA 125 nadir ≤ 10 U/mL or if CA $125 \geq 2 \times$ nadir on two consecutive occasions for patients with nadir more than 10 U/mL. This proposal, which essentially applies the GCIG CA-125 disease progression criterion, lowering however the upper normal limit from 35 to 10 U/mL, obtained a positive predictive value of 93 % (95 % CI, 88–97 %).

To analyze the prognostic value of the CA-125 nadir in the normal range (<35 U/mL), Prat et al. [69] included in their retrospective analysis patients with CA-125>35 U/mL at time of diagnosis, treated with optimal cytoreductive surgery and perioperative platinum/taxane-based chemotherapy. By dividing patients that have achieved a complete biochemical (<35 U/mL) and radiological response after primary treatment into the following arbitrary groups, group A ≤ 10 U/mL; and group B, 11–35 U/mL, they have found that the outcome were significantly improved for group A as compared to group B. Similarly to previous findings, also results from this study, with a 96.4 % positive predictive value, demonstrated that the CA-125 nadir value is a strong independent prognostic factor for subsequent disease relapse and overall survival. All together, these results suggest that variations in the CA- 125 levels after primary surgery and, more importantly, the nadir value of the CA-125 after primary chemotherapy, are associated with patient outcome. An appropriate use of CA 125 and a careful evaluation of the variations from CA 125 nadir may be useful to oncologist to early detect ovarian cancer relapse.

14.5 Other Serum Markers for Pancreatic Cancer

14.5.1 HE4

Human epididymis protein 4 (HE4) is another ovarian cancer marker intensely studied in the last years and recently introduced in clinical use. HE4 is a small secretory protein, encoded by the *WFDC2* gene, which resides on human chromosome 20q12-13.1, a region that harbors a locus of 14 genes encoding protein domains that have homology with whey acidic protein (WAP) [70]. This protein is also designated WAP four-disulfide core domain protein 2 (WFDC2) because it contains two WAP domains and a "four disulfide core" made up of eight cysteine residues. The WAP domain is a conserved motif, containing eight cysteines found in a characteristic 4-disulphide core arrangement, that is present in a number of otherwise unrelated proteins. These proteins typically are secreted and are protease inhibitors, although this function has not been ascribed to HE4, and its exact physiologic role has not been characterized.

HE4 protein was initially discovered, by using microarrays, to be overexpressed in epididymal tissue and later in ovarian cancer tissue [71, 72]. Generation of the monoclonal antibodies 2H5 and 3D8 to epitopes on HE4 has allowed development of a sandwich ELISA and measurement of HE4 serum, test which has become available for the routine laboratory repertoire. Subsequent studies have shown that HE4 is not specific for ovarian tumors, although its expression is however restricted to the normal tissue of the reproductive tracts and respiratory epithelium. It has been observed also in a subset of lung tumour cell lines [73].

In the serum of patients with epithelial ovarian cancer, HE4 is overexpressed in 93 % of serous histologic subtype and in 100 % of endometrioid epithelial ovarian cancers, but only in 50 % of clear cell carcinomas and not in mucinous or germ-cell ovarian cancers.

14.5.1.1 Clinical Applications of HE4

At an HE4 concentration of 150 pM, 95 % of healthy women were below this cutoff, while 79 % of women with ovarian cancer were above this cutoff. Elevations in other subjects include breast (13 %), endometrial (26 %), gastrointestinal (16 %), and lung cancers (42 %), as well as benign gynecologic disease (7 %) and other benign disease (24 %). A recent study revising the available literature on biological and lifestyle factors affecting HE4 concentrations in serum highlights that, in contrast to CA-125, higher HE4 concentrations are reported in the elderly, with a strong difference in biomarker biological intra-individual variation according to the fertility status is reported. In addition, the evaluation of HE4 results may be problematic when patients suffer from additional conditions that may alter HE4 level. Other factors, such as smoking and decreased renal function also show a substantial impact on HE4 values, which should be considered in each patient [74].

The great interest aroused by HE4 is motivated primarily by better specificity that this protein seems to have compared with CA125 in discriminating benign diseases. Recent studies demonstrated that the more prominent differences among them are observed in patients with some benign ovarian diseases, such as endometriosis, who showed the 67 % of increased CA 125 values compared with 3 % of HE4 [75]. It has been reported that mean serum concentration of HE4 was significantly higher in serum samples of patients with both endometrial (99.2 pM, $P<0.001$) and ovarian (1125.4 pM, $P<0.001$) cancer but not with ovarian endometriomas (46.0 pM) or other types of endometriosis (45.5 pM) as compared with healthy controls (40.5 pM) [76].

At present, although several studies comparing HE4 and CA 125 performance demonstrated that HE4 is a more specific marker for ovarian cancer than CA 125 [75, 76], the clinical use of HE4 in differentiation of ovarian cancer from other benign gynecologic diseases continues to be evaluated. Certainly, measuring both HE4 and

CA125 serum concentrations may allow more accurate prediction of cancer than use of the individual markers, thus providing valuable information to discriminate ovarian tumours from ovarian endometriotic cysts. Furthermore, the HE4 assay is FDA cleared for monitoring recurrence or progressive disease in patients with epithelial ovarian cancer. Similarly to CA 125, a prompt reduction and subsequent normalization of HE4 levels reflects a response to primary surgery and chemotherapy. But HE4 values that remains elevated are important indicator of the recurrence of the disease. Interestingly, the study by Anastasi et al. [77] showed that, in the follow-up of patients with ovarian cancer, the increased expression of HE4 is detected 5–8 months before CA125 increment, suggesting that HE4 might be a better marker for monitoring disease progression. Hynninen et al. [78] in evaluating response of patients treated with primary surgery and six cycles of chemotherapy demonstrated that HE4 correlated with PET/CT results better than CA 125. Similarly, the study of Manganaro et al. [79] confirmed that HE4 may serve as marker of epithelial ovarian cancer relapse and, more importantly, its values, measured within three time intervals after surgery and adjuvant chemotherapy, were found to increase early compared with CA 125. A percentage of elevated HE4 levels were detected already in patients within the first time interval, while positivity for CA-125 was found later at time interval III and only in 44 % of patients. Combining then HE4 serum evaluation with CE CT imaging may improve the monitoring management of women affected by ovarian cancer.

About the diagnostic test performance, available data are rather limited and still insufficient to conclude that HE4 alone or in combination with CA-125 has significantly better diagnostic performance than CA-125 alone. Moreover, there is not sufficient evidence from prospective or controlled studies demonstrating that HE4 is an effective screening tool for identifying ovarian cancer in asymptomatic women.

14.6 Multiple-Marker Based Algorithms

Due to well-known limitations associated to the use of a single marker, for some years oncologic research has turned to evaluate clinical utility of the combined use of multiple biomarkers associated with ovarian cancers, including biochemical, ultrasound and other imaging techniques. Two algorithms, ROMA and OVA1, have been recently approved by FDA and are used to assess ovarian cancer risk for premenopausal or postmenopausal women with a pelvic mass.

ROMA (Risk of Ovarian Malignancy Algorithm) is a qualitative serum test that generates a numerical score (from 0.0 to 10.0) by incorporating the results of CA-125 (the most widely accepted biomarker for ovarian cancer) and HE4 blood tests, plus menopausal status, to identify patients presenting with an adnexal mass as being at high or low likelihood for having malignancy. Results must be interpreted in conjunction with an independent clinical and radiological assessment (https://www.accessdata.fda.gov/cdrh_docs/reviews/K103358.pdf)

Data from a combined population of pre- and postmenopausal women, published in the instructions for use of ROMA [80], showed for this algorithm a sensitivity of 88.4 %, a specificity of 67.2 %, and an NPV of 96.2 %. The high accuracy and reproducibility characteristic of this regression model in stratifying patients into a high or low ovarian cancer risk is independently confirmed in a number of publications, some of which indicated increased benefit with ROMA vs traditionally measured CA-125 and HE4 [81–83]. It may, furthermore, be improved with inclusion of supplemental data, such as age and ultrasound findings. The performance and clinical utility of ROMA has been described in detail by Chudecka-Głaz [84] in her exhaustive review.

Based on the proteomics biomarker discovery approach using mass spectrometry, Zhang and coworkers [55, 85] identified several proteins that, when combined with CA 125, provide diagnostic value for ovarian cancer. Data were submitted to the FDA and were cleared for clinical use as the OVA1 test the first in vitro diagnostic multivariate index assay proteomic diagnostic for cancer.

The OVA1 Test is a qualitative serum test that combines the values for 5 analytes (Prealbumin, Apo A-1, β2M, Transferrin, and CA 125) from separately run immunoassays into a single numerical score between 0.0 and 10.0 to indicate the likelihood that the pelvic mass is benign or malignant. The algorithm was derived using two independent training data sets from preoperative serum samples. Two cutoffs, 5.0 and 4.4 for pre- and post-menopausal patients respectively, were identified based on the training data. The cutoff score classifies a patient based on her OVA1™ Test score as low probability or high probability for presence of ovarian malignancy [86]. The FDA reviewed a study of 516 patients, collected from 27 clinical sites and including 269 evaluated by non-gynecological oncologists, which compared OVA1 results with biopsy results. When combined with pre-surgical information, such as radiography and other laboratory tests, results from the OVA1 tests identified additional patients, not identified using pre-surgical information alone, who might benefit from oncology referral (https://www.accessdata.fda.gov/cdrh_docs/reviews/K081754.pdf).

The effectiveness of OVA1 in the preoperative assessment of ovarian tumors has been investigated in a study of Ueland and coworkers [87], who assessed its clinical performance in a prospective, double-blind clinical study of 524 subjects (29 % with ovarian cancer) at 27 demographically diverse collection sites throughout the U.S. The authors reported high sensitivity (93 %) and NPV (93 %) but low specificity (43 %) and low PPV (42 %), demonstrating for OVA1 a higher sensitivity and lower specificity compared with physician assessment and CA 125 in detecting ovarian malignancies. Similar results were reported by Bristow et al. [88], who evaluated the effectiveness of a multivariate index assay in identifying ovarian malignancy compared to clinical assessment and CA125-II. Data from a prospective, multi-institutional trial, enrolling a total of 494 women, scheduled to undergo surgery for an adnexal mass from 27 non-gynecologic oncology practices, showed that, when combined with clinical impression, the sensitivity for OVA1 was 95.7 %, validating its usefulness as a preoperative cancer referral test. Investigators concluded that OVA1 demonstrated higher sensitivity and negative predictive value (98.1 %) for ovarian malignancy compared to clinical impression and CA125-II in an intended

In conclusion, OVA1 test is not intended for ovarian cancer screening or for a definitive diagnosis of ovarian cancer. It should be used as an adjunctive test to complement, not replace, other diagnostic and clinical procedures. Furthermore, interpreting the test result requires to know whether the woman is pre- or post-menopausal.

More recently, Grenache et al. [89] evaluated the clinical performance of OVA1 and ROMA for the prediction of malignancy in women with an adnexal mass, reporting a sensitivity of OVA1 and ROMA of 97 % and 87 %, respectively ($p=0.25$). Results indicated that ROMA was more specific than OVA1 (83 % vs. 55 %, respectively; $p<0.0001$), while the negative predictive values of both tests were similar (98.4 % and 96.0 %, respectively). A sequential testing strategy may improve overall performance, producing a positive predictive value of 69 % when ROMA is performed on all patients identified as high risk by OVA1. The authors concluded that the use of these tests to appropriately triage women with an adnexal mass should be gauged within the context of their respective limitations.

14.7 Conclusions

Although the role of CA 125 in the screening is controversial, CA 125 serum measurement is useful in the differential diagnosis of ovarian masses, and in monitoring response to therapeutic treatment and in detecting residual or recurrent disease during the follow up women with epithelial ovarian cancer. However, due to its limited specificity and sensitivity, CA 125 alone cannot still be an ideal biomarker. From all these considerations arises the need to identify complementary biomarkers which may be used in association with CA 125, to improve diagnostic performance. HE4 is another ovarian cancer marker intensely studied in the last years and recently introduced in clinical use as marker of epithelial ovarian cancer relapse. Considerable efforts have been applied to the development of multiplexed biomarker-based tests and more than 200 potential markers of ovarian cancer has been proposed so far [90]. Several significant advancements have been achieved recently, including the introduction of FDA-approved HE4, ROMA and OVA1 tests to evaluate the risk of ovarian cancer for patients with a pelvic mass. Results from recent studies are encouraging, in demonstrating that a multi-marker approach seems guarantee a better sensitivity than CA 125 alone, although their real clinical contribution is still under accurate investigations in properly designed clinical trials. Meanwhile major efforts are underway to detect biomarkers capable of recognizing disease in its preclinical phase, in an attempt to improve ovarian cancer risk stratification by identifying populations at greatest risk of disease. It is a very difficult challenge, but the considerable advances in high-throughput technologies over the past decade and their intense use in identifying a characteristic disease-related markers profile clearly indicates that a new era in screening is underway.

References

1. Senapati S, Das S, Batra SK (2010) Mucin-interacting proteins: from function to therapeutics. Trends Biochem Sci 35:236–245
2. Rose MC, Voynow JA (2006) Respiratory tract mucin genes and mucin glycoproteins in health and disease. Physiol Rev 86:245–278
3. Gendler SJ, Burchell JM, Duhig T et al (1987) Cloning of partial cDNA encoding differentiation and tumor-associated mucin glycoproteins expressed by human mammary epithelium. Proc Natl Acad Sci U S A 84:6060–6064
4. Gupta R, Jentoft N (1989) Subunit structure of porcine submaxillary mucin. Biochemistry 28:6114–6121
5. Timpte CS, Eckhardt AE, Abernethy JL, Hill RL (1988) Porcine submaxillary gland apomucin contains tandemly repeated, identical sequences of 81 residues. J Biol Chem 263:1081–1088
6. Lang T, Hansson GC, Samuelsson T (2007) Gel-forming mucins appeared early in metazoan evolution. Proc Natl Acad Sci U S A 104:16209–16214
7. Hollingsworth MA, Swanson BJ (2004) Mucins in cancer: protection and control of the cell surface. Nat Rev Cancer 4:45–60
8. Chen Y, Zhao YH, Kalaslavadi TB et al (2004) Genome-wide search and identification of a novel gel-forming mucin MUC19/Muc19 in glandular tissues. Am J Respir Cell Mol Biol 30:155–165
9. Corfield AP (2015) Mucins: a biologically relevant glycan barrier in mucosal protection. Biochim Biophys Acta 1850:236–252
10. Kufe DW (2009) Mucins in cancer: function, prognosis and therapy. Nat Rev Cancer 9:874–885
11. Carraway KL, Ramsauer VP, Haq B, Carothers Carraway CA (2003) Cell signaling through membrane mucins. Bioessays 25:66–71
12. Jepson S, Komatsu M, Haq B et al (2002) Muc4/sialomucin complex, the intramembrane ErbB2 ligand, induces specific phosphorylation of ErbB2 and enhances expression of p27(kip), but does not activate mitogen-activated kinase or protein kinaseB/Akt pathways. Oncogene 21:7524–7532
13. Levitin F, Stern O, Weiss M et al (2005) The MUC1 SEA module is a self-cleaving domain. J Biol Chem 280:33374–33386
14. Gendler SJ, Spicer AP (1995) Epithelial mucin genes. Annu Rev Physiol 57:607–634
15. Singh AP, Moniaux N, Chauhan SC et al (2004) Inhibition of MUC4 expression suppresses pancreatic tumor cell growth and metastasis. Cancer Res 64:622–630
16. Chan AK, Lockhart DC, von Bernstorff W (1999) Soluble MUC1 secreted by human epithelial cancer cells mediates immune suppression by blocking T-cell activation. Int J Cancer 82:721–726
17. Argueso P, Guzman-Aranguez A, Mantelli F et al (2009) Association of cell surface mucins with galectin-3 contributes to the ocular surface epithelial barrier. J Biol Chem 284:23037–23045
18. Seelenmeyer C, Wegehingel S, Lechner J, Nickel W (2003) The cancer antigen CA125 represents a novel counter receptor for galectin-1. J Cell Sci 116:1305–1318
19. Patankar MS, Jing Y, Morrison JC et al (2005) Potent suppression of natural killer cell response mediated by the ovarian tumor marker CA125. Gynecol Oncol 99:704–713
20. Belisle JA, Gubbels JA, Raphael CA et al (2007) Peritoneal natural killer cells from epithelial ovarian cancer patients show an altered phenotype and bind to the tumour marker MUC16 (CA125). Immunology 122:418–429
21. Gubbels JA, Belisle J, Onda M et al (2006) Mesothelin-MUC16 binding is a high affinity, N-glycan dependent interaction that facilitates peritoneal metastasis of ovarian tumors. Mol Cancer 5:50
22. Rump A, Morikawa Y, Tanaka M (2004) Binding of ovarian cancer antigen CA125/MUC16 to mesothelin mediates cell adhesion. J Biol Chem 279:9190–9198

23. Bergan L, Gross JA, Nevin B et al (2007) Development and in vitro validation of antimesothelin biobodies that prevent CA125/Mesothelin-dependent cell attachment. Cancer Lett 255:263–274
24. Kaneko O, Gong L, Zhang J et al (2009) A binding domain on mesothelin for CA125/MUC16. J Biol Chem 284:3739–3749
25. Bast RC Jr, Feeney M, Lazarus H et al (1981) Reactivity of a monoclonal antibody with human ovarian carcinoma. J Clin Invest 68:1331–1337
26. Bast RC Jr, Klug TL, St. John E et al (1983) A radioimmunoassay using a monoclonal antibody to monitor the course of epithelial ovarian cancer. N Engl J Med 309:883
27. Bast RC Jr, Xu FJ, Yu YH et al (1998) CA 125: the past and the future. Int J Biol Markers 13:179–187
28. Sturgeon CM, Duffy MJ, Stenman UH et al (2008) National academy of clinical biochemistry laboratory medicine practice guidelines for use of tumor markers in testicular, prostate, colorectal, breast, and ovarian cancers. Clin Chem 54:e11–e79
29. Davelaar EM, van Kamp GJ, Verstraeten RA, Kenemans P (1998) Comparison of seven immunoassays for the quantification of CA 125 antigen in serum. Clin Chem 44:1417–1422
30. Shih Ie M, Sokoll L, Chan DW (2002) Ovarian cancer. In: Diamandis EP, Fritsche HA, Lilja H, Chan DW, Schwartz MK (eds) Tumor markers: physiology, pathobiology, technology and clinical applications. AACC Press, Washington, DC, pp 239–252
31. Masahashi T, Matsuzawa K, Ohsawa M et al (1988) Serum CA 125 levels in patients with endometriosis: changes of CA 125 levels during menstruation. Obstet Gynecol 72:328
32. Bergmann JF, Beaugrand M, Labadie H et al (1986) CA 125 (ovarian tumour-associated antigen) in ascitic liver diseases. Clin Chim Acta 155:163
33. Molina R, Ballesta AM, Casals E et al (1984) Value of CA 125 antigen as tumor marker: preliminary results. In: Peeters H (ed) Protides of the biological fluids. Proceedings of the 32nd Colloquium, Brussels, p 613
34. Ruibal A, Encabo G, Miralles EM et al (1984) CA 125 seric levels in non ovarian pathologies. In: Peeters H (ed) Protides of the biological fluids. Proceedings of the 32nd Colloquium, Brussels, p 605
35. Giudice LC, Jacobs A, Pineda J et al (1986) Serum levels of CA 125 in patients with endometriosis: a preliminary report. Fertil Steril 45(6):876
36. Malkasian GD Jr, Podratz KC, Stanhope CR et al (1986) CA 125 in gynecologic practice. Am J Obstet Gynecol 155:515
37. Haga Y, Sakamoto K, Egami H et al (1986) Evaluation of serum CA 125 values in healthy individuals and pregnant women. Am J Med Sci 292:25
38. Halila H, Stenman UH, Seppala M (1986) Ovarian cancer antigen CA 125. Levels in pelvic inflammatory disease and pregnancy. Cancer 57:1327
39. Pittaway DE, Fayez JA, Douglas JW (1987) Serum CA 125 in the evaluation of benign adnexal cysts. Am J Obstet Gynecol 157:1426
40. Niloff JM, Knapp RC, Schaetzl E et al (1984) CA 125 antigen levels in obstetric and gynecologic patients. Obstet Gynecol 64:703
41. Haga Y, Sakamoto K, Egami H et al (1986) Clinical significance of serum CA 125 values in patients with cancers of the digestive system. Am J Med Sci 292:30
42. Duk JM, Aalders JG, Fleuren GJ et al (1986) CA 125: a useful marker in endometrial carcinoma. Am J Obstet Gynecol 155:1097
43. Bertholf RL, Johannsen L, Guy B (2002) False elevation of serum CA-125 level caused by human anti-mouse antibodies. Ann Clin Lab Sci 32:414–418
44. Boerman OC, Segers MF, Poels LG et al (1990) Heterophilic antibodies in human sera causing falsely increased results in the CA 125 immunofluorometric assay. Clin Chem 36:888–891
45. Young RH, Clement PB, Scully RE, Sternberg SS (1999) The ovary: diagnostic surgical pathology, vol 3. Lippincott Williams & Wilkins, Philadelphia, pp 2307–2394
46. Scully RE (ed) (1999) Histological typing of ovarian tumours, 2nd edn, Sobin LH and pathologists in 5 countries, collaborators. Springer, New York, p 136
47. Seidman JD, Horkayne-Szakaly I, Haiba M et al (2004) The histologic type and stage distribution of ovarian carcinomas of surface epithelial origin. Int J Gynecol Pathol 23:41–44
48. Ferlay J, Steliarova-Foucher E, Lortet-Tieulent J et al (2013) Cancer incidence and mortality patterns in Europe: estimates for 40 countries in 2012. Eur J Cancer 49:1374–1403
49. Fleisher M, Dnistrian A, Sturgeon C, Lamerz R, Witliff J (2002) Practice guidelines and recommendations for use of tumor markers in the clinic. Tumor markers: physiology, pathobiology, technology and clinical applications. AACC Press, Washington, DC, pp 33–63
50. NCCN [National Comprehensive Cancer Network] Clinical Practice Guidelines in Oncology (2008) Ovarian cancer. Version 1. http://www.nccn.org/professionals/physician_gls/PDF/ovarian.pdf. Accessed Nov 2008
51. Vasey PA, Herrstedt J, Jelic S (2005) ESMO minimum clinical recommendations for diagnosis, treatment and follow-up of epithelial ovarian carcinoma. Ann Oncol 16(Suppl 1):i13–i15
52. Skates SJ, Xu FJ, Yu YH et al (1995) Toward an optimal algorithm for ovarian cancer screening with longitudinal tumor markers. Cancer 76:2004–2010
53. Bast RC Jr, Brewer M, Zou C et al (2007) Prevention and early detection of ovarian cancer: mission impossible? Recent Results Cancer Res 174:91–100
54. Bast RC Jr, Urban N, Shridhar V et al (2002) Early detection of ovarian cancer: promise and reality. Cancer Treat Res 107:61–97
55. Zhang Z, Bast RC Jr, Yu Y et al (2004) Three biomarkers identified from serum proteomic analysis for the detection of early stage ovarian cancer. Cancer Res 64:5882–5890
56. Kobayashi H, Yamada Y, Sado T et al (2008) A randomized study of screening for ovarian cancer: a mul-

ticenter study in Japan. Int J Gynecol Cancer 18:414–420
57. Buys SS, Partridge E, Black A et al (2011) Effect of screening on ovarian cancer mortality: the Prostate, Lung, Colorectal and Ovarian (PLCO) cancer screening randomized controlled trial. JAMA 305:2295–2303
58. Menon U, Gentry-Maharaj A, Hallett R et al (2009) Sensitivity and specificity of multimodal and ultrasound screening for ovarian cancer, and stage distribution of detected cancers: results of the prevalence screen of the UK Collaborative Trial of Ovarian Cancer Screening (UKCTOCS). Lancet Oncol 10:327–340
59. Menon U, Griffin M, Gentry-Maharaj A (2014) Ovarian cancer screening-current status, future directions. Gynecol Oncol 132:490–495
60. Duffy MJ, Bonfrer JM, Kulpa J et al (2005) CA125 in ovarian cancer: European group on tumor markers guidelines for clinical use. Int J Gynecol Cancer 15:679–691
61. Gronlund B, Hogdall C, Hilden J et al (2004) Should CA-125 response criteria be preferred to response evaluation criteria in solid tumors (RECIST) for prognostication during second-line chemotherapy of ovarian carcinoma? J Clin Oncol 22:4051–4058
62. Su Z, Graybill WS, Zhu Y (2013) Detection and monitoring of ovarian cancer. Clin Chim Acta 415:341–345
63. Rustin GJ, Vergote I, Eisenhauer E et al (2011) Definitions for response and progression in ovarian cancer clinical trials incorporating RECIST 1.1 and CA 125 agreed by the Gynecological Cancer Intergroup (GCIG). Int J Gynecol Cancer 21:419–423
64. Gadducci A, Fuso L, Cosio S et al (2009) Are surveillance procedures of clinical benefit for patients treated for ovarian cancer?: a retrospective Italian multicentric study. Int J Gynecol Cancer 19:367–374
65. Nadal RM, Ojeda BM, Artigas V et al (2006) Stratification of the normal range of CA-125 after chemotherapy as a predictive factor in carcinoma of the ovary. J Clin Oncol 24:270 s (suppl; abstr 5059)
66. Tanabe H, Katsumata N, Matsumoto K et al (2006) CA-125 nadir as a prognostic factor in advanced ovarian carcinoma: a retrospective study of 84 patients achieving clinical CR. J Clin Oncol 24:270 s (suppl; abstr 5060)
67. Markman M, Liu PY, Rothenberg ML et al (2006) Pretreatment CA-125 and risk of relapse in advanced ovarian cancer. J Clin Oncol 24:1454–1458
68. Liu PY, Alberts DS, Monk BJ et al (2007) An early signal of CA-125 progression for ovarian cancer patients receiving maintenance treatment after complete clinical response to primary therapy. J Clin Oncol 25:3615–3620
69. Prat A, Parera M, Peralta S et al (2008) Nadir CA-125 concentration in the normal range as an independent prognostic factor for optimally treated advanced epithelial ovarian cancer. Ann Oncol 19:327–331
70. Clauss A, Lilja H, Lundwall A (2002) A locus on human chromosome 20 contains several genes expressing protease inhibitor domains with homology to whey acidic protein. Biochem J 368:233–242
71. Hellstrom I, Raycraft J, Hayden-Ledbetter M et al (2003) The HE4 (WFDC2) protein is a biomarker for ovarian carcinoma. Cancer Res 63:3695–3700
72. Li J, Dowdy S, Tipton T et al (2009) HE4 as a biomarker for ovarian and endometrial cancer management. Expert Rev Mol Diagn 9:555–566
73. Bingle L, Singleton V, Bingle CD (2002) The putative ovarian tumour marker gene HE4 (WFDC2), is expressed in normal tissues and undergoes complex alternative splicing to yield multiple protein isoforms. Oncogene 21:2768–2773
74. Ferraro S, Schiumarini D, Panteghini M (2015) Human epididymis protein 4: factors of variation. Clin Chim Acta 438:171–177
75. Moore RG, Miller MC, Eklund EE (2012) Serum levels of the ovarian cancer biomarker HE4 are decreased in pregnancy and increase with age. Am J Obstet Gynecol 206(349):e1–e7
76. Huhtinen K, Suvitie P, Hiissa J et al (2009) Serum HE4 concentration differentiates malignant ovarian tumours from ovarian endometriotic cysts. Br J Cancer 100:1315–1319
77. Anastasi E, Marchei GG, Viggiani V et al (2010) HE4: a new potential early biomarker for the recurrence of ovarian cancer. Tumour Biol 31:113–119
78. Hynninen J, Auranen A, Dean K et al (2011) Serum HE4 profile during primary chemotherapy of epithelial ovarian cancer. Int J Gynecol Cancer 21:1573–1578
79. Manganaro L, Michienzi S, Vinci V et al (2013) Serum HE4 levels combined with CE CT imaging improve the management of monitoring women affected by epithelial ovarian cancer. Oncol Rep 30:2481–2487
80. ROMA™ (HE4 EIA + ARCHITECT CA 125 IITM) Prescribing Information (2011) Fujirebio Diagnostics, Inc.
81. Kalapotharakos G, Asciutto C, Henic E et al (2012) High preoperative blood levels of HE4 predicts poor prognosis in patients with ovarian cancer. J Ovarian Res 5:20
82. Sandri MT, Bottari F, Franchi D et al (2013) Comparison of HE4, CA125 and ROMA algorithm in women with a pelvic mass: correlation with pathological outcome. Gynecol Oncol 128:233–238
83. Wang J, Gao J, Yao H et al (2014) Diagnostic accuracy of serum HE4, CA125 and ROMA in patients with ovarian cancer: a meta-analysis. Tumour Biol 35:6127–6138
84. Chudecka-Głaz AM (2015) ROMA, an algorithm for ovarian cancer. Clin Chim Acta 440:143–151
85. Zhang Z, Chan DW (2010) The road from discovery to clinical diagnostics: lessons learned from the first FDA-cleared in vitro diagnostic multivariate index assay of proteomic biomarkers. Cancer Epidemiol Biomarkers Prev 19:2995–2999

86. Fung ET (2010) A recipe for proteomics diagnostic test development: the OVA1 test, from biomarker discovery to FDA clearance. Clin Chem 56:327–329
87. Ueland FR, Desimone CP, Seamon LG et al (2011) Effectiveness of a multivariate index assay in the preoperative assessment of ovarian tumors. Obstet Gynecol 117:1289–1297
88. Bristow RE, Smith A, Zhang Z et al (2013) Ovarian malignancy risk stratification of the adnexal mass using a multivariate index assay. Gynecol Oncol 128:252–259
89. Grenache DG, Heichman KA, Werner TL, Vucetic Z (2015) Clinical performance of two multi-marker blood tests for predicting malignancy in women with an adnexal mass. Clin Chim Acta 438:358–363
90. Lokshin AE (2012) The quest for ovarian cancer screening biomarkers: are we on the right road? Int J Gynecol Cancer 22(Suppl 1):S35–S40

Part VII

Tumor Markers – A Critical Revision: Blood Group Antigens

CA 19-9: Biochemical and Clinical Aspects

15

Salvatore Scarà, Patrizia Bottoni, and Roberto Scatena

Abstract

CA19-9 (carbohydrate antigen 19-9, also called cancer antigen 19-9 or sialylated Lewis a antigen) is the most commonly used and best validated serum tumor marker for pancreatic cancer diagnosis in symptomatic patients and for monitoring therapy in patients with pancreatic adenocarcinoma. Normally synthesized by normal human pancreatic and biliary ductal cells and by gastric, colon, endometrial and salivary epithelia, CA 19-9 is present in small amounts in serum, and can be over expressed in several benign gastrointestinal disorders. Importantly, it exhibits a dramatic increase in its plasmatic levels during neoplastic disease. However, several critical aspects for its clinical use, such as false negative results in subjects with Lewis $^{a-b-}$ genotype and false positive elevation, occasional and transient, in patients with benign diseases, together with its poor positive predictive value (72.3 %), do not make it a good cancer-specific marker and renders it impotent as a screening tool. In the last years a large number of putative biomarkers for pancreatic cancer have been proposed, most of which is lacking of large scale validation. In addition, none of these has showed to possess the requisite sensitivity/specificity to be introduced in clinical use. Therefore, although with important limitations we well-know, CA 19-9 continues being the only pancreatic cancer marker actually in clinical use.

Keywords

Biomarker • CA 19-9 • CA 19-9 biochemical structure • CA 19-9 measurement • Clinical interferences • DUPAN-2 • Follow-up pancreatic cancer • K-ras • Methodological interferences • MIC-1 • MicroRNA • Pancreatic cancer • REG-4 • Serum tumor markers • Sialylated Lewis a antigen

S. Scarà • P. Bottoni (✉) • R. Scatena
Institute of Biochemistry and Clinical Biochemistry,
School of Medicine, Catholic University,
Largo Gemelli 8, 00168 Rome, Italy
e-mail: patrizia.bottoni@rm.unicatt.it

R. Scatena (ed.), *Advances in Cancer Biomarkers*, Advances in Experimental Medicine and Biology 867, DOI 10.1007/978-94-017-7215-0_15

15.1 Introduction

CA 19-9 (carbohydrate antigen 19-9, also called cancer antigen 19-9) is the most widely used and best validated marker for pancreatic cancer [1]. First described in 1979 by Koprowski et al. [2] in colorectal carcinoma cell line SW1116 using the mouse monoclonal antibody 1116-NS-19-9, this molecule was then discovered in the serum of patients with colon and pancreatic cancer in 1981 [3] and was later found also to be a component of glycoproteins and mucins [4–6]. It belongs to the large family of mucinous markers: glycoproteins with a transmembrane protein skeleton and the extracellular side consisting of oligosaccharides chains extensively glycosylated, which are a normal component of the glandular secretions of mucous type. In particular, CA 19-9 is synthesized by normal human pancreatic and biliary ductal cells and by gastric, colon, endometrial and salivary epithelia. Normally present in small amounts in serum, in which it exists as mucin, a high molecular mass (200–1000 kDa) glycoprotein complex, CA 19-9 is over expressed in certain inflammatory conditions as pancreatitis and other benign gastrointestinal diseases. Moreover, it exhibits an increase in its plasmatic levels in course of neoplastic disease, during which several processes regulating both the passage of these molecules in the bloodstream and their metabolization appear altered [7]. Sialyl Lewis a is not found at high levels in normal tissues, whereas it is found at elevated levels in patients with pancreatic, hepatobiliary, gastric, hepatocellular, colorectal and breast cancer.

15.2 Biochemical Structure

CA 19-9 antigen is a tetrasaccharide carbohydrate termed sialyl Lewis a (part of the Lewis family of blood group antigens) with the sequence Neu5Aca2,3Galb1,3 (Fuca1,4) GlcNAc. Sialyl Lewis a is synthesized by glycosyltransferases which sequentially bind the monosaccharide precursors onto both N-linked and O-linked glycans. The expression of the antigen requires the Lewis gene product, 1,4-fucosyltransferase, and subjects who are genotypically Le^{a-b-}, approximately 6 % of Caucasian and about 22 % of non-Caucasican population, do not synthesize the molecule. The Lewis blood group system comprises a set of fucosylated glycosphingolipids that are synthesized by exocrine epithelial cells and subsequently adsorbed onto the surface of the erythrocyte, giving rise to their Lewis phenotype and thus circulating in body fluid as red cell antigens. The Lewis antigen system is based on expression of genes members of the fucosyltransferase family, which catalyzes the addition of α-fucose residue to precursor polysaccharides in the last step of Lewis antigen biosynthesis. In particular, enzymes with $\alpha\ 1\rightarrow3$ fucosyltransferase and $\alpha\ 1\rightarrow4$ fucosyltransferase activities, encoded by Le or FUT3 gene, add an α-fucose residue to the precursor oligosaccharide substrate in subterminal position, converting it to the Le^a antigen. The α-fucose residue linked to terminal β-galactose through $1\rightarrow2$ linkage is synthesized by the $\alpha1\rightarrow2$ fucosyltransferase, encoded by FUT2 (Se) gene, and can be added only if an α-fucose has already been added by the Le gene product. Therefore, the addition of a second fucose to the Le^a antigen produces the Le^b antigen.

Besides Le^a and Le^b, also two minor antigens exist, Le^c and Le^d, and several sialylated or sulfated forms of antigens whose identification has been facilitated by the use of monoclonal antibodies, started on a large scale about 30 years ago. Le^{a-b+} phenotypes are present with a frequency of 72 % among Europeans and white American populations, followed by Le^{a+b-} (22 %), and Le^{a-b-} (6 %), while the percentage of Le^{a-b-} is as high as 22 % in Afro-Americans [8]. The Le^{a+b+} phenotype is more frequent among people of East Asia and the Pacific rim region, due to the presence of *Se* genes encoding less efficient $\alpha1\rightarrow2$ fucosyltransferase [9].

Le^a and Le^b antigens start to appear after birth, the first develops soon, the second much later, till it reach the adult level at 6 years of age. It has long been known that Le^a and Le^b glycolipid antigens are mainly synthesized by intestinal epithelial cells, secreted into the blood stream, and adsorbed at the surface of RBCs. This process can be affected by abnormalities in serum lipoprotein composition during pregnancy or malignant disorders, thus resulting in a considerable decrease of Le^a and Le^b antigen expression on RBCs.

15.3 Physiology and Pathophysiology

It is well known that immune cells express specific recognition molecules for cell surface glycans, such as galectins, sialic acid binding Ig-like lectins (siglecs), and selectins [9–11]. Such recognition molecules seem to be essential in cell-cell interaction processes, but the exact mechanism that involve glycan-mediated cell-cell interactions in mucosal immunity are still to be clarified.

It has also long be known that cell surface glycans undergo remarkable changes during malignant transformation, an altered expression ascribable to a process already defined 'incomplete synthesis' of complex carbohydrate determinants, with the resulting expression of structurally less complicated carbohydrate molecules [12–15].

The sialyl Lewis a antigen is just one of these carbohydrate determinants. It has recently been shown that, besides this determinant, linked to a single molecule of sialic acid, there is another form, tied to two molecules of sialic acid (the second sialic acid residue attached at the C6-position of penultimate GlcNAc in sialyl Lewis a), which is prevalently expressed in non-malignant epithelial cells (disialyl Lewis a). This 'normal' molecule, whose expression decreases significantly during malignant transformation, functions as a ligand for immunosuppressive receptors and contributes to maintaining immunological homeostasis of the gastrointestinal mucous membranes. In particular, studies conducted by Miyazaki et al. [16] indicate that the glycans expressed in normal epithelial cells serves as ligands for sialic acid-binding immunoglobulin-like lectin-7 (Siglec-7) and sialic acid-binding immunoglobulin-like lectin-9 (Singlec-9), the immunosuppressive carbohydrate-recognition receptors expressed mainly on leukocytes, whereas the cancer-associated glycans do not. The downregulated transcription of a gene encoding the $\alpha\, 2 \rightarrow 6$ sialyltransferase in cancer cells produces initially a partial synthesis of incomplete bond of the second sialic acid residue then a gradual transition of carbohydrate determinants from disialyl Lewis a-dominant status to sialyl Lewis a-dominant status, with a resulting accumulation of this last. Important functional consequences are evident, such as the loss of right cell-cell recognition between mucosal epithelial cells and lymphoid cells and the gain of E-selectin binding activity. Similarly, impairment of 6-sulfation seems to occur on malignant transformation of colonic epithelial cells, leading to the loss of sialyl 6-sulfo Lewis x determinant and gain of sialyl Lewis x in cancer cells, another ligand for E-selectin [17]. Therefore, the expression of these siglec-7/-9 ligands that was impaired upon carcinogenesis were replaced by cancer-associated glycans sialyl Lewis a and sialyl Lewis x, which have no siglec ligand activity. If normal glycans of epithelial cells exert a suppressive effect on cyclooxygenase-2 expression by resident macrophages, thus maintaining immunological homeostasis in colonic mucosal membranes, their loss caused by impaired glycosylation can enhance inflammatory mediator production [18]. Subsequently, hypoxic conditions that arise in the course of neoplastic disease, in inducing the transcription of several genes responsible for glycosylation involved in the synthesis of sialyl Lewis a, further accelerate the expression of this determinant in hypoxia-resistant cells with a high degree of malignancy, which become the predominant clones in advanced tumors with high frequency of hematogenous metastases [19].

15.4 Measurement of CA 19-9

15.4.1 Clinical Interferences with the Assay

Initial enthusiasm for applying sialyl Lewis a for serum diagnosis of cancers has waned in part when the presence of false-positives in patients suffering from intra- and extra-cholestatic diseases as well as liver dysfunction have been reported [20–22]. Since then, it appeared to be clear that clinical interpretation of CA 19.9 measurement requires a careful evaluation of important interfering situations which render difficult the use of this tumor marker in clinical practice. Now, in the light of more recent data analyzing the diagnostic accuracy in patients with pancreatic cancer, appear evident that the diagnostic utility of CA 19.9 presents important limitations above all related to a low sensitivity in sympthomatic patients and a low PPV. In particular for the following:

- Impossibility to detect CA 19-9 in subjects that have a fucosyltransferase deficiency, approximately of 5–10 % of the Caucasian population, who cannot synthesize the Ca-19-9 epitope. Therefore, in these genotypically Lewis $^{a-b-}$ patients, false negative results for CA 19-9 serum levels can be obtained even in the presence of advanced pancreatic cancer. It follows that the maximum achievable sensitivity of CA 19-9 for pancreatic cancer in Caucasian populations is 90–95 % [23];
- Appearance of sialyl Lewis a in the serum is not specific to malignant disorders, and patients with benign disorders sometimes show elevated serum levels of sialyl Lewis a.
- The occasional and transient elevation of CA 19.9 serum levels in a wide variety of benign conditions limits its diagnostic utility, showing as sialyl Lewis a is not a cancer-specific marker in a strict sense. The determinant is expressed by a small number of ductal epithelial cells in the normal pancreas, and its serum levels exhibit an increase, sometimes dramatic [24], in several non-malignant disorders such as inflammatory diseases, including chronic and acute pancreatitis, liver cirrhosis, cholangitis and obstructive jaundice [25]. Other benign conditions, including ovarian cyst, heart failure, hashimoto's thyroiditis, rheumatoid arthritis and diverticulitis have been reported to cause an increase of CA 19-9 serum levels [26–31];
- Possibility to detect elevated CA 19-9 levels in multiple types of adenocarcinoma, especially in advanced gastrointestinal cancers [1,7,26]. In an overview study, Steinberg [26] reported an elevation percentage, which sometimes may be significant, of CA 19-9 in patients with bile duct cancer, gastric and colorectal cancer, and with hepatocellular carcinoma;
- Lacking in CA 19-9 sensitivity for early or small-diameter pancreatic cancers. Because of serum CA 19-9 concentration is highly correlated to the tumor size in most, if not in all, patients with pancreatic cancer [32], just 50 % of patients with pancreatic cancers less that 3 cm in diameter presents elevated levels of CA 19-9 [26], thus it is difficult to use CA 19-9 as a marker for early diagnosis of pancreatic cancer [33,34];
- Poor correlation between the degree of cell differentiation of the tumor and the serum level of CA 19-9 (National health Insurance Corporation [35]). Poorly differentiated pancreatic cancers appear to express less CA 19-9 than either moderately or well differentiated cancers [26].

Given all these limitations, it is evident the CA 19-9 is a marker that should be used carefully, particularly in the initial diagnostic approach, during which its use may at worst aid diagnosis, but of course cannot replace histological proof of pancreatic cancer, even when imaging is indicative [1]. Moreover, if false-positive results in a given population of patients with benign disorders are inevitable, however the possibility to simultaneously determinate serum levels of sialyl- and disialyl Lewis a and to calculate the monosialyl/disialyl Lewis a ratio is very important to limit these false positives. In particular, during the course of cancer progression, the expression of sialyl Lewis a determinant is accelerated, with consequent increase of sialyl Lewis a/disialyl Lewis a ratio, which tends to be higher in serum of cancer patients while maintaining low in patients with benign disorders. In this way it is possible to distinguish pathological forms more severe than the benign, thus reducing the number of patients who are sometimes subjected to long hospitalization periods, and undergo unnecessary further clinical examinations, including diagnostic imaging techniques, for have differential diagnosis.

15.4.2 Methodological Interferences with the Assay

Almost all assays for CA 19-9 detection depend on the use of the monoclonal antibody 1116-NS-19-9, which recognizes a carbohydrate epitope expressed on circulating antigen. An important aspect must be considered about CA 19.9 assays. In fact, although assays for the quantitative detection of CA 19-9 have been available for almost 30 years, its measurement is still somewhat problematic, reflecting primarily the lack of an international standard for CA 19-9 and differences in assay design. A comparative analysis of different assays for CA19-9 carried out extensively over the last few years has clearly demonstrated that different assays may give different results [36–38]. Also a recent study, undertaken to compare the results obtained by two widespread commercial methods, showed that the two assays were comparable in diagnostic accuracy and had a good correlation, but are not interchangeable [39]. The poor comparability of CA 19-9 results obtained using different methods complicates their clinical interpretation. It is therefore fundamental that patients who undergo serial determination of CA 19-9 levels are monitored for this marker using a single method and that each report states the method used for analysis [40].

Another problem in measuring of CA 19.9 is represented by the possibility of obtaining false results caused by the presence of interference methodology. Although interferences in the CA 19-9 assay are not frequent, this phenomenon, common to all immunoassays, must therefore always be considered. It has been reported that the presence of rheumatoid factor (RF) and of heterophilic antibodies are the most important causes of interference in the determination of CA 19-9. First described by Biguet et al. in [41], the possible interference of RF in the determination of CA 19-9 has been afterwards evaluated by Berth and co-workers in an RF-positive population, with RF concentrations exceeding 100 kIU/L, using four different immunoassay platforms [42]. The Authors reported that, among the eight discrepant results probably related to method dependent differences, only one, obtained with an assay for CA 19-9 (Centaur, Siemens Healthcare) but not with three others (ARCHITECT and AxSYM, Abbott, and Vidas, Biomerieux), is clearly referable to a interference problem of RF, with high level positivity for high RF (900 kU/L) associated with a very high positivity of CA 19-9 (80,000 U/L).

Contrarily, in a case report of a patient with a history of biliary polyp, Liang et al. [43] exclude that RF is responsible for the falsely elevated carbohydrate antigen 19-9 level, attributing instead this false-positivity to the presence of heterophilic antimouse antibody interference. Regarding the possible interference by heterophilic antibodies in serum CA 19-9 determination, Passerini et al. [39] demonstrated that both immunoassays considered in their study appeared to be affected by such interference, because a reduction of values below the proposed diagnostic cut-off was seen in 40–46 % of discrepant specimens after these antibodies were removed.

15.4.3 Sensitivity, Specificity

Some scientific publications have been carried out on the diagnostic accuracy of CA 19-9 in patients with pancreatic cancer and have been recently revised by Duffy et al. [1] in their exhaustive and comprehensive review. In all these works, in which serum CA 19-9 levels in pancreatic cancer patients have been compared with different control groups, has been used 37 kU/l as cut-off point for CA 19-9 and, with this cut off, CA 19-9 has been shown to have an overall mean sensitivity of 81 % and a mean specificity of 90 % for pancreatic cancer. Increasing the cut-off point improved considerably the specificity, but reduced gradually the sensitivity [26]. Data from 1990 to 2005, analyzed by Goonnetilleke and Siriwardena in a recent review, showed a median sensitivity of CA 19-9 for pancreatic cancer of the 79 % and a median specificity of 82 % [7]. Moreover, CA 19-9 sensitivity varies with the stage of pancreatic cancer, and only 50 % of patients with pancreatic cancers of <3 cm diameter will have an elevated CA 19-9 level. As reported in a document of the Association for Clinical Biochemistry [44], sensitivity for other malignancies is the following: 70 % for hepatobiliary, 40–50 % for gastric cancer, 30–50 % for hepatocellular carcinoma, 30 % for colorectal cancer and 15 % for breast cancer.

15.5 Clinical Indications

15.5.1 Pancreatic Cancer

According to American Cancer Society, in 2014 there will be 46,420 new cases of pancreatic cancer and an estimated 39,590 people will die of this disease. Rates of pancreatic cancer have been increasing slightly over the past decade, accounting for about 3 % of all cancers in the United States, and for about 7 % of cancer deaths. Compared to other cancers, pancreatic cancer is relatively rare, with an average lifetime risk of developing it of about 1.5 %. Although only the 12th most frequent malignancy, cancer of the pancreas was the fifth most frequent cause of cancer-related mortality in the Europe [1] and the fourth leading cause of cancer death in the US. With increasing age, this cancer type becomes more common and slightly more common in men than women.

Cancer stage at diagnosis addresses to chemotherapy or chemoradiotherapy treatment options and early detection has a strong influence on the patient survival. In general, the earlier pancreas cancer is caught, the better chance a person has of surviving 5 years after being diagnosed. The 5-year survival for localized pancreas cancer (approximately 9 % of the total) is of 25.8 %. Moreover, only 20 % of patients who have diagnosis of pancreas cancer are considered eligible for surgery and, of these, about a half undergoes successful resection. For the remaining 80 % of patients, suffering from locally advanced or metastatic disease, no curative therapy currently exists, and the median survival times estimated for them are of the order of 8–12 months and 5–8 months, respectively [1]. This poor prognosis is attributable to late pancreas cancer detection, that renders often ineffective the therapeutic treatments, to its early recurrence and, above all, to the absence of clinically useful biomarker(s) which can detect pancreatic cancer in its precursor form(s) or earliest stages [45]. Therefore, the prognosis continues to be poor, despite some improvements, mainly due to a more specialized surgery treatment and to the application of specific chemotherapy protocol, have been made in recent years. Yet, the large number of new putative pancreatic biomarkers that have been recently proposed needs to a large scale clinical validation, which at present still lacks.

15.5.2 CA 19-9 as a Screening and Diagnostic Biomarker for Pancreatic Cancer

The role of CA 19-9 as a screening tool for pancreatic cancer in asymptomatic individuals has been extensively evaluated, demonstrating that it has no utility as a screening marker given its very low positive predictive value [27,28]. In particular, Kim et al. [27] have drawn this conclusion, analyzing data from our study in which 70,940 asymptomatic subjects were screened using CA19-9. Only four cases of pancreatic cancer were detected along with 1059 false-positives, yielding a positive predictive value of only 0.9 %, although the sensitivity and specificity were 100 % and 98.5 % respectively. Similarly, Chang et al. [28], in illustrating results of our screening study on a group of 5343 subjects, reported that only two, among the 385 patients with CA 19-9 serum level >37 U/ml, were suffering from pancreatic cancer. The PPV of an elevated serum CA 19-9 level in the asymptomatic population in this study was only 0.5 %. False positive elevation of the CA 19-9 serum levels was noted in 325 patients (6.1 %) and a total of 58 other cancers were identified. Moreover, in screening high-risk populations, serum CA19-9 level is often normal also when many preinvasive pancreatic lesions are detected by imaging [46–48]. Based on these evidences, according to American Society of Clinical Oncology (ASCO) guidelines, CA 19-9 should not be used as screening in asymptomatic subjects. Currently, a multimodality screening combining various evaluative imaging techniques appears to be the most effective way to detect precancerous pancreatic lesions, even though it is an issue still controversial in some its aspects (the age to initiate screening, the optimal screening modalities as well as the intervals for follow-up imaging). In 2013, International Cancer of the Pancreas Screening (CAPS) consortium state that "initial screening should include endoscopic ultrasonography (EUS) and/or magnetic resonance imaging (MRI)/magnetic resonance cholangiopancreatography (MRCP), not computed tomography (CT) or endoscopic retrograde cholangiopancreatography (ERCP)" [49,50].

In addition to screening, early detection of pancreatic cancer is important for a differential diagnosis and a timely management of this malignancy. The utility of serum CA19-9 in the diagnosis of pancreatic cancer has been extensively evaluated, as well as the diagnostic cutoff value of CA19-9. Results from a study performed in 1999, enrolling 20,035 asymptomatic subjects, 160 patients with pancreatic diseases and 322 with biliary tract diseases, showed a mean serum concentration of CA19-9 in asymptomatic individuals of 9.42 ± 9.95 U/ml. Levels above 37 U/mL were determined to be most accurate for discriminating pancreatic cancer from benign pancreatic diseases (sensitivity and specificity of 77 % and 87 %, respectively) [29]. The diagnostic utility of CA 19-9 has been investigated also in the already mentioned review by Goonnetilleke and Siriwardena [7], who analyzed pooled data from 2283 symptomatic subjects. The Authors reported a median sensitivity of serum CA 19-9 level for pancreatic cancer of 79 % and a median specificity of 82 % with a PPV and NPV of 72 % and 81 % respectively. Among patients with symptoms suspicious for pancreatic cancer, elevated CA 19-9 is a poor predictor of pancreatic cancer with a predictive value of 0.5–0.9 %. Based on this evidence of poor sensitivity for early lesions, the European Group on Tumor Marker (EGTM) guidelines affirms that CA 19-9 has limited value in the diagnosis of pancreatic cancer, especially for early forms of the disease. Similarly, the National Academy of Clinical Biochemistry (NACB; USA) does not recommend measurement of CA 19-9 in the diagnosis of pancreatic cancer, but states that the marker could be used in aiding diagnosis, in conjunction with results from accurate radiological procedures, such as computed tomography (CT) or endoscopic ultrasound (EUS) and can guide further invasive testing such as endoscopic retrograde cholangiopancreatography, laparoscopy or EUS fine-needle aspiration [1].

15.5.3 CA 19-9 Serum Levels as a Biomarker of Prognosis in Patients with Pancreatic Cancer

Measuring serum CA 19-9 levels provides significant prognostic information and allows patient stratification (survival groups) and determination of resectability of pancreatic cancer. For example, based on pre-operative CA 19-9 levels, Berger et al. stratified 129 surgically resected pancreatic cancer patients into four groups [(undetectable, normal (<37 U/ml), 38–200 U/ml, and >200 U/mL)], demonstrating an inverse correlation between CA 19-9 levels and median survival of patients [51]. Preoperative CA19-9 levels ($p = 0.030$) and lymph node ratio ($p = 0.042$) emerged as independent predictors of survival on multivariate analysis conducted by Smith et al. [52] in patients with resected pancreatic ductal adenocarcinoma. Data from study of Zhang et al. [53] showed that preoperative serum CA19-9 level is a useful marker for evaluating the resectability of pancreatic cancer, while the multivariate analysis of factors predicting survival, conducted by Waraya et al. [54] in 117 pancreatic cancer individuals undergoing surgical resection, demonstrated the prognostic value of preoperative Ca 19-9, in conjunction with dissected peripancreatic tissue margin, and confirmed that at higher preCA19-9 corresponds a worse prognosis.

Moreover, several Authors investigate which prognostic value, if the pre- or post-operative serum CA19-9 level, is more useful in predicting survival. Besides correlating preCA 19-9 levels with stage of disease, Ferrone and coworkers [55], showed that both a postoperative decrease in CA19-9 and a postoperative CA19-9 value of less than 200 U/mL are strong independent predictors of survival. In analyzing data of pre- and postoperative serum CA19-9 levels from 109 patients who underwent surgical resection for pancreatic cancer, Kondo et al. [56] considered significant the differences in overall survival between groups divided on the basis of four postoperative CA19-9 cutoff values (37, 100, 200, and 500 U/ml) but not significant those between groups divided on the basis of the same four preoperative CA19-9 cutoff values. They conclude that postoperative CA19-9 level is a better prognostic factor than preoperative CA19-9 level. All together, results from these studies suggest that: (i) preoperative CA 19-9 correlates with stage of disease; (ii) a median of pre operative CA 19-9 serum level <100 U/ml correlates with resectability (41–80 %) whereas levels >100 U/ml suggest advanced or metastatic pancreatic cancer (60–85 %) [30, 57]; (iii) postoperative normalization or a downward trend of the CA 19-9 serum level is associated with prolonged survival whereas elevated or failure of the CA 19-9 to decrease following pancreatic resection reflects residual disease or occult metastasis and portends a poor survival [58].

15.5.4 CA 19-9 Serum Levels as a Biomarker for Chemotherapy Response in Pancreatic Cancer Patients

Several studies have been performed investigating the utility of CA 19-9 for assessing the efficacy of chemotherapy for advanced pancreatic cancer. Willett et al. [59] measured serum CA 19-9 levels in 42 individuals before and following chemotherapy treatment with 5-flourouracil and irradiation, to define the potential role of this tumor marker in preoperative management of these patients. In comparing these CA 19-9 values with findings of restaging computed tomography (CT) scan and laparotomy, the Authors showed a correlation, statistically significant ($P=0.009$), between increased or decreased CA 19-9 levels and disease progression. Results suggest that monitoring of CA 19-9 appears useful for the identification of patients who manifest progressive tumor growth and metastasis in spite of this treatment. In analyzing data of CA 19-9 levels in 36 subjects receiving gemcitabine treatment, Halm et al. [60] demonstrated the utility of serial measurements of this marker, to evaluate the response to chemotherapy. Authors showed that patients with a decrease of CA 19-9 >20 % after 8 weeks of treatment ($n=25$) have a significantly better median survival compared to patients with a rise or a decrease < or = 20 % ($n=11$) $P<0.001$. Other more recent studies analyzing prospective trials showed similar results, suggesting that CA 19-9 is a prognostic and predictive biomarker in patients with advanced pancreatic cancer who receive gemcitabine-containing chemotherapy [61–63]. Moreover, on the basis of data, from 1997 to 2002, of 96 patients who underwent pancreatectomy without adjuvant chemotherapy as the control arm of a large randomized prospective adjuvant therapy trial, Hernandez et al. [64] concluded that CA 19-9 velocity predicts disease-free survival and overall survival after pancreatectomy of curative intent. According to previous results, Reni et al. [65], plotting the survival curves on a pre-defined decline in CA 19-9 serum levels of 247 advanced pancreatic cancer patients enrolled in five consecutive chemotherapy trials, illustrated that a higher percent decline in CA 19-9 serum levels following treatment corresponds to an improved overall survival. In spite of all these evidences, however, the NACB Panel recommends that serial CA 19-9 measurements during palliative chemotherapy should be used in conjunction with imaging tests to determine the efficacy of treatment. Serial CA19-9 monitoring is also recommended in the follow-up of patients after potentially curative surgery. Moreover, according to 2006 ASCO update of recommendations for the use of tumor markers in gastrointestinal cancer, CA 19-9 should not be used to define disease recurrence if not with the support of accurate evaluative imaging techniques.

15.6 Other Serum Markers for Pancreatic Cancer

Early detection of pancreatic cancer is an ever prominent problem, considering the high death rate for this disease. A wide range of potential new markers, including serum, pancreatic juice and tissue-based markers, have been proposed for early detection, as reported by the European Group on Tumor Markers (EGTM) [1]. Among these, duke pancreatic monoclonal antigentype 2 (DUPAN-2), macrophage inhibitory cytokine (MIC-1) and regenerating islet derived (REG-4), being unaffected by Lewis blood group status, may be more effective for detecting the presence of pancreatic cancer in sialyl Lewis negative population [66]. Additional tissue-based markers have been object of a series of studies, reporting initially promising results. For example, among possible oncogene/oncosuppressor mutations, which occur at various stages during proceeding of neoplastic disease, the most important are: K-ras, EGF e EFGR (precocious), of p16 and p53 (intermediate in the neoplastic evolution), and of SMAD and BRCA2 (more tardy). The KRAS is an oncogene that encodes a small GTPase transductor protein called p21, which participates in intracellular signal transduction and is involved in the regulation of cell division. Activating mutations in the KRAS gene impair the ability of the KRAS protein to switch between active and inactive states, inducing the active state. The resulting aberrant forms of p21 have a profound effect on the downstream effector pathways, resulting in much higher proliferation rates, enhanced cell survival and resistance to apoptosis that may evolve toward neoplastic process. K-ras mutations are frequently observed in human cancers [67] and are reported to be present in about 90 % of pancreatic ductal carcinomas, appearing in the relatively early stages of carcinogenesis [68]. The mutations found most frequently in the KRAS gene of cancer cells are located at positions 12 and 13 in exon 1, and less frequently in codons 61, 63, 117, 119, and 146 [69]. In particular, mutations in codons 12 or 13, which are present with high frequency in pancreatic cancer, are known to lead to conformational changes in the KRAS protein. The majority studies analyzing the potential biomarker role of KRAS mutations in pancreatic adenocarcinoma show those mutations as an adverse prognostic indicator, others, however, does not found significant relationship between the presence of mutant K-ras and poor outcome. The resulting data, obtained moreover by using methods with varying sensitivities and specificities to determine K-ras mutant, are still conflicting, as reported in a systematic review of the literature of Garcea et al. [68]. The available evidence do not sustain till now the use of K-ras for routinely determining prognosis in patients with pancreatic cancer. Of similar limitations suffer studies that related p53 mutation/overexpression to outcome in patients with pancreatic cancer [68]. As well known, p53 tumor suppressor gene encodes a transcription factor which is involved in regulating cell cycle, apoptosis, and has been defined "the guardian of genome" [70], because of its role in conserving stability by preventing genome mutation [71]. Mutations in the p53 gene are frequently found in human cancer, and are present in a percentage ranging from 50 % to 70 % of pancreatic cancers, appearing relatively late in the genesis of this malignancy. However, available conflicting data does not permit to establish a strict association between p53 status and patient outcome.

Also mucins are extensively studied in relationship with pancreatic cancer [72]. As well known, mucins are high molecular weight glycoproteins widely expressed by specialized epithelial cells of the gastrointestinal, respiratory, and urinogenital tracts. Under normal circumstances, mucins are known to play a protective role for epithelial tissues. However, in numerous pathologic situations, their aberrant expression is known to have multiple implications in development, progression, metastasis and a poor prognosis of cancer [73,74]. In particular, MUC1, MUC2, MUC4 and MUC5AC are key mucins in pathological diagnosis of pancreatic neoplasm. In 2007, Wang and coworkers, in immunohistochemically confirming the aberrant expression as well as changed in the level and distribution pattern of mucins (MUC1, MUC2 and MUC5AC) in pancreatic cancer, furthermore observed that the combined implementation of conventional imaging technique and molecular diagnostic approaches may provide improved sensitivity and specificity of diagnosis of pancreatic cancer and mucinous neoplasms. In particular, the Authors reported that the combination test of MUC1 + cytology and MUC5AC + cytology could improve sensitivity (respectively 85 % versus 65 %, 100 % versus 65 % of cytology alone) and accuracy (89 % versus 73 %, 91 % versus 72 % of cytology alone) for pancreatic cancer diagnosis. Also the combination test of MUC2+cytology and MUC5AC + cytology could achieve higher sensitivity (78 % versus 39 %, 100 % versus 39 % of cytology alone), specificity (97 % versus 60 %, 71 % versus 60 %) and accuracy for mucinous neoplasm diagnosis. Recently, Yokoyama et al. [75] showed that three mucin genes (MUC1, MUC2 and MUC4) expression in cancer cell line was regulated by DNA methylation and analyzed the DNA methylation status of mucin genes by a 'methylation-specific electrophoresis' method to high sensitivity and resolution. Results from pancreatic juice samples from 45 patients with various pancreatic lesions indicated that the DNA methylation status of MUC1, MUC2 and MUC4 in pancreatic juice with the mucin expression in tissue. Analyses of the DNA methylation status of MUC1, MUC2 and MUC4 of human pancreatic juice may provide useful information for differential diagnosis of human pancreatic neoplasms, with specificity and sensitivity of 87 % and 80 % for PDAC. In an attempt to define the cellular and molecular mechanisms through which MUC4 contributes to the metastasis of pancreatic cancer cells, Senapati et al. demonstrated that MUC4-NIDO domain interaction may play a role in promoting the breaching of basement membrane integrity and spreading of cancer cells [76].

More recently, the discovery of miRNA, small non-protein-coding RNA molecules that negatively regulate gene expression at the post-transcriptional level, seems to open new ways not only in oncology research but also in cancer therapeutics. A growing number of direct and indirect evidence demonstrates that miRNAs expression is profoundly altered in human cancer or strongly modulated during carcinogenesis. Moreover, the peculiar features of miRNAs, including their tissue- and disease-specific expression and their high stability in tissue and fluids, together with the possibility to detect them in very low amount of samples, may provide important advantages for supporting the possible use of miRNA as diagnostic and prognostic/predictive biomarkers and therapeutic targets. Following the first report in 2007 by Lee and coworkers [77], who identified a differential miRNAs expression profile in clinical specimens of pancreatic adenocarcinoma and pancreatic cancer cell lines, Wang et al. [78], 2 years later, detected miRNA in the blood of patients with PC. They showed that plasma profiling of four miRNAs (miR-21, miR-210, miR-196a and miR-155) can differentiate cancer patients from healthy controls, revealing a sensitivity of 64 % and a specificity of 89 % for pancreatic cancer. Afterwards, a series of researches have been performed for characterizing the miRNAs expression profile, highlighting a clear discrimination between pancreatic cancer, chronic pancreatic and normal pancreas. From all these translational studies, a panel of miRNAs whose expression results profoundly altered in PC is emerging [79]. Interestingly, a series of miRNA which are either upregulated (e.g. miR-146) or silenced (e.g. miR-205 and miR-7) was recently identified in advanced pancreatic cancer clinical samples as well as in pure populations of CSCs isolated from pancreatic cancer cell line resistant to gemcitabine [80]. In their recently published miRNA analysis from plasma of 140 pancreatic cancer patients, Liu et al. [81] support the diagnostic utility of the combination of plasma miRNAs (miR-155, 181a, 181b and 196a) with serum CA19-9 for early detection of pancreatic cancer. Using logistic modeling analysis, they proved that major effectiveness in combining miR-16, miR-196a and CA19-9 for discriminating PCa from non-PCa (normal+CP) (AUC-ROC, 0.979; sensitivity, 92.0 %; specificity, 95.6 %), and for discriminating PCa from CP (AUC-ROC, 0.956; sensitivity, 88.4 %; specificity, 96.3 %) compared with the miRNA panel (miR-16+miR-196a) or CA19-9 alone. Importantly, the combination was reported to be effective at identification of tumors in Stage 1 (85.2 %). Similarly, Wang et al. [82] identifying in peripheral blood mononuclear cells (PBMC) specific microRNAs whose levels might facilitate diagnosis of pancreatic cancer, evaluated their predictive value by logistic regression models, showing that a combination of PBMC miR-27a-3p and serum CA19-9 levels provided a higher diagnostic accuracy with a sensitivity of 85.3 % and specificity of 81.6 % (AUC=0.886; 95 % CI, 0.837–0.923 %). Last, to assess the diagnostic value of the serum miRNA profiling, Liu et al. [83] identified a panel of seven miRNA (miR-20a, miR-21, miR-24, miR-25, miR-99a, miR-185, and miR-191), which appear to have an high sensitivity and specificity for distinguishing various stages of PaC from cancer-free controls and to accurately discriminate PaC patients from chronic pancreatitis patients. The diagnostic accuracy rate of the 7-miRNA profile was 83.6 % in correctly classifying 55 cases with clinically suspected PaC.

All these evidences suggest that miRNAs profiling may be used as potential tool for the early stage PC diagnosis, monitoring cancer progression and efficacy of the treatment. Another interesting aspect that is attracting the attention of oncologic research is the therapeutic potential of miRNAs. Recent studies demonstrate that microRNAs may soon translate into clinical applications not only as screening tools but also as therapeutic targets for this cancer. In fact, the possibility to modulate the miRNAs expression, by activating tumor suppressive miRNAs and by inhibiting oncogenic miRNAs with small molecules or gene transfer, seems to open new ways for the development of cancer therapeutics. This potential therapeutic aspect is very intriguing. At present, however, this application remains still a challenge and requires further in depth studies.

15.7 Conclusions

A large number of putative biomarkers derived from serum, tissue, bile, pancreatic juice and saliva has been proposed and are currently undergoing evaluation for pancreatic cancer detection. At present, most of them lacks large scale validation and however none of them has showed to possess the sensitivity and specificity required to be employed individually in early detection of pancreatic cancer. Therefore, although with important limitations we well-know, ranging from false negative results in sialyl Lewis negative subjects to false positive results in the presence of obstructive jaundice, CA 19-9 continues being the only pancreatic cancer marker of actual clinical use. However, because of its low positive predictive value, serum CA 19-9 determination cannot be used as screening marker, while it can be used in aiding diagnosis, in conjunction with results from accurate radiological procedures, in symptomatic patients. Measuring preoperative serum CA19-9 level is useful for evaluating the resectability of pancreatic cancer and for predicting the disease course. The inverse correlation existing between CA 19-9 levels and median survival of patients renders serum CA 19-9 a good marker for estimating overall survival of the patient and for evaluating the possible presence of residual disease after pancreatic resection. Serial CA 19-9 monitoring can be useful in the follow-up of patients during chemotherapy for appraising the efficacy of treatment.

Poor prognosis of pancreatic cancer patients makes the research of new sensitive and specific markers necessary to identify this malignancy at early stages of development. The possibility of a timely therapeutic intervention should assure a more effective treatment and could translate in a real improvement in the patients' survival but also in their of quality of life during the course of the illness.

References

1. Duffy MG, Sturgeon C, Lamerz R et al (2010) Tumor markers in pancreatic cancer: a European Group on Tumor Markers (EGTM) status report. Ann Oncol 21:441–447
2. Koprowski H, Steplewski Z, Mitchell K et al (1979) Colorectal carcinoma antigens detected by hybridoma antibodies. Somatic Cell Genet 5:957–971
3. Koprowski H, Herlyn M, Steplewski Z, Sears HF (1981) Specific antigen in serum of patients with colon carcinoma. Science 212:53–55

4. Magnani JL, Brockhaus M, Smith DF et al (1981) A monosialoganglioside is a monoclonal antibody-defined antigen of colon carcinoma. Science 212:55–56
5. Magnani JL, Steplewski Z, Koprowski H, Ginsburg V (1983) Identification of the gastrointestinal and pancreatic cancer-associated antigen detected by monoclonal antibody 19-9 in the sera of patients as a mucin. Cancer Res 43:5489–5492
6. Uhlenbruck G, van Meensel-Maene U, Hanisch FG, Dienst C (1984) Unexpected occurrence of the Ca 19-9 tumor marker in normal human seminal plasma. Hoppe Seylers Z Physiol Chem 365:613–617
7. Goonetilleke KS, Siriwardena AK (2007) Systematic review of carbohydrate antigen (CA 19–9) as a biochemical marker in the diagnosis of pancreatic cancer. Eur J Surg Oncol 33:266–270
8. Daniels G (1995) Human blood groups. Blackwell Science Ltd., Oxford
9. Kannagi R (2002) Regulatory roles of carbohydrate ligands for selectins in the homing of lymphocytes. Curr Opin Struct Biol 12:599–608
10. Liu FT, Rabinovich GA (2010) Galectins: regulators of acute and chronic inflammation. Ann N Y Acad Sci 1183:158–182
11. Crocker PR, Paulson JC, Varki A (2007) Siglecs and their roles in the immune system. Nat Rev Immunol 7:255–266
12. Hakomori S (1983) Tumor-associated glycolipid antigens defined by monoclonal antibodies. Bull Cancer 70:118–126
13. Hakomori S (1986) Tumor-associated glycolipid antigens, their metabolism and organization. Chem Phys Lipids 42:209–233
14. Hakomori S, Kannagi R (1983) Glycosphyngolipids as tumor-associated and differentiation markers. J Natl Cancer Inst (Bethesda) 71:231–251
15. Itai S, Nishikata J, Yoneda T et al (1991) Tissue distribution of sialyl 2–3 and 2–6 Lewis a antigens and the significance of serum 2-3/2-6 sialyl Lewis a antigen ratio for the differential diagnosis of malignant and benign disorders of the digestive tract. Cancer (Phila) 67:1576–1587
16. Miyazaki K, Ohmori K, Izawa M et al (2004) Loss of disialyl Lewis a, the ligand for lymphocyte inhibitory receptor siglec-7, associated with increased sialyl Lewis a expression on human colon cancers. Cancer Res 64:4498–4505
17. Izawa M, Kumamoto K, Mitsuoka C et al (2000) Expression of sialyl 6-sulfo Lewis x is inversely correlated with conventional sialyl Lewis x expression in human colorectal cancer. Cancer Res 60:1410–1416
18. Miyazaki K, Sakuma K, Kawamura YI et al (2012) Colonic epithelial cells express specific ligands for mucosal macrophage immunosuppressive receptors siglec-7 and -9. J Immunol 188:4690–4700
19. Galli C, Basso D, Plebani M (2013) CA 19-9: handle with care. Clin Chem Lab Med 51:1369–1383
20. Basso D, Fabris C, Del Favero G et al (1990) How does liver dysfunction influence serum CA 19-9 in pancreatic cancer? Ital J Gastroenterol 22:1–6
21. Fabris C, Basso D, Piccoli A et al (1991) Role of local and systemic factors in increasing serum glycoprotein markers of pancreatic cancer. J Med 22:145–156
22. Basso D, Meggiato T, Fabris C et al (1992) Alterations in bilirubin metabolism during extra- and intrahepatic cholestasis. Clin Investig 70:49–54
23. Rothenberg ML, Abbruzzese JL, Moore M et al (1996) A rationale for expanding the endpoints for clinical trials in advanced pancreatic carcinoma. Cancer 78:627–632
24. Albert MB, Steinberg WM, Henry JP (1988) Elevated serum levels of tumor marker CA 19-9 in acute cholangitis. Dig Dis Sci 33:1223–1225
25. Duffy MJ (2007) Role of tumor markers in patients with solid cancers: a critical review. Eur J Intern Med 18:175–184
26. Steinberg W (1990) The clinical utility of the CA 19-9 tumor associate antigen. Am J Gastroenterol 85:350–355
27. Kim JE, Lee KT, Lee JK et al (2004) Clinical usefulness of carbohydrate antigen 19-9 as a screening test for pancreatic cancer in an asymptomatic population. J Gastroenterol Hepatol 19:182–186
28. Chang CY, Huang SP, Chiu HM et al (2006) Low efficacy of serum levels of CA 19-9 in prediction of malignant diseases in asymptomatic population in Taiwan. Hepatogastroenterology 53:1–4
29. Kim HR, Lee CH, Kim YW et al (2009) Increased CA 19-9 level in patients without malignant disease. Clin Chem Lab Med 47:750–754
30. Kim YC, Kim HJ, Park JH et al (2009) Can preoperative CA19-9 and CEA levels predict the resectability of patients with pancreatic adenocarcinoma? J Gastroenterol Hepatol 24:1869–1875
31. Ventrucci M, Pozzato P, Cipolla A, Uomo G (2009) Persistent elevation of serum CA 19-9 with no evidence of malignant disease. Dig Liver Dis 41:357–363
32. Sakahara H, Endo K, Nakajima K et al (1986) Serum CA 19-9 concentrations and computed tomography findings in patients with pancreatic carcinoma. Cancer 57:1324–1326
33. Frebourg T, Bercoff E, Manchon N et al (1988) The evaluation of CA 19-9 antigen level in the early detection of pancreatic cancer. A prospective study of 866 patients. Cancer 62:2287–2290
34. Fabris C, Del Favero G, Basso D et al (1988) Serum markers and clinical data in diagnosing pancreatic cancer: a contrastive approach. Am J Gastroenterol 83:549–553
35. National Health Insurance Corporation (2000) National health insurance statistical yearbook 1999, 21:350–563
36. La'ulu SL, Roberts WL (2007) Performance characteristics of five automated CA 19-9 assays. Am J Clin Pathol 127:436–440
37. Hotakainen K, Tanner P, Alfthan H et al (2009) Comparison of three immunoassays for CA 19–9. Clin Chim Acta 400:123–127

38. Deinzer M, Faissner R, Metzger T et al (2010) Comparison of two different methods for CA19-9 antigen determination. Clin Lab 56:319–325
39. Passerini R, Cassatella MC, Boveri S et al (2012) The pitfalls of CA 19–9: routine testing and comparison of two automated immunoassays in a reference oncology center. Am J Clin Pathol 138:281–287
40. Sturgeon C, Dati F, Duffy MJ et al (1999) Quality requirements and control: EGTM recommendations. Anticancer Res 19:2785–2820
41. Biguet B, Habersetzer F, Beaudonnet A et al (1995) Discordant CA 19.9 serum results by microparticle enzyme immunoassay and immunoradiometric assay. Clin Chem 41:1057–1058
42. Berth M, Bosmans E, Everaert J et al (2006) Rheumatoid factor interference in the determination of carbohydrate antigen 19-9 (CA 19-9). Clin Chem Lab Med 44:1137–1139
43. Liang Y, Yang Z, Ye W et al (2009) Falsely elevated carbohydrate antigen 19-9 level due to heterophilic antibody interference but not rheumatoid factor: a case report. Clin Chem Lab Med 47:116–117
44. Troup S (2012) Analyte monographs alongside the National Laboratory Medicine Catalogue. The Association for Clinical Biochemistry and Laboratory Medicine, London
45. Gillen S, Schuster T, Meyer zum Büschenfelde C et al (2010) Preoperative/neoadjuvant therapy in pancreatic cancer: a systematic review and meta-analysis of response and resection percentages. PLoS Med 7, e1000267
46. Brentnall TA, Bronner MP, Byrd DR et al (1999) Early diagnosis and treatment of pancreatic dysplasia in patients with a family history of pancreatic cancer. Ann Intern Med 131:247–255
47. Canto MIGM, Yeo CJ, Griffin C, Axilbund JE et al (2003) Screening for pancreatic neoplasia in high risk individuals. Clin Gastroenterol Hepatol 2:606–621
48. Canto MI, Hruban RH, Fishman EK et al (2012) Frequent detection of pancreatic lesions in asymptomatic high-risk individuals. Gastroenterology 142:796
49. Canto MI, Harinck F, Hruban RH et al (2013) International Cancer of the Pancreas Screening (CAPS) Consortium summit on the management of patients with increased risk for familiar pancreatic cancer. Gut 62:339
50. Konstantinou F, Syrigos KN, Saif MW (2013) Pancreatic cancer: what about screening and detection? Highlights from the "2013 ASCO Annual Meeting", Chicago, 30 May–4 June 2013
51. Berger AC, Meszoely IM, Ross EA et al (2004) Undetectable preoperative levels of serum CA 19-9 correlate with improved survival for patients with resectable pancreatic adenocarcinoma. Ann Surg Oncol 11:644–649
52. Smith RA, Bosonnet L, Ghaneh P et al (2008) Preoperative CA19-9 levels and lymph node ratio are independent predictors of survival in patients with resected pancreatic ductal adenocarcinoma. Dig Surg 25:226–232
53. Zhang S, Wang YM, Sun CD et al (2008) Clinical value of serum CA19-9 levels in evaluating resectability of pancreatic carcinoma. World J Gastroenterol 14:3750–3753
54. Waraya M, Yamashita K, Katagiri H et al (2009) Preoperative serum CA19-9 and dissected peripancreatic tissue margin as determiners of long-term survival in pancreatic cancer. Ann Surg Oncol 16:1231–1240
55. Ferrone CR, Finkelstein DM, Thayer SP et al (2006) Perioperative CA19-9 levels can predict stage and survival in patients with resectable pancreatic adenocarcinoma. J Clin Oncol 24:2897–2902
56. Kondo N, Murakami Y, Uemura K et al (2010) Prognostic impact of perioperative serum CA 19-9 levels in patients with resectable pancreatic cancer. Ann Surg Oncol 17:2321–2329
57. Schlieman MG, Ho HS, Bold RJ et al (2003) Utility of tumor markers in determining resectability of pancreatic cancer. Arch Surg 138:951–955
58. Montgomery RC, Hoffman JP, Riley LB et al (1997) Prediction of recurrence and survival by post resection CA 19-9 values in patients with adenocarcinoma of the pancreas. Ann Surg Oncol 4:551–556
59. Willett CG, Daly WJ, Warshaw AL (1996) CA 19-9 is an index of response to neoadjunctive chemoradiation therapy in pancreatic cancer. Am J Surg 172:350–352
60. Halm U, Schumann T, Schiefke I et al (2000) Decrease of CA 19-9 during chemotherapy with gemcitabine predicts survival time in patients with advanced pancreatic cancer. Br J Cancer 82:1013–1016
61. Maisey NR, Norman AR, Hill A et al (2005) CA19-9 as a prognostic factor in inoperable pancreatic cancer: the implication for clinical trials. Br J Cancer 93:740–743
62. Takahashi H, Ohigashi H, Ishikawa O et al (2010) Serum CA19-9 alterations during preoperative gemcitabine-based chemoradiation therapy for resectable invasive ductal carcinoma of the pancreas as an indicator for therapeutic selection and survival. Ann Surg 251:461–469
63. Bauer TM, El-Rayes BF, Li X et al (2013) Carbohydrate antigen 19-9 is a prognostic and predictive biomarker in patients with advanced pancreatic cancer who receive gemcitabine-containing chemotherapy: a pooled analysis of 6 prospective trials. Cancer 119:285–292
64. Hernandez JM, Cowgill SM, Al-Saadi S et al (2009) CA 19-9 velocity predicts disease-free survival and overall survival after pancreatectomy of curative intent. J Gastrointest Surg 13:349–353
65. Reni M, Cereda S, Balzano G et al (2009) Carbohydrate antigen 19-9 change during chemotherapy for advanced pancreatic adenocarcinoma. Cancer 115:2630–2639
66. Ballehaninna UK, Chamberlain RS (2012) The clinical utility of serum CA 19-9 in the diagnosis, prognosis and management of pancreatic adenocarcinoma: an evidence based appraisal. J Gastrointest Oncol 3:105–119

67. Jancík S, Drábek J, Radzioch D, Hajdúch M (2010) Clinical relevance of KRAS in human cancers. J Biomed Biotechnol 2010:150960
68. Garcea G, Neal CP, Pattenden CJ et al (2005) Molecular prognostic markers in pancreatic cancer: a systematic review. Eur J Cancer 41:2213–2236
69. Er TK, Chen CC, Bujanda L, Herreros-Villanueva M (2014) Clinical relevance of KRAS mutations in codon 13: where are we? Cancer Lett 343:1–5
70. Lane DP (1992) Cancer. p53, guardian of the genome. Nature 358:15–16
71. Talar-Wojnarowska R, Malecka-Panas E (2006) Molecular pathogenesis of pancreatic adenocarcinoma: potential clinical implications. Med Sci Monit 12:RA186–RA193
72. Wang Y, Gao J, Li Z et al (2007) Diagnostic value of mucins (MUC1, MUC2 and MUC5AC) expression profile in endoscopic ultrasound-guided fine-needle aspiration specimens of the pancreas. Int J Cancer 121:2716–2722
73. Ringel J, Lohr M (2003) The MUC gene family: their role in diagnosis and early detection of pancreatic cancer. Mol Cancer 2:9
74. Moniaux N, Andrianifahanana M, Brand RE, Batra SK (2004) Multiple roles of mucins in pancreatic cancer, a lethal and challenging malignancy. Br J Cancer 91:1633–1638
75. Yokoyama S, Kitamoto S, Higashi M et al (2014) Diagnosis of pancreatic neoplasms using a novel method of DNA methylation analysis of mucin expression in pancreatic juice. PLoS One 9, e93760
76. Senapati S, Gnanapragassam VS, Moniaux N (2012) Role of MUC4-NIDO domain in the MUC4-mediated metastasis of pancreatic cancer cells. Oncogene 31:3346–3356
77. Lee EJ, Gusev Y, Jiang J et al (2007) Expression profiling identifies microRNA signature in pancreatic cancer. Int J Cancer 120:1046–1054
78. Wang J, Chen J, Chang P et al (2009) MicroRNAs in plasma of pancreatic ductal adenocarcinoma patients as novel blood-based biomarkers of disease. Cancer Prev Res (Phila) 2:807–813
79. Humeau M, Torrisani J, Cordelier P (2013) miRNA in clinical practice: pancreatic cancer. Clin Biochem 46:933–936
80. Singh S, Chitkara D, Kumar V, Behrman SW, Mahato RI (2013) miRNA profiling in pancreatic cancer and restoration of chemosensitivity. Cancer Lett 334:211–220
81. Liu J, Gao J, Du Y et al (2012) Combination of plasma microRNAs with serum CA19-9 for early detection of pancreatic cancer. Int J Cancer 131:683–691
82. Wang WS, Liu LX, Li GP et al (2013) Combined serum CA19-9 and miR-27a-3p in peripheral blood mononuclear cells to diagnose pancreatic cancer. Cancer Prev Res (Phila) 6:331–338
83. Liu R, Chen X, Du Y et al (2012) Serum microRNA expression profile as a biomarker in the diagnosis and prognosis of pancreatic cancer. Clin Chem 58:610–618

Part VIII

Tumor Markers – A Critical Revision: Genetic Markers

Non Coding RNA Molecules as Potential Biomarkers in Breast Cancer

16

Kim De Leeneer and Kathleen Claes

Abstract

The pursuit of minimally invasive biomarkers is a challenging but exciting area of research. Clearly, such markers would need to be sensitive and specific enough to aid in the detection of breast cancer at an early stage, would monitor progression of the disease, and could predict the individual patient's response to treatment. Unfortunately, to date, markers with such characteristics have not made it to the clinic for breast cancer. Past years, many studies indicated that the non-coding part of our genome (the so called 'junk' DNA), may be an ideal source for these biomarkers. In this chapter, the potential use of microRNAs and long non-coding RNAs as biomarkers will be discussed.

Keywords

BC200 • Circulating miRNAs • Her2neu/ERBB2 • let-7 miRNA • Long non coding RNA • microRNA • miR-10b • miR-145 • miR-16 • miR-195 • miR-200 family • miR-21 • miR-21 • miR-29 • miR-31 • miR-335 • miR-451 • miR-9 • MiRNAS and breast cancer

16.1 Introduction

Despite worldwide research on detection and therapy, breast cancer remains the leading cause of cancer death in women. Early detection of breast cancer is essential for survival and efficient treatment, yet current methods of detection, such as mammography, lack the sensitivity to sufficiently detect occult cancer and differentiate indolent from aggressive breast cancer. This deficiency may result in mortality due to a missed diagnosis or require additional invasive testing, which can result in unnecessary distress or overtreatment. Biomarkers that could function as an adjunct to mammography to detect breast cancer at an early stage, to identify aggressive disease or predict metastasis, could have a major impact on the management and outcome of this disease.

Currently, standard clinical parameters such as tumor size, grade, lymph node involvement and tumor-node-metastasis staging correlate with

K. De Leeneer (✉) • K. Claes
Center for Medical Genetics Ghent, Ghent University, Ghent, Belgium
e-mail: Kim.deleeneer@ugent.be

R. Scatena (ed.), *Advances in Cancer Biomarkers*, Advances in Experimental Medicine and Biology 867, DOI 10.1007/978-94-017-7215-0_16

outcome and serve to stratify patients with respect to (neo)adjuvant chemotherapy and/or radiotherapy. Furthermore, molecular breast cancer markers of which the best known are estrogen receptor overexpression or HER2 amplification are used to predict the response to hormone therapy. However, stage-matched tumors grouped by histological or molecular subtypes can respond differently to the same treatment, so there is an additional need for tumor classifying molecular biomarkers. Emerging players in genetics are classes of non coding RNA molecules (like miRNAs and lncRNAs), due to their key roles in almost every developmental and cellular process, there for the possibility they could function as biomarkers in (breast) cancer is not unthinkable.

16.2 MicroRNAs

The first microRNAs (miRNAs) were characterized in the early 1990s [1]. However, miRNAs were not recognized as a distinct class of biological regulators with conserved functions until the early 2000s. MicroRNAs are small (ca. 22 nucleotides) non-coding RNA molecules found in plants and animals, which function in transcriptional and post-transcriptional regulation of gene expression [2]. Encoded by eukaryotic nuclear DNA, a miRNA will translationally repress or degrade his target through base-pairing with complementary sequences within mRNA molecules [3, 4]. The human genome may encode over 1000 miRNAs, which may target about 60 % of mammalian genes and are present in many human cell types [5–8].

Most microRNA genes are found in intergenic regions or in anti-sense orientation to certain genes and hence contain their own miRNA gene promoter and regulatory units [9–12]. However, probably 40 % is situated in introns of protein and non-protein coding genes or even rarely in exons. These are usually, though not exclusively, found in a sense orientation and thus show a concurrent transcription and regulation expression profile originating from a common promoter with their host genes [13, 14].

Mature miRNAs are produced through a multistage process that starts in the nucleus, where primary (pri-)miRNAs (several hundred to a thousand nucleotides in length) are transcribed by RNA polymerase II [12, 15, 16]. Pri-miRNAs are then processed to shorter (70–85 nucleotide) precursor (pre-)miRNAs mediated by Drosha, an RNase III enzyme, and its cofactor DGCR8 [17, 18]. Subsequently, pre-miRNAs are exported to the cytoplasm by exportin 5 [18, 19] and then cleaved by Dicer, another RNase III enzyme, to produce a ~22 nucleotide double-stranded miRNA duplex [20–22]. The strand containing less stable hydrogen-bonding at its 5′ end is a mature miRNA and is integrated into the RNA-induced silencing complex, while the other strand is degraded [23, 24]. The microRNA/RISC complex attaches to the messenger RNA (mRNA) in one of two ways: when the sequences are perfectly complementary, the microRNA/ RISC complex binds tightly to the mRNA and, with the help of the enzyme Ago2, the mRNA is degraded [23, 25]. More commonly, when the sequences are imperfectly complementary, the microRNA/ RISC complex binds and inhibits translation of the mRNA without degradation. The final outcome of either of these pathways is a decrease in the protein level of the target gene.

miRNAs are thought to have a key role in gene regulation although mostly they exhibit only partial complementarity to their mRNA targets [26, 27]. A 'seed region' of about 6–8 nucleotides long at the 5′ end of a miRNA is an important determinant of target specificity [8, 28]. It has been shown that gene regulation by miRNAs is a complex network, a given miRNA may have multiple different mRNA targets and a given target might similarly be targeted by multiple miRNAs [29, 30].

16.2.1 MiRNAS and Breast Cancer

Three important observations in the early history of miRNAs suggested a potential role in human cancer:

1. The miRNAs discovered in *C. elegans* and *Drosophila* were shown to be involved in cell proliferation and apoptosis, hence their deregulation may therefore contribute to proliferative diseases such as cancer [1, 31].

2. When human miRNAs were discovered, it was noticed that many miRNA genes were located at loci in the genome that are frequently amplified or deleted in human cancer [32]. A specific example of this is the polycistron cluster miR-17–92 at the *c13orf25* locus on chromosome 13q31. This locus is known to undergo loss of heterozygosity in a number of different cancer types, including breast cancer [33]. Similarly, miR-125b, which is underexpressed in breast cancer, is located at chromosome 11q23-24, one of the regions most frequently deleted in breast, ovarian, and lung tumors [33].
3. Malignant tumors and tumor cell lines were found to have widespread deregulated miRNA expression compared to normal tissues [34–36]. The question remains whether the altered miRNA expression observed in cancer is a cause or consequence of malignant transformation.

In 2002, Calin et al. [37] reported the first direct evidence of miRNAs playing a role in human cancer; they found that miR-15 and miR-16 contribute to chronic lymphocytic leukemia. They discovered that this specific miRNA cluster was deleted in a significant portion of chronic lymphocytic leukemia cases. It was found that normally these miRNAs had a direct repressive effect on Bcl-2, a well-characterized anti-apoptotic protein. In these CLL cases with low miR-15a/16-1 expression, it was found that Bcl-2 levels were increased, leading to an increased ability to avoid apoptosis, cell-death and tumor suppressor mechanism.

Subsequently, more examples of miRNAs involved in human cancer were discovered. Iorio and colleagues [38] first demonstrated miRNA deregulation in human breast cancer by miRNA microarray analysis; they identified a set of 15 miRNAs that was able to correctly predict the nature of the sample analyzed (i.e., tumor or normal breast tissue) with 100 % accuracy. These results leave few doubts that aberrant expression of miRNA is indeed involved in human breast cancer. They found that miR-10b, miR-125b, and miR-145 were down regulated, while miR-21 and miR-155 were up regulated, suggesting that these miRNAs may have potential tumor suppressor genes or oncogenes as targets. In addition, miRNA expression was correlated with biopathologic features such as estrogen receptor (ER), progesterone receptor status and tumor stage [38]. Measurement of miRNA levels demonstrates a global decrease in miRNA expression in breast tumours compared to adjacent normal tissue and a gradual decline with increased tumour grade [39].

The differential expression of miRNAs in breast tumor compared with normal breast tissue, and the indication of associations between miRNAs and tumor subtypes, suggest a potential role for such molecules in diagnostic biomarker panels.

16.2.2 miRNAs and Breast Tumor Tissue Profiling

To date, commonly three markers are established in the routine evaluation of breast tumors: estrogen and progesterone receptors (ER/PR: for predicting response to endocrine therapies) and HER2/neu (for predicting response to Trastuzumab) [40]. The most commonly employed technique to evaluate the hormone receptor status of breast tumors is immunohistochemistry, which relies on recognition of the receptor protein by specific antibodies. Although technically easy to perform and cost effective, this method is subjective and time consuming. If miRNAs prove useful for clinical diagnosis, their key advantage might be their high stability. In contrast to most messenger RNAs, they are long-lived in vivo and very stable in vitro, which might allow analysis of paraffin-embedded samples for routine diagnostic applications [24, 41].

miRNA profiling can be used to cluster cancer types with the cell of origin [42], so miRNA profiling may provide useful information to classify and diagnose metastases of unknown origin. This type of classification represents an important application in the diagnosis of patients with metastases (late-stage disease) without an established primary tumor (i.e., a site where a therapeutically curative or palliative intervention can be performed).

miRNA expression profiles have been used to differentiate tumor tissue from surrounding normal tissue for tumor classification and for prognostication. The capacity of miRNA expression profiles to classify breast tumors according to clinicopathologic variables currently used to predict disease progression highlights the potential of miRNA signatures as novel prognostic indicators which may contribute to the improved selection of patients for adjuvant therapy.

There are large-scale molecular differences between estrogen receptor (ER) α-positive and ERα-negative breast cancers [43, 44]. Endocrine therapy has become the most important treatment option for women with ERα-positive breast cancer, and approximately 70 % of primary breast cancers express ERα. ERα is essential for estrogen-dependent growth, and its level of expression is a crucial determinant of response to endocrine therapy and prognosis in ERα-positive breast cancer [45–47]. Of all histopathological clinical parameters, ER status has the largest effect on the miRNA expression profiles (Dvinge et al. 2013). Multiple studies now have shown that **ERα-expression** is regulated by miRNAs. For example, miRNAs, miR-18a, miR-18b, miR-22, miR-193b, miR-302c, and miR-221/222, as well as miR-206, directly target ERα in 3'UTR reporter assays. Adams et al. [48] investigated the relationship between miR-206, and the expression of ERα. The authors identified and verified two specific miR-206 binding sites in the ERα 3′-UTR. Transfection of MCF-7 breast cancer cells with synthetic pre–miR-206 induced a dose-dependent repression of ERα mRNA levels. Conversely, MCF-7 cell transfection with antagomiR-206 resulted in increased ERα mRNA, indicating that miR-206 regulates endogenous ERα mRNA levels. Furthermore, treatment with ERα-selective agonists decreased miR-206 levels within MCF-7 cells. Notably, this study detected at least 65 putative miRNA target sites in the 3′-UTR of the ERα transcript, confirming that multiple miRNAs may play a role in regulation of ERα expression. The existence of a feedback loop between miR-206 and estradiol has considerable implications for our understanding of the endocrine influence on breast cancer, and the mechanisms involved in hormonal therapy resistance. Another interesting observation is that the expression of various *let-7* miRNA isoforms is associated with features like progesterone receptor status, lymph node metastasis, or high proliferation index in breast tumor samples. The human **let-7 miRNA** family consists of 13 members located in 8 genomic locations frequently deleted in human cancers [49]. Nine distinct mature let-7 miRNAs with identical seed sequences are produced from 12 precursor sequences [50]. A reduced expression of let-7a in breast cancer was associated with larger tumor size and higher proliferative status, indicative that reduced let-7a expression may contribute to tumor growth.

mRNA profiles have identified distinct molecular subclasses of breast cancer, predictive of prognosis, based on their ER and **Her2neu/ ERBB2 classification** (luminal A, luminal B, basal-like, Her2-overexpressing, normal-like) [44]. A comprehensive study of the breast cancer subclasses through miRNA expression profiling could probably further characterize the molecular basis underlying these subtypes, perhaps define more precise subsets of breast cancer. Blenkiron et al. [51] performed an integrated analysis of miRNA expression, mRNA expression and genomic changes in breast cancer and found that many miRNAs were differentially expressed between the different molecular subclasses of breast tumors. They identified a miRNA signature that differentiated basal from luminal subtypes and found nine miRNAs that were differentially expressed between luminal A and luminal B tumors (miR-100, miR-99a, miR-130a, miR-126, miR-136, miR-146b, miR-15b, miR-107 and miR-103). Similar to mRNA profiling, Mattie et al. [52] could show clustering of breast cancer tumors according to Her2/neu/ ErBB2 status or ER/progesterone receptor status by miRNA profiling, Her-2neu/ERBB2–overexpressing breast tumors exhibit aggressive growth and unpredictable response to therapy; enhanced understanding of the regulation of ERBB2 expression has the potential to greatly improve the management of these aggressive tumors and miRNA profiles may have superior accuracy to mRNA profiling in this regard [35].

Dvinge et al. found that the mRNA-miRNA landscape is dominated by positive associations, suggesting that downregulation of target mRNA levels by miRNAs across the global breast tumour cohort is minor. They postulated that rather than acting as on-off switches of particular mRNAs, most miRNAs exert their effect by modulating the relationship between effector and target mRNAs, conceptually acting as co-repressors or.

16.2.3 Circulating miRNAs

A number of circulating tumor markers (for example: carcinoembryonic antigen and carbohydrate antigen 15–3) can be used in the management of breast cancer, but the sensitivity of these markers is low [53–55]. Therefore, they are not well suited to monitor disease progression or recurrence. Current challenges in the management of breast cancer include an ongoing search for sensitive and specific biomarkers that can be used to detect early neoplastic changes to facilitate the detection of breast cancer at an early stage. Furthermore, biomarkers are needed to monitor the progress of patients with breast cancer and their response to treatments. Existing diagnostic tools and biomarkers for breast cancer have many deficiencies. Mammography is currently the golden standard as diagnostic tool however it is not without limitations, including its use of ionizing radiation and a false positive rate of 8–10 % [56].

MiRNA presence in serum was described in patients with diffuse large B-cell lymphoma a few years ago [57]. Subsequently, a number of studies have reported similar findings on the presence of circulating miRNAs and have illustrated the potential of these miRNAs as novel biomarkers for diseases [58, 59]. Circulating miRNAs have many of the essential characteristics of good biomarkers. They are stable in the circulation and resistant to storage handling. Serum miRNAs are resistant to RNase digestion and other harsh conditions such as extreme pH, boiling, extended storage, and multiple freeze-thaw cycles. Further, most miRNAs sequences are conserved across species and third in some cases, changes in miRNA levels in circulation have been associated with different diseases as well as certain biological or pathological stages [60–63].

Although the exact mechanisms on how the small RNAs enter the plasma/serum and whether or not they are biologically functional need further investigations, it is possible that circulating miRNAs, compared to 'tissue' miRNAs are a unique diagnostic system. There is little doubt that plasma/serum miRNAs are cancer related, but the releasing mechanisms may be complicated. While the majority of miRNAs are found intracellularly, a significant number of miRNAs have been observed outside of cells, including various body fluids [64–68]. Given the instability of most RNA molecules in the extracellular environment, the presence and apparent stability of miRNAs here is surprising. Serum and other body fluids are known to contain ribonuclease, which suggests that secreted miRNAs are likely packaged in some manner to protect them against RNase digestion [69]. Tumor-derived microvesicles/exosomes are probably involved in the way miRNAs enter the circulation, rather than a simply leaking from cancer cells. One may hypothesize that at least some of the exported miRNAs are used for cell-to-cell communication, although further investigations are needed to determine how miRNAs are specifically targeted for secretion, recognized for uptake, and what information can be transmitted via this process [61].

Before this relatively new source of biomarkers can make it to the clinic, certain points remain to be explored. An important issue is the suitability of different sample types for miRNA detection. While Mitchell et al. [70] found no significant differences when comparing serum and plasma levels of miRNAs this result was limited to only four miRNAs and might not reflect the general image [71]. Studies have been performed in non-enriched or enriched whole blood, serum and plasma, without clear data being available on the distribution of miRNAs in these different blood compartments. It is acceptable that only a selection of miRNAs is, actively or passively, shed from circulating tumor cells.

A variety of independent studies have successfully proved the use of circulating miRNAs as diagnostic tools. Wu and colleagues [72] found that **miR-21** and **miR-29** were significantly up regulated in the serum of breast cancer patients and may be useful biomarkers for breast cancer detection [72, 73]. Heneghan et al. [74] surveyed a panel of 7 candidate miRNAs in whole blood RNAs from 148 breast cancer patients and 44 age-matched and disease free controls. They found that the expression of **miR-195** was significantly elevated in breast cancer patients. Additionally, they observed a significant reduction in miR-195 in post-operative whole blood compared to the pre-operative samples of the same patients. However, Zhao et al. [75] could not confirm differential expression of miR-195 between cases and controls. The discrepancy between two studies might be due to different study materials. The first study used whole blood for detection of miRNAs, while the second one used plasma. Whole blood contains different types of cells, so the detected miRNAs may be circulating miRNAs as well as cellular miRNAs from additional cell types. Another explanation is that the discrepancy may reflect the heterogeneity of breast cancer. Different molecular pathways are involved in different subtypes of breast cancer, with different molecular characteristics between luminal A, luminal B, and basal like subtypes. In the Heneghan study, 59 % of breast cancers were stage I and II, 71 % were invasive ductal cancer, and 82 % were ER positive versus all stage I and II invasive ductal cancers, and only 55 % ER positive in the second study.

Ng et al. [76] identified significant increase of **miR-16, miR-21**, and **miR-451** and significant decrease of **miR-145** in the plasma of breast cancer patients. Intriguingly, the combination of plasma miR-145 and miR-451 levels provided the best markers for breast cancer prediction. The optimal sensitivity was 90 % and optimal specificity was 92 % in discriminating breast cancer from control subjects including all other types of cancers recruited in their study. The odds ratio for the cases with combined miR-145 and miR-451 level being associated with breast cancer was 44.2. In the blind validation, the positive predictive value was 88 % and the negative predictive value was 92 %.

Another drawback on the breakthrough of circulating miRNAs as biomarkers is the scarcity of data on the occurrence and expression levels of circulating miRNAs in healthy individuals. Expansion of this data set can be done either by testing selected panels of miRNAs in a large cohort of gender- and otherwise matched healthy controls in parallel with cancer patients and will help in the quest to determine new circulating biomarkers.

16.2.4 miRNA and Metastasis

A major complication of breast cancer is its metastatic potential. Metastasis is a process characterized by local invasion, intravasion, transport of tumor cells to the parenchyma of other organs, extravasation and establishment of secondary lesions [77]. There is evidence that metastasis can originate from genetic and epigenetic alterations in the molecular profile of a subpopulation of cells within the primary tumor, whose behavior is modulated towards a more aggressive phenotype [78]. Mutations occur primarily in the DNA sequence whereas epigenetic changes are related to the structure of the chromatin and might involve DNA methylation, histone modifications and non-coding RNAs [79]. Hence many studies have focused on identifying the critical regulatory molecules involved in the malign transformation of cells, and both proteins and miRNAs are believed to play a key role [80, 81].

miRNAs can function as suppressors or promoters of metastasis according to their mRNA targets [81]. In the next paragraphs we provide a brief overview of a handful of well-known examples of miRNAs believed to suppress or promote metastasis. Many more miRNAs are hypothesized to be involved in the metastatic process.

One of the first miRNAs identified as playing a role in metastasis, despite some conflicting evidence, was **miR-10b**. Functional studies have demonstrated that miR-10b overexpression promotes cell migration and invasion in vitro, and initiates tumor invasion and metastasis in vivo [82].

Upstream of mir-10b activation, the transcription factor Twist was found, which has been previously shown to be associated with invasive lobular carcinoma [82]. Downstream, it appears miR-10b inhibits translation of *homeobox D10* (HOXD10) ensuring increased expression of *ras homolog gene family, member C*, a gene that promotes cell migration and invasion. In the same study breast carcinomas from metastasis-free patients showed low levels of miR-10b expression, whereas high levels of miR-10b expression were detected in 50 % of metastasis-positive patients. Gee et al. [83] studied miR-10b expression in patients with primary tumors and nodal metastases versus primary tumors without nodal metastases, but could not confirm a significant association between miR-10b levels and metastasis or prognosis. Added to these findings, miR-10b expression has been associated with the prognostically favorable luminal A subtype [51]. Further investigations and large scale studies will be required to fully elucidate the role of miR-10b in breast cancer metastasis.

Huang et al. [84] found a negative correlation between **miR-21** and the expression of *phosphatase and tensin homolog deleted on chromosome* 10 (*PTEN*), which suggests PTEN is a potential target of miR-21. In the same study, the authors compared miR-21 expression to markers of aggressive phenotype. They found a correlation between increased expression and lymph node positivity, higher proliferation index and advanced TNM stage. Since the tumor suppressor gene *PTEN* is also implicated in cell migration and invasion [85, 86], mir-21 may also have a role in invasion and metastasis. This supports the results of two other studies, which also identified a correlation between increased miR-21 expression and poor disease-free survival in early-stage patients and advanced clinical stage, lymph node metastases and shortened survival [87, 88]. According to Zhu et al. [89] miR-21 may promote tumor invasion and metastasis by simultaneously down regulating multiple metastasis-related tumor suppressor genes operating at distinct steps of tumor progression. Given that a miRNA can target over 100 genes [25], additional miR-21 targets which have a role in invasion and metastasis may be identified.

The miR-200 family contains 5 members (miR-200a, miR-200b, miR-200c, miR-141 and miR-429) clustered in 2 genomic loci (200b-200a-429 and 200c-141) which target members of the Zeb family of transcriptional repressors [90]. The miR-200 family is believed to play an essential role in tumor suppression by inhibiting epithelial-mesenchymal transition (EMT), the initiating step of metastasis [91]. During EMT, cells lose adhesion and increase in motility [92]. Epithelial cells typically have normal cell-to-cell junction and adhesion, while mesenchymal cells have weaker cell wall adhesion, making them more motile and likely to enhance invasive characteristics. EMT has been found to play an essential role in tumor invasion, metastatic dissemination, and the acquisition of resistance to current cancer therapies (reviewed in [77]). Studies indicate that the miRNA-200 family could regulate the EMT process by targeting specific molecular markers of EMT [93]. In the pioneering work by Gregory et al. [94], it was suggested that the entire miR-200 family is down regulated upon exposure to transforming growth factor-β (TGF-β). TGF-β is a cytokine that is known to induce the EMT phenotype [95–97]. Re-expression of the miR-200 family significantly inhibited EMT that was induced by TGF-β, while inhibition of the miR-200 family resulted in the induction of EMT phenotype. Furthermore, there were increased levels of ZEB1 and ZEB2 following the induction of EMT, which suggests that the miR-200 family is a negative regulator of the mesenchymal markers, ZEB1 and ZEB2. Down regulation of miR-200b and miR-200c has been demonstrated to be associated with loss of E-cadherin expression in breast cancer cells with mesenchymal phenotype, as a result of a consequential up regulation of the E-cadherin transcriptional repressor, ZEB1 [98]. Conversely, miR-200b or miR-200c restoration induced E-cadherin expression, therefore inhibiting EMT and causing a less aggressive phenotype in the cancer cells. Another study [99] focused on the miRNAs suppressed by ZEB1 and showed that the affected miRNAs were members of the miR-200 family. It was revealed that ZEB1 can bind to highly conserved sites in the promoter and directly suppress transcription of the complete cluster of the miR-200 family. Furthermore, ZEB1 is also a target of miR-200c (as mentioned above), which indicates that there is an EMT-inducing feed-forward cycle. Thus, evidence from all these studies suggests that the miR-200 family acts as a central regulator in tumorigenesis, metastasis and aggressiveness.

miR-31 has been identified as an inhibitor of multiple steps of the invasion-metastasis cascade in breast cancer [100, 101]. miR-31 is encoded by a single genomic locus and is expressed in a variety of human tissues [102, 103] and this miRNA is one of the pleiotropically cancer-relevant miRNAs. Valastyan et al. [101] identified miR-31 as a regulator of metastatic progression in human breast cancer. The authors demonstrated an inverse correlation between miR-31 expression and the invasive capability in 15 different breast epithelial cell lines. Additionally, miR-31 levels in primary human breast tumors were revealed to be inversely associated with the propensity of clinically detectable distant metastases.

miR-335 was found to inhibit metastasis through the targeting of a set of metastasis genes, including the transcription factor SOX4 and the extracellular matrix protein Tenascin-C, however, its expression is down regulated in the majority of primary breast tumors from patients who subsequently relapse [104]. The combined genetic and epigenetic targeting of the miR-335 locus in all metastatic derivatives obtained from distinct patients highlights the significance of this molecule as a barrier to metastatic progression in breast cancer. The observation that miR-335 is often silenced in the primary tumor has led to the identification of this miRNA as an inhibitor of tumor re-initiation in addition to its established role as a suppressor of invasion and metastatic colonization [105]. This miRNA, like let-7, can suppress tumor initiation in breast cancer. Interestingly, while let-7 also suppresses proliferation and tumor growth, miR-335 selectively abolishes tumor re-initiation without inhibiting proliferation or tumor growth [106].

miR-9 is up regulated in breast cancer cells through activation by MYC and MYCN, and it directly targets E-cadherin-encoding mRNA and CDH1, leading to increased cell motility and invasiveness [107]. miR-9 levels correlate with grade in primary breast tumors and are significantly elevated in those patients with metastases compared with those without. These findings are consistent with the observation that miR-9 expression is higher in breast cancer patients with local relapse. The higher expression of miR-9 in cancer cells may indicate a more aggressive tumor, also suggested by the association with higher stage in the study of Zhou et al. [108].

Many examples of a correlation of miRNA expression and metastasis are present in literature. The challenge of selecting the ones usable in the clinic remains.

16.3 Long Non Coding RNA Molecules

Long non-coding RNAs (lncRNAs) are a heterogeneous group of non-coding transcripts longer than 200 nucleotides that are involved in many biological processes. This class of ncRNA makes up the largest portion of the mammalian non-coding transcriptome [109]. Long non-coding RNAs provide a new opportunity to identify both functional drivers and cancer-type-specific biomarkers. As the knowledge about lncRNAs grows, studies concluded that lncRNAs tend to show more tissue-specific expression than protein-coding genes [110]. This property of makes them highly attractive as tissue-specific biomarkers.

Very little is known about lncRNA biogenesis, in contrast with miRNAs, pre-processing mechanisms are not necessary. Until recently, very few lncRNAs were annotated within the human genome. Now, various groups have developed independent catalogs of human lncRNAs [110–112]. Despite the thousands of human lncRNAs now predicted, only a handful of lncRNAs have been well characterized to date, little is known about the expression patterns of most lncRNAs in different cell types.

Various mechanisms of transcriptional regulation of gene expression by lncRNAs have been suggested. lncRNAs utilize a large arsenal of mechanisms to regulate gene expression. lncRNAs act as co-activators, binding to transcription factors and enhancing their transcriptional activity [113–115]. Another mechanism is transcriptional interference, where the act of transcribing a lncRNA interferes with transcription initiation, elongation or termination of another gene [116]. lncRNAs can also affect transcription by binding to transcription factors and shuttling them into the cytoplasm to keep them away from their nuclear targets [117]. Recent evidence also suggests that some lncRNAs may have enhancer-like function [118], activating expression of nearby genes by an unknown mechanism.

While the study of lncRNA function is still in its infancy, a role for a number of these transcripts has recently been established in cancer, in general, as well as specifically in breast cancer. Like protein-coding genes and miRNAs, lncRNAs play key roles in tumorigenesis. They have been shown to play a functional role in a number of fundamental processes associated with cancer including cell cycle regulation, apoptosis, the DNA damage response, and metastasis. Similar to mRNA profiling and miRNA profiling one may hypothesize that lncRNA profiling could serve as a signature to divide breast cancer tumors in clinically relevant subtypes.

Since the functions of most lncRNA still need to be unraveled or confirmed (although it is clear they can function, like miRNAs, as oncogenes or tumor suppressor genes) the focus in this chapter lies on two well known examples (HOTAIR and BC-200), both with great potential as breast cancer biomarkers.

Gupta et al. [119] found that lncRNA in the *HOX* loci become deregulated during breast cancer progression. This study identified a distinct set of *HOX* lncRNA to be overexpressed in primary tumors and very frequently overexpressed in metastases. One such lncRNA, *HOTAIR*, was increased in primary tumors and metastases and its expression level in primary tumors was a predictor of eventual metastasis and death. Enforced expression of HOTAIR in epithelial cancer cells induced genome-wide re-targeting of Polycomb Repressive Complex 2 (PRC2) to an occupancy pattern more resembling embryonic fibroblasts, leading to altered histone H3 lysine 27 methylation, gene expression, and increased cancer invasiveness and metastasis in a manner dependent on PRC2. Conversely, loss of HOTAIR can inhibit cancer invasiveness, particularly in cells that possess excessive PRC2 activity [119, 120]. Chisholm et al. [121] provided evidence that expression levels of lncRNA in the HOX loci do tend to cluster with some clinicopathologic data, such that increased ncHoxA1 trends with proliferation rate, and ncHoxD4 trends with positive PR receptor status.

BC200, also known as BCYRN1 (brain cytoplasmic RNA 1), is a 200 nucleotide long ncRNA selectively expressed in the nervous system and usually not detected in somatic cells other than neurons. It is, however, overexpressed in several solid cancers including breast cancer [122]. BC200 RNA is expressed at high levels in invasive breast carcinomas, but is barely detectable in normal tissue or in benign tumors [123]. Interestingly, in ductal carcinomas in situ (DCIS), significant BC200 expression is associated with high nuclear grade. This suggests that BC200 may be a useful marker for early detection of breast cancer and that the presence of BC200 RNA in early lesions might have utility as a prognostic indicator of tumor progression.

In conclusion, this overview clearly suggest that non coding RNAs have great potential to be used as biomarkers in breast cancer. Various applications (tumor profiling, risk of relapse, detection of early stage breast cancer) are possible but many aspects still need to be explored before these RNA molecules will be transferred from bench to bedside.

References

1. Lee RC, Feinbaum RL, Ambros V (1993) The C. elegans heterochronic gene lin-4 encodes small RNAs with antisense complementarity to lin-14. Cell 75(5):843–854
2. Chen K, Rajewsky N (2007) The evolution of gene regulation by transcription factors and microRNAs. Nat Rev Genet 8(2):93–103

3. Bartel DP (2009) MicroRNAs: target recognition and regulatory functions. Cell 136(2):215–233
4. Kusenda B et al (2006) MicroRNA biogenesis, functionality and cancer relevance. Biomed Pap Med Fac Univ Palacky Olomouc Czech Repub 150(2):205–215
5. Homo sapiens miRNAs in the miRBase at Manchester University. http://www.mirbase.org/
6. Bentwich I et al (2005) Identification of hundreds of conserved and nonconserved human microRNAs. Nat Genet 37(7):766–770
7. Friedman RC et al (2009) Most mammalian mRNAs are conserved targets of microRNAs. Genome Res 19(1):92–105
8. Lewis BP, Burge CB, Bartel DP (2005) Conserved seed pairing, often flanked by adenosines, indicates that thousands of human genes are microRNA targets. Cell 120(1):15–20
9. Lagos-Quintana M et al (2001) Identification of novel genes coding for small expressed RNAs. Science 294(5543):853–858
10. Lau NC et al (2001) An abundant class of tiny RNAs with probable regulatory roles in Caenorhabditis elegans. Science 294(5543):858–862
11. Lee RC, Ambros V (2001) An extensive class of small RNAs in Caenorhabditis elegans. Science 294(5543):862–864
12. Lee Y et al (2004) MicroRNA genes are transcribed by RNA polymerase II. EMBO J 23(20):4051–4060
13. Baskerville S, Bartel DP (2005) Microarray profiling of microRNAs reveals frequent coexpression with neighboring miRNAs and host genes. RNA 11(3):241–247
14. Rodriguez A et al (2004) Identification of mammalian microRNA host genes and transcription units. Genome Res 14(10A):1902–1910
15. Lee Y et al (2002) MicroRNA maturation: stepwise processing and subcellular localization. EMBO J 21(17):4663–4670
16. Cai X, Hagedorn CH, Cullen BR (2004) Human microRNAs are processed from capped, polyadenylated transcripts that can also function as mRNAs. RNA 10(12):1957–1966
17. Denli AM et al (2004) Processing of primary microRNAs by the Microprocessor complex. Nature 432(7014):231–235
18. Gregory RI et al (2004) The Microprocessor complex mediates the genesis of microRNAs. Nature 432(7014):235–240
19. Lund E et al (2004) Nuclear export of microRNA precursors. Science 303(5654):95–98
20. Grishok A et al (2001) Genes and mechanisms related to RNA interference regulate expression of the small temporal RNAs that control C. elegans developmental timing. Cell 106(1):23–34
21. Hutvagner G et al (2001) A cellular function for the RNA-interference enzyme Dicer in the maturation of the let-7 small temporal RNA. Science 293(5531):834–838
22. Ketting RF et al (2001) Dicer functions in RNA interference and in synthesis of small RNA involved in developmental timing in C. elegans. Genes Dev 15(20):2654–2659
23. Gregory RI et al (2005) Human RISC couples microRNA biogenesis and posttranscriptional gene silencing. Cell 123(4):631–640
24. Lin SL, Chang D, Ying SY (2005) Asymmetry of intronic pre-miRNA structures in functional RISC assembly. Gene 356:32–38
25. Brennecke J et al (2005) Principles of microRNA-target recognition. PLoS Biol 3(3), e85
26. Kren BT et al (2009) MicroRNAs identified in highly purified liver-derived mitochondria may play a role in apoptosis. RNA Biol 6(1):65–72
27. Tanzer A, Stadler PF (2004) Molecular evolution of a microRNA cluster. J Mol Biol 339(2):327–335
28. Lewis BP et al (2003) Prediction of mammalian microRNA targets. Cell 115(7):787–798
29. Krek A et al (2005) Combinatorial microRNA target predictions. Nat Genet 37(5):495–500
30. Rajewsky N (2006) microRNA target predictions in animals. Nat Genet 38(Suppl):S8–S13
31. Brennecke J et al (2003) Bantam encodes a developmentally regulated microRNA that controls cell proliferation and regulates the proapoptotic gene hid in Drosophila. Cell 113(1):25–36
32. Calin GA et al (2004) Human microRNA genes are frequently located at fragile sites and genomic regions involved in cancers. Proc Natl Acad Sci U S A 101(9):2999–3004
33. Negrini M et al (1995) Definition and refinement of chromosome 11 regions of loss of heterozygosity in breast cancer: identification of a new region at 11q23.3. Cancer Res 55(14):3003–3007
34. Calin GA, Croce CM (2006) MicroRNA signatures in human cancers. Nat Rev Cancer 6(11):857–866
35. Lu J et al (2005) MicroRNA expression profiles classify human cancers. Nature 435(7043): 834–838
36. Gaur A et al (2007) Characterization of microRNA expression levels and their biological correlates in human cancer cell lines. Cancer Res 67(6):2456–2468
37. Calin GA et al (2002) Frequent deletions and down-regulation of micro- RNA genes miR15 and miR16 at 13q14 in chronic lymphocytic leukemia. Proc Natl Acad Sci U S A 99(24):15524–15529
38. Iorio MV et al (2005) MicroRNA gene expression deregulation in human breast cancer. Cancer Res 65(16):7065–7070
39. Dvinge H et al (2013) The shaping and functional consequences of the microRNA landscape in breast cancer. Nature 497(7449):378–382
40. Piccart-Gebhart MJ (2006) Adjuvant trastuzumab therapy for HER2-overexpressing breast cancer: what we know and what we still need to learn. Eur J Cancer 42(12):1715–1719

41. Tang F et al (2006) MicroRNA expression profiling of single whole embryonic stem cells. Nucleic Acids Res 34(2):e9
42. Jiang J et al (2005) Real-time expression profiling of microRNA precursors in human cancer cell lines. Nucleic Acids Res 33(17):5394–5403
43. Perou CM et al (2000) Molecular portraits of human breast tumours. Nature 406(6797):747–752
44. Sorlie T et al (2003) Repeated observation of breast tumor subtypes in independent gene expression data sets. Proc Natl Acad Sci U S A 100(14):8418–8423
45. Dowsett M, Dunbier AK (2008) Emerging biomarkers and new understanding of traditional markers in personalized therapy for breast cancer. Clin Cancer Res 14(24):8019–8026
46. Harvey JM et al (1999) Estrogen receptor status by immunohistochemistry is superior to the ligand-binding assay for predicting response to adjuvant endocrine therapy in breast cancer. J Clin Oncol 17(5):1474–1481
47. Yamashita H et al (2006) Immunohistochemical evaluation of hormone receptor status for predicting response to endocrine therapy in metastatic breast cancer. Breast Cancer 13(1):74–83
48. Adams BD, Furneaux H, White BA (2007) The micro-ribonucleic acid (miRNA) miR-206 targets the human estrogen receptor-alpha (ERalpha) and represses ERalpha messenger RNA and protein expression in breast cancer cell lines. Mol Endocrinol 21(5):1132–1147
49. Boyerinas B et al (2010) The role of let-7 in cell differentiation and cancer. Endocr Relat Cancer 17(1):F19–F36
50. Griffiths-Jones S et al (2008) miRBase: tools for microRNA genomics. Nucleic Acids Res 36(Database issue):D154–D158
51. Blenkiron C et al (2007) MicroRNA expression profiling of human breast cancer identifies new markers of tumor subtype. Genome Biol 8(10):R214
52. Mattie MD et al (2006) Optimized high-throughput microRNA expression profiling provides novel biomarker assessment of clinical prostate and breast cancer biopsies. Mol Cancer 5:24
53. Harris L et al (2007) American Society of Clinical Oncology 2007 update of recommendations for the use of tumor markers in breast cancer. J Clin Oncol 25(33):5287–5312
54. O'Hanlon DM et al (1995) An evaluation of preoperative CA 15–3 measurement in primary breast carcinoma. Br J Cancer 71(6):1288–1291
55. Uehara M et al (2008) Long-term prognostic study of carcinoembryonic antigen (CEA) and carbohydrate antigen 15–3 (CA 15–3) in breast cancer. Int J Clin Oncol 13(5):447–451
56. Taplin S et al (2008) Mammography facility characteristics associated with interpretive accuracy of screening mammography. J Natl Cancer Inst 100(12):876–887
57. Lawrie CH et al (2008) Detection of elevated levels of tumour-associated microRNAs in serum of patients with diffuse large B-cell lymphoma. Br J Haematol 141(5):672–675
58. Chen X et al (2008) Characterization of microRNAs in serum: a novel class of biomarkers for diagnosis of cancer and other diseases. Cell Res 18(10):997–1006
59. Gilad S et al (2008) Serum microRNAs are promising novel biomarkers. PLoS One 3(9), e3148
60. Corsten MF et al (2010) Circulating microRNA-208b and microRNA-499 reflect myocardial damage in cardiovascular disease. Circ Cardiovasc Genet 3(6):499–506
61. Etheridge A et al (2011) Extracellular microRNA: a new source of biomarkers. Mutat Res 717(1–2):85–90
62. Huang Z et al (2010) Plasma microRNAs are promising novel biomarkers for early detection of colorectal cancer. Int J Cancer 127(1):118–126
63. Park NJ et al (2009) Salivary microRNA: discovery, characterization, and clinical utility for oral cancer detection. Clin Cancer Res 15(17):5473–5477
64. Hanson EK, Lubenow H, Ballantyne J (2009) Identification of forensically relevant body fluids using a panel of differentially expressed microRNAs. Anal Biochem 387(2):303–314
65. Wang K et al (2010) Export of microRNAs and microRNA-protective protein by mammalian cells. Nucleic Acids Res 38(20):7248–7259
66. Weber JA et al (2010) The microRNA spectrum in 12 body fluids. Clin Chem 56(11):1733–1741
67. Zen K, Zhang CY (2012) Circulating microRNAs: a novel class of biomarkers to diagnose and monitor human cancers. Med Res Rev 32(2):326–48
68. Zubakov D et al (2010) MicroRNA markers for forensic body fluid identification obtained from microarray screening and quantitative RT-PCR confirmation. Int J Legal Med 124(3):217–226
69. Weickmann JL, Glitz DG (1982) Human ribonucleases. Quantitation of pancreatic-like enzymes in serum, urine, and organ preparations. J Biol Chem 257(15):8705–8710
70. Mitchell PS et al (2008) Circulating microRNAs as stable blood-based markers for cancer detection. Proc Natl Acad Sci U S A 105(30):10513–10518
71. Kroh EM et al (2010) Analysis of circulating microRNA biomarkers in plasma and serum using quantitative reverse transcription-PCR (qRT-PCR). Methods 50(4):298–301
72. Wu Q et al (2011) Next-generation sequencing of microRNAs for breast cancer detection. J Biomed Biotechnol 2011:597145
73. Asaga S et al (2011) Direct serum assay for microRNA-21 concentrations in early and advanced breast cancer. Clin Chem 57(1):84–91
74. Heneghan HM et al (2010) Systemic miRNA-195 differentiates breast cancer from other malignancies and is a potential biomarker for detecting noninvasive and early stage disease. Oncologist 15(7):673–682

75. Zhao H et al (2010) A pilot study of circulating miRNAs as potential biomarkers of early stage breast cancer. PLoS One 5(10), e13735
76. Ng EK et al (2013) Circulating microRNAs as specific biomarkers for breast cancer detection. PLoS One 8(1), e53141
77. Gupta GP, Massague J (2006) Cancer metastasis: building a framework. Cell 127(4):679–695
78. Nguyen DX, Bos PD, Massague J (2009) Metastasis: from dissemination to organ-specific colonization. Nat Rev Cancer 9(4):274–284
79. Sawan C et al (2008) Epigenetic drivers and genetic passengers on the road to cancer. Mutat Res 642(1–2):1–13
80. Ma L, Weinberg RA (2008) Micromanagers of malignancy: role of microRNAs in regulating metastasis. Trends Genet 24(9):448–456
81. Nicoloso MS et al (2009) MicroRNAs–the micro steering wheel of tumour metastases. Nat Rev Cancer 9(4):293–302
82. Ma L, Teruya-Feldstein J, Weinberg RA (2007) Tumour invasion and metastasis initiated by microRNA-10b in breast cancer. Nature 449(7163):682–688
83. Gee HE et al (2008) MicroRNA-10b and breast cancer metastasis. Nature 455(7216):E8–E9, author reply E9
84. Huang GL et al (2009) Clinical significance of miR-21 expression in breast cancer: SYBR-Green I-based real-time RT-PCR study of invasive ductal carcinoma. Oncol Rep 21(3):673–679
85. Bandyopadhyay S et al (2004) PTEN up-regulates the tumor metastasis suppressor gene Drg-1 in prostate and breast cancer. Cancer Res 64(21):7655–7660
86. Varga AE et al (2005) Silencing of the Tropomyosin-1 gene by DNA methylation alters tumor suppressor function of TGF-beta. Oncogene 24(32):5043–5052
87. Qian B et al (2009) High miR-21 expression in breast cancer associated with poor disease-free survival in early stage disease and high TGF-beta1. Breast Cancer Res Treat 117(1):131–140
88. Yan LX et al (2008) MicroRNA miR-21 overexpression in human breast cancer is associated with advanced clinical stage, lymph node metastasis and patient poor prognosis. RNA 14(11):2348–2360
89. Zhu Q et al (2012) miR-21 promotes migration and invasion by the miR-21-PDCD4-AP-1 feedback loop in human hepatocellular carcinoma. Oncol Rep 27(5):1660–1668
90. Gibbons DL et al (2009) Contextual extracellular cues promote tumor cell EMT and metastasis by regulating miR-200 family expression. Genes Dev 23(18):2140–2151
91. Adams BD, Guttilla IK, White BA (2008) Involvement of microRNAs in breast cancer. Semin Reprod Med 26(6):522–536
92. Liu C, Tang DG (2011) MicroRNA regulation of cancer stem cells. Cancer Res 71(18):5950–5954
93. Ahmad A et al (2011) Phosphoglucose isomerase/autocrine motility factor mediates epithelial-mesenchymal transition regulated by miR-200 in breast cancer cells. Cancer Res 71(9):3400–3409
94. Gregory PA et al (2008) The miR-200 family and miR-205 regulate epithelial to mesenchymal transition by targeting ZEB1 and SIP1. Nat Cell Biol 10(5):593–601
95. Corcoran C et al (2011) Intracellular and extracellular microRNAs in breast cancer. Clin Chem 57(1):18–32
96. Maitah MY et al (2011) Up-regulation of sonic hedgehog contributes to TGF-beta1-induced epithelial to mesenchymal transition in NSCLC cells. PLoS One 6(1), e16068
97. Zavadil J, Bottinger EP (2005) TGF-beta and epithelial-to-mesenchymal transitions. Oncogene 24(37):5764–5774
98. Tryndyak VP, Beland FA, Pogribny IP (2010) E-cadherin transcriptional down-regulation by epigenetic and microRNA-200 family alterations is related to mesenchymal and drug-resistant phenotypes in human breast cancer cells. Int J Cancer 126(11):2575–2583
99. Burk U et al (2008) A reciprocal repression between ZEB1 and members of the miR-200 family promotes EMT and invasion in cancer cells. EMBO Rep 9(6):582–589
100. Valastyan S et al (2011) Activation of miR-31 function in already-established metastases elicits metastatic regression. Genes Dev 25(6):646–659
101. Valastyan S et al (2009) A pleiotropically acting microRNA, miR-31, inhibits breast cancer metastasis. Cell 137(6):1032–1046
102. Stuelten CH, Salomon DS (2010) miR-31 in cancer: location matters. Cell Cycle 9(23):4608–4609
103. Valastyan S, Weinberg RA (2010) miR-31: a crucial overseer of tumor metastasis and other emerging roles. Cell Cycle 9(11):2124–2129
104. Tavazoie SF et al (2008) Endogenous human microRNAs that suppress breast cancer metastasis. Nature 451(7175):147–152
105. Png KJ et al (2011) MicroRNA-335 inhibits tumor reinitiation and is silenced through genetic and epigenetic mechanisms in human breast cancer. Genes Dev 25(3):226–231
106. Yu F et al (2007) Let-7 regulates self renewal and tumorigenicity of breast cancer cells. Cell 131(6):1109–1123
107. Ma L et al (2010) miR-9, a MYC/MYCN-activated microRNA, regulates E-cadherin and cancer metastasis. Nat Cell Biol 12(3):247–256
108. Zhou X et al (2012) MicroRNA-9 as potential biomarker for breast cancer local recurrence and tumor estrogen receptor status. PLoS One 7(6):e39011

109. Katayama S et al (2005) Antisense transcription in the mammalian transcriptome. Science 309(5740):1564–1566
110. Cabili MN et al (2011) Integrative annotation of human large intergenic noncoding RNAs reveals global properties and specific subclasses. Genes Dev 25(18):1915–1927
111. Derrien T, Guigo R, Johnson R (2011) The long non-coding RNAs: a new (P)layer in the "Dark Matter". Front Genet 2:107
112. Guttman M et al (2010) Ab initio reconstruction of cell type-specific transcriptomes in mouse reveals the conserved multi-exonic structure of lincRNAs. Nat Biotechnol 28(5):503–510
113. Caretti G et al (2006) The RNA helicases p68/p72 and the noncoding RNA SRA are coregulators of MyoD and skeletal muscle differentiation. Dev Cell 11(4):547–560
114. Feng J et al (2006) The Evf-2 noncoding RNA is transcribed from the Dlx-5/6 ultraconserved region and functions as a Dlx-2 transcriptional coactivator. Genes Dev 20(11):1470–1484
115. Lanz RB et al (1999) A steroid receptor coactivator, SRA, functions as an RNA and is present in an SRC-1 complex. Cell 97(1):17–27
116. Mazo A et al (2007) Transcriptional interference: an unexpected layer of complexity in gene regulation. J Cell Sci 120(Pt 16):2755–2761
117. Willingham AT et al (2005) A strategy for probing the function of noncoding RNAs finds a repressor of NFAT. Science 309(5740):1570–1573
118. Orom UA et al (2010) Long noncoding RNAs with enhancer-like function in human cells. Cell 143(1):46–58
119. Gupta RA et al (2010) Long non-coding RNA HOTAIR reprograms chromatin state to promote cancer metastasis. Nature 464(7291):1071–1076
120. Rinn JL et al (2007) Functional demarcation of active and silent chromatin domains in human HOX loci by noncoding RNAs. Cell 129(7):1311–1323
121. Chisholm KM et al (2012) Detection of long non-coding RNA in archival tissue: correlation with polycomb protein expression in primary and metastatic breast carcinoma. PLoS One 7(10):e47998
122. Chen W et al (1997) Expression of neural BC200 RNA in human tumours. J Pathol 183(3): 345–351
123. Iacoangeli A et al (2004) BC200 RNA in invasive and preinvasive breast cancer. Carcinogenesis 25(11):2125–2133

Urinary Prostate Cancer Antigen 3 as a Tumour Marker: Biochemical and Clinical Aspects

17

Marianne Schmid, Jens Hansen, and Felix K.-H. Chun

Abstract

Due to low specificity of Prostate-Specific Antigen (PSA) we face a certain risk of overdiagnosis and overtreatment of Prostate Cancer (PCa). The benefits and harms of PSA-screening are controversially discussed. To overcome this weakness of PSA novel PCa biomarkers and detection tools are required.

The urine-based biomarker Prostate Cancer Antigen 3 (PCA3) has been shown to be highly PCa-specific. Application of PCA3 was tested in the diagnostic setting and staging. Several studies pointed out the additional value of PCA3 for further stratification of men selected for biopsy (BX) based on an elevated PSA and/or an abnormal digital rectal examination (DRE). Its combined use with established clinical risk factors for positive prostate BX, particularly within nomograms or risk calculators, may represent a valid and helpful aid for clinicians in patient counselling and BX indication confirmation.

When it comes to prediction of favourable or unfavourable histopathological features, respectively, such as tumour volume or PCa significance, PCA3's value remains controversial. Based on relatively small patient numbers, PCA3 has been identified to independently predict small-volume and insignificant PCa. However, in other studies PCA3 was not associated with advanced disease and its ability of predicting PCa aggressiveness in men undergoing radical prostatectomy is limited.

PCA3's value may be best given for BX outcome prediction. Finally, the implementation of the PCA3 promoter in developing new highly PCa-specific gene therapies represents a promising perspective in the near future.

M. Schmid, MD • J. Hansen, MD
F.K.-H. Chun, MD, FEBU (✉)
Department of Urology, University Medical Center Hamburg-Eppendorf, Martinistrasse 52, 20246 Hamburg, Germany
e-mail: mschmid@uke.de; j.hansen@uke.de; chun@uke.de

R. Scatena (ed.), *Advances in Cancer Biomarkers*, Advances in Experimental Medicine and Biology 867, DOI 10.1007/978-94-017-7215-0_17

Keywords

5a-reductase inhibitor • AMACR • Circulating tumour cells • Diagnosis • Gene therapy • Gleason score • GOLM1 • PCA3 • PCA3 nomogram • Performance characteristics • Prostate biopsy • Prostate cancer • Prostate cancer antigen 3 score • PSA • SPINK1 • Transmembrane-serine protease • Urine analysis

Abbreviations

%fPSA	Percent-free PSA
AMACR	A-methylacyl-coenzyme racemase
AS	Active surveillance
AUC	Area under the curve
BPH	Benign prostate hyperplasia
CE	Conformiteé européenne
CTC	Circulating tumour cell
DHT	Dihydrotestosterone
DRE	Digital rectal examination
EAU	European Association of Urology
ECE	Extracapsular extension
ERG	V-ets erythroblastosis virus E26 oncogene
ERSPC	European Randomised Study of Screening for Prostate Cancer
FDA	US Food and Drug Administration
GOLM1	Golgi membrane protein 1
GS	Gleason score
IL	Interleukin
mRNA	Messenger Ribonucleic Acid
PCa	Prostate cancer
PCA3	Prostate Cancer Antigen 3
PCPT-RC	Prostate Cancer Prevention Trial risk calculator
PSA	Prostate Specific Antigen
REDUCE	Reduction by Dutasteride of Prostate Cancer Events – trial
RP	Radical prostatectomy
RT-PCR	Reverse transcriptase polymerase chain reaction
SPINK1	Serine peptidase inhibitor Kazal type 1
TMPRSS2	Transmembrane-serine protease gene
TV	Tumour volume

17.1 Introduction

Prostate Cancer (PCa) represents the most common disease affecting men, with 238.590 estimated new cases diagnosed in 2013 in the United States (US) [1]. Due to the implementation of total serum Prostate-Specific Antigen (tPSA) in clinical practice for PCa screening and detection, incidence rates of PCa have increased dramatically over time [2]. The rationale behind PCa screening is to reduce the prevalence of advanced disease and PCa-related mortality. However, due to the heterogeneity of PCa cancer subtypes most patients have slow-growing tumours and have minimal risk of dying from the disease [3–5]. On the other hand, there are aggressive tumours resulting in significant morbidity and death. During the decision-making process of biopsy (BX) indication for PCa diagnosis or active PCa treatment after histologically confirmed PCa, the treating physician as well as the patient have to be aware of this dilemma. The challenge in managing clinically localized disease is to distinguish between men with aggressive cancers who would truly need immediate therapy, and those with less aggressive disease who can be safely managed by e.g. active surveillance (AS). As a consequence efforts are made to improve PCa detection performance, risk assessment and surveillance. It is known that PSA testing shows limited specificity mainly in lower PSA ranges [3]. However, increased PSA levels do not reflect PCa exclusively, but also indicate benign prostate enlargement (BPH) and/or inflammatory reactions [6]. In this setting, novel biomarkers represent a promising component to increase the specificity of PCa detection [7]. One of these novel biomarkers is Prostate Cancer Antigen 3 (PCA3). PCA3 messenger Ribonucleic Acid (mRNA) is highly overexpressed in prostatic tumours [8] and represents a urine-based biomarker that has been widely examined and shown to keep up to its promise. When the third-generation of urinary PCA3 assay (Progensa® PCA3; Hologic Gen-Probe Inc., Bedford, MA, USA) [9] attained Conformiteé européenne (CE) approval in 2006, several clinical studies were conducted to evaluate PCA3 as a novel diagnostic marker, to counsel patients or to confirm BX indications and/or to rule out aggressive cancer at BX, respectively. Beside BX endpoints, the clinical staging significance of preoperative urinary PCA3 was assessed to identify respectively favourable and/or unfavourable histopathological features, such as small tumour volume/insignificant PCa vs. locally advanced disease and aggressive disease. Based on promising findings from previous studies, the novel marker was further evaluated in its ability as a first-line diagnostic test in prescreened men [10–19]. In these studies, specificities range between 71 % and 93 % for prediction of PCa at BX in men with elevated PSA levels, whereas the corresponding sensitivities range from 47 % to 75 % when PCA3 is used in isolation. The observed differences are due to the different PCA3 cut-offs that are used. A plethora of PCA3 cut-offs have been tested, still leaving the question of the "best" cut-off unsolved, even though the U.S. Food and Drug Administration (FDA) has recently approved a PCA3 score cut-off of 25 as justification for a repeat BX [20]. In contrast to the PCA3 score cut-off of 25, Auprich et al. conclude that PCA3 may be most clinically relevant in the repeat BX setting, when using a cut-off of 35 to confirm repeat prostate BX indication [21]. However, so far no cut-off seems to provide a reasonable trade-off for sensitivity and specificity when PCA3 is used in isolation. Furthermore, it has to be considered that biomarkers should ideally be used as a continuous variable instead of using cut-offs, since risk levels are not truly discrete but represent a continuum of risk [22, 23]. Nonetheless, according to the European Association of Urology (EAU) Guidelines 2011 [24] the use of PCA3 in the detection setting of PCa is not any more classified as experimental. Integrated in novel BX nomograms, PCA3 can be a useful aid for patient counselling and BX indication confirmation, and it may also be used to determine whether a men needs a repeat BX after an initially negative BX outcome (evidence level 2A).

Concerning usefulness of PCA3 in men undergoing active surveillance (AS) so far no evidence has been presented [21].

Beyond these clinical implications, further research was also directed at evaluating its potential use in combination with other new biomarkers, and as a novel target for PCa therapy.

17.2 Prostate Cancer Antigen 3

17.2.1 History

By comparing PCa tissue with non-malignant prostatic tissue, Bussemakers et al. firstly identified the DD3 (later called *PCA3*) gene in 1999 (Fig. 17.1), functioning as non-coding RNA and mapping to chromosome 9q21–22. Using a reverse transcriptase polymerase chain reaction (RT-PCR) method, they detected that PCA3 was overexpressed in cancerous tissue and low expressed in benign prostatic tissue and not measurable in the normal tissue of numerous organs such as the testis, bladder, kidney, seminal vesicles, brain and lung. PCR3 is highly prostate specific and was overexpressed in 95 % of tumour lesions, but in only 1 of 7 human PCa cell lines (lymph node carcinoma of the prostate) and in none of 18 non-malignant prostate samples [8]. A multitude of studies further implicated significantly higher PCR3-mRNA expression in prostatic tumours in comparison to non-malignant prostatic tissue [19, 21–23, 25] (Fig. 17.2). These findings promoted the idea of developing a PCA3 diagnostic test.

17.2.2 Urine Analysis

There are several urinary assays measuring PCA3 mRNA, which is highly upregulated in neoplastic prostate tissue [9, 26, 27]. The assays

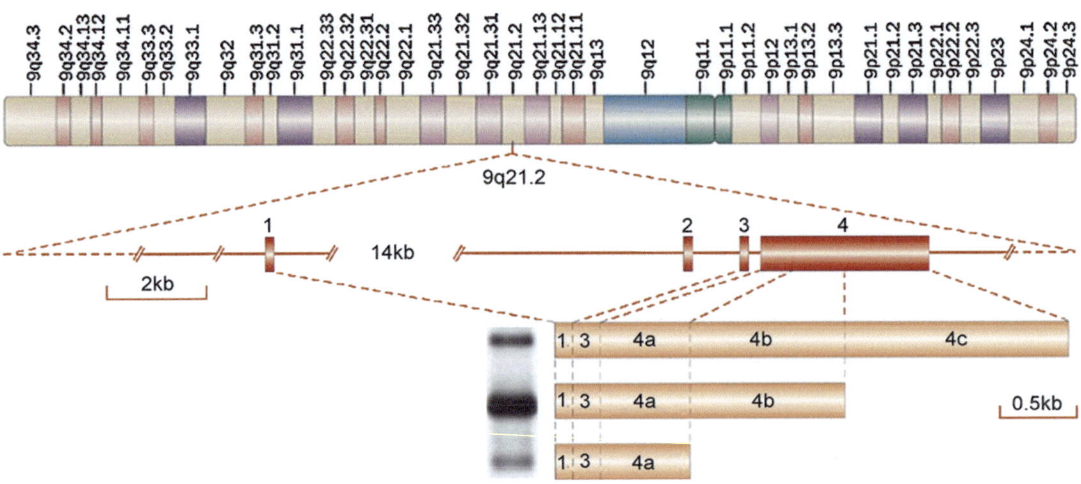

Fig. 17.1 The prostate cancer antigen 3 (PCA3) gene, located at chromosome 9q21-22, consists of four exons, and exon 2 is often skipped by alternative splicing. Three alternative polyadenylations can occur in exon 4 (4a, 4b, and 4c). Most frequently, the transcript contains exons 1, 3, 4a, and 4b (Reprinted with permission from Nature Publishing Group: Hessels et al. Nature Reviews Urology, copyright 2009 [62])

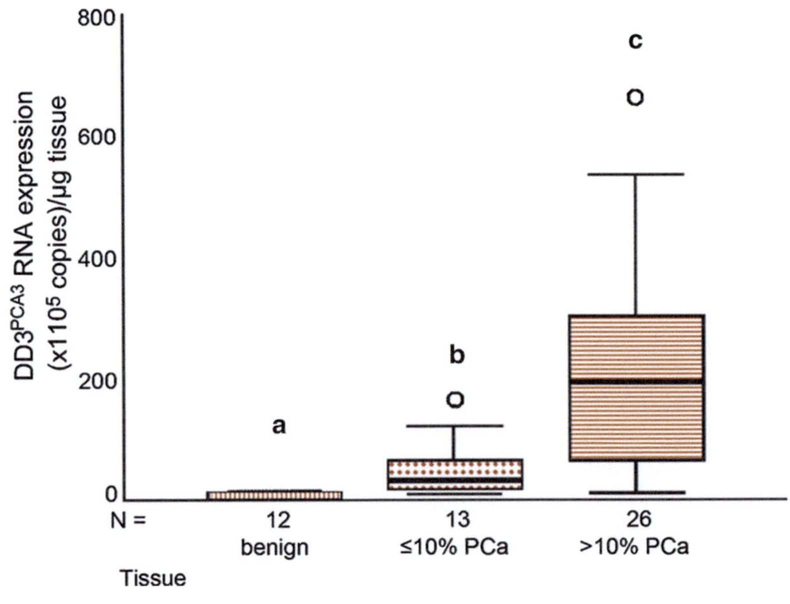

Fig. 17.2 Prostate cancer antigen 3 (PCA3) messenger RNA (mRNA) expression in prostatic tissue. *Box plots* representing the expression of PCA3 mRNA comparing (**a**) benign prostatic tissue (median: 2.4 T 105; range: 0.2 T 105–10.1 T 105); (**b**) prostate tumour containing = 10 % prostate cancer (PCa) cells (median: 25.3 T 105; range: 66.0 T 105–166.0 T 105), and (**c**) prostate tumour containing >10 % PCa cells (median: 158.4 T 105; range: 7.0 T 105–994.0 T 105) (Reprinted with permission from Elsevier: Hessels et al. European Urology, copyright 2003 [26])

measure PCA3 mRNA out of prostate cells shed into urine after digital rectal examination (DRE). Hessels et al. were the first to report of PCA3 mRNA measurement in sedimented urine. PSA mRNA was used to normalise for the amount of prostate specific RNA in the molecular test sample. Although PSA expression is constant in normal cells and 1.5 fold lower in PCa cells, the ratio between PCA3 mRNA over PSA mRNA multiplied by 1000, was presented as a new diagnostic tool – the "**PCA3 score**". In 108 patients, undergoing prostate BX for PCa suspicion based on a PSA level >3 ng/ml, test sensitivity of 67 % and specificity of 83 % were achieved using a determined PCA3-PSA cut-off of 200×10^3 [26].

Tinzl et al. validated the second-generation PCA3 test (uPM3™ assay) comparing urinary

PCA3 to PSA in men undergoing initial and repeat BX for an elevated PSA. In this study the informative rate of 79 % was inferior to current third-generation assays. However, PCA3 achieved a sensitivity and specificity of 82 % and 76 % compared to PSA of 87 % and 16 %, respectively [30]. Using the same assay, the diagnostic superiority of PCA3 was confirmed by Fradet et al. in the first multicenter study including 443 men undergoing prostate BX for elevated PSA. PCA3 vs. PSA revealed an area under the curve (AUC) of 81 % vs. 40 % [28].

In 2006, the prototype of a new quantitative, validated PCA3-based urine test using post-DRE whole-urine specimens further processed in a single-tube format, was presented by Groskopf et al. Urine samples were stored at either 4 °C or 30 °C. The PCA3-to-PSA ratio at 4 °C remained within a 20 % range of the initial values after 2 weeks, but at 30 °C a significant degradation of PCA3 reflected its instability at room temperature. Comparing 52 healthy, 52 BX-negative and 16 BX-positive men, again, median PCA3 mRNA to PSA mRNA ratio values showed significant differences (4.5 vs. 27.0 vs. 81.8; $p<0.01$) [9]. The analytic value oft the new assay was further tested in a multicenter study ($n=179$) conducted by Sokoll et al. Once again, they confirmed the need of an attentive DRE, performed with three or eight strokes ($p=0.85$), to provide high informative test rates up to 95.5 % with total (>18 %), intra-assay (>15 %) and inter-assay (<10 %) variations, respectively. PCA3 scores of BX-positive men showed high correlation when two different research sites were compared (97 %; $p<0.0001$) [29]. Overall, the informative rate of 94–100 % [9, 12, 29–33] of the third-generation PCA3 assay (Progensa®, Hologic Gen-Probe Inc., Bedford, MA, USA) was significantly improved compared to the previously reported ones [27].

The CE approved the PCA3 test in 2006 and finally, the U.S. Food and Drug Administration (FDA) followed in February 2012, to "help clinicians in counselling and determine initial and repeat biopsy indications".

17.3 Clinical Applicability of Prostate Cancer Antigen 3

17.3.1 Early Detection of Prostate Cancer: Initial and Repeat Prostate Biopsy

A main limitation of early PCa detection due to elevated PSA levels remains the high proportion of men detected with non-malignant findings at first or subsequent BX [5, 34]. One of the most important clinical rationales of PCA3 application therefore is the reduction of potentially unnecessary BXs.

Marks et al. evaluated the diagnostic ability of PCA3 in 226 men subjected to repeat BX. They demonstrated PCA3's superiority over PSA in predicting positive BX outcome (AUC: 0.68 vs. 0.52; $p=0.008$). Using 35 as PCA3 score cut-off, a sensitivity, specificity and odds ratio of 58 %, 72 % and 3.6, respectively, was obtained. But, compared to earlier studies [25, 26] median PCA3 scores in aggressive PCa (Gleason score (GS)<7 vs. GS>7) were not significantly different [11]. In contrast, de la Taille et al. have shown in the initial BX setting that the PCA3 score was significantly higher in men with GS 7 or greater vs. GS less than 7 [35].

Consequently, prospective U.S. and European multicentre trials were conducted in patients undergoing initial or repeat BX [10, 13] (Fig. 17.3). As a result comparable diagnostic accuracies of U.S. and European men at first and repeat BX were reported (AUC: 0.68 vs. 0.65). Despite some conflicting results, both studies demonstrated that a combination of PCA3 with established BX risk factors such as age, PSA, DRE, prostate volume and Percent free PSA (%fPSA) improved the predictive accuracy in multivariable regression models. Ploussard et al. performed a subgroup analyses of the European multicenter study and confirmed the superiority of PCA3 over %fPSA in univariable analysis as a predictor of repeat BX outcome (AUC: 0.69 vs. 0.57) [36].

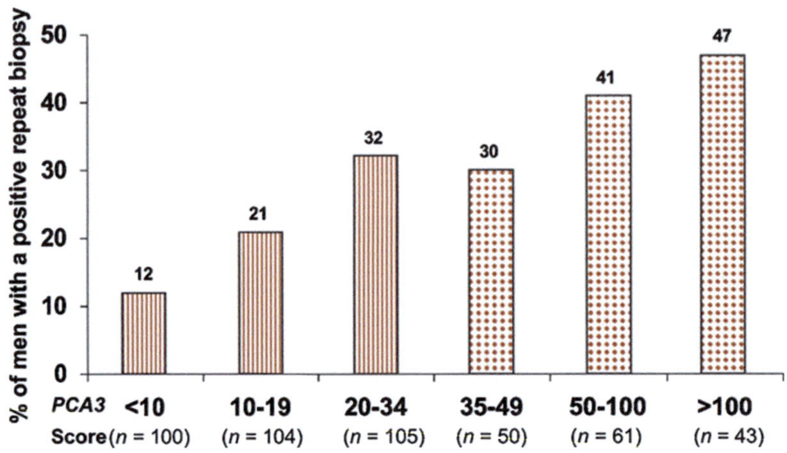

Fig. 17.3 The correlation of prostate cancer antigen 3 (PCA3) to repeat biopsy outcome. *Bars* represent the probability of a positive repeat biopsy expressed in percentages according to different PCA3 score ranges (Reprinted with permission from Elsevier: Haese et al. European Urology, copyright 2008 [10])

The incorporation of PCA3 in the Prostate Cancer Prevention Trial risk calculator (PCPT-RC) improved the diagnostic accuracy compared with the established BX risk factors (AUC: 0.65 vs. 0.70) [37]. In a large mixed BX patient cohort from Europe and Northern America ($n=809$), Chun et al. following Kattan criteria [38, 39] demonstrated that PCA3 independently predicted PCa, and its addition to established risk factors (age, PSA, DRE, prostate volume, BX history) significantly improved predictive AUC of the base model between 2 % and 5 % [14] (Fig. 17.4). The PCA3 based BX nomogram was further externally validated, showing a comparable gain in predictive accuracy [40]. In the specific initial BX setting, an initial BX-specific nomogram has been developed, showing similar findings (AUC 78.1–80.7 %). However, unlike the mixed BX nomogram, the latter initial-BX specific nomogram has also been tested in terms of its ability to avoid unnecessary biopsies without missing high grade PCa. At an exemplary nomogram-derived probability cut-off of 20 %, only 2 % of men with high-grade PCa would be missed, while avoiding up to 55 % of unnecessary prostate BXs [41]. A similar predictive accuracy gain in multivariable analysis has been previously reported by de la Taille et al. where inclusion of PCA3 in multivariable models increased the predictive accuracy by up to 5.5 % [35].

Perdona et al. compared the updated PCPT-RC, including PCA3 and Chun's PCA3-based nomogram. A significantly better discriminative power (AUC: 0.80 vs. 0.72; $p=0.04$) and superior calibration was demonstrated. Decision curve analysis revealed a higher net benefit for Chun's nomogram, resulting in up to 21 % of avoided unnecessary repeat BXs at the expense of missing up to 6.8 % of cancers [42].

Regarding health care expenses and different reimbursement systems in different European countries, at the moment urinary PCA3 measurement is more expensive than PSA measurement. Up-to-date costs for urinary PCA3 testing may be up to 15-fold higher. But, due to PCA3's use to avoid up to 67 % of repeat BXs compared with PSA [10] the avoided BX expenses and further follow-up diagnostic interventions should be considered. Moreover, BX-related anxiety, discomfort and complications may be spared [43].

In conclusion, PCA3 performs as a reliable predictor of PCa at BX, demonstrating superiority over PSA and %fPSA. In combination with established risk factors, PCA3 showed improved accuracy and applicability of new diagnostic tools to assist clinicians in BX decision-making in men who already met established criteria for BX (e.g. elevated PSA, abnormal DRE).

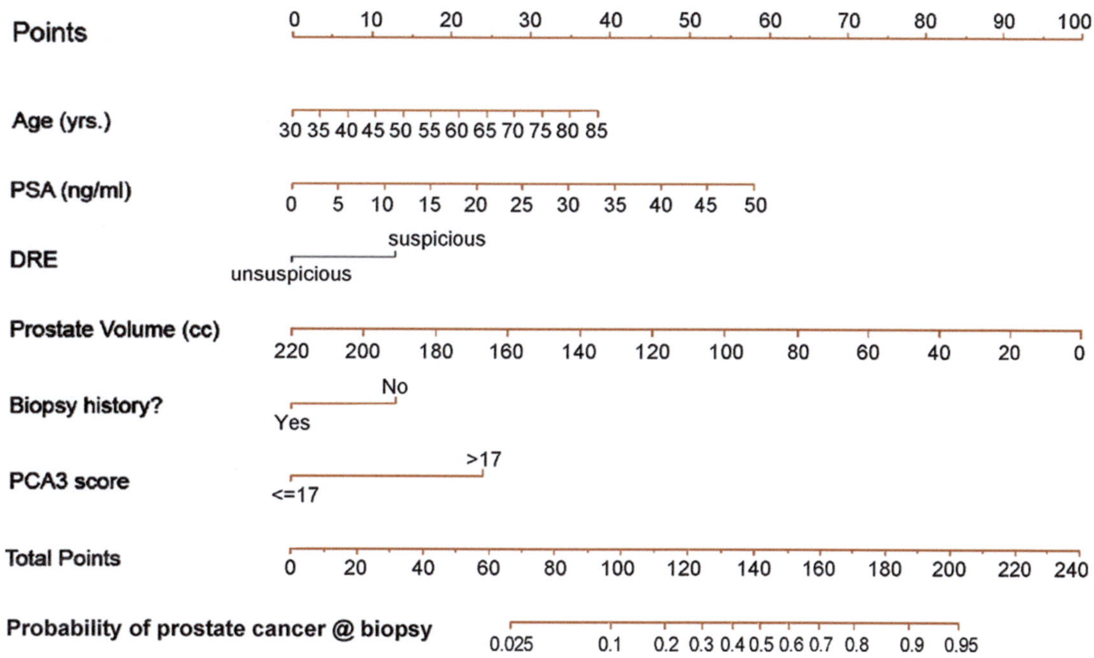

Fig. 17.4 The prostate cancer antigen 3 (PCA3) biopsy nomogram. This recently externally validated nomogram combines established biopsy risk factors such as age, digital rectal examination (DRE), total serum prostate-specific antigen (PSA), prostate volume, and history of previous biopsy together with PCA3 score to predict cancer on prostate initial and repeat biopsy. Instructions for physicians: To obtain nomogram-predicted probability of prostate cancer, locate patient values at each axis. Draw a *vertical line* to the "Point" axis to determine how many points are attributed for each variable value. Sum the points for all variables. Locate the sum on the "Total Points" line to be able to assess the individual probability of cancer on prostate biopsy on the "Probability of prostate cancer at biopsy" line (Reprinted with permission from Elsevier: Chun et al. European Urology, copyright 2009 [14])

17.3.2 Screening and Active Surveillance

PCA3 was assessed as a first-line screening test within the European Randomised Study of Screening for Prostate Cancer (ERSPC) trial. A PCA3 score ≥10 demonstrated a positive predictive value of 17.1 compared with 18.8 for a PSA value ≥3.0 ng/ml. Interestingly, PCA3 versus PSA missed substantially fewer cancers (32 % vs. 65 %) and serious cancers (26 % vs. 58 %). Because this unique study evaluated a PSA-prescreened cohort (third round or more; 33 % had a negative first BX), a consecutive study in unscreened patients, avoiding attribution bias, should be conducted to further assess PCA3 as a potential screening marker [19].

Recently, Tosoian et al. assessed PCA3's ability to rule out clinically significant PCa in men undergoing AS according to the criteria for clinically significant PCa defined by Epstein et al. [44]. A trend towards higher median PCA3 scores in patients with GS upgrading at follow-up BX (72 vs. 50.8; $p=0.08$) was recorded. However, at adjusted multivariable Cox regression analysis, PCA3 did not represent an independent risk factor of BX progression ($p=0.15$) [12]. Considering the limitations that the number of events was small ($n=38$) and that PCA3 was assessed only once at the time of first diagnosis but not repeated during the follow-up biopsies, so far no evidence for the usefulness of PCA3 in AS programs has been presented. Since PCA3 does not appear to represent a useful marker to monitor PCa aggressiveness at biopsies [11, 13] its role in risk assessment during AS needs to be tested in larger studies with repeated PCA3 score measures.

17.3.3 Prediction of Pathological Tumour Volume, Stage and Grade

Du to the fact that PCA3 is highly overexpressed in PCa tissue and improves the prediction of BX outcome, several studies have focused on its potential ability to predict pathological PCa stage and aggressiveness: Bostwick et al. at first reported on 24 patients undergoing radical prostatectomy (RP) for PCa based on a suspicious uPM3™ test. The assessed RP specimens demonstrated no difference in cancer volume, location, stage, and GS compared with RP specimens of men diagnosed with PCa based on PSA or suspicious DRE findings [45].

Using the Progensa® PCA3 assay, Nakanishi et al. analysing 83 RP samples, reported that the urinary PCA3 score significantly correlated with tumour volume (TV), GS, and independently predicted small-volume diseases (TV < 0.5 ml) (AUC: 0.76). Using 25 as a PCA3 score cut-off to predict small-volume tumours in combination with low grade (GS < 7) resulted in a sensitivity and specificity of 70 % and 73 %, respectively. However, it is important to note that the number of events was limited ($n = 10$) [15]. Similarly, Whitman et al. confirmed PCA3's correlation to TV and identified it as an independent predictor ($p < 0.01$) of extracapsular extension (ECE) resulting in a multivariable AUC of 0.90 when combined with PSA and BX GS [16]. In contrast to Nakanishi, Whitman et al. could not find a significant association of PCA3 with pathologic GS [16]. Hessels et al. and van Gils et al. demonstrated neither a significant correlation of PCA3 to pathologic grading nor to TV and pathologic stage in a cohort combining 132 patients [17, 46].

At present, the largest ($n = 305$) published series on urinary PCA3's correlation to clinicopathologic features demonstrated that the multivariable AUC of low-volume disease (+2.4 % to +5.5 %) and insignificant PCa models (+3 % to +3.9 %) improved when PCA3 was added to standard clinical risk factors (Fig. 17.5). On the other side, there was no significant correlation between PCA3 and adverse features such as ECE and seminal vesicle invasion, and its significance on aggressive PCa (RP GS ≥ 7) was reported to be limited [18]. Similar results were reported on

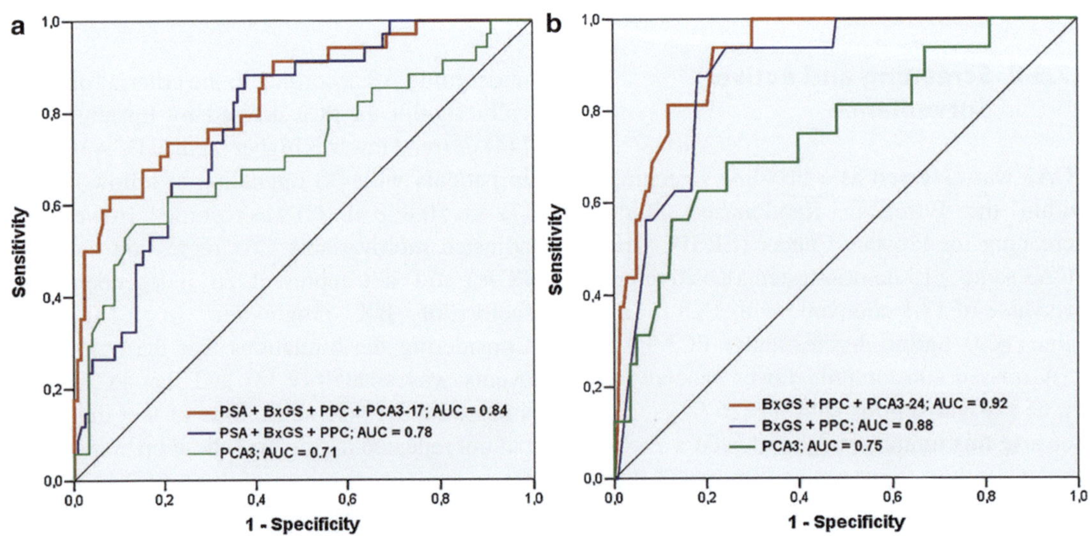

Fig. 17.5 Prediction of small-volume and insignificant prostate cancer with preoperative prostate cancer antigen 3 (PCA3). Receiver operating characteristic curve analyses and area under the curve (AUC) for predicting (**a**) tumour volume <0.5 ml and (**b**) pathologically confirmed insignificant prostate cancer. B × GS = biopsy Gleason score; PPC = percentage of positive cores; PSA = prostate-specific antigen (Reprinted by permission from Elsevier: Auprich et al. European Urology, copyright 2011 [18])

106 consecutive men undergoing RP due to clinically low-risk disease (PSA < 10 ng/ml, T1c–T2a, and biopsy GS < 7). Low urinary PCA3 scores and favourable BX criteria (<33 % or 3-mm tumour; <3 positive cores) independently predicted small TV (<0.5 ml) and insignificant PCa. Again, the urinary PCA3 score, combined with established risk factors in multivariable logistic regression models, was not significantly associated with high-grade and locally advanced disease [47].

Higher PCA3 scores are supposed to be associated with more aggressive cancer, which is based on the hypothesis that with increasing dedifferentiation, PCa cells become more invasive and could therefore more easily be shed into the ductal system of the prostatic gland after DRE or that larger tumours simply have more surface area left to shed PCA3 [46, 47]. Most studies, especially in RP cohorts, failed to confirm this hypothesis [16–18, 46, 47]. But, following GS system [48], some authors suggest that tumours with pattern 4 and 5 increasingly lose their glandular differentiation and lumina, disabling cells to be shed into urine after DRE in correlation with their TV. Therefore, potentially higher PCA3 mRNA tissue levels, resulting from larger tumour masses, might not be adequately measured by the urinary test [18].

In conclusion, evaluations on the potential prognostic role of PCA3, which are currently based on a relatively small number of patients, revealed that it independently predicts small-volume and insignificant PCa. However, PCA3 is not significantly associated with locally advanced disease and has limited value in the prediction of aggressive tumours.

17.3.4 Prostate Cancer Antigen 3 Score Alterations Over Time and Consequence for Bioptic or Medical Intervention

Within the placebo arm of the Reduction by Dutasteride of Prostate Cancer Events (REDUCE) trial, urinary PCA3, PSA and %fPSA were available at the year 2 and year 4 follow-up BX in 1072 men (age: 50–75 years; PSA: 2.5–10 ng/ml; one previous negative 6- to 12-core BX). On univariable analyses for the prediction of year 4 BX outcome based on year 2 biomarker values, PCA3 score was exclusively found as a significant predictor for a positive follow-up BX at year 4. Interestingly, PCA3 scores in BX-positive men only slightly increased (+15.7 %) within the study period [33].

Urinary PCA3 scores before and 2 h after BX, showed no significant difference of measured PCA3 scores, neither in all men (18 %; $p > 0.05$) nor in PCa-positive men (1.5 %; $p > 0.05$) [49]. Sokoll et al. [29] suggest a certain robustness of PCA3 towards interventional effects on the prostatic tissue. In this context, the influence of Dutasteride (5a-reductase inhibitor [5-ARI]) on prostatic markers was assessed by van Gils et al.: In 16 men with BPH and 9 men with clinically localised PCa (all treated with 5-ARI), PSA, testosterone, dihydrotestosterone (DHT), and urinary PCA3 were measured at baseline and after 1, 2 and 3 months. As expected, Dutasteride reduced DHT (>90 %), halved PSA levels, decreased prostate volume (10–16 %), and increased testosterone (20–30 %). In contrast, 5-ARI treatment had a widely variable effect on PCA3 scores, which increased (75–284 %) and decreased (14–77 %) over time, irrespective of whether patients with or without PCa were observed [50]. This needs to be taken into account when counselling patients on Dutasteride who are designated for a PCA3 test.

17.4 New Perspectives

17.4.1 Combination of Prostate Cancer Antigen 3 with New Biomarkers

Since PCA3 is highly PCa specific and a clinically useful marker to predict BX outcome, its combined use with other new tumour markers may further improve its diagnostic accuracy. Therefore, transcripts of a fusion between the transmembrane-serine protease gene (TMPRSS2) and the v-ets erythroblastosis virus E26 oncogene

(ERG) were evaluated in combination with PCA3 in the post-DRE urine of 108 patients undergoing BX. In this study TMPRSS2-ERG fusion transcripts were only found in 59 % of the primary PCa tissue specimens and the included patients did not represent a typical BX cohort because PCa detection rate was quite high with 72 % due to PSA levels ranging from 1.1 to 1619 ng/ml. Urine sediments of men diagnosed with PCa were positive for TMPRSS2-ERG fusion transcripts and PCA3 (cut-off: 48) in 37 % and 62 %, respectively. Combining both markers improved the sensitivity to 73 %, yet a considerable decreased specificity of 63 %, compared with 93 % of TMPRSS2-ERG fusion alone [51].

Laxman et al. further evaluated Golgi membrane protein 1 (GOLM1), serine peptidase inhibitor Kazal type 1 (SPINK1), PCA3 and TMPRSS2-ERG fusion in sedimented urine of men before BX ($n=216$) or RP ($n=60$). A multivariable regression model for the detection of PCa including these four biomarkers improved the diagnostic AUC from 0.66 (for PCA3 alone) to 0.76, respectively [52]. When a-methylacyl-coenzyme racemase (AMACR) and PCA3 from post-DRE urine was assessed in patients undergoing BX due to suspicion of PCa, both markers demonstrated an improved AUC over PSA (0.65 vs. 0.67 vs. 0.59). Using AMACR (cut-off: 10.7) and PCA3 (cut-off: 19.9) within a combined model resulted in a high sensitivity and specificity of 81 % and 84 % vs. 70 % and 71 % vs. 72 % and 59 % for AMACR vs. PCA3 alone, respectively [53]. Rigau et al. using PCA3 together with prostate-specific demonstrated comparable findings G-protein coupled receptor in urine sediments after prostatic massage from 215 patients presented for BX. An increased specificity of 44 % at an assumed sensitivity of 90 % was reported for the combined test compared with each biomarker used as a stand-alone test (25 % vs. 24 %) [54]. Despite the fact that the reported studies used PCA3 cut-off values (19.9, 48) different from the more established cut-off value of 35 reported in previous studies [10, 11, 13, 14, 36, 40], a substantial improvement in the prediction of BX outcome was demonstrated by combining PCA3 and new biomarkers in a limited number of patients. If these promising results could be confirmed by further studies, combinations of new biomarkers including PCA3 may potentially offer an interesting new perspective on the early detection and staging of PCa. However, because to date most of the markers combined with PCA3 are still in their experimental phase, it remains to be assessed which marker panel has the greatest potential to improve predictive ability compared to established markers.

17.4.2 Detection of Prostate Cancer Antigen 3 in Circulating Tumour Cells

In PCa patients, the presence of circulating tumour cells (CTCs) appears to be correlated with a poor prognosis [55]. For this reason detection of specific biomarkers found in prostatic CTCs could potentially indicate an advanced and aggressive stage of disease. In 2008, Väänänen et al. described a quantitative RT-PCR assay for the detection of PCA3 mRNA in peripheral blood and evaluated 67 patients with locally advanced ($n=23$) and metastatic disease ($n=9$), respectively. Interestingly, only two patients were found positive for PCA3 mRNA in peripheral blood samples [56]. In contrast, Marangoni et al. detected PCA3 mRNA expression in 25 (62.5 %) of 40 patients with PCa compared with 15 (37.5 %) of 40 BPH patients by evaluating preoperative peripheral blood samples [57]. Patients presenting with progressive castrate-resistant PCa demonstrated significantly overexpressed levels of PCA3 in CTCs from peripheral blood [58]. Similar findings have been reported by Jost et al. using an immuno-magnetic CTC enrichment method to assess peripheral blood from 67 PCa patients. Although none of the androgen-dependent patients has been tested positive for PCA3, 5 (31 %) of 16 androgen-independent patients were found positive for CTC-PCA3 [59]. In summary, detection of PCA3 mRNA expression in CTCs from peripheral blood samples has been proved to be feasible, although its value in identifying patients with poor prognosis is still unclear due to limited data. Therefore, further studies are needed.

17.4.3 Prostate Cancer Antigen 3 as a Novel Gene Therapy Target

Van der Poel et al. have demonstrated the high PCa specificity of PCA3 and highlighted its potential use as a precursor to suicide gene therapy by using a specific diphtheria toxin model [60]. A combination of PCA3's promoter region driving the expression of a suicide gene could be used to process novel PCa therapies. In theory, this combined therapeutic construct would bind, interact and finally induce cell death in PCa tissue, and non-malignant and non-prostatic cells would not be affected by this highly specific therapeutic cascade. Based on this concept, Fan et al. developed an oncolytic adenovirus (Ad.DD3-E1A-IL-24), in which replication is driven by the $PCA3^{DD3}$ promoter, carrying the therapeutic gene interleukin (IL)-24. Its in vitro and in vivo effects have been investigated in DU-145 cell lines and in DU-145 xenograft tumours in nude mice. In five of six treated mice, tumours have been completely eliminated within 50 days. Most remarkably, all mice have survived until the end of observation [61]. Despite non- negligible discrepancies regarding the therapeutic effect of Ad.DD3-E1A-IL-24 in vitro and in vivo, this study has demonstrated "Gene-ViroTherapy's" excellent antitumoural efficacy in an initial small single tumour model study in mice. Therefore further investigations on PCA3's potential role in PCa gene therapy should be intensively promoted in the future.

17.5 Conclusions

PCA3 has shown its potential to assist clinicians in patient counselling and BX indication confirmation in men at risk for PCa based on elevated serum tPSA levels and/or suspicious DRE. Ideally, PCA3 would be used in combination with other established PCa risk factors to combine each marker's strengths to focus on detection of significant disease that is more likely to be cured if detected early. The value of PCA3 for prediction of PCa significance remains controversial. It does not appear to be associated with advanced disease and PCa aggressiveness in men undergoing RP, and its use as a follow-up marker for AS patients does not seem to be given. The main current indication of the PCA3 urine test may be to determine whether a man needs a (repeat) BX after an initially negative BX outcome, albeit its cost-effectiveness remains to be shown. Finally, the implementation of the PCA3 promoter in developing new highly PCa-specific gene therapies represents a promising perspective in the near future.

References

1. National Cancer Institute (2013) Prostate cancer 2013. http://www.cancer.gov/types/prostate. Accessed 27 Mar 2013
2. Siegel R, Naishadham D, Jemal A (2012) Cancer statistics, 2012. CA Cancer J Clin 62:10–29
3. Etzioni R, Penson DF, Legler JM, di Tommaso D, Boer R, Gann PH et al (2002) Overdiagnosis due to prostate-specific antigen screening: lessons from U.S. prostate cancer incidence trends. J Natl Cancer Inst 94:981–990
4. Schroder FH, Hugosson J, Roobol MJ, Tammela TL, Ciatto S, Nelen V et al (2009) Screening and prostate-cancer mortality in a randomized European study. N Engl J Med 360:1320–1328
5. Telesca D, Etzioni R, Gulati R (2008) Estimating lead time and overdiagnosis associated with PSA screening from prostate cancer incidence trends. Biometrics 64:10–19
6. Huber PR, Schnell Y, Hering F, Rutishauser G (1987) Prostate specific antigen. Experimental and clinical observations. Scand J Urol Nephrol Suppl 104:33–39
7. Madu CO, Lu Y (2010) Novel diagnostic biomarkers for prostate cancer. J Cancer 1:150–177
8. Bussemakers MJ, van Bokhoven A, Verhaegh GW, Smit FP, Karthaus HF, Schalken JA et al (1999) DD3: a new prostate-specific gene, highly overexpressed in prostate cancer. Cancer Res 59:5975–5979
9. Groskopf J, Aubin SM, Deras IL, Blase A, Bodrug S, Clark C et al (2006) APTIMA PCA3 molecular urine test: development of a method to aid in the diagnosis of prostate cancer. Clin Chem 52:1089–1095
10. Haese A, de la Taille A, van Poppel H, Marberger M, Stenzl A, Mulders PF et al (2008) Clinical utility of the PCA3 urine assay in European men scheduled for repeat biopsy. Eur Urol 54:1081–1088

11. Marks LS, Fradet Y, Deras IL, Blase A, Mathis J, Aubin SM et al (2007) PCA3 molecular urine assay for prostate cancer in men undergoing repeat biopsy. Urology 69:532–535
12. Tosoian JJ, Loeb S, Kettermann A, Landis P, Elliot DJ, Epstein JI et al (2010) Accuracy of PCA3 measurement in predicting short-term biopsy progression in an active surveillance program. J Urol 183: 534–538
13. Deras IL, Aubin SM, Blase A, Day JR, Koo S, Partin AW et al (2008) PCA3: a molecular urine assay for predicting prostate biopsy outcome. J Urol 179: 1587–1592
14. Chun FK, de la Taille A, van Poppel H, Marberger M, Stenzl A, Mulders PF et al (2009) Prostate cancer gene 3 (PCA3): development and internal validation of a novel biopsy nomogram. Eur Urol 56:659–667
15. Nakanishi H, Groskopf J, Fritsche HA, Bhadkamkar V, Blase A, Kumar SV et al (2008) PCA3 molecular urine assay correlates with prostate cancer tumor volume: implication in selecting candidates for active surveillance. J Urol 179:1804–1809; discussion 9–10
16. Whitman EJ, Groskopf J, Ali A, Chen Y, Blase A, Furusato B et al (2008) PCA3 score before radical prostatectomy predicts extracapsular extension and tumor volume. J Urol 180:1975–1978; discussion 8–9
17. Hessels D, van Gils MP, van Hooij O, Jannink SA, Witjes JA, Verhaegh GW et al (2010) Predictive value of PCA3 in urinary sediments in determining clinico-pathological characteristics of prostate cancer. Prostate 70:10–16
18. Auprich M, Chun FK, Ward JF, Pummer K, Babaian R, Augustin H et al (2011) Critical assessment of pre-operative urinary prostate cancer antigen 3 on the accuracy of prostate cancer staging. Eur Urol 59:96–105
19. Roobol MJ, Schroder FH, van Leeuwen P, Wolters T, van den Bergh RC, van Leenders GJ et al (2010) Performance of the prostate cancer antigen 3 (PCA3) gene and prostate-specific antigen in prescreened men: exploring the value of PCA3 for a first-line diagnostic test. Eur Urol 58:475–481
20. US Food and Drug Administration (2012) P100033: Progensa® PCA3 assay
21. Auprich M, Bjartell A, Chun FK, de la Taille A, Freedland SJ, Haese A et al (2011) Contemporary role of prostate cancer antigen 3 in the management of prostate cancer. Eur Urol 60:1045–1054
22. Thompson IM, Ankerst DP, Chi C, Lucia MS, Goodman PJ, Crowley JJ et al (2005) Operating characteristics of prostate-specific antigen in men with an initial PSA level of 3.0 ng/ml or lower. JAMA 294:66–70
23. Shariat SF, Semjonow A, Lilja H, Savage C, Vickers AJ, Bjartell A (2011) Tumor markers in prostate cancer I: blood-based markers. Acta Oncol 50(Suppl 1):61–75
24. Heidenreich A, Bellmunt J, Bolla M, Joniau S, Mason M, Matveev V et al (2011) EAU guidelines on prostate cancer. Part 1: screening, diagnosis, and treatment of clinically localised disease. Eur Urol 59:61–71
25. de Kok JB, Verhaegh GW, Roelofs RW, Hessels D, Kiemeney LA, Aalders TW et al (2002) DD3(PCA3), a very sensitive and specific marker to detect prostate tumors. Cancer Res 62:2695–2698
26. Hessels D, Klein Gunnewiek JM, van Oort I, Karthaus HF, van Leenders GJ, van Balken B et al (2003) DD3(PCA3)-based molecular urine analysis for the diagnosis of prostate cancer. Eur Urol 44:8–15; discussion 15–6
27. Tinzl M, Marberger M, Horvath S, Chypre C (2004) DD3PCA3 RNA analysis in urine--a new perspective for detecting prostate cancer. Eur Urol 46:182–186; discussion 7
28. Fradet Y, Saad F, Aprikian A, Dessureault J, Elhilali M, Trudel C et al (2004) uPM3, a new molecular urine test for the detection of prostate cancer. Urology 64:311–315; discussion 5–6
29. Sokoll LJ, Ellis W, Lange P, Noteboom J, Elliott DJ, Deras IL et al (2008) A multicenter evaluation of the PCA3 molecular urine test: pre-analytical effects, analytical performance, and diagnostic accuracy. Clinica Chim Acta; Int J Clin Chem 389:1–6
30. Shappell SB, Fulmer J, Arguello D, Wright BS, Oppenheimer JR, Putzi MJ (2009) PCA3 urine mRNA testing for prostate carcinoma: patterns of use by community urologists and assay performance in reference laboratory setting. Urology 73:363–368
31. Wang R, Chinnaiyan AM, Dunn RL, Wojno KJ, Wei JT (2009) Rational approach to implementation of prostate cancer antigen 3 into clinical care. Cancer 115:3879–3886
32. Nyberg M, Ulmert D, Lindgren A, Lindstrom U, Abrahamsson PA, Bjartell A (2010) PCA3 as a diagnostic marker for prostate cancer: a validation study on a Swedish patient population. Scand J Urol Nephrol 44:378–383
33. Aubin SM, Reid J, Sarno MJ, Blase A, Aussie J, Rittenhouse H et al (2010) PCA3 molecular urine test for predicting repeat prostate biopsy outcome in populations at risk: validation in the placebo arm of the dutasteride REDUCE trial. J Urol 184: 1947–1952
34. Andriole GL, Crawford ED, Grubb RL 3rd, Buys SS, Chia D, Church TR et al (2009) Mortality results from a randomized prostate-cancer screening trial. N Engl J Med 360:1310–1319
35. de la Taille A, Irani J, Graefen M, Chun F, de Reijke T, Kil P et al (2011) Clinical evaluation of the PCA3 assay in guiding initial biopsy decisions. J Urol 185:2119–2125
36. Ploussard G, Haese A, Van Poppel H, Marberger M, Stenzl A, Mulders PF et al (2010) The prostate cancer gene 3 (PCA3) urine test in men with previous negative biopsies: does free-to-total prostate-specific antigen ratio influence the performance of the PCA3 score in predicting positive biopsies? BJU Int 106:1143–1147
37. Ankerst DP, Groskopf J, Day JR, Blase A, Rittenhouse H, Pollock BH et al (2008) Predicting prostate cancer risk through incorporation of prostate cancer gene 3. J Urol 180:1303–1308; discussion 8

38. Kattan MW (2003) Judging new markers by their ability to improve predictive accuracy. J Natl Cancer Inst 95:634–635
39. Kattan MW (2004) Evaluating a new marker's predictive contribution. Clin Cancer Res 10:822–824
40. Auprich M, Haese A, Walz J, Pummer K, de la Taille A, Graefen M et al (2010) External validation of urinary PCA3-based nomograms to individually predict prostate biopsy outcome. Eur Urol 58:727–732
41. Hansen J, Auprich M, Ahyai SA, de la Taille A, van Poppel H, Marberger M et al (2013) Initial prostate biopsy: development and internal validation of a biopsy-specific nomogram based on the prostate cancer antigen 3 assay. Eur Urol 63:201–209
42. Perdona S, Cavadas V, Di Lorenzo G, Damiano R, Chiappetta G, Del Prete P et al (2011) Prostate cancer detection in the "grey area" of prostate-specific antigen below 10 ng/ml: head-to-head comparison of the updated PCPT calculator and Chun's nomogram, two risk estimators incorporating prostate cancer antigen 3. Eur Urol 59:81–87
43. Katz DA, Jarrard DF, McHorney CA, Hillis SL, Wiebe DA, Fryback DG (2007) Health perceptions in patients who undergo screening and workup for prostate cancer. Urology 69:215–220
44. Epstein JI, Walsh PC, Carmichael M, Brendler CB (1994) Pathologic and clinical findings to predict tumor extent of nonpalpable (stage T1c) prostate cancer. JAMA 271:368–374
45. Bostwick DG, Gould VE, Qian J, Susani M, Marberger M (2006) Prostate cancer detected by uPM3: radical prostatectomy findings. Mod Pathol 19:630–633
46. van Gils MP, Hessels D, Hulsbergen-van de Kaa CA, Witjes JA, Jansen CF, Mulders PF et al (2008) Detailed analysis of histopathological parameters in radical prostatectomy specimens and PCA3 urine test results. Prostate 68:1215–1222
47. Ploussard G, Durand X, Xylinas E, Moutereau S, Radulescu C, Forgue A et al (2011) Prostate cancer antigen 3 score accurately predicts tumour volume and might help in selecting prostate cancer patients for active surveillance. Eur Urol 59:422–429
48. Gleason DF, Mellinger GT (1974) Prediction of prognosis for prostatic adenocarcinoma by combined histological grading and clinical staging. J Urol 111:58–64
49. Larre S, Ronsin C, Irani J (2010) Immediate impact of ultrasound-guided prostate biopsies on PCA3 score. Eur Urol 57:1121–1122
50. van Gils MP, Hessels D, Peelen WP, Vergunst H, Mulders PF, Schalken JA (2009) Preliminary evaluation of the effect of dutasteride on PCA3 in post-DRE urine sediments: a randomized, open-label, parallel-group pilot study. Prostate 69:1624–1634
51. Hessels D, Smit FP, Verhaegh GW, Witjes JA, Cornel EB, Schalken JA (2007) Detection of TMPRSS2-ERG fusion transcripts and prostate cancer antigen 3 in urinary sediments may improve diagnosis of prostate cancer. Clin Cancer Res 13:5103–5108
52. Laxman B, Morris DS, Yu J, Siddiqui J, Cao J, Mehra R et al (2008) A first-generation multiplex biomarker analysis of urine for the early detection of prostate cancer. Cancer Res 68:645–649
53. Ouyang B, Bracken B, Burke B, Chung E, Liang J, Ho SM (2009) A duplex quantitative polymerase chain reaction assay based on quantification of alpha-methylacyl-CoA racemase transcripts and prostate cancer antigen 3 in urine sediments improved diagnostic accuracy for prostate cancer. J Urol 181:2508–2513; discussion 13–4
54. Rigau M, Morote J, Mir MC, Ballesteros C, Ortega I, Sanchez A et al (2010) PSGR and PCA3 as biomarkers for the detection of prostate cancer in urine. Prostate 70:1760–1767
55. Danila DC, Heller G, Gignac GA, Gonzalez-Espinoza R, Anand A, Tanaka E et al (2007) Circulating tumor cell number and prognosis in progressive castration-resistant prostate cancer. Clin Cancer Res 13:7053–7058
56. Vaananen RM, Rissanen M, Kauko O, Junnila S, Vaisanen V, Nurmi J et al (2008) Quantitative real-time RT-PCR assay for PCA3. Clin Biochem 41:103–108
57. Marangoni K, Araujo TG, Neves AF, Goulart LR (2008) The -786 T>C promoter polymorphism of the NOS3 gene is associated with prostate cancer progression. BMC Cancer 8:273
58. Shaw G, Price AM, Ktori E, Bisson I, Purkis PE, McFaul S et al (2008) Hedgehog signalling in androgen independent prostate cancer. Eur Urol 54:1333–1343
59. Jost M, Day JR, Slaughter R, Koreckij TD, Gonzales D, Kinnunen M et al (2010) Molecular assays for the detection of prostate tumor derived nucleic acids in peripheral blood. Mol Cancer 9:174
60. van der Poel HG, McCadden J, Verhaegh GW, Kruszewski M, Ferrer F, Schalken JA et al (2001) A novel method for the determination of basal gene expression of tissue-specific promoters: an analysis of prostate-specific promoters. Cancer Gene Ther 8:927–935
61. Fan JK, Wei N, Ding M, Gu JF, Liu XR, Li BH et al (2010) Targeting Gene-ViroTherapy for prostate cancer by DD3-driven oncolytic virus-harboring interleukin-24 gene. Int J Cancer 127:707–717
62. Hessels D, Schalken JA (2009) The use of PCA3 in the diagnosis of prostate cancer. Nat Rev Urol 6: 255–261

Part IX

Tumor Markers – A Critical Revision: Various Protein Markers

Biomarker in Cisplatin-Based Chemotherapy for Urinary Bladder Cancer

18

Thorsten H. Ecke

Abstract

The treatment of metastasized bladder cancer has been evolving during recent years. Cisplatin based chemotherapy combinations are still gold standard in the treatment of advanced and metastasized bladder cancer. But new therapies are approaching. Based to this fact biological markers will become more important for decisions in bladder cancer treatment. A systematic MEDLINE search of the key words "cisplatin", "bladder cancer", "DNA marker", "protein marker", "methylation biomarker", "predictive marker", "prognostic marker" has been made. This review aims to highlight the most relevant clinical and experimental studies investigating markers for metastasized transitional carcinoma of the urothelium treated by cisplatin based regimens.

Keywords

Adjuvant chemotherapy • Bax • Bcl-2 • Biomarker • Bladder cancer • CD40 • Chemotherapy • Cisplatin • C-reactive protein (CRP) • Emmprin • ERCC1 • HER2/neu • Human epidermal growth factor receptor 2 (HER-2) • Ki-67 • MDR1 • Metallothionein (MT) • p53 • Smac/DIABLO • Survivin • Tissue polypeptide antigen (TPA) • TLX3 gene • Transcription factor TFAP2α

18.1 Introduction

Bladder cancer is a potentially curable malignancy, but for patients with muscle-invasive disease, there is a high risk of metastases and cancer-related death [1]. The gold standard treatment of muscle-invasive bladder cancer (pT2+) is still an early radical cystectomy [2].

Adjuvant chemotherapy for locally advanced urinary bladder cancer is still a problem [3, 4].

T.H. Ecke (✉)
Department of Urology, HELIOS Hospital Bad Saarow, Pieskower Str. 33, D-15526 Bad Saarow, Germany
e-mail: thorsten.ecke@helios-kliniken.de

R. Scatena (ed.), *Advances in Cancer Biomarkers*, Advances in Experimental Medicine and Biology 867, DOI 10.1007/978-94-017-7215-0_18

New biomarkers could help to stratify risk groups and find out which patients benefit from adjuvant strategies after surgery [5–7].

Common sites of metastasis include regional lymph nodes, bone, lung and liver. From the low cure rates achieved with radical cystectomy, there is strong evidence that bladder cancer is a systemic disease. The limitations of local treatment are well-documented: a local control rate of 30 % with radiation treatment, and 50–70 % with radical cystectomy [5]. Since the initial reports of the effectiveness of cisplatin in the treatment of advanced bladder cancer, there has been a steady flow of chemotherapeutic agents shown to be effective. While response rates and complete response (CR) rates have increased with the use of combination chemotherapy, this has not translated into survival in advanced disease of more than 16 months [8]. While searching for more effective agents and combinations attention has been given to the roles of neoadjuvant and adjuvant chemotherapy in an effort to improve the cure rate achieved with surgery alone.

18.2 Part One: Cisplatin as Therapy in Cancer

18.2.1 In General

Cis-diamminedichloroplatinum (II) is the first of a group of platinum coordination complexes with antineoplastic activity to be studied in humans [9]. In 1969, Rosenberg was the first who demonstrated that platinum compounds inhibit cell division in *Escherichia coli* [10].

Especially cisplatin exerts its cytotoxic as well as radiosensitizing potential when cells proliferation into the S/G2/M phases. This effect may be less operative, and radiotherapy less effective, when cells are in the G0 phase, as indicated by a low Ki-67 index [11].

18.2.2 In Bladder Cancer

Advanced transitional cell carcinoma of the urothelium is moderately sensitive to chemotherapy, and there are a number of agents that produce response rates in the 10–40 % range [12–14].

Methotrexate and cisplatin have long been considered the most active agents [8]. In phase II studies, single-agent cisplatin produces response rates of about 35 % overall, with a range of 26–65 %. Complete responses are unusual [15, 16].

In the past decade, several new chemotherapeutic agents have shown activity against advanced transitional cell carcinoma, including the taxanes paclitaxel and docetaxel [17], and gemcitabine [18]. Nowadays gemcitabine and cisplatin are gold standard for metastasized urothelial cancer [2]. New substances like vinflunine maybe could have the power to bring change in the second-line treatment of metastasized bladder cancer [19].

Since information about predictive factors for response and survival are needed for selection of patients who are likely to benefit from new combinations and for stratification purposes in randomized trials, an analysis of the predictive factors for response and survival with the regimen containing PCG has been performed [20]. The factors that were associated with decreased survival in univariate analysis were performance status >0, presence of visceral metastasis, and more than one site of malignant disease.

It was hypothesized that cisplatin-based chemotherapy applied before or after surgery for locally advanced bladder cancer would increase survival in high-risk patient population. Although several randomized trials have been conducted, none of them conclusively demonstrated a significant survival benefit. However, improved progression-free survival was observed after adjuvant MVAC compared with observation [21].

Chemotherapy has been used in two phases of treatment: as radiosensitizers, given concurrently with radiation treatment and as adjuvant treatment, recognizing that survival will only be improved by the successful treatment of micrometastases [5].

18.2.3 Adjuvant and Neo-adjuvant Chemotherapy

In the randomized multicenter phase III study of Lehmann et al. the MVEC standard therapy failed to outperform the less toxic CM regimen [22]. Unfortunately due to the lack of an observation arm the CM regimen could not recommended as standard for adjuvant bladder cancer.

Neo-adjuvant cisplatin combination chemotherapy has a modest survival benefit, with those patients achieving a complete response after chemotherapy having the best outcome. There are several potential benefits to the use of perioperative chemotherapy in the neo-adjuvant rather than the adjuvant setting [23]. First, administration of chemotherapy before surgery avoids the potential for postoperative recovery and complications that might affect the ability to receive a maybe more needed adjuvant chemotherapy. In a trial of 140 patients with localized bladder cancer randomized to RC with plus adjuvant chemotherapy vs. RC with chemotherapy before and afterward, nine assigned to immediate surgery never received chemotherapy [24]. Second, the use of neo-adjuvant chemotherapy allows for in vivo drug sensitivity testing, which might also provide important prognostic information [25]. Third, chemotherapy might lead to tumor down staging and allow for less morbid surgery or potentially convert unresectable to resectable disease. Surgery after chemotherapy appears to provide a benefit in patients who achieve a major response after chemotherapy for unresectable or regionally metastatic bladder cancer [26]. Finally, the ability to monitor the primary tumor during treatment allows for discontinuation of ineffective chemotherapy if there is evidence of disease progression. But most trials of chemotherapy given before radical cystectomy or radiotherapy have failed to improve survival significantly; many of these studies had sample sizes that were too small for important changes in survival to be detected [27]. A systematic review and meta-analysis from 10 randomized trials has shown that neo-adjuvant platinum-based combination chemotherapy is associated with a 5 % benefit in overall survival at 5 years and a 13 % reduction in the risk of death ($p=0.016$) [28]. In the report of Sonpavde et al. about neo-adjuvant chemotherapy was described that conventional first-line platinum-based combination chemotherapy with gemcitabine/cisplatin and standard methotrexate, vinblastine, doxorubicin and cisplatin yields high response rates, but suboptimal long-term outcomes for advanced urothelial cancer. The emergence of novel biological agents offers the promise of improved outcomes. Neo-adjuvant therapy preceding cystectomy for muscle-invasive bladder cancer provides an important paradigm and an interesting approach in developing novel agents [3]. But in this report also new agents for metastatic bladder cancer are described. Neo-adjuvant therapy with cisplatin-based regimens (GC, MVAC) has been shown to be safe and does not increase the risk of postoperative complications [29].

In the review of Sawhney et al. randomized clinical trials of neo-adjuvant cisplatin-based combination chemotherapy for locally advanced bladder cancer has shown a survival benefit over cystectomy alone [30].

The major advantage for the use of adjuvant chemotherapy is treatment based upon pathological criteria, with the ability to select those patients at high risk of recurrence, who are likely to benefit the most from chemotherapy, and to avoid unnecessary treatment of patients with low-risk disease [23].

There have been several prospective trials designed to evaluate adjuvant chemotherapy, but all have been fraught with problems, leading to significant limitations in interpretation [4, 31]. In an early trial evaluating single-agent cisplatin, 77 patients with invasive, non-metastatic bladder cancer were randomly assigned to either observation or three courses of postoperative cisplatin chemotherapy [4]. Although there was no significant difference in survival between the two arms, in the cisplatin group, 24 % required dose reduction and 19 % refused treatment. Skinner et al. [31] reported a prospective comparative trial of adjuvant chemotherapy or observation in patients with invasive or node positive disease. In that study there was a significant delay in time to progression with adjuvant chemotherapy, with 70 % of patients assigned to chemotherapy free of disease at 3 years, vs. 46 % in the observation group ($p=0.001$).

In the meta-analyses of Vale analyses were based on 498 patients from six trials, representing 90 % of all patients randomized in cisplatin-based combination chemotherapy trials and 66 % of patients from all eligible trials [32]. The overall hazard ratio for survival of 0.75 suggests a 25 % relative reduction in the risk of death for chemotherapy compared to that on control.

In general, the problem of these studies regarding adjuvant chemotherapy is mostly the low number of included patients, use of substandard chemotherapy, early stopping of patient entry, irrelevant end points or a lack of recommendations concerning salvage chemotherapy for relapse or metastases [33]. Following the EAU guidelines for invasive bladder cancer adjuvant chemotherapy is not recommended for clinical routine use [2]. Although the role of adjuvant chemotherapy for invasive bladder cancer is not fully confirmed, it represents a reasonable treatment for patients who have not received neo-adjuvant chemotherapy and for those with extravesical extension and/or node-positive disease after radical cystectomy [23].

18.2.4 Combinations

In the early 1980s, cisplatin and methotrexate were combined in several different schedules designed to minimize the nephrotoxicity of the combination [8]. Randomized multicenter trials have demonstrated superior progression-free survival after treatment with three to four courses of MVAC/MVEC [34]. The prognosis of patients with metastatic transitional cell carcinoma remains poor, with a median survival of only 12–14 months [1]. Furthermore the MVAC regimen is relatively toxic, especially in elderly patients and for patients who have a poor performance status. In general, no benefit in overall survival could be found.

Gemcitabine is a pyramidine antimetabolite that has activity against urothelial cancer with an overall response rate of 30 % in previously treated and untreated patients [35]. In particular, in metastatic urothelial cancer, gemcitabine alone yielded response rates of 23–29 % with a complete response rate of 4–13 %, in both previously treated and untreated patients [14].

GC was compared with MVAC in a large, multicenter, randomized phase III study with 405 included patients [1]. It was powered to detect a 33 % difference in survival, which it failed to do. No apparent difference was observed in survival, with median survivals of 13.8 months (GC) and 14.8 months (MVAC). GC was better tolerated than MVAC, with a lower toxic death rate, less neutropenic fever, mucositis and alopecia, and less hospitalization.

Well known clinical prognostic factors, such as performance status, level of plasma alkaline phosphatase, and presence or absence of visceral metastases, are reported to correlate well with outcome of treatment [1, 36] and are presently included in the decision about treatment strategies for the individual patient. The study of Niegisch et al. carried out several prognostic factors. This group randomized 102 patients receiving gemcitabin/cisplatin and 357 patients receiving vinflunine. In a multivariate analyses the factors only lymph nodes involved, alkaline phosphatase, low hemoglobin, Karnofsky performance index, interval between end of first-line and start of second-line chemotherapy were prognostical important [37].

Nevertheless it can be pointed out that chemotherapy in advanced bladder cancer has reached a plateau with no evidence of survival improvement using new combinations [1]. Therefore it is a coming interested in the development of new treatment strategies for these patients. Better understanding of the genetic basis of chemotherapy response may offer promise in better treatment strategies [13, 20, 38].

18.3 Part Two: Based on the Mechanism

For bladder cancer, genome-wide expression profiling has been used to identify genes predictive of response in a neo-adjuvant setting [39]. In the past, several genes and gene products have been described to modify the cellular response to chemotherapeutic agents in vitro and in vivo. Bladder cancer cells can stimulate more angiogenesis than normal urothelium, and increased micro vessel density is an independent prognostic indicator of recurrence and poor survival. In muscle-invasive bladder cancer, micro vessel count correlates significantly with the presence of occult lymph-node metastases [8].

As cisplatin is still regarded the main active drug in urothelial bladder cancer treatment, it is biologically plausible that the expression of an established modifier of the cellular platin response correlates with treatment efficacy [7]. The cytotoxic effect of cisplatin-based chemotherapy has been attributed to the formation of bulky platinum DNA adducts. Cisplatin resistance appears to be associated with the removal of these adducts by the nucleotide excision repair (NER) system, which plays a major part in cisplatin resistance [40].

The major DNA lesions induced by cisplatin are intrastrand DNA crosslinks between two guanines or guanine and adenine, accounting together for ~90 % of the platination lesions [41]. In contrast, interstrand crosslinks (ICLs) between the two DNA strands are minor lesions, accounting for less than 5 % of all cisplatin lesions [42].

A report from Sidransky et al. demonstrated the clonality of multiple bladder tumors from different sites [43]. Miayo showed concordant genetic alterations in asynchronous tumors from individual patients [44]. These studies suggest that urothelial bladder cancer appearing at different times and sites may be derived from the same neoplastic clone.

Miura et al. tried to clarify the molecular mechanisms underlying cisplatin resistance in bladder cancer. The bladder cancer cell line HT1376, and conducted large-scale analyses of the expressed proteins using two-dimensional gel electrophoresis was coupled with mass spectrometry. In that very experimental study the authors could find adseverin (SCIN) and its binding to voltage-depended channels (VDAC) as inhibitor of mitochondria-mediated apoptosis in cisplatin-resistant cells. Targeting the VDAC-SCIN interaction may offer a new therapeutic strategy for cisplatin-resistant bladder cancer [45].

In fact, there are only few studies that found chemotherapy response modifiers. Several gene products have been described to modify the cellular response to chemotherapeutic agents in vitro and to correlate with clinical outcome in vivo. For example, excision repair cross-complementing 1 (*ERCC1*) is a component of nucleotide excision repair (NER) pathway, a major repair mechanism of DNA damage induced by platin compounds reacting with DNA and forming inter- and intra-strand cross links. The balance of DNA damage to DNA repair dictates tumor cell death or survival after cisplatin therapy [46]. *ERCC1* expression as detected by immunochemistry as well as gene expression has been linked to response and survival in other studies with platin-based therapies [7, 47, 48]. ERCC1 is the lead enzyme in the NER process. High ERCC1 levels are associated with increased removal of platinum-induced DNA adducts and relative platinum resistance [49].

Another important example is the multidrug resistance gene 1 (*MDR1*). It encodes an integral membrane protein named P-glycoprotein (Pgp) or an ATP-binding cassette subfamily B which acts as an energy-dependent cellular efflux pump [50]. Anticancer drugs were found to induce *MDR1* gene [51]. Although cisplatin is not considered as a substrate of Pgp, some studies have suggested an altered expression of MDR1 after cisplatin administration, possibly resulting in decreased cytotoxic efficacy [52–54]. Hoffmann et al. wrote that the positive correlation of his and other studies between high MDR1 expression and inferior survival and progression-free survival after adjuvant cisplatin-based chemotherapy does not automatically imply a causative role of Pgp [7].

18.4 Part Three: Cisplatin Based Chemotherapy in Bladder Cancer and Protein Markers

Most tumor markers are protein markers. Predictive as well as prognostic markers will become important in future in decision making for clinical work. This part is an overview about protein based markers who will answer questions for invasive bladder cancer patients receiving cisplatin based chemotherapy.

Cell lines often can help in the beginning of experimental studies to identify key proteins for further work. Many studies have to begin with cell lines to identify the most interesting proteins.

An important point to evaluate a study in this review is to describe whether a marker is prognostic or predictive factor. Predictive factors can make a decision which therapy is better; prognostic factors can make a decision if a therapy is necessary or useful.

Another point is that many studies combine cell lines and clinical samples in one study. In Table 18.1 there is an overview about the most important studies, Table 18.2 shows some important studies in detail. At last Table 18.3 gives an overview for all important markers of this review.

18.4.1 Emmprin and Survivin

Another very interesting protein is emmprin (*BSG*) that has been used in many studies, two of them focus on the question of emmprin as marker in cisplatin based therapy for bladder cancer [55, 56]. Emmprin is a 46.6-kDa membrane protein mapped to 19p13.3. It is a modulator of metalloproteinases and is up-regulated in bladder cancer compared with normal urothelium [57]. Studies showed that emmprin enhances growth and resistance to chemotherapy via the phosohatidylinositol 3-kinase/Akt pathway in a hyaluron-dependent manner [38, 58].

Survivin (*BIRC5*) is localized to 17q25 and is a 16.6-kDa protein present in the cytoplasm and nucleus. Several slica variants have been reported [59, 60]. The variant 3B is described to be in the cytoplasm and is functionally relevant as it is described to inhibit apoptosis via cytoplasmic caspases [61]. High levels of surviving have been associated with poor prognosis in bladder cancer [61]. Survivin has also been described to be a predictor of cisplatin resistance in gastric cancer, as well as in different cell lines [62, 63].

Table 18.1 Protein based markers

Marker	Chemotherapy	Cell line	Clinical	N	Prognostic	Predictive	Reference
Bax	Cisplatin based radiatio	No	Yes	62	No	Yes	[74]
Bcl-2	Cisplatin based radiatio	No	Yes	62	No	Yes	[74]
CRP	Cisplatin + Radiatio	No	Yes	88	Yes	No	[93]
EGFR	MCV + Radiatio	No	Yes	73	Yes	Yes	[96]
Emmprin	cisplatin-based	Yes	Yes	124	Yes	No	[55]
Emmprin	MVAC	No	Yes	27	No	Yes	[56]
ERCC1	MVEC vs. CM	No	Yes	108	Yes	No	[7]
ERCC1	GC vs. GCT	No	Yes	57	Yes	Yes	[47]
ERCC1	Cisplatin-based	No	Yes	89	No	Yes	[48]
Galectin-7	Cisplatin-based	Yes	No	17	No	Yes	[92]
HER-2	MCV + Radiatio	No	Yes	55	Yes	Yes	[96]
HER-2	MVEC	No	Yes	114	Yes	No	[6]
Ki-67	Cisplatin based radiatio	No	Yes	136	No	No	[11]
Ki-67	Cisplatin based radiatio	No	Yes	62	No	Yes	[74]
Lapatinib	GTC	Yes	No	n.d.	No	Yes	[120]
MDR1	MVEC vs. CM	No	Yes	108	Yes	No	[7]
MIB-1	Cisplatin-based	No	Yes	118	No	Yes	[101]
Metallothionein	Cisplatin-based	No	Yes	118	No	Yes	[101]
P-glycoprotein	Cisplatin-based	No	Yes	118	No	Yes	[101]
Smac/DIABLO	Cisplatin-based	Yes	Yes	84	Yes	No	[97]
Survivin	cisplatin-based	No	Yes	124	Yes	No	[55]
Survivin	MVAC	No	Yes	27	No	Yes	[56]
TFAP2α	Cisplatin-based	Yes	Yes	282	No	Yes	[91]
TPA	MVEC	No	Yes	58	Yes	No	[76]

Table 18.2 Selected studies with results

Study	Patients	Marker	Chemo regimen	Median follow-up	End point	Result
Matsumoto et al. [74]	$n=62$ T1: 12 T2: 20 T3: 25 T4: 5 G1: 0 G2: 15 G3: 53 N+: 1 N0 61	Bax/Bcl-2 ratio Ki-67 P53 Apoptosis index (AI)	CRT with cisplatin	34	Survival	Survival rate with Ki-67-positive tumors significantly lower than those of Ki-67-negative tumors ($P<0.05$)
Matsumoto et al. [114]	$n=67$ T1G3: 12 T2: 22 T3: 28 T4: 5 N+: 0 N0: 67	P53 P73	CRT with cisplatin	32.6	Survival	TP73 as independent predictive factor of poor survival ($P=0.0002$)
Bellmunt et al. [47]	$n=57$ Metastatic or locally advanced bladder cancer ECOG 0: 23 ECOG 1: 34	ERCC1 BRCA1 RRM1 Caveolin-1	GC ($n=14$) vs. GCT ($n=43$)	19	Survival Progress	Median survival higher in low ERCC1 levels ($P=0.03$)
Hoffmann et al. [7]	$n=108$ T1: 4 T2: 18 T3: 68 T4: 8 N+: 66 N0: 42	ERCC1 MDR1	CM ($n=56$) vs. M-VEC ($n=52$)	~60	Survival Progress	Expressions of MDR1 and ERCC1 independently associated with overall PFS ($P=0.001$) Median OS higher in low ERCC1 levels ($P=0.19$)
Kim et al. [48]	$n=89$ Advanced urothelial cancer	ERCC1	Cisplatin-based	53.7	Survival Progress	Longer PFS associated with ERCC-1-negative patients ($p=0.03$); median OS not associated mit ERCC1 levels ($p=0.73$); no independent prognostic factor for PFS

(continued)

Table 18.2 (continued)

Study	Patients	Marker	Chemo regimen	Median follow-up	End point	Result
Yoshida et al. [93]	$n=88$	CRP	Cisplatin + RT	33	Survival	High CRP level before therapy was associated with cancer-specific survival ($P=0.003$)
						CRP and cT stage were independent prognostic indicators for CSS ($P=0.046$)
Siu et al. [101]	$n=118$ G1: 2 G2: 17 G3: 90 ECOG 0: 12 ECOG 1: 78 ECOG 2: 20 ECOG 3: 6	P53 MT P-glycoprotein MIB-1	M-VAC ($n=69$) vs. CMV ($n=45$)	~12	Survival	Overexpression of MT in patients with metastatic disease was associated with a shorter survival ($P=0.04$)
Weiss et al. [11]	$n=136$ T1: 28 T2: 81 T3/4: 27 G1: 5 G2: 60 G3: 71	Ki-67	Cisplatin + RT ($n=86$) vs. RT alone ($n=50$)	43	Progress	Association between high Ki-67 index and CR for patients receiving RCT (93 % vs. 66 %; $p=0.001$)
Tsai et al. [6]	$n=114$	HER2	MVEC ($n=30$) vs. surgery alone ($n=26$)	27	Survival Progress	HER2 was associated with PFS ($p=0.02$) and disease-specific OS ($p=0.005$); HER2 was a significant prognostic factor for PFS in chemotherapy receiving patients ($p=0.03$) and disease-specific OS ($p=0.02$)
Nordentoft et al. [91]	$n=282$ pT2-T4b N0: 124 N+: 158	TFAP2α	Cisplatin-based	n.d.	Survival	Low TFAP2α was associated with increased OS ($p=0.048$)
						TFAP2α as strong independent predictive marker for a good response and survival after cisplatin-containing chemotherapy

(continued)

Table 18.2 (continued)

Study	Patients	Marker	Chemo regimen	Median follow-up	End point	Result
Als et al. [55]	$n=124$ T4b N2-3 or M1	Survivin Emmprin	MVAC or GC	56.5	Survival	Emmprin and survivin are independent prognostic factors for response and survival after chemotherapy: emmprin expression ($P<0.0001$), survivin expression ($P<0.0001$)
Pollard et al. [56]	$n=27$	Survivin Emmprin GGH DBI	MVAC	n.d.	Survival	DBI as significant marker for survival ($p=0.046$)
Schmidt et al. [76]	$n=58$	TPA	MVEC	n.d.	Survival Progress	High sensitivity: 96.6 %
						No predictive marker
Chakravati et al. [96]	$n=73$ T2-T4a	HER-2 EGFR P53 pRB p16	CRT with cisplatin	n.d.	Survival CR	EGFR positivity was associated with improved OS ($p=0.044$), disease-specific survival (DSS) ($p = 0.042$)

Als et al. performed a study to identify molecular markers for survival in locally advanced and/or metastatic bladder cancer following cisplatin-based chemotherapy [55]. In their study the protein products emmprin and survivin were validated using immunohistochemistry. Multivariate analysis identified emmprin expression and survivin expression as independent prognostic markers for poor outcome, together with the presence of visceral metastases. In the clinical good prognostic group of patients without visceral metastases, both markers showed significant discriminating power as supplemental risk factors ($p<0.0001$). Protein expression assessed by immunohistochemistry was strongly correlated to response to chemotherapy. Also in that study two different cisplatin-based regimens have been performed. Nevertheless this is one of the important data presenting novel molecular factors of independent prognostic significance for the outcome of cisplatin-based chemotherapy in advanced bladder cancer. The study group proposed that after testing in an independent prospective randomized study survivin and emmprin may help to identify patients with either a high or a low probability of benefit from cisplatin containing chemotherapy.

Another study about emmprin and survivin was performed by Pollard et al. This group evaluated an approach that combines genomic, proteomic, and therapeutic outcome datasets to identify novel putative urinary biomarkers of clinical outcome after neoadjuvant MVAC. Using this method, they identified gamma-glutamyl hydrolase (GGH), emmprin, survivin, and diazepam-binding inhibitor (DBI). Using disease-free survival as a marker for clinical outcome, this group evaluated the ability of GGH, emmprin, survivin, and DBI expression in tumor tissue to stratify 27 patients treated with neoadjuvant MVAC. DBI ($p=0.046$) but not GGH ($p=0.190$), emmprin ($p=0.066$), or survivin ($p=0.393$) successfully stratified patients. The authors supposed that methotrexate and also the

Table 18.3 Overview of all used markers

Marker	Characteristic	Protein	Other	Therapeutic	Reference
AQ4N	Prodrug	No	Yes	Yes	[116]
Bax	Protein	Yes	No	No	[74]
Bcl-2	Protein	Yes	No	No	[74]
BRCA1	Gene	Yes	No	No	[47]
Caveolin-1	Gene	Yes	No	No	[47]
CD40	Tumor necrosis factor	Yes	No	Yes	[89, 90]
CRP	Protein	Yes	No	No	[93]
EGFR	Membrane-bound receptor	Yes	Yes	Yes	[96]
Emmprin	Protein	Yes	Yes	Yes	[55, 56]
ERCC1	Gene	Yes	Yes	No	[7, 41, 47, 48]
Galectin-7	Protein	Yes	No	No	[92]
HER-2	Protein	Yes	Yes	Yes	[88, 96, 105]
Ki-67	Nuclear protein	Yes	No	No	[11, 74]
Lapatinib	Tyrosin kinase inhibitor	No	Yes	Yes	[120]
MDR1	Gene	Yes	Yes	No	[7]
MIB-1	Gene	No	Yes	No	[101]
Metallothionein	Cytosolic protein	No	Yes	No	[101]
P-glycoprotein	Integral membrane protein	Yes	No	No	[101]
pRB	Gene	No	Yes	No	[96]
TP53	Tumor suppressor gene	Yes	Yes	No	[74, 101, 105, 106, 114]
TP73	Tumor suppressor gene	Yes	Yes	No	[114]
RRM1	Gene	Yes	No	No	[47]
S100P	Calcium-binding protein	Yes	No	Yes	[104]
Smac/DIABLO	Protein	Yes	No	No	[97]
Survivin	Protein	Yes	Yes	Yes	[55, 56]
TFAP2α	Protein	No	Yes	Yes	[91]
TLX3	Gene	No	Yes	Yes	[118]
TPA	Tumor associated antigen	Yes	No	No	[76, 80]
XAF1	Apoptosis-associated gene	No	Yes	Yes	[113]
XIAP	Apoptosis-associated gene	No	Yes	Yes	[113]

other agents in the MVAC regimen may have the ability to diminish the effects of GGH activity inside the cell, thus increasing the viability of methotrexate within the cell, or they are more efficacious than methotrexate and thus drive the clinical outcome to a higher degree. Although these predictive results were obtained on tumor tissues, the presence of GGH and DBI in urine serves as a rationale for developing them as urinary markers of clinical outcomes for patients treated with neo-adjuvant MVAC [56].

18.4.2 Bax and Bcl-2

It is known that Bax and Bcl-2 regulate apoptosis downstream of p53 [64]. Bcl-1 blocks cell death following various stimuli, demonstrating a death spearing effect [65]; however, overexpression of Bax has a pro-apoptotic effect and Bax also counters the anti-apoptotic activity of Bcl-2 [66]. It has been proposed that the ratio of Bcl-2 to Bax or other members of the Bcl-2 family may govern the sensitivity of cells to apoptotic stimuli [67, 68].

Recent studies have suggested that the indexes for p53, Bcl-2, Bax and Ki-67 may correlate with the grade, stage or prognosis of bladder cancer [69]. The bcl-2 family of proteins is also involved in the regulation of apoptosis. Bcl-2 expression has been linked to poorer survival in patients with invasive bladder cancer treated with synchronous chemo-radiotherapy [70] and its overexpression with poorer survival in a group of patients with bladder cancer treated with neo-adjuvant chemotherapy [71].

18.4.3 Ki-67

The study of Weiss et al. [11] was performed to investigate whether the addition of chemotherapy to radiotherapy (RT) is beneficial in bladder tumors with rapid proliferation. Ki-67 recognizes a nuclear protein forming part of the DNA replicase complex [72] and is widely used to determine the proliferation activity of tumors. The Ki-67 index was evaluated by immunohistochemistry on pretreatment biopsies from 136 patients treated by transurethral tumor resection and RT or cisplatin-based radiochemotherapy. Ki-67 expression was correlated with response to RT/RCT and long-term local control rates. A statistically significant association between high Ki-67 index and CR was noted for patients receiving RCT ($p=0.001$), but not for patients treated with RT alone ($p=0.12$). They found out that increased pretreatment proliferation is an independent predictor for tumor response and local control when chemotherapy was given in conjunction with radiotherapy. The Ki-67 index reflects the biological aggressiveness of tumors and has been shown to correlate with known prognostic factors such as tumor grade and stage [72, 73].

Another study about biomarkers and radiochemotherapy in bladder cancer was performed by Matsumoto et al. Local advanced bladder cancer was treated by radiation combined with cisplatin therapy. A retrospective analysis was conducted to predict the clinical response to radio-chemotherapy based on the immunohistochemistry of apoptosis-related proteins. Mucosal biopsy was performed before and after therapy. Paraffin-embedded tumor specimens were examined for Ki-67, p53, Bcl-2 and Bax; the Bax/Bcl-2 ratio and apoptosis index (AI). The survival rate of patients with Ki-67-positive tumors was significantly lower than those of patients with Ki-67-negative tumors ($p<0.05$). No significant correlation was observed between the expression of any protein, the AI and the clinical response. However, the Bax/Bcl-2 ratio showed a significant association with the CR rate ($p=0.0289$). The results of this study suggest that the combined assessment of Bcl-2 and Bax protein expression may be used to predict a clinical response to CRT based on the Bax/Bcl-2 ratio determined before therapy. The Ki-67 index may be a useful predictor of prognosis in patients treated by CRT [74].

18.4.4 Tissue Polypeptide Antigen (TPA)

Another classic tumor marker for bladder cancer as tumor-associated antigen is TPA [75]. Schmidt et al. used TPA for monitoring bladder cancer patients after cisplatin-based chemotherapy [76]. In that study 58 patients with advanced bladder cancer were treated with MVEC chemotherapy. TPA was registered before each course of chemotherapy and 3 months after the last application. The sensitivity for locally advanced tumors was 90.9 %, for tumors with lymph node metastases 100 % and for tumors with distant metastases 100 % also, overall 96.6 %. No statistically significant different values between each tumor group were found. In 85.7 % a concordant reaction of TPA values and clinical status was notable. In conclusion, this study could not show any predictive power of this marker, though the sensitivity and specificity is higher than in several other studies [77–79]. Nevertheless, the authors conclude that TPA is a valuable and a reliable marker for monitoring therapeutic efficacy of chemotherapy for advanced bladder cancer.

The use of TPA is well known in bladder cancer [78, 79]. The group of van der Gaast et al. evaluated the use of TPA in serum for monitoring disease activity of bladder cancer during chemotherapy [80]. They found that in most patients with elevated TPA levels who responded to chemotherapy, TPA levels rapidly returned to normal. It is concluded that serial measurement of TPA for monitoring disease activity has limited value because of the low sensitivity of TPA, especially for patients with early-stage cancer, and because of the occurrence of false positive results.

18.4.5 MDR1 and ERCC1

In a study of Hoffmann et al. from 2010 interesting results have been presented. They hypothesized that assessing the gene expression of the chemotherapy response modifiers multidrug resistance gene 1 (*MDR1*) and excision repair cross-complementing 1 (*ERCC1*) may help identify the group of patients benefiting from cisplatin-based adjuvant chemotherapy [7]. Formalin-fixed paraffin-embedded tumor samples from 108 patients with locally advanced bladder cancer, who had been enrolled in AUO-AB05/95, a phase III trial randomizing a maximum of three courses of adjuvant CM versus MVEC, were included in the study. Tumor cells were analyzed for MDR1 and ERCC1 expression using a quantitative real-time RT-PCR assay. Expressions of MDR1 and ERCC1 were independently associated with overall progression-free survival. The correlation of high MDR1 expression with inferior outcome was stronger in patients receiving MVEC, whereas ERCC1 analysis performed equally in the CM and MVEC groups. High MDR1 and ERCC1 gene expressions are associated with inferior outcome after cisplatin-based adjuvant chemotherapy for locally advanced bladder cancer. A major limitation in this study is the fact that because of the lack of observation in one study arm, it is impossible to decide whether expressions of MDR1 and ERCC1 are prognostic or predictive markers [7]. Years before Petrylak et al. reported that MVAC treatment of bladder leads to transactivation and significantly increased expression of MDR1, although this result was not obtained in an outcome-driven study [81].

Bellmunt et al. has performed a study about ERCC1 as prognostic marker for bladder cancer patients receiving cisplatin-based chemotherapy. Messenger RNA expression levels of ERCC1, breast cancer 1 (BRCA1), ribonucleotide reductase subunit M1 (RRM1) and caveolin-1 were determined by RT-PCR in tumor DNA from 57 advanced and metastatic bladder cancer patients treated with either GC or PCG polychemotherapy. Levels were correlated with survival, time to disease progression and chemotherapy response. Median survival was significantly higher in patients with low ERCC1 levels ($p=0.03$). A trend towards longer time to progression was observed in patients with tumors expressing low levels of all markers. On multivariate analysis with pretreatment prognostic factors, ERCC1 emerged as an independent predictive factor for survival. The results of the study indicate that ERCC1 may predict survival in bladder cancer treated by platinum-based therapy [47]. Concluding this study includes also two different cisplatin-based regimens with a low number of patients and a low follow-up; a demonstration of a relationship between molecular marker level and chemotherapy response could not be presented. At the moment there is one recruiting study in www.clinicaltrials.gov measuring ERCC1 and BRCA1 in a cisplatin containing regimen for urinary bladder cancer. In this phase I study with the protocol number NCT01182168 gemcitabine and cisplatin plus everolimus the safety of this regimen at different dose levels will be evaluated (http://www.clinicaltrials.gov/ct2/show/NCT01182168).

As it is known that cell lines derived from metastasized germ cell tumors are hypersensitive to cisplatin reflecting the clinical response

Usanova et al. performed a study to investigate the formation and repair of intrastrand and interstrand crosslinks (ICLs) induced by cisplatin in testis tumor cells and resistant bladder cancer cells. Their data indicate that downregulation of ERCC1-XPF increased the sensitivity to cisplatin, as shown by the higher level of apoptosis. The increase in sensitivity was statistically significant but small, perhaps due to the relatively long cultivation period following after siRNA transfection, and variations in transfection efficiency [41].

Another study about ERCC1 was performed by Kim et al. to find out if immunohistochemical expression of ERCC1 can predict objective tumor response and cancer-specific survival in patients with advanced urothelial carcinoma treated with cisplatin-based chemotherapy. In this retrospective analysis pretherapeutic samples of 89 patients with urothelial cancer has been examined. ERCC1 expression was assessed by immunohistochemistry. This group found a statistical significance ($p=0.03$) comparing the progression-free survival of ERCC-1-negative and ERCC-1-positive patients. They concluded that this result suggest a negative contribution by ERCC1 expression to PFS in metastatic urothelial carcinoma patients treated with cisplatin-based chemotherapy [48].

18.4.6 Human Epidermal Growth Factor Receptor 2 (HER-2)

Tsai et al. evaluated the impact of HER-2 immunoreactivity on clinical outcome in locally advanced urothelial carcinoma patients who received surgery alone, or MVEC as adjuvant chemotherapy. The group studied 114 formalin-fixed paraffin-embedded specimens obtained from locally advanced urothelial carcinoma patients receiving surgery alone or adjuvant MVEC. The authors evaluated HER-2 immunoreactivity using immunohistochemical staining and explored the influence of pathological parameters and HER-2 immunoreactivity on PFS and disease-specific OS. In their results they could show that urothelial carcinoma of the bladder had a significantly higher frequency of HER-2 immunoreactivity than that of the upper urinary tract. Overall, nodal status was a strong and independent prognostic indicator for clinical outcome. HER-2 immunoreactivity was significantly associated with PFS ($p=0.02$) and disease-specific OS ($p=0.005$) in advanced urothelial carcinoma patients. As for patients with adjuvant MVEC, HER-2 immunoreactivity was a significant prognostic factor for PFS ($p=0.03$) and disease-specific OS ($p=0.02$) using univariate analysis, but not multivariate analysis, and not for patients receiving watchful waiting. They concluded that HER-2 immunoreactivity might have a limited prognostic value for advanced urothelial carcinoma patients with adjuvant MVEC [6]. Also other studies could show the important role of HER-2 in urinary bladder cancer, muscle-invasive carcinomas had higher HER-2 levels and nearly all HER-2-positive tumors have HER-2-positive metastases [82, 83]. The study group of Kruger et al. could show in a cohort of 138 samples that HER-2 status was an independent predictor for disease related survival [84].

A Phase II trial was carried out by Hussain et al. in which 59 patients with HER-2/neu-positive metastatic urothelial cell cancer were treated with the human anti HER-2/neu monoclonal antibody trastuzumab in combination with carboplatin, gemcitabine, and paclitaxel. HER-2/neu overexpression rates were prospectively evaluated by IHC, gene amplification and/or elevated serum HER-2/neu. 52.3 % of registered patients were HER-2/neu positive. HER-2/neu-positive patients had more metastatic sites and visceral metastasis than did HER-2/neu negative patients. Median time to progression and survival were 9.3 and 14.1 months, respectively [85].

HER-2 expression in bladder cancer has been extensively studied, but reports referring to its prognostic value have been mixed. A recent cohort study demonstrated HER-2 expression in 45 % of bladder tumors and showed a statistically significant correlation with higher grade, tumor recurrence, and survival [86]. In patients with muscle-invasive bladder cancer, a retrospective IHC study has shown HER-2 overexpression to be an independent predictor of reduced cancer-specific survival [84]. In contrast, another prospective study found that HER-2 overexpression in the context of paclitaxel-based chemotherapy significantly decreased the risk of death [87]. The usefulness of HER-2 overexpression was described in a case report by Amsellem-Ouazana [88].

18.4.7 CD40

CD40, a tumor necrosis factor receptor family member, is an emerging target for cancer therapy being best appreciated as an important regulator of the anti-tumor immune response. Vardouli et al. reported the development of a replication-defective recombinant adenovirus (RAd) vector expressing human CD40 ligand and showed that sustained engagement of the CD40 pathway in malignant cells results in direct anti-proliferative and pro-apoptotic effects. Transduction of CD40-positive carcinoma cell lines with RAd-hCD40L potently inhibits their proliferation in vitro, whereas CD40-negative lines remain unresponsive. The results implicated in understanding the multifaceted anti-tumor activities of the CD40 pathway in carcinomas, which thus offer an attractive option for future clinical application, and a direct therapeutic effect due to gene transfer could be shown [89].

Another experimental study was performed by Ghamade et al. who could show in mice that recombinant CD40 ligand therapy has significant antitumor effects on CD40-positive ovarian tumor and demonstrates an augmented effect with cisplatin [90].

18.4.8 Others

Nordentoft et al. published 2011 an interesting study to find another prognostic factor. After cell line analyses (T24 and SW780) the transcription factor TFAP2α was identified. Expression and localization was assessed by immunohistochemistry using a tissue microarray (TMA) containing 282 bladder cancer tumors from patients with locally advanced (pT2-T4b and N1-3) or metastatic disease. All patients had received cisplatin containing chemotherapy. TFAP2α was identified as a strong independent predictive marker for a good response and survival after cisplatin-containing chemotherapy in patients with advanced bladder cancer. Strong TFAP2α nuclear and cytoplasmic staining predicted good response to chemotherapy in patients with lymph node metastasis, whereas weak TFAP2α nuclear staining predicted good response in patients without lymph node metastasis. High levels of nuclear and cytoplasmic TFAP2a protein were a predictor of increased overall survival and progression free survival in patients with advanced bladder cancer treated with cisplatin based chemotherapy [91].

In the study of Matsui et al. they assessed the possibility of galectin-7 to accelerate cisplatin-induced cell killing in vitro and also to predict chemosensitivity against cisplatin in urothelial cancer patients. The expression of galectin-7 was analyzed in five bladder cancer cell lines with different p53 status after treatment with cisplatin. The relationship between the expression of galectin-7 and the response to neoadjuvant chemotherapy was analyzed in a small number of 17 bladder cancer specimens. In clinical samples, the expression levels of galectin-7 were significantly lower in urothelial carcinomas compared with normal urothelium. When chemosensitivity was tested, its expression levels were higher in the chemosensitive group than in the chemo resistant group. Galectin-7 is a candidate for a predictive marker of chemo sensitivity against cisplatin [92].

An unusual study was performed by Yoshida et al. They investigated the effect of C-reactive protein (CRP) level on the prognosis of patients with muscle-invasive bladder cancer treated with radio-chemotherapy, as it is increasingly recognized that the presence of a systemic inflammatory response is associated with poor survival in various malignancies. In this retrospective study ($n=88$) radio-chemotherapy comprised external beam radiotherapy to the bladder (40 Gy) with two cycles of cisplatin [93]. CRP is a classic parameter for infections [94] and there are so many interactions in tumor patients that it seems not very sensitive [95]. Nevertheless, multivariate analysis of Yoshida et al. showed that CRP and tumor stage were independent prognostic indicators for cancer-specific survival [93].

Chakravarti et al. found out that EGFR expression was intriguingly associated with improved response to radio-chemotherapy [96]. Nevertheless, the group could not specifically address the issue of tumor cell proliferation. But the published results from 73 patients could show a strong association between EGFR expression and cell proliferation in bladder cancer and appears to correlate significantly with improved outcome in bladder cancer, whereas HER-2 expression is significantly associated only with reduced CR rates after radio-chemotherapy. In combination with the results of Weiss et al. [11], it could be hypothesized that EGFR may be a molecular marker of enhanced proliferation which in turn renders cells more responsive to radio-chemotherapy.

Mizutani et al. performed a study to evaluate the relationship between progression of disease and caspase (Smac/DIABLO) expression by clinical pathological analysis of patients with bladder cancer. Patients with invasive bladder cancer expressing Smac/DIABLO had a longer postoperative disease-specific survival than those without Smac/DIABLO expression after radical cystectomy in the 5-year follow-up. The cisplatin-resistant bladder cancer cell line (T24/CDDP) and the adriamycin-resistant cell line (T24/ADR) showed lower level of Smac/DIABLO expression, compared with the T24 parental line. In conclusion, the study demonstrates for the first time that Smac/DIABLO expression was down-regulated in bladder cancer, especially in high grade muscle-invasive bladder cancer, and that lower Smac/DIABLO expression in bladder cancer predicted a worse prognosis. In addition, the cisplatin-resistant T24/CDDP line and the adriamycin-resistant T24/ADR line expressed lower level of Smac/DIABLO expression. These results suggest that Smac/DIABLO expression in bladder cancer may be used as a prognostic parameter, and that low Smac/DIABLO expression in bladder cancer may be associated with resistance to chemotherapy [97].

Another attempt to find out a prognostic marker in blood was performed by Soygür et al. [98]. They wanted to assess the prognostic value of peripheral blood lymphocyte subsets in patients with bladder cancer who were treated with neo-adjuvant chemotherapy. Peripheral blood samples were assessed in both groups using monoclonal antibodies. Patients with bladder cancer who achieved complete or partial responses and those who had progression of the disease after MVEC chemotherapy were compared according to the pretreatment values of the peripheral blood lymphocyte subsets. There were no significant differences in B lymphocyte levels between the groups. In patients with bladder cancer, the percentages of T lymphocytes ($p<0.01$), natural killer (NK) cells ($p<0.05$) and the CD4+/CD8+ ratio ($p<0.05$) were significantly lower than in the control group. In patients who responded to the chemotherapy regimen, the pretreatment values of T lymphocytes ($p<0.001$), the CD4+/CD8+ ratio ($p<0.01$) and NK cell levels ($p<0.01$) were significantly higher than in the patients who did not. In patients with invasive bladder carcinoma, cell-mediated immunity may have a role in the resistance to this malignancy and in these patients the pretreatment levels of T lymphocyte subsets may be an indicator of the potential response to chemotherapy.

Metallothionein (MT) is the last presented marker in that section of the review. MTs are a family of cytosolic proteins rich in sulfhydryl-containing cysteine residues, whose major physiological function seems to involve the absorption, transport, and metabolism of essential trace metals such as copper and zinc [99]. They are normally found at low concentrations in various tissues but are readily inducible by a variety of stimuli, including steroids, heavy metals, and lymphokines. Experimental evidence has linked the overexpression of cellular MT with resistance to alkylating agents and cisplatin [100], but the precise mechanism of action is unknown. Although the results of this study are interesting, it is confusing that more than three different cisplatin-based chemotherapy regimens have been performed. In the study of Siu et al. tissue from primary tumors was analyzed for 118 patients with urothelial cancer who subsequently received cisplatin-based chemotherapy. Immunohistochemical staining was performed for nuclear p53 reactivity, MT, P-glycoprotein, and for the cell proliferation marker MIB-1. ECOG performance status ($p=0.0025$), tumor grade ($p=0.03$), percentage of MT staining ($p=0.01$), and percentage-intensity index of MT staining ($p=0.04$) were significant predictors of response to chemotherapy. Expression of p53, P-glycoprotein, and MIB-1 did not predict for survival. Overexpression of MT was associated with a poorer outcome from chemotherapy, possibly due to cisplatin resistance [101]. In this study MT was the only biomarker demonstrated to be an independent predictor for tumor response.

A cell line study of Mizutani et al. could show that combination treatment with anti-Fas mAb and cisplatin resulted in a synergistic cytotoxicity against acquired and natural cisplatin-resistant bladder cancer cells. This synergistic effect was not restricted to established cell lines but was also observed in freshly derived cancer cells. These findings suggest that the therapeutic use of cisplatin in combination with Fas-mediated immunotherapy might be useful in patients with cisplatin-resistant or immunotherapy-resistant bladder cancer [102].

Zhang et al. investigated the short-term effects of TNP-470 in combination with cisplatin in a rat model of bladder cancer. Treatment of TNP-470 with or without cisplatin was performed, the states of angiogenesis, apoptosis and cell proliferation were evaluated in rat bladder cancer. In comparison with untreated tumors, they noted a significantly decreased microvessel density (MVD) in the rat bladder cancer treated by TNP-470, and a significantly increased apoptotic index (AI) when treated by cisplatin. In TNP-470 plus cisplatin-treated tumors, both significantly decreased MVD and increased AI were observed in rat bladder cancers [103].

Another protein that has been evaluated was the calcium-binding protein S100P. The group of Shiota et al. found a cisplatin resistance for that protein. With cDNA microarrays using two pairs of cisplatin-resistant bladder cancer cell lines they could show that S100P mRNA expression was significantly reduced in cisplatin-resistant cells. The over-expression of the protein S100P in cisplatin resistant cells resulted in an increased sensitivity to cisplatin [104].

18.5 Part Five: Cisplatin Based Chemotherapy in Bladder Cancer and DNA Markers

It seems to be difficult to separate the markers into protein, DNA and methylation markers, because most of the studies have examined markers from different fields. That's why a mixture of markers in the different sections is possible.

Tsai et al. performed a study about the prognostic values of p53 and HER2/neu co-expression for muscle-invasive bladder cancer. They could show that in invasive bladder cancer, p53 was an important prognostic factor since its expression correlated with tumor grade and stage, even nodal status, whereas HER-2/neu did not show prognostic significance. Tumors with p53 and HER-2/neu coexpression were associated with nodal metastases, probably resulting in decreased progression-free survival [105]. These results might imply that p53- and HER-2/neu co-expressing tumors had a more aggressive behavior.

Konstantakou et al. examined the apoptosis-related cellular responses to cisplatin exposure in two bladder cancer cell lines (RT4 and T24) characterized by different malignancy grade and *p53* genetic status. Both RT4 and T24 cell types proved to be vulnerable to cisplatin apoptotic activity. The differential resistance of RT4 and T24 cells to cisplatin-induced apoptosis was associated with an RT4-specific phosphorylation (Ser15; Ser392) pattern of p53. The results strongly support the role of p53-dependent and p53-independent transcriptional responses in cisplatin-induced apoptosis of bladder cancer cells [106].

p53 initiates the effectors of apoptosis, and can induce either apoptosis or DNA repair [107]. Its overexpression or accumulation has been shown to predict for a better outcome for patients with bladder cancer after radiotherapy [108] or systemic chemotherapy [109]. P53 is the most intensively studied tumor suppressor gene, but in retrospective analyses on whether a mutation of *TP53* confers an increased responsiveness or an increased resistance to chemotherapy or radiation gives conflicting data [110].

Many tumor suppressor gene modifications, including those of p53, pRB, p16, p21, thrombospondin-1, glutathione, and factors controlling the expression and function of the epidermal growth factor receptor (EGFR) have been shown in retrospective analyses to influence the outcomes of patients with bladder cancer following various treatments [110–112].

Pinho et al. performed a study to investigate whether mRNA expression of the apoptosis-associated genes, XAF1 and XIAP, in bladder cancer patients correlates with response to neoadjuvant treatment. In a small sample size of 14 bladder cancer patients the authors found that the clinical response in the XAF1-high subset was remarkably higher compared with the XAF1-low subset. Although the number of patients was so low this study should be pointed out because it is one of the few studies to address the role of XAF1 in a clinical setting. The data presented here identify XAF1 as a novel predictive and prognostic factor in bladder cancer patients [113].

Matsumoto performed a study to find a marker for predicting patient outcome as well as clinical response after chemoradiation therapy (CRT) by investigating allelic loss of apoptosis-related genes. They investigated allelic imbalances at 14 loci on chromosomes 17p13 and 1p36 including the p53 and p73 gene regions by fluorescent multiplex PCR based on DNA from paraffin-embedded tumor specimens and peripheral blood. There was no statistical correlation between treatment response and clinical parameters, such as tumor grade, stage, radiation dose, or CDDP dose. The frequencies of allelic imbalance for TP53 and TP73 were 21 % and 56 %, respectively; neither was correlated with clinical treatment response and tumor stage or grade. There was no statistical correlation between treatment response and allelic imbalance at the other 12 loci. An allelic imbalance of TP73 was the most remarkable independent predictive factor of poor patient survival ($p=0.0002$). The authors suggested that the allelic loss of the TP73 gene predicts a clinical outcome of locally advanced bladder cancer when treated by CRT [114].

Williams et al. presented a in vivo study about the hypoxia-targeted cytotoxin AQ4N (banoxantrone). AQ4N is a prodrug that is enzymatically converted to the cytotoxic DNA-binding agent AQ4 [115]. The aim of the study was to quantify tumor exposure to AQ4 following treatment with AQ4N, and to relate exposure to outcome of treatment. The bladder cancer cell line RT112 was used in the experiments. This is the first demonstration that AQ4N will increase the efficacy of chemoradiotherapy in preclinical models [116].

18.6 Part Six: Cisplatin Based Chemotherapy in Bladder Cancer and Methylation Markers

Beside protein and DNA markers nowadays methylation markers will change some thoughts of the development and recurrence of bladder cancer [117]. It seems difficult to find studies with methylation markers in studies with bladder cancer treated with cisplatin based therapies. In our pubmed search of the literature only one interesting study concerning this question could be found.

Tada et al. presented the gene TLX3 that is unmethylated in cisplatin sensitive cells and methylated in resistant cells. 21 % of the measured samples of bladder cancer showed the methylated pattern in TLX3. Cisplatin sensitivity was closely associated with the methylation status of TLX3. This could be an interesting and useful novel biomarker for cisplatin resistance. As many other markers that are important in diagnostics, it could also be used to design therapies to counteract the resistance against cisplatin in bladder cancer [118].

18.7 Part Seven: New Alternatives for Therapy

Because of the availability of the tissue before and after chemotherapy, it might be possible to determine molecular and biological characteristics that predict chemo sensitivity. However, it is possible that activity in early disease might not translate to efficacy in advanced disease [3].

Ongoing research aims to individualize patient treatment by identifying biomarkers that predict a pathological complete response to neo-adjuvant treatment, and to incorporate novel molecular target therapies into the preoperative plan [23].

High expression of vascular endothelial growth factor (VEGF) mRNA is significantly associated with early recurrence, progression to invasion and a high expression of p53 protein. The key roles of angiogenesis and its controlling factors in the initiation of bladder cancer and its subsequent progression and invasion make it a strong candidate for targeting for therapeutic manipulation [108].

Shiota et al. concluded in their study that S100P might thus represent a molecular marker predicting cisplatin sensitivity and a molecular therapeutic target for cisplatin-based chemotherapy [104].

McHugh et al. presented several studies investigating the potential utility of lapatinib as an adjunct to chemotherapy in human bladder cancer cell lines. Lapatinib is a dual inhibitor of ErbB-1/-2 receptors. The bladder cancer cell lines RT112 and J82 were used to determine the growth inhibitory effects of lapatinib and the clinically relevant combination of gemcitabine and cisplatin chemotherapy. Lapatinib cooperates with clinically relevant cytotoxic agents and may have therapeutic utility in the management of chemotherapy-naive metastatic bladder cancer. Lapatinib may also enable reduced-dose chemotherapy, a potential toxicity-sparing strategy [119]. Though this is very experimental and difficult to translate to clinical practice because of the cytotoxic effect of triple agent chemotherapies [1, 13], another study of the same group indicated that a combinatorial approach involving gemcitabine, paclitaxel, and cisplatin, and lapatinib may have therapeutic potential in a subset of bladder tumors depending on the genetic context [120].

In the study of Mita et al. only one patient with bladder cancer was included. This patient receiving AMG 386 plus C/P for bladder cancer refractory to gemcitabine/cisplatin had a complete response at week 8. Concluding weekly administration of AMG 386 in combination with three common chemotherapy regimens was well tolerated in patients with advanced solid tumors. No pharmacokinetic interactions between AMG 386 and any of the tested chemotherapy regimens were noted [121].

The prognostic significance of alterations in the mediators of cell adhesion has been less clearly defined. One family of matrix-degrading proteases, the human matrix metalloproteinases, is of great interest as a therapeutic target, but early clinical trials have been disappointing [8].

The development of novel biologic agents targeted against tumor specific growth factor pathways or against angiogenesis has resulted in positive studies in a variety of solid tumors [5]. Two classes of agents that have received great attention are inhibitors of EGFR, including EGFR1 and EGFR2 (HER-2/neu), and inhibitors of VEGF or its receptors [122]. It is known that many bladder tumors express products of the EGFR family, that over-expression correlates with an unfavorable outcome, and that inhibition of these pathways may have an antitumor effect [83, 123–126]. The mechanisms underlying EGFR overexpression in bladder cancer are not clear, but, despite the absence of altered gene copy numbers or chromosomal translocations, elevated levels of EGFR mRNA have been detected in tumor compared with normal urothelium [124]. Overexpression of growth-signal receptors, such as EGFR, may make tumor cells hyper-responsive to normal tissue levels of growth factors. EGFR expression in bladder cancer is associated with high tumor stage and grade, and with rapid tumor proliferation. Expression of TGFα, which is considered to be the more important ligand for EGFR in bladder tumors, correlates strongly with death from bladder cancer. The mitogen-activated protein kinase (MAPK) pathway is involved in the transduction of signals from membrane-bound receptors, such as EGFR, which makes its therapeutic manipulation an attractive subject for research [127].

With technique of double transgenic mice, overexpression of EGFR alone or in cooperation with Ha-ras expression, derived specifically in the urothelium by the uroplakin-II gene promoter, can promote urothelial hyperplasia, but not tumorigenesis. In cooperation with p53 dysfunction, bound and inactivated by SV40 T antigen, EGFR overexpression can promote bladder tumor growth and convert carcinoma in situ into high-grade bladder carcinoma [128].

Both p53 and HER-2/neu are associated with topoisomerase IIα (TopoIIα) gene, a target gene from many cytotoxic drugs, such as anthracycline (e.g. doxorubicin). TopoIIα amplification and deletion may account for both relative chemo sensitivity and resistance to anthracycline therapy depending on the specific genetic defect at the TopoIIα locus, which is adjacent to the HER-2/neu locus at 17q12-q21 [129]. P53 can regulate the minimal promoter of the human TopoIIα gene and stimulate its catalytic activity by enhancing the rate of ATP hydrolysis [130]. Therefore, the TopoIIα gene could be affected by either p53 or HER-2/neu. Further, HER-2/neu-mediated chemo resistance to DNA-damaging agents (e.g. etoposide) may require the activation of Akt and PI3K, then Mdm phosphorylation which could degrade p53 [131].

Another way is the inhibition of angiogenetic inducers, which are frequently present in bladder tumors [5]. Several studies have correlated elevated VEGF levels or cyclooxygenase-2 (COX-2) expression with disease recurrence or progression [132, 133]. This is the basis for combining in prospective clinical trials, anti-VEGF therapy or various COX-2 inhibitors with other forms of cytotoxic therapy [5].

Early work with TKIs assessed the potential as primary chemotherapeutic agents. They have been shown to be capable of inhibiting the growth of bladder cancer cells in vitro [134], as well as inhibiting other cancer cell lines [135]. In vivo work assessing the inhibitory effect of small molecule TKIs, using subcutaneous inoculation of human tumor cell lines in athymic nude mice, has confirmed earlier in vitro results [136]. Gefitinib has been shown to be well tolerated in Phase I testing, involving patients with a range of EGFR-expressing malignancies [137].

Targeting surviving as an anticancer strategy by antisense oligonucleotides has been investigated in several cancer types [61].

The long-term follow-up of patients in clinical trials has enabled us to identify clinical prognostic indicators that allow selection of patients most likely to benefit from treatment and also to stratify future studies. The developments in the understanding of the molecular biology of urothelial cancer carry the promise that they will enable us to refine prognostic predictions, select individually appropriate treatments and develop targeted treatments that exploit genetic differences between normal and malignant urothelial cells [8].

The major challenge for clinical and translational investigators is to design appropriate prospective trials that will identify which molecular tumor markers will be prognostic of outcome and be predictive of whether a patient will be better treated by surgery, radiation or chemotherapy or a combination of these. Only then can molecular tumor markers be incorporated into clinical decision-making and allow physicians to make better treatment choices on behalf of their patients [5].

The other major challenge in the treatment of advanced bladder cancer is to increase survival. Systemic chemotherapy has had a disappointing impact on survival when used as an adjunct to radical cystectomy or radiotherapy. Regimens incorporating novel agents are needed [122].

18.8 Summary

In conclusion, all studies working on this important and interesting field have limitations like small amount of patients, inhomogenous groups, different chemotherapy regimens, a short follow-up time, and/or an insufficient definition of the start and end points as well as an insufficient follow-up schedule. Relatively low patient numbers and a brief follow-up in these studies could also explain the lack of measurable survival benefit from adjuvant chemotherapy. In general, it is important to analyze tumor samples from patients receiving uniform adjuvant chemotherapy in a large randomized multicenter trial. This could increase the ability to identify truly predictive biomarkers.

References

1. von der Maase H, Hansen SW, Roberts JT et al (2000) Gemcitabine and cisplatin versus methotrexate, vinblastine, doxorubicin, and cisplatin in advanced or metastatic bladder cancer: results of a large, randomized, multinational, multicenter, phase III study. J Clin Oncol 18:3068–3077
2. Stenzl A, Cowan NC, De Santis M et al (2011) Treatment of muscle-invasive and metastatic bladder cancer: update of the EAU guidelines. Eur Urol 59:1009–1018
3. Sonpavde G, Sternberg CN (2008) Treatment of metastatic urothelial cancer: opportunities for drug discovery and development. BJU Int 102:1354–1360
4. Studer UE, Bacchi M, Biedermann C et al (1994) Adjuvant cisplatin chemotherapy following cystectomy for bladder cancer: results of a prospective randomized trial. J Urol 152:81–84
5. Kaufman DS (2006) Challenges in the treatment of bladder cancer. Ann Oncol 17(Suppl 5):v106–v112
6. Tsai YS, Tzai TS, Chow NH (2007) Does HER2 immunoreactivity provide prognostic information in locally advanced urothelial carcinoma patients receiving adjuvant M-VEC chemotherapy? Urol Int 79:210–216
7. Hoffmann AC, Wild P, Leicht C et al (2010) MDR1 and ERCC1 expression predict outcome of patients with locally advanced bladder cancer receiving adjuvant chemotherapy. Neoplasia 12:628–636
8. Roberts JT (2005) Chemotherapy for metastatic bladder cancer. Clin Oncol 17:514–523
9. DeConti RC, Toftness BR, Lange RC, Creasey WA (1973) Clinical and pharmacological studies with cis-diamminedichloroplatinum (II). Cancer Res 33:1310–1315
10. Rosenberg B, VanCamp L, Trosko JE, Mansour VH (1969) Platinum compounds: a new class of potent antitumour agents. Nature 222:385–386
11. Weiss C, Rodel F, Ott O et al (2007) Pretreatment proliferation and local control in bladder cancer after radiotherapy with or without concurrent chemotherapy. Strahlentherapie und Onkologie 183:552–556
12. Loehrer PJ Sr, Einhorn LH, Elson PJ et al (1992) A randomized comparison of cisplatin alone or in combination with methotrexate, vinblastine, and doxorubicin in patients with metastatic urothelial carcinoma: a cooperative group study. J Clin Oncol 10:1066–1073
13. Bellmunt J, Guillem V, Paz-Ares L et al (2000) Phase I-II study of paclitaxel, cisplatin, and gemcitabine in advanced transitional-cell carcinoma of the urothelium. Spanish Oncology Genitourinary Group. J Clin Oncol 18:3247–3255
14. Sternberg CN (2000) Gemcitabine in bladder cancer. Semin Oncol 27:31–39
15. Herr HW (1980) Cis-diamminedichloride platinum II in the treatment of advanced bladder cancer. J Urol 123:853–855
16. Soloway MS, Ikard M, Ford K (1981) Cis-diamminedichloroplatinum (II) in locally advanced and metastatic urothelial cancer. Cancer 47:476–480
17. de Wit R, Kruit WH, Stoter G et al (1998) Docetaxel (Taxotere): an active agent in metastatic urothelial cancer; results of a phase II study in non-chemotherapy-pretreated patients. Br J Cancer 78:1342–1345
18. Moore MJ, Tannock IF, Ernst DS et al (1997) Gemcitabine: a promising new agent in the treatment of advanced urothelial cancer. J Clin Oncol 15:3441–3445
19. Gerullis H, Ecke T, Eimer C et al (2011) Vinflunine as second-line treatment in platin-resistant metastatic urothelial carcinoma: a review. Anticancer Drugs 22:9–17
20. Bellmunt J, Albanell J, Paz-Ares L et al (2002) Pretreatment prognostic factors for survival in patients with advanced urothelial tumors treated in a phase I/II trial with paclitaxel, cisplatin, and gemcitabine. Cancer 95:751–757
21. Lehmann J, Franzaring L, Thuroff J et al (2006) Complete long-term survival data from a trial of adjuvant chemotherapy vs control after radical cystectomy for locally advanced bladder cancer. BJU Int 97:42–47
22. Lehmann J, Retz M, Wiemers C et al (2005) Adjuvant cisplatin plus methotrexate versus methotrexate, vinblastine, epirubicin, and cisplatin in locally advanced bladder cancer: results of a randomized, multicenter, phase III trial (AUO-AB 05/95). J Clin Oncol 23:4963–4974
23. Milowsky MI, Stadler WM, Bajorin DF (2008) Integration of neoadjuvant and adjuvant chemotherapy and cystectomy in the treatment of muscle-invasive bladder cancer. BJU Int 102:1339–1344
24. Millikan R, Dinney C, Swanson D et al (2001) Integrated therapy for locally advanced bladder cancer: final report of a randomized trial of cystectomy plus adjuvant M-VAC versus cystectomy with both preoperative and postoperative M-VAC. J Clin Oncol 19:4005–4013
25. Rosenberg JE, Carroll PR, Small EJ (2005) Update on chemotherapy for advanced bladder cancer. J Urol 174:14–20
26. Herr HW, Donat SM, Bajorin DF (2001) Post-chemotherapy surgery in patients with unresectable or regionally metastatic bladder cancer. J Urol 165:811–814

27. (1999) Neoadjuvant cisplatin, methotrexate, and vinblastine chemotherapy for muscle-invasive bladder cancer: a randomised controlled trial. International collaboration of trialists. Lancet 354: 533–540
28. (2003) Neoadjuvant chemotherapy in invasive bladder cancer: a systematic review and meta-analysis. Lancet 361: 1927–1934
29. Grossman HB, Natale RB, Tangen CM et al (2003) Neoadjuvant chemotherapy plus cystectomy compared with cystectomy alone for locally advanced bladder cancer. N Engl J Med 349:859–866
30. Sawhney R, Bourgeois D, Chaudhary UB (2006) Neo-adjuvant chemotherapy for muscle-invasive bladder cancer: a look ahead. Ann Oncol 17:1360–1369
31. Skinner DG, Daniels JR, Russell CA et al (1991) The role of adjuvant chemotherapy following cystectomy for invasive bladder cancer: a prospective comparative trial. J Urol 145:459–464, discussion 464–457
32. (2005) Adjuvant chemotherapy in invasive bladder cancer: a systematic review and meta-analysis of individual patient data Advanced Bladder Cancer (ABC) meta-analysis collaboration. Eur Urol 48:189–199; discussion 199–201
33. Sylvester R, Sternberg C (2000) The role of adjuvant combination chemotherapy after cystectomy in locally advanced bladder cancer: what we do not know and why. Ann Oncol 11:851–856
34. Sternberg CN, Yagoda A, Scher HI et al (1985) Preliminary results of M-VAC (methotrexate, vinblastine, doxorubicin and cisplatin) for transitional cell carcinoma of the urothelium. J Urol 133:403–407
35. Boven E, Schipper H, Erkelens CA et al (1993) The influence of the schedule and the dose of gemcitabine on the anti-tumour efficacy in experimental human cancer. Br J Cancer 68:52–56
36. Bajorin DF, Dodd PM, Mazumdar M et al (1999) Long-term survival in metastatic transitional-cell carcinoma and prognostic factors predicting outcome of therapy. J Clin Oncol 17:3173–3181
37. Niegisch G, Fimmers R, Siener R et al (2011) Prognostic factors in second-line treatment of urothelial cancers with gemcitabine and paclitaxel (German Association of Urological Oncology trial AB20/99). Eur Urol 60:1087–1096
38. Nawroth R, Stohr R, Hartmann A et al (2008) EMMPRIN (CD147). A new key protein during tumor progression in bladder cancer. Der Urologe Ausg A 47:1152–1156
39. Takata R, Katagiri T, Kanehira M et al (2005) Predicting response to methotrexate, vinblastine, doxorubicin, and cisplatin neoadjuvant chemotherapy for bladder cancers through genome-wide gene expression profiling. Clin Cancer Res 11:2625–2636
40. Rosell R, Taron M, Ariza A et al (2004) Molecular predictors of response to chemotherapy in lung cancer. Semin Oncol 31:20–27
41. Usanova S, Piee-Staffa A, Sied U et al (2010) Cisplatin sensitivity of testis tumour cells is due to deficiency in interstrand-crosslink repair and low ERCC1-XPF expression. Mol Cancer 9:248
42. Eastman A (1986) Reevaluation of interaction of cis-dichloro(ethylenediamine)platinum(II) with DNA. Biochemistry 25:3912–3915
43. Sidransky D, Frost P, Von Eschenbach A et al (1992) Clonal origin bladder cancer. N Engl J Med 326:737–740
44. Miyao N, Tsai YC, Lerner SP et al (1993) Role of chromosome 9 in human bladder cancer. Cancer Res 53:4066–4070
45. Miura N, Takemori N, Kikugawa T et al (2012) Adseverin: a novel cisplatin-resistant marker in the human bladder cancer cell line HT1376 identified by quantitative proteomic analysis. Mol Oncol 6:311–322
46. Metzger R, Leichman CG, Danenberg KD et al (1998) ERCC1 mRNA levels complement thymidylate synthase mRNA levels in predicting response and survival for gastric cancer patients receiving combination cisplatin and fluorouracil chemotherapy. J Clin Oncol 16:309–316
47. Bellmunt J, Paz-Ares L, Cuello M et al (2007) Gene expression of ERCC1 as a novel prognostic marker in advanced bladder cancer patients receiving cisplatin-based chemotherapy. Ann Oncol 18:522–528
48. Kim KH, Do IG, Kim HS et al (2010) Excision repair cross-complementation group 1 (ERCC1) expression in advanced urothelial carcinoma patients receiving cisplatin-based chemotherapy. APMIS 118:941–948
49. Li Q, Yu JJ, Mu C et al (2000) Association between the level of ERCC-1 expression and the repair of cisplatin-induced DNA damage in human ovarian cancer cells. Anticancer Res 20:645–652
50. Simon G, Sharma A, Li X et al (2007) Feasibility and efficacy of molecular analysis-directed individualized therapy in advanced non-small-cell lung cancer. J Clin Oncol 25:2741–2746
51. Pastan I, Willingham MC, Gottesman M (1991) Molecular manipulations of the multidrug transporter: a new role for transgenic mice. FASEB J 5:2523–2528
52. Demeule M, Brossard M, Beliveau R (1999) Cisplatin induces renal expression of P-glycoprotein and canalicular multispecific organic anion transporter. Am J Physiol 277:F832–F840
53. Takara K, Tsujimoto M, Kokufu M et al (2003) Up-regulation of MDR1 function and expression by cisplatin in LLC-PK1 cells. Biol Pharm Bull 26:205–209
54. van den Broek GB, Wildeman M, Rasch CR et al (2009) Molecular markers predict outcome in squamous cell carcinoma of the head and neck after concomitant cisplatin-based chemoradiation. Int J Cancer (J Int du Cancer) 124:2643–2650
55. Als AB, Dyrskjot L, von der Maase H et al (2007) Emmprin and survivin predict response and survival

following cisplatin-containing chemotherapy in patients with advanced bladder cancer. Clin Cancer Res 13:4407–4414
56. Pollard C, Nitz M, Baras A et al (2009) Genoproteomic mining of urothelial cancer suggests {gamma}-glutamyl hydrolase and diazepam-binding inhibitor as putative urinary markers of outcome after chemotherapy. Am J Pathol 175:1824–1830
57. Muraoka K, Nabeshima K, Murayama T et al (1993) Enhanced expression of a tumor-cell-derived collagenase-stimulatory factor in urothelial carcinoma: its usefulness as a tumor marker for bladder cancers. Int J Cancer 55:19–26
58. Misra S, Ghatak S, Zoltan-Jones A, Toole BP (2003) Regulation of multidrug resistance in cancer cells by hyaluronan. J Biol Chem 278:25285–25288
59. Zaffaroni N, Pennati M, Daidone MG (2005) Survivin as a target for new anticancer interventions. J Cell Mol Med 9:360–372
60. Moussa O, Abol-Enein H, Bissada NK et al (2006) Evaluation of survivin reverse transcriptase-polymerase chain reaction for noninvasive detection of bladder cancer. J Urol 175:2312–2316
61. Akhtar M, Gallagher L, Rohan S (2006) Survivin: role in diagnosis, prognosis, and treatment of bladder cancer. Adv Anat Pathol 13:122–126
62. Tran J, Master Z, Yu JL et al (2002) A role for survivin in chemoresistance of endothelial cells mediated by VEGF. Proc Natl Acad Sci U S A 99:4349–4354
63. Nakamura M, Tsuji N, Asanuma K et al (2004) Survivin as a predictor of cis-diamminedichloroplatinum sensitivity in gastric cancer patients. Cancer Sci 95:44–51
64. Miyashita T, Krajewski S, Krajewska M et al (1994) Tumor suppressor p53 is a regulator of bcl-2 and bax gene expression in vitro and in vivo. Oncogene 9:1799–1805
65. Vaux DL, Cory S, Adams JM (1988) Bcl-2 gene promotes haemopoietic cell survival and cooperates with c-myc to immortalize pre-B cells. Nature 335:440–442
66. Oltvai ZN, Milliman CL, Korsmeyer SJ (1993) Bcl-2 heterodimerizes in vivo with a conserved homolog, bax, that accelerates programmed cell death. Cell 74:609–619
67. Gazzaniga P, Gradilone A, Vercillo R et al (1996) Bcl-2/bax mRNA expression ratio as prognostic factor in low-grade urinary bladder cancer. Int J Cancer 69:100–104
68. Thomas A, El Rouby S, Reed JC et al (1996) Drug-induced apoptosis in B-cell chronic lymphocytic leukemia: relationship between p53 gene mutation and bcl-2/bax proteins in drug resistance. Oncogene 12:1055–1062
69. Wu TT, Chen JH, Lee YH, Huang JK (2000) The role of bcl-2, p53, and ki-67 index in predicting tumor recurrence for low grade superficial transitional cell bladder carcinoma. J Urol 163:758–760
70. Hussain SA, Ganesan R, Hiller L et al (2003) BCL2 expression predicts survival in patients receiving synchronous chemoradiotherapy in advanced transitional cell carcinoma of the bladder. Oncol Rep 10:571–576
71. Cooke PW, James ND, Ganesan R et al (2000) Bcl-2 expression identifies patients with advanced bladder cancer treated by radiotherapy who benefit from neoadjuvant chemotherapy. BJU Int 85:829–835
72. Bush C, Price P, Norton J et al (1991) Proliferation in human bladder carcinoma measured by Ki-67 antibody labelling: its potential clinical importance. Br J Cancer 64:357–360
73. Mulder AH, Van Hootegem JC, Sylvester R et al (1992) Prognostic factors in bladder carcinoma: histologic parameters and expression of a cell cycle-related nuclear antigen (Ki-67). J Pathol 166:37–43
74. Matsumoto H, Wada T, Fukunaga K et al (2004) Bax to Bcl-2 ratio and Ki-67 index are useful predictors of neoadjuvant chemoradiation therapy in bladder cancer. Jpn J Clin Oncol 34:124–130
75. Bjorklund B (1978) Tissue polypeptide antigen (TPA): biology, biochemistry, improved assay methodology, clinical significance in cancer and other conditions, and future outlook. Antibiot Chemother 22:16–31
76. Schmidt A, Bub P, Ruther U, Eisenberger F (1992) Tissue polypeptide antigen for monitoring of advanced bladder cancer after MVEC chemotherapy. Eur Urol 21(Suppl 1):10–12
77. Sanchez-Carbayo M, Herrero E, Megias J et al (1999) Comparative sensitivity of urinary CYFRA 21–1, urinary bladder cancer antigen, tissue polypeptide antigen, tissue polypeptide antigen and NMP22 to detect bladder cancer. J Urol 162:1951–1956
78. Maulard C, Toubert ME, Chretien Y et al (1994) Serum tissue polypeptide antigen (S-TPA) in bladder cancer as a tumor marker. A prospective study. Cancer 73:394–398
79. Ecke TH, Lenk SV, Schlechte HH, Loening SA (2003) Tissue polypeptide antigen (TPA) in comparison with mutations of tumour suppressor gene P53 (TP53) in patients with bladder cancer. Anticancer Res 23:957–962
80. van der Gaast A, Kirkels WJ, Blijenberg BG, Splinter TA (1992) Evaluation of tissue polypeptide antigen serum levels for monitoring disease activity during chemotherapy in patients with transitional carcinoma of the urinary tract. J Cancer Res Clin Oncol 118:626–628
81. Petrylak DP, Scher HI, Reuter V et al (1994) P-glycoprotein expression in primary and metastatic transitional cell carcinoma of the bladder. Ann Oncol/ESMO 5:835–840
82. Latif Z, Watters AD, Dunn I et al (2003) HER2/neu overexpression in the development of muscle-invasive transitional cell carcinoma of the bladder. Br J Cancer 89:1305–1309

83. Jimenez RE, Hussain M, Bianco FJ Jr et al (2001) Her-2/neu overexpression in muscle-invasive urothelial carcinoma of the bladder: prognostic significance and comparative analysis in primary and metastatic tumors. Clin Cancer Res 7:2440–2447
84. Kruger S, Weitsch G, Buttner H et al (2002) HER2 overexpression in muscle-invasive urothelial carcinoma of the bladder: prognostic implications. Int J Cancer 102:514–518
85. Hussain MH, MacVicar GR, Petrylak DP et al (2007) Trastuzumab, paclitaxel, carboplatin, and gemcitabine in advanced human epidermal growth factor receptor-2/neu-positive urothelial carcinoma: results of a multicenter phase II National Cancer Institute trial. J Clin Oncol 25:2218–2224
86. Chow NH, Chan SH, Tzai TS et al (2001) Expression profiles of ErbB family receptors and prognosis in primary transitional cell carcinoma of the urinary bladder. Clin Cancer Res 7:1957–1962
87. Gandour-Edwards R, Lara PN Jr, Folkins AK et al (2002) Does HER2/neu expression provide prognostic information in patients with advanced urothelial carcinoma? Cancer 95:1009–1015
88. Amsellem-Ouazana D, Beuzeboc P, Peyromaure M et al (2004) Management of primary resistance to gemcitabine and cisplatin (G-C) chemotherapy in metastatic bladder cancer with HER2 overexpression. Ann Oncol/ESMO 15:538
89. Vardouli L, Lindqvist C, Vlahou K et al (2009) Adenovirus delivery of human CD40 ligand gene confers direct therapeutic effects on carcinomas. Cancer Gene Ther 16:848–860
90. Ghamande S, Hylander BL, Oflazoglu E et al (2001) Recombinant CD40 ligand therapy has significant antitumor effects on CD40-positive ovarian tumor xenografts grown in SCID mice and demonstrates an augmented effect with cisplatin. Cancer Res 61:7556–7562
91. Nordentoft I, Dyrskjot L, Bodker JS et al (2011) Increased expression of transcription factor TFAP2alpha correlates with chemosensitivity in advanced bladder cancer. BMC Cancer 11:135
92. Matsui Y, Ueda S, Watanabe J et al (2007) Sensitizing effect of galectin-7 in urothelial cancer to cisplatin through the accumulation of intracellular reactive oxygen species. Cancer Res 67:1212–1220
93. Yoshida S, Saito K, Koga F et al (2008) C-reactive protein level predicts prognosis in patients with muscle-invasive bladder cancer treated with chemoradiotherapy. BJU Int 101:978–981
94. Mortensen RF, Rudczynski AB (1982) Prognostic significance of serum CRP levels and lymphoid cell infiltrates in human breast cancer. Oncology 39:129–133
95. Nicolini A, Carpi A, Rossi G (2007) Relationship of cellular immunity, cytokines and CRP with clinical course in breast cancer patients with endocrine-dependent distant metastases treated with immunotherapy. Cancer Lett 251:330–338
96. Chakravarti A, Winter K, Wu CL et al (2005) Expression of the epidermal growth factor receptor and Her-2 are predictors of favorable outcome and reduced complete response rates, respectively, in patients with muscle-invading bladder cancers treated by concurrent radiation and cisplatin-based chemotherapy: a report from the Radiation Therapy Oncology Group. Int J Radiat Oncol Biol Phys 62:309–317
97. Mizutani Y, Katsuoka Y, Bonavida B (2010) Prognostic significance of second mitochondria-derived activator of caspase (Smac/DIABLO) expression in bladder cancer and target for therapy. Int J Oncol 37:503–508
98. Soygur T, Beduk Y, Baltaci S et al (1999) The prognostic value of peripheral blood lymphocyte subsets in patients with bladder carcinoma treated using neoadjuvant M-VEC chemotherapy. BJU Int 84:1069–1072
99. Hamer DH (1986) Metallothionein. Annu Rev Biochem 55:913–951
100. Kelley SL, Basu A, Teicher BA et al (1988) Overexpression of metallothionein confers resistance to anticancer drugs. Science 241:1813–1815
101. Siu LL, Banerjee D, Khurana RJ et al (1998) The prognostic role of p53, metallothionein, P-glycoprotein, and MIB-1 in muscle-invasive urothelial transitional cell carcinoma. Clin Cancer Res 4:559–565
102. Mizutani Y, Yoshida O, Bonavida B (1998) Sensitization of human bladder cancer cells to Fas-mediated cytotoxicity by cis-diamminedichloroplatinum (II). J Urol 160:561–570
103. Zhang X, Yamashita M, Uetsuki H, Kakehi Y (2002) Short-term effects of TNP-470 in combination with cisplatin in the rat model of bladder cancer. In Vivo 16:293–297
104. Shiota M, Tsunoda T, Song Y et al (2011) Enhanced S100 calcium-binding protein P expression sensitizes human bladder cancer cells to cisplatin. BJU Int 107:1148–1153
105. Tsai YS, Tzai TS, Chow NH et al (2003) Prognostic values of p53 and HER-2/neu coexpression in invasive bladder cancer in Taiwan. Urol Int 71:262–270
106. Konstantakou EG, Voutsinas GE, Karkoulis PK et al (2009) Human bladder cancer cells undergo cisplatin-induced apoptosis that is associated with p53-dependent and p53-independent responses. Int J Oncol 35:401–416
107. Spruck CH 3rd, Rideout WM 3rd, Olumi AF et al (1993) Distinct pattern of p53 mutations in bladder cancer: relationship to tobacco usage. Cancer Res 53:1162–1166
108. Qureshi KN, Griffiths TR, Robinson MC et al (2001) Combined p21WAF1/CIP1 and p53 overexpression predict improved survival in muscle-invasive bladder cancer treated by radical radiotherapy. Int J Radiat Oncol Biol Phys 51:1234–1240

109. Qureshi KN, Griffiths TR, Robinson MC et al (1999) TP53 accumulation predicts improved survival in patients resistant to systemic cisplatin-based chemotherapy for muscle-invasive bladder cancer. Clin Cancer Res 5:3500–3507
110. Cote RJ, Esrig D, Groshen S et al (1997) p53 and treatment of bladder cancer. Nature 385:123–125
111. Sarkis AS, Bajorin DF, Reuter VE et al (1995) Prognostic value of p53 nuclear overexpression in patients with invasive bladder cancer treated with neoadjuvant MVAC. J Clin Oncol 13:1384–1390
112. Rodel C, Grabenbauer GG, Rodel F et al (2000) Apoptosis, p53, bcl-2, and Ki-67 in invasive bladder carcinoma: possible predictors for response to radiochemotherapy and successful bladder preservation. Int J Radiat Oncol Biol Phys 46:1213–1221
113. Pinho MB, Costas F, Sellos J et al (2009) XAF1 mRNA expression improves progression-free and overall survival for patients with advanced bladder cancer treated with neoadjuvant chemotherapy. Urol Oncol 27:382–390
114. Matsumoto H, Matsuyama H, Fukunaga K et al (2004) Allelic imbalance at 1p36 may predict prognosis of chemoradiation therapy for bladder preservation in patients with invasive bladder cancer. Br J Cancer 91:1025–1031
115. Patterson LH (2002) Bioreductively activated antitumor N-oxides: the case of AQ4N, a unique approach to hypoxia-activated cancer chemotherapy. Drug Metab Rev 34:581–592
116. Williams KJ, Albertella MR, Fitzpatrick B et al (2009) In vivo activation of the hypoxia-targeted cytotoxin AQ4N in human tumor xenografts. Mol Cancer Ther 8:3266–3275
117. Esteller M (2008) Epigenetics in cancer. N Engl J Med 358:1148–1159
118. Tada Y, Yokomizo A, Shiota M et al (2011) Aberrant DNA methylation of T-cell leukemia, homeobox 3 modulates cisplatin sensitivity in bladder cancer. Int J Oncol 39:727–733
119. McHugh LA, Kriajevska M, Mellon JK, Griffiths TR (2007) Combined treatment of bladder cancer cell lines with lapatinib and varying chemotherapy regimens–evidence of schedule-dependent synergy. Urology 69:390–394
120. McHugh LA, Sayan AE, Mejlvang J et al (2009) Lapatinib, a dual inhibitor of ErbB-1/-2 receptors, enhances effects of combination chemotherapy in bladder cancer cells. Int J Oncol 34:1155–1163
121. Mita AC, Takimoto CH, Mita M et al (2010) Phase 1 study of AMG 386, a selective angiopoietin 1/2-neutralizing peptibody, in combination with chemotherapy in adults with advanced solid tumors. Clin Cancer Res 16:3044–3056
122. McHugh LA, Griffiths TR, Kriajevska M et al (2004) Tyrosine kinase inhibitors of the epidermal growth factor receptor as adjuncts to systemic chemotherapy for muscle-invasive bladder cancer. Urology 63:619–624
123. Neal DE, Sharples L, Smith K et al (1990) The epidermal growth factor receptor and the prognosis of bladder cancer. Cancer 65:1619–1625
124. Wood DP Jr, Fair WR, Chaganti RS (1992) Evaluation of epidermal growth factor receptor DNA amplification and mRNA expression in bladder cancer. J Urol 147:274–277
125. Lipponen P, Eskelinen M (1994) Expression of epidermal growth factor receptor in bladder cancer as related to established prognostic factors, oncoprotein (c-erbB-2, p53) expression and long-term prognosis. Br J Cancer 69:1120–1125
126. Mellon JK, Lunec J, Wright C et al (1996) C-erbB-2 in bladder cancer: molecular biology, correlation with epidermal growth factor receptors and prognostic value. J Urol 155:321–326
127. Bryan RT, Hussain SA, James ND et al (2005) Molecular pathways in bladder cancer: part 1. BJU Int 95:485–490
128. Cheng J, Huang H, Zhang ZT et al (2002) Overexpression of epidermal growth factor receptor in urothelium elicits urothelial hyperplasia and promotes bladder tumor growth. Cancer Res 62:4157–4163
129. Jarvinen TA, Liu ET (2000) Effects of HER-2/neu on chemosensitivity of tumor cells. Drug Resist Updat 3:319–324
130. Sandri MI, Isaacs RJ, Ongkeko WM et al (1996) p53 regulates the minimal promoter of the human topoisomerase IIalpha gene. Nucleic Acids Res 24:4464–4470
131. Zhou BP, Liao Y, Xia W et al (2001) HER-2/neu induces p53 ubiquitination via Akt-mediated MDM2 phosphorylation. Nat Cell Biol 3:973–982
132. Williams SG, Buscarini M, Stein JP (2001) Molecular markers for diagnosis, staging, and prognosis of bladder cancer. Oncology 15:1461–1470, 1473–1484, 1476; discussion 1476–1484
133. Kim SI, Kwon SM, Kim YS, Hong SJ (2002) Association of cyclooxygenase-2 expression with prognosis of stage T1 grade 3 bladder cancer. Urology 60:816–821
134. Sion-Vardy N, Vardy D, Rodeck U et al (1995) Antiproliferative effects of tyrosine kinase inhibitors (tyrphostins) on human bladder and renal carcinoma cells. J Surg Res 59:675–680
135. Ciardiello F, Caputo R, Bianco R et al (2001) Inhibition of growth factor production and angiogenesis in human cancer cells by ZD1839 (Iressa), a selective epidermal growth factor receptor tyrosine kinase inhibitor. Clin Cancer Res 7:1459–1465
136. Sirotnak FM, Zakowski MF, Miller VA et al (2000) Efficacy of cytotoxic agents against human tumor xenografts is markedly enhanced by coadministration of ZD1839 (Iressa), an inhibitor of EGFR tyrosine kinase. Clin Cancer Res 6:4885–4892
137. Ranson M, Hammond LA, Ferry D et al (2002) ZD1839, a selective oral epidermal growth factor receptor-tyrosine kinase inhibitor, is well tolerated and active in patients with solid, malignant tumors: results of a phase I trial. J Clin Oncol 20:2240–2250

A Critical Approach to Clinical Biochemistry of Chromogranin A

19

Patrizia Bottoni, Teresa De Michele, and Roberto Scatena

Abstract

Chromogranin A (CGA) is a member of the granin family of proteins which are widespread in endocrine, neuroendocrine, peripheral, and central nervous tissues, where they are typically found in secretory granules. It is well accepted that CGA cooperates to regulate synthesis and secretion of these various granule signaling molecules.

Because of its ubiquitous distribution within neuroendocrine tissues, CGA can be a useful diagnostic marker for neuroendocrine neoplasms, including carcinoids, pheochromocytomas, neuroblastomas, medullary thyroid carcinomas (MTC), some pituitary tumors, functioning and non-functioning islet cell tumors and other amine precursor uptake and decarboxylation (APUD) tumors. It is also useful as a prognostic marker for detection of recurrence and monitoring of response to different treatments. As other tumor markers, it is imperative to know its physiology and pathophysiology, its sensitivity and specificity in different neuroendocrine tumors (NETs), and carefully integrate these data with the clinical data of the single patient, to maximize its diagnostic/prognostic index.

Keywords

Amine precursor uptake and decarboxylation (APUD) tumors • Androgen deprivation therapy • Carcinoids • Catestatin • Chromacin • Chromofungin • GE25 • Hook effect • Medullary thyroid carcinomas • Methods • Multiple endocrine neoplasia type 2 • Neuroblastomas • Neuroendocrine tumors (NETs) • Pancreastatin • Parastatin • Pheochromocytomas • Serpinin • Vasostatin I • Vasostatin II • WE14

P. Bottoni • R. Scatena (✉)
Institute of Biochemistry and Clinical Biochemistry, Faculty of Medicine, UCSC – Catholic University of Rome, Gemelli Hospital 8, Largo Gemelli, 00168 Rome, Italy
e-mail: r.scatena@rm.unicatt.it

T. De Michele
Institute of Biochemistry and Clinical Biochemistry, Faculty of Medicine, UCSC – Catholic University of Rome, Gemelli Hospital 8, Largo Gemelli, 00168 Rome, Italy

R. Scatena (ed.), *Advances in Cancer Biomarkers*, Advances in Experimental Medicine and Biology 867, DOI 10.1007/978-94-017-7215-0_19

19.1 Biochemistry

Chromogranin A (CGA), a member of the granin family of acidic proteins (which contain an high percentage of acidic amino acids), present in the secretory granules of a wide variety of endocrine and neuro-endocrine cells. In particular CGA is a 439-amino acid protein – its premature form contains 457 amino acids- with a molecular weight ranging from 48 to 60 kDa, depending on the levels of glycosylation and phosphorylation and with a pI of 4.9. Tipically, human CGA presents 10 dibasic sites, which are potential points for proteolytic cleavage, a particular heat stability due to its high hydrophilic nature and the ability to bind calcium and to form aggregates [1–3].

19.2 Physiology

The exact functions of chromogranins family is not yet fully understood. They possess a typical biophysical aggregation characteristics suggesting a function in the formation of secretory granules. They are precursors of some biologically active peptides and/or they may act as helper proteins in large dense-core vesicle biogenesis and regulated secretion of LDCV (large dense-core vesicle) which package various peptide hormones and neuropeptides. On these molecular basis plasma CgA concentrations seem to be linked with level of catecholamine release and consequent blood pressure. Importantly, at the CNS level, CgA seems to influence the secretion of peptides derived from proopiomelanocortin, so directly and indirectly influencing a lot of endocrine functions and thereby physiological activities (cardiovascular functions, immune responses, tissue remodeling, calcium and glucose metabolism). Moreover, at this level CGA induces microglia to release TNF-α and other neurotoxic cytokines which may promote apoptosis in neurons. On the other side, patients affected by amyotrophic lateral sclerosis show low level of CGA with respect to controls [3–5].

Considering its function as precursor peptide, it is valuable to note that the human CGA gene, located on chromosome 14q32.12 and spans 12192 bp, is organized in eight exons and seven introns. These exons encode for peptides with tangled and diversified biological activities, like:

- The vasorelaxant and cardiosuppressive peptides vasostatin I and II (other biological activities: antimicrobial and antifungal, PTH secretion inhibitor, cell adhesion promoter, intracellular calcium regulator, apoptosis inducer, endothelial cell proliferation/migration inhibitor).
- Chromofungin, which tipically accumulates in the microorganism, and inhibits calcineurin activity.
- Chromacin, which also possesses bacteriostatic activities for Gram-negative and gram-positive bacteria;
- The dysglycemic hormone pancreastatin (which strongly inhibits glucose- induced insulin release from the pancreas, glucose uptake, PTH release, and glycogenolysis; on the other side it stimulates glucagon and histamine release).
- The catecholamine release-inhibitory and antihypertensive peptide catestatin (which inhibits nAchR, reduces cardiac contractility, and acts as vasodilator and inducer of endothelial cell proliferation/migration); moreover, it acts as inducer of pro-inflammatory cytokines and chemotaxis. From this point of view, intriguingly, CgA is a significant component of the plaques in Alzheimer's disease and catestatin seems to have a chemotactic effect on the monocytes that invade and surround the plaques. Lastly, this peptide may directly inhibit growth of fungi, yeast, and bacteria because of its highly cationic nature.
- The autoantigen for type 1 diabetes, WE14 (a modulator of histamine release at the level of mast cells);
- Serpinin which binds to a G protein-coupled receptor to increasing the transcription and biosynthesis of protease nexin-1 (PN-1) which in turn inhibits granule proteins degradation and stimulate LDCV formation;
- GE25 typically expressed by the pituitary gland, gut and pancreas, and
- Parastatin mainly expressed by parathyroids where it inhibits PTH and CgA release [3, 6, 7].

In conclusion, all these physiological functions confirm that CGA and CGA derived peptides prominently function in metabolic and glucose homeostasis, emotional behavior, pain pathways, and blood pressure modulation, and seem to suggest an utility of CGA as potential new biomarker in various diseases and not only in cancer.

19.3 Pathophysiology

Considering the physiological diversified role of CgA and its derivative peptides, it could be possible to hypothesize a pathogenic role of this granin in different diseases, like: cancer, cardiovascular, inflammatory and neurologic diseases. Just as example, it is interesting to note that CgA has a role in neuroinflammation associated to Alzheimer disease. Specifically, it has been reported, in AD brain, highly activated microglia surrounding CGA-positive plaques more frequently than Aβ-positive plaques [8]. Also a mechanistic role in some psychiatric disorders is under evaluation [9–11]. Considering CVD, CgA concentrations correlate with severe diseases like acute coronary syndromes or chronic heart failure. For these conditions both CgA and its peptide derivative catestatin were studied as possible diagnostic and prognostic markers [3, 12, 13].

Interestingly, genetic studies on single-nucleotide polymorphism (SNP) characterization of CgA are consistent with an important functional contribution of this granin to hypertension. These diversified pathophsiological roles, however, impair specificity and sensitivity of CgA as tumor markers and should be carefully evaluated in clinical settings. Therefore, interpretation of CgA results must be in the context of these confounding factors [14, 15].

19.4 Clinical Applications

The chromogranins are ubiquitous components of secretory vesicles; their widespread presence among endocrine tissues has led to their measurement in plasma as useful, albeit relatively nonspecific, markers of neuroendocrine tumors (NETs), including pheochromocytomas and carcinoid tumors. At present, CgA is considered the most useful biomarker of both non-functioning and functioning NETs (being elevated in 60–80 % of patients with NETs) including carcinoids, pheochromocytomas, neuroblastomas, medullary thyroid carcinomas (MTC), some pituitary tumors, functioning and nonfunctioning islet cell tumors and other amine precursor uptake and decarboxylation (APUD) tumors. Interestingly, increased serum chromogranin levels are detected in epithelial cancers with neuroendocrine differentiation, including prostate, breast, ovary, pancreas, and colon and small cell lung carcinoma [16]. In particular, in prostate cancer with a significant neuroendocrine cell subpopulation, Cga may have a role in outcome prediction and follow-up of patients. Importantly, prostate cancer patients with elevated CGA levels, are often resistant to antiandrogen therapy and have a worse prognosis [17, 18].

Considering the main clinical indication, i.e. carcinoid tumors, it is important to stress that these tumors often secrete CGA along with various other substances (serotonin and/or 5-hydroxytryptamine and different peptides, just foregut carcinoids show, at least at initial stages, a low frequency of CgA secretion). Thereby, serum CgA and urine 5-hydroxyindolacetic acid (5-HIAA) are considered the most useful biochemical markers and are first-line tests in disease surveillance of most patients with carcinoid tumors. In this setting, it has been reported a sensitivity of 75–85 % and a specificity of 84–95 % for carcinoid tumors, but some other studies showed much more lower level of specificity/sensitivity [19, 20].

Importantly, the level of CgA showed a good linear correlation with the mass of carcinoid [21, 22].

In pheocromocytomas, elevated levels of CgA are present in about 80 % of patients. However, serum CgA is less sensitive and specific than direct measurement of catecholamine and metabolites serum levels [23, 24].

Recently, CgA showed a strong correlation with 5-years survival of patients with gastroenteropancreatic neuroendocrine tumors [25].

Thereby, CgA is also used together to other biochemical and clinical parameters, to monitor efficacy of various anticancer treatments in NETS [26–29]. Moreover, it seems to represent a sensitive marker for residual or recurrent neuroendocrine neoplasm in already treated patients as well [30, 31].

Interestingly, de Laat et al. [32] showed a low specificity and sensitivity (sensitivity 0.33 and a specificity 0.73) of serum CgA for diagnosing pancreatic neuroendocrine tumors in Multiple Endocrine Neoplasia Type 1 Patients (MEN1). In a similar study, Qiao et al. [33] showed that a CgA cut off values of 74 ng/ml may discriminate patients with non-insulinoma pancreatic NETs from healthy controls, with a sensitivity and specificity of 65.6 % and 91.9 %, respectively.

Recently, Guillemot et al. [34] analyzed the diagnostic sensitivity of CgA-derived peptide WE-14 in patients with pheochromocytoma with respect to CgA and EM66. However results did not show real significant advantages.

As already stressed some non-neuroendocrine tumors (prostate, breast, testicular, ovary, pancreas, and colon and small cell lung carcinoma) might show elevations, usually modest, in serum CGA concentrations. This not only reduce specificity of such a marker for NETs, but it must induce a careful evaluation of clinical picture in patients with apparently unjustified elevations of sCgA.

Intriguingly, Isshiki et al. [35] and Tricoli et al. [36] showed that higher levels of serum CgA are associated with poorly differentiated prostate cancer. Moreover, CgA is also increased after continuous androgen deprivation therapy (ADT) and systemic radionucleotide therapy [37, 38] due to a secondary hyperactivation of neuroendocrine cells . Furthermore, an association between increased CgA and prostate cancer metastasis has been observed as well [39]. Differently, intermittent ADT seems to reduce the levels of CgA, and thus the neuroendocrine differentiation of prostate cancer [35].

Medullary Thyroid Carcinoma (MTC) originates from C Cells of the thyroid. The precursor lesion of the familial variety of MTC is a C-cell hyperplasia. Patients with MEN types 2A and 2B who are at risk for MTC are generally monitored by measurements of serum calcitonin, CEA and chromogranin as well. When the serum concentrations of these biomarkers increases, total thyroidectomy may be considered [40, 41].

19.5 Interfering Clinical Factors

Considering clinical influences, most importantly, CgA is mainly eliminated by kidney, after an hepatic metabolism. The effect of hepatic insufficiency is negligible, while even mild renal impairment can induce significant elevation of sCgA, making single serum CGA measurements, like other biochemical parameters (e.g. high sensitivity troponin assays) interpretable with some difficulty. Serial measurements may have some value in selected patients if the impaired renal function remains stable [42]. Just as example, Canale and Bravo [43] showed that in pheochromocytoma hypertensive patients with CrCl less than 80 mL/min, overall sensitivity, specificity, and accuracy and positive and negative predictive values of serum CgA dropped to 85 %, 50 %, 59 %, 38 %, and 90 %, respectively. Importantly, end-stage renal failure makes single serum CGA measurements uninterpretable.

Moreover sCgA levels can be elevated in patients with hypergastrinemia, and also in atrophic gastritis and pernicious anemia, in these latter conditions the misleading increment depends on a lack of feedback inhibition of gastrin production due to gastric achlorhydria. A similar mechanism is at the basis of the wide range of artifactual CGA elevations in patients treated with proton pump inhibitors (e.g., omeprazole; PPI). It is important to stress that PPI should be discontinued for at least 2 weeks before CGA measurements. Noteworthy, H2-receptor antagonists at modest doses can substitute PPI without a significant risk of false-elevations in CGA. Significant serum elevations of CgA can also be related to corticosteroids administration [44, 45].

19.6 Interfering Methodological Factors

First of all, one of the main difficulties related to CgA measurements arise from the low correlation between different CgA immunoassays. This depends on both the lack of a universal calibration standard and the use of different antibodies which display different cross-reactivity for the various CGA fragments. Hence, results and reference intervals differ significantly among various CGA assays and cannot be directly compared [46, 47]. All that hampers the value of comparisons among patients obtained in different laboratories and also clinical studies comparison realized to validate data on sensitivity/specificity of CgA as tumor marker [22, 24].

Moreover, for CgA assay as with all immunometric assays there is a low, but definite, possibility of false-positive results in patients with heterophilic antibodies, as well. Clinicians and not only laboratorists should know the possibility of such an artifact and evaluate it in the specific clinical setting (concomitant infections and/or autoimmune diseases and/or previous sensitization to rodent proteins and so on) [24].

Also for CgA determinations there is the possibility of an "Hook Effect". It is a well known phenomenon that can occur at extremely high CGA serum concentrations, resulting in a false lower measured CGA levels [46, 47].

19.7 Conclusions

Chromogranin A is the most widely used generic biomarker in monitoring secretory/nonsecretory sympathetic/parasympathetic neuroendocrine tumors. Its diagnostic accuracy depends on the type of tumor, differentiation level and disease extension but also by the method adopted. The sensitivity varies between 52 % and 90 % [30]. Importantly, the possibility of false positives related to athrophic gastritis, Helicobacter pylori infection, PPI therapy, chronic inflammatory diseases and uncontrolled arterial hypertension must be always considered. Therefore, interpretation of CgA results must be in the context of these clinical and methodological confounding factors. These considerations, applicable to the majority of the current tumor markers, are more stringent for chromogranin because of its particular physiology and pathophysiology.

Interestingly, CgA plays an important role in pathologic diagnosis of NETs, while its role as circulating tumor marker is less defined. Moreover, the relationship between immunohistochemistry (IHC) expression and serum levels of CgA has not been yet sufficiently investigated. All that hampers partly the value of CgA for evaluating treatment response and prognosis in neuroendocrine tumors.

Just as example, it could be interesting to cite the recent study of Jilesen et al. [31] which evaluated the diagnostic accuracy of CgA in patients with nonfunctioning pancreatic neuroendocrine tumors and low tumor burden. Results showed that CgA was elevated preoperatively in only 27 % of patients. Moreover, in metastases detection, the positive predictive value for CgA was 50 % and negative predictive value was 81 %. Importantly, in 50 % of the patients with an elevated CgA during follow-up, this test result was false-positive. The conclusion of this research confirmed the moderate diagnostic and prognostic value of CgA in patients with nonfunctioning pancreatic neuroendocrine tumors.

In conclusion, the moderate value of CgA should not induce an underestimation of this marker, as well as other tumor markers, but it must stress the value of an accurate integration of biochemical markers with the clinical picture to maximize their diagnostic/prognostic accuracy.

References

1. Simon JP, Aunis D (1989) Biochemistry of the chromogranin A protein family. Biochem J 262:1–13
2. Sokoll LJ, Rai AJ, Chan DW (2012) Tumor markers. In: Burtis CA, Ashwood ER, Bruns DE (eds) Tietz textbook of clinical chemistry and molecular diagnostics. Elsevier-Saunders, St.Louis, p 650
3. D'Amico MA, Ghinassi B, Izzicupo P, Manzoli L, Di Baldassarre A (2014) Biological function and clinical relevance of chromogranin A and derived peptides. Endocr Connect 3:R45–R54

4. Bartolomucci A, Possenti R, Mahata SK et al (2011) The extended granin family: structure, function, and biomedical implications. Endocr Rev 32: 755–797
5. Borges R, Dominguez N, Smith CB, Bandyopadhyay GK, O'Connor DT, Mahata SK, Bartolomucci A (2013) Granins and catecholamines: functional interaction in chromaffin cells and adipose tissue. Adv Pharmacol 68:93–113
6. Gerdes HH, Glombik MM (2000) Signal-mediated sorting of chromogranins to secretory granules. Adv Exp Med Biol 482:41–54
7. Aunis D, Metz-Boutigue MH (2000) Chromogranins: current concepts. Structural and functional aspects. Adv Exp Med Biol 482:21–38
8. Wu Z, Sun L, Hashioka S, Yu S, Schwab C, Okada R, Hayashi Y, McGeer PL, Nakanishi H (2013) Differential pathways for interleukin-1β production activated by chromogranin A and amyloid β in microglia. Neurobiol Aging 34:2715–2725
9. Jakobsson J, Stridsberg M, Zetterberg H, Blennow K, Ekman CJ, Johansson AG, Sellgren C, Landén M (2013) Decreased cerebrospinal fluid secretogranin II concentrations in severe forms of bipolar disorder. J Psychiatry Neurosci 38:E21–E26
10. Plá V, Paco S, Ghezali G, Ciria V, Pozas E, Ferrer I, Aguado F (2013) Secretory sorting receptors carboxypeptidase E and secretogranin III in amyloid β-associated neural degeneration in Alzheimer's disease. Brain Pathol 23:274–284
11. Guest PC, Schwarz E, Krishnamurthy D, Harris LW, Leweke FM, Rothermundt M, van Beveren NJ, Spain M, Barnes A, Steiner J, Rahmoune H, Bahn S (2011) Altered levels of circulating insulin and other neuroendocrine hormones associated with the onset of schizophrenia. Psychoneuroendocrinology 36:1092–1096
12. Goetze JP, Alehagen U, Flyvbjerg A, Rehfeld JF (2013) Making sense of chromogranin A in heart disease. Lancet Diab Endocrinol 1:7–8
13. Goetze JP, Alehagen U, Flyvbjerg A, Rehfeld JF (2014) Chromogranin A as a biomarker in cardiovascular disease. Biomark Med 8:133–140
14. Zhang K, Rao F, Wang L, Rana BK, Ghosh S, Mahata M, Salem RM, Rodriguez-Flores JL, Fung MM, Waalen J, Tayo B, Taupenot L, Mahata SK, O'Connor DT (2010) Common functional genetic variants in catecholamine storage vesicle protein promoter motifs interact to trigger systemic hypertension. J Am Coll Cardiol 55:1463–1475
15. Yu L, Jiang L, Zhou XJ, Zhu L, Zhang H (2010) Common genetic variants in the chromogranin a promoter are associated with renal injury in IgA nephropathy patients with malignant hypertension. Ren Fail 32:41–46
16. Wu JT, Erickson AJ, Tsao KC, Wu TL, Sun CF (2000) Elevated serum chromogranin A is detectable in patients with carcinomas at advanced disease stages. Ann Clin Lab Sci 30:175–178
17. Sciarra A, Abrahamsson PA, Brausi M, Galsky M, Mottet N, Sartor O, Tammela TL, Calais da Silva F (2013) Intermittent androgen-deprivation therapy in prostate cancer: a critical review focused on phase 3 trials. Eur Urol 64:722–730
18. Sciarra A, Monti S, Gentile V, Mariotti G, Cardi A, Voria G, Lucera R, Di Silverio F (2003) Variation in chromogranin A serum levels during intermittent versus continuous androgen deprivation therapy for prostate adenocarcinoma. Prostate 55:168–179
19. Kocha W, Maroun J, Kennecke H, Law C, Metrakos P, Ouellet JF, Reid R, Rowsell C, Shah A, Singh S, Van Uum S, Wong R (2010) Consensus recommendations for the diagnosis and management of well-differentiated gastroenterohepatic neuroendocrine tumours: a revised statement from a Canadian National Expert Group. Curr Oncol 17:49–64
20. Grimaldi F, Fazio N, Attanasio R, Frasoldati A, Papini E, Angelini F, Baldelli R, Berretti D, Bianchetti S, Bizzarri G, Caputo M, Castello R, Cremonini N, Crescenzi A, Davì MV, D'Elia AV, Faggiano A, Pizzolitto S, Versari A, Zini M, Rindi G, Oberg K (2014) Italian Association of Clinical Endocrinologists (AME) position statement: a stepwise clinical approach to the diagnosis of gastroenteropancreatic neuroendocrine neoplasms. J Endocrinol Invest 37:875–909
21. Boudreaux JP, Klimstra DS, Hassan MM et al (2010) The NANETS consensus guideline for the diagnosis and management of neuroendocrine tumors-well-differentiated neuroendocrine tumors of the jejunum, ileum, appendix, and cecum. Pancreas 39:753–766
22. Anthony LB, Stosberg JR, Klimstra DS et al (2010) The NANETS consensus guideline for the diagnosis and management of neuroendocrine tumors – well-differentiated NETs of the distal colon and rectum. Pancreas 39:767–774
23. Algeciras-Schimnich A, Preissner CM, Young WF et al (2008) Plasma chromogranin A or urine fractionated metanephrines follow-up testing improves the diagnostic accuracy of plasma fractionated metanephrines for pheochromocytomas. J Clin Endocrinol Metab 93:91–95
24. Kullke MH, Benson AB, Bergsland E et al (2012) National Comprehensive Cancer Network Clinical Practice Guidelines in Oncology (NCCN Guidelines): NCCN Guidelines version 1.2012 – neuroendocrine tumors, pp 1–94, E-Pub Date 20 Mar 2012. URL: http://www.nccn.org/professionals/physician_gls/pdf/neuroendocrine.pdf
25. van Adrichem RC, Hofland LJ, Feelders RA, De Martino MC, van Koetsveld PM, van Eijck CH, de Krijger RR, Sprij-Mooij DM, Janssen JA, de Herder WW (2013) Chromogranin A, Ki-67 index and IGF-related genes in patients with neuroendocrine tumors. Endocr Connect 2:172–177
26. Moore AR, Boyce M, Steele IA, Campbell F, Varro A, Pritchard DM (2013) Netazepide, a gastrin receptor antagonist, normalises tumour biomarkers and causes

regression of type 1 gastric neuroendocrine tumours in a nonrandomised trial of patients with chronic atrophic gastritis. PLoS One 8, e76462
27. Ito T, Okusaka T, Nishida T, Yamao K, Igarashi H, Morizane C, Kondo S, Mizuno N, Hara K, Sawaki A, Hashigaki S, Kimura N, Murakami M, Ohki E, Chao RC, Imamura M (2013) Phase II study of sunitinib in Japanese patients with unresectable or metastatic, well-differentiated pancreatic neuroendocrine tumor. Invest New Drugs 31:1265–1274
28. Kratochwil C, López-Benítez R, Mier W, Haufe S, Isermann B, Kauczor HU, Choyke PL, Haberkorn U, Giesel FL (2011) Hepatic arterial infusion enhances DOTATOC radiopeptide therapy in patients with neuroendocrine liver metastases. Endocr Relat Cancer 18:595–602
29. Lubner SJ, Kunnimalaiyaan M, Holen KD, Ning L, Ndiaye M, Loconte NK, Mulkerin DL, Schelman WR, Chen H (2011) A preclinical and clinical study of lithium in low-grade neuroendocrine tumors. Oncologist 16:452–457
30. Wang YH, Yang QC, Lin Y, Xue L, Chen MH, Chen J (2014) Chromogranin A as a marker for diagnosis, treatment, and survival in patients with gastroentero-pancreatic neuroendocrine neoplasm. Medicine 93, e247
31. Jilesen AP, Busch OR, van Gulik TM, Gouma DJ, Nieveen van Dijkum EJ (2015) Standard pre- and postoperative determination of chromogranin A in resectable non-functioning pancreatic neuroendocrine tumors – diagnostic accuracy: NF-pNET and low tumor burden. Dig Surg 31:407–414
32. de Laat JM, Pieterman CR, Weijmans M, Hermus AR, Dekkers OM, de Herder WW, van der Horst-Schrivers AN, Drent ML, Bisschop PH, Havekes B, Vriens MR, Valk GD (2013) Low accuracy of tumor markers for diagnosing pancreatic neuroendocrine tumors in multiple endocrine neoplasia type 1 patients. J Clin Endocrinol Metab 98:4143–4151
33. Qiao XW, Qiu L, Chen YJ, Meng CT, Sun Z, Bai CM, Zhao DC, Zhang TP, Zhao YP, Song YL, Wang YH, Chen J, Lu CM (2014) Chromogranin A is a reliable serum diagnostic biomarker for pancreatic neuroendocrine tumors but not for insulinomas. BMC Endocr Disord 14:64
34. Guillemot J, Guérin M, Thouënnon E, Montéro-Hadjadje M, Leprince J, Lefebvre H, Klein M, Muresan M, Anouar Y, Yon L (2014) Characterization and plasma measurement of the WE-14 peptide in patients with pheochromocytoma. PLoS One 9, e88698
35. Isshiki S, Akakura K, Komiya A, Suzuki H, Kamiya N, Ito H (2002) Chromogranin aconcentration as a serum marker to predict prognosis after endocrine therapy for prostate cancer. J Urol 167:512–515
36. Tricoli JV, Schoenfeldt M, Conley BA (2004) Detection of prostate cancer and predicting progression: current and future diagnostic markers. Clin Cancer Res 10:3943–3953
37. Ferrero-Poüs M, Hersant AM, Pecking A, Brésard-Leroy M, Pichon MF (2001) Serum chromogranin-A in advanced prostate cancer. BJU Int 88:790–796
38. Hirano D, Hasegawa R, Satoh K, Mochida J, Yamanaka Y, Hirakata H, Yamaguchi K, Sugimoto S, Kawata N, Takahashi S (2014) Prospective study on the relationship between clinical efficacy of secondary hormone therapy with flutamide and neuroendocrine differentiation in patients with relapsed prostate cancer after first line hormone therapy. Scand J Urol 48:436–444
39. Tarle M, Ahel MZ, Kovacić K (2002) Acquired neuroendocrine-positivity during maximal androgen blockade in prostate cancer patients. Anticancer Res 22:2525–2529
40. Moline J, Eng C (2011) Multiple endocrine neoplasia type 2: an overview. Genet Med 13:755–764
41. Taïeb D, Kebebew E, Castinetti F, Chen CC, Henry JF, Pacak K (2014) Diagnosis and preoperative imaging of multiple endocrine neoplasia type 2: current status and future directions. Clin Endocrinol (Oxf) 81:317–328
42. Bech PR, Ramachandran R, Dhillo WS et al (2012) Quantifying the effects of renal impairment on plasma concentrations of the neuroendocrine neoplasia biomarkers chromogranin A, chromogranin B, and cocaine- and amphetamine-regulated transcript. Clin Chem 58:941–943
43. Canale MP, Bravo EL (1994) Diagnostic specificity of serum chromogranin-A for pheochromocytoma in patients with renal dysfunction. J Clin Endocrinol Metab 78:1139–1144
44. Korse CM, Muller M, Taal BG (2011) Discontinuation of proton pump inhibitors during assessment of chromogranin A levels in patients with neuroendocrine tumors. Br J Cancer 32:1173–1175
45. Mosli HH, Dennis A, Kosha W, Asher LJ, Van Uum SH (2012) Effect of short-term proton pump inhibitor treatment and its discontinuation on chromogranin A in healthy subjects. J Clin Endocrinol Metab 97:E1731–E1735
46. Glinicki P, Kapuścińska R, Jeske W (2013) Improved diagnostic accuracy for neuroendocrine neoplasms using two chromogranin A assays: the importance of protein matrix effects. Clin Endocrinol (Oxf) 79:295–296
47. Gruson D, Lepoutre T, Smits F (2015) Chromogranin-A levels measured with automated immunoassay. Int J Biol Markers 30:e132–e135

Part X

Receptors as Biomarkers

The Actual Role of Receptors as Cancer Markers, Biochemical and Clinical Aspects: Receptors in Breast Cancer

20

Matthew Brennan and Bora Lim

Abstract

A biomarker is a characteristic that is objectively measured and evaluated as an indicator of normal biological processes, pathogenic processes, or pharmacologic responses to a therapeutic intervention. The discovery and development of proper biomarkers is a critical part of modern oncology. Among the many different types of biomarkers, cell receptors have demonstrated important roles as diagnostic, prognostic, and predictive biomarkers in cancer research and therapy, leading to their integration into drug development trials. In breast cancer, Estrogen/Progesterone receptors and HER2/neu receptors are two good examples of biomarkers that are prognostic of outcomes, as well as predictive of response to certain therapies. Limitations exist, however, such as the invasive procedures required obtaining tissue, and the difficulty measuring the actual distribution of the receptors. Thus, continued efforts to develop receptors as comprehensive cancer biomarkers with novel approaches is mandated to further advance the modern oncology.

Keywords

Biomarker • Cancer prognosis • Cancer thserapy • Circulating free DNA • Clinical response • EGFR mutations • Estrogen receptor • HER2/neu • Hormonal therapy • Hormone receptor status • Novel therapeutics • Nuclear receptors • Predictive marker • Progesteron receptor • Receptor • Type 1 biomarkers • Type 2 biomarkers

M. Brennan
Hematology/Oncology Division, Department of Internal Medicine, Penn State Hershey Cancer Institute, Penn State Hershey Medical Center, Hershey, PA 17033, USA

B. Lim (✉)
Breast Medical Oncology, The University of Texas MD Anderson Cancer Center, Unit 1354, Houston TX 77030, USA
e-mail: naborala@gmail.com

R. Scatena (ed.), *Advances in Cancer Biomarkers*, Advances in Experimental Medicine and Biology 867, DOI 10.1007/978-94-017-7215-0_20

20.1 Definition, Categorization, and Role of Biomarkers

20.1.1 Definition and Classification

In 1998, the National Institutes of Health (NIH) Biomarkers Definitions Working Group defined a biomarker as "a characteristic that is objectively measured and evaluated as an indicator of normal biological processes, pathogenic processes, or pharmacologic responses to a therapeutic intervention" [1]. The NIH's 'Biomarkers and Surrogate Endpoint Working Group' classifies biomarkers based on their differences into three distinct types based on plausibility, correlation/association, prognostic value, predictive power, and cause [2, 3].

Type 0 biomarkers are diagnostic or prognostic and measure the natural history of a disease and correlate with known clinical indices, such as clinical findings or symptoms. Type 1 markers measure the outcome or the effect of an intervention in accordance with the mechanism of the drug, whether or not the underlying correlation between the two is known. Type 2 markers are recognized as surrogate endpoints, which can provide prediction of the clinical benefit [4]. A simpler classification suggested by Simon et al. narrowed biomarkers into two categories – the prognostic and the predictive [5]. In this review, we will use the classification by the working group.

The type 0 biomarkers include both diagnostic and prognostic markers. Diagnostic biomarkers are used to verify the presence of disease, or define the category of disease. For example, the existence of the chromosomal translocation Bcr/Abl (Philadelphia chromosome) detected in either blood, or bone marrow aspiration confirms the diagnosis of a hematologic malignancy – Chronic Myeloid Leukemia [6]. Prognostic biomarkers, on the other hand, offer insight into the expected behavior of the disease. For example, hypermethylation of the MGMT (O6-methylguanine-DNA methyltransferase) promoter gene in Glioblastoma Multiforme, is associated with a better survival [7], while high serum LDH levels in lymphoma [8] and a FLT3-ITD mutation in Acute Myeloid Leukemia are associated with poorer outcomes [9]. It is important to note most times a prognostic marker does not necessarily support the correlation between an intervention and a clinical outcome, which can cause confusion in interpreting a study or planning a treatment. Therefore, causal relationship between the biomarker and the clinical outcome is established, offering a more aggressive therapy to a patient because of one's poor prognostic marker, may not result in an improved outcome [10]. A predictive biomarker that can detect such a relationship, and support the choice of therapy will be discussed below.

The type 1 biomarkers are the biomarkers that are based on the understanding of mechanisms-thus, called as mechanistic markers. Pharmacodynamic, pharmacokinetic markers are good examples [11]. Pharmacodynamic biomarkers measure how targeting agents effect their target (i.e. the effect of the drug on the body), and are useful as a surrogate endpoint in early phase clinical trials for drug development [11, 12]. Pharmacokinetic markers, on the other hand, measure how the body affects the drug, allowing treatment optimization, and are thus vital to the success of early drug development. The importance of pharmacodynamics and pharmacokinetic biomarkers is illustrated in the failure of early stage clinical trials during the 1990s. For example in 1991, about 40 % of phase I/II clinical trials had to stop early due to the shortcomings of pharmacokinetic or pharmacodynamic biomarkers, perhaps eliminating effective drugs from trial. Furthermore, trial size and budget increase without the integration of these biomarkers.

Type 2 biomarkers are one of the most important as they measure a characteristic of the disease that is predictive of a response to certain treatment. This attribute relies on an understanding of a direct correlation between the target biomarker and the drug, which is in contrast to type 0 biomarkers which give prognostic information. The two are not mutually exclusive, and a good example is in breast cancer. Hormone (Estrogen/Progesterone) and HER2/neu receptors [13, 14] are prognostic of the natural history of the disease (type 0), but are also predictive of a response to treatment – aromatase inhibitors and trastuzumab, for example.

Developing good biomarkers for novel drug discovery and development is both the greatest challenge and the most essential component of bridging the gap between pre-clinical science and the clinical application [13, 14]. The task is large given the heterogeneity among different biomarkers in regards to quality and validity. The discovery and development of 'ideal biomarkers' from the large pool of biomarkers is a critical task, and various biomarker working groups as well as researchers have tried to achieve this goal. The most commonly recognized qualities of 'ideal biomarkers' include the following: accuracy, reproducibility, standardization, and analytic stability (being robust) [15].

20.1.2 The Importance of Biomarkers in Modern Cancer Research

The importance of biomarkers in the modern era of cancer research has grown over time. The AACR-FDA-NCI (American Association for Cancer Research-Food and Drug Administration-National Cancer Institute) Cancer Biomarkers Collaborative meeting illustrates the increasing recognition of the significance biomarkers play in cancer research. This meeting brings more than 120 experts world wide – including academia, the pharmaceutical and diagnostic industries, government agencies, regulators, and patient advocates – together – to set up action plans and collaborate in an effort to develop standardized, safe, and effective biomarkers [16].

The emerging importance of biomarker development in cancer research parallels the need for novel drug discovery and development in the field. Translational research that leads to novel drug discovery and development is the main vehicle that brings these paramount scientific discoveries into the clinic, thus changing the nature of disease [17]. Two of the most important qualities biomarkers must achieve for novel drug development include (1) an ability to recognize the target population of patients who will respond to the new treatment, and (2) an ability to avoid toxicity by discerning which patients will not benefit from the intervention [18]. The category of biomarker that is critical for proper delivery of translational cancer research, however, has changed over time [2]. As reviewed earlier, in the 1990s when the importance of translational research took its first baby steps, pharmacokinetic and pharmacodynamic markers were the critical markers that decided either the success or failure of the trials.

More recently, predictive biomarkers play an increasingly important role in the success of clinical trials in recent years, since the lack of efficacy of the new drug, as well as it's toxicities [2] cause many trials to fail. The 'lack of efficacy' could be due to many factors, including not only a lack of pre-clinical rationale, but also an inability to find the proper predictive biomarkers – even with a well-reasoned trial design. Thus, identifying the proper group of patients who harbor the target of a novel drug enables the trial to achieve proof-of-concept, improved efficacy, and diminished risk of toxicity which can lead to phase III trials [19, 20]. Taken together, the discovery and the integration of proper pharmacodynamics, predictive, and prognostic measuring biomarkers, along with careful planning of trial design in the modern era of oncology, cannot be emphasized enough.

20.1.3 Receptors as Cancer Biomarkers

A receptor is a protein located either on a cell surface or within the cell cytoplasm or nucleus that binds to a specific ligand, initiating signal transduction and a change in cellular activity [21]. In cancer therapeutic development, the receptors can serve as not only important diagnostic markers, but as prognostic/predictive markers as well. Hormone (Estrogen/Progesterone), and HER2/neu receptors help diagnose the site of origin, as well as prognosticate the course of disease [22–24], EGFR positive non-small cell lung cancer (NSCLC) patients have a much better prognosis compared to those who are receptor negative [25, 26]. Since the receptors are often targets of novel therapy, detection of the receptors can direct researchers and physicians to select the correct population of patients who will benefit from targeted therapy, as predictive marker [27]. In the proof-of-concept trials, the receptors can act as surrogate endpoints, enabling an assessment of the targeting drug's efficacy [14].

20.1.4 Technical Challenges of Receptor as Cancer Biomarkers

Most tests use tissue-based techniques to detect receptors in cancer. This necessity of accessible tissue limits the ability to use receptors as monitoring biomarkers, especially given the poor condition and suffering of cancer patients at baseline. Thus, researchers developed novel techniques to measure the receptors using non- invasive measures [28]. These techniques include analyzing either Circulating Tumor Cells (CTC's) or DNA to detect receptors. For example, several groups of researchers were able to detect the EGFR mutation from CTC's in NSCLC patients [29, 30]. Another example of a surrogate marker is the truncated form of the HER2 receptor which will be discussed below [31, 32]. A new approach is a functional imaging technique. PET/CT scan using specific antibodies like trastuzumab or ABY-002 that are bind to nuclear isotope that bind specifically to HER2/neu receptor allows the visualization of receptors in situ, and currently developed in clinical trials [33, 34].

20.2 Examples of Receptors as Cancer Biomarkers in Breast Cancer

20.2.1 Hormone (Estrogen/Progesterone) Receptors in Breast Cancer

Since the 1980s, the nuclear hormone receptor for Estrogen has been recognized as one of the most powerful prognostic and predictive cancer biomarkers in breast cancer [35] (citation 39). Female estrogen – estradiol (E2), serves to enrich and stimulate breast cancer cell growth [36]. Despite this well established prognostic value and many speculations as to the underlying scientific background, the tumorigenesis in human breast cancer caused by estrogen receptors is poorly understood [37]. The metabolism of estrogen within the mammalian cells may contribute to carcinogenesis by DNA damage [38]. In any case, breast cancer patients with positive estrogen receptor expression have better disease free survival, as well as overall survival [39]. Estrogen receptor positivity of the primary tumor also predicts the prevalence of the receptor status in a contralateral breast cancer if it occurs [40]. Nulliparity, early menarche, and absence of breastfeeding have been shown to all correlate with higher incidence of hormone receptor positive breast cancers [41].

Two forms of estrogen receptors – ER α, and β have been identified. ER α plays a crucial role in the progression and proliferation of breast cancer, and ER β appears to correlate with a more aggressive nature of breast cancer [42]. This aggressive feature of the ER β positive tumors may be due to the activation of the PI3K/Akt pathway [43]. Activated Akt at the time of diagnosis in the ER positive breast cancer correlates with a worse clinical outcome [44]. ER β breast cancers show enhanced activity of PI3K (Phosphatidylinositol 3-kinase), which promotes PIP3 (3,4,5 phosphatidylinositol triphosphate) generation, and leads to serine/threonine kinase activity of Akt [45]. Therefore, ER β may have prognostic and negative predictive value. Unfortunately, ER β can also give false positive signal of ER α [46], and the importance of ER β still requires further investigation, and to date, the testing of ER β has not been integrated into clinical practice.

The Progesterone receptor (PR) is another nuclear hormone receptor that is routinely examined along with the Estrogen receptor in breast cancer. In both humans, progesterone binds to the progesterone receptor and promotes the proliferation of epithelial cells during the menstrual cycle or pregnancy [47]. Over the years, there has been debate over whether the combined testing of

PR with ER is mandatory to define hormone receptor positivity in breast cancer. For example, Olivotto et al. suggested the lack of utility of PR testing in clinical decision-making given the fact that most ER positive tumors are also PR positive [48]. In response, several other publications emphasized the importance of PR detection [49, 50]. Important arguments point out the cases that are PR positive but ER negative. Furthermore, among tumors that are ER positive, the ones that are PR positive are more sensitive to hormonal therapies, thus defining two clinically relevant subgroups of ER positive tumors [51]. Thus PR still remains an important biomarker in conjunction with ER [52].

Estrogen and Progesterone receptors have been tested by several different methods since their initial recognition as important biomarkers in 1980 s [53–55]. Most recently, the standard of practice is the immunohistochemistry (IHC) testing method [54]. Challenges remain despite standardized methods of detection globally. For example, the discordance among different labs and a debate as to the appropriate cut-off defining ER positivity still exist [56]. Collaborative efforts to minimize the noise and discordance of standardized detection and reporting systems of ER positivity are still ongoing [56, 57]. In 2010, the American Society of Clinical Oncology (ASCO) and the College of American Pathologist (CAP) convened an international expert panel to conduct a systematic review and evaluation of the literature in collaboration with Cancer Care Ontario. Not surprisingly from this systematic review, the experts recognized up to a 20 % inaccuracy in current IHC detection methods. The panel set as the threshold for a positive result 1 % nuclei expression or more in the presence of expected reactivity of normal epithelial cells and external controls [58].

Perhaps the greatest biomarker role the ER and PR receptors possess in breast cancer is their predictive value for hormonal receptor blockage – so called hormone therapy/endocrine therapy. Hormone therapy in breast cancer was first adapted in risk reduction of women with the precancerous lesion, Ductal Carcinoma In Situ (DCIS). Selective Estrogen-Receptor Modulators (SERMs) including tamoxifen, raloxifen, and toremifen have demonstrated a successful risk reduction in developing either an ipsilateral or contralateral invasive breast cancer in both pre- and post-menopausal women [59–61]. SERMs were also applied as secondary preventive methods [62], decreasing the rate of recurrence in early breast cancer patients with hormone receptor positivity. Overall, both SERMs, and aromatase inhibitor (AIs) decrease recurrence rates of breast cancer when used over 5 years, with a relative risk reduction between 50 % and 66 % [63, 64], reducing the rate of secondary cancer more than any other agents known to modern oncology.

Recently, data suggest 10 years of estrogen receptor blocking therapy gives additional survival benefit compared to 5 years of therapy [65–67]. More intriguingly, in early stage node negative breast cancer, ER/PR status in combination with genomic profiling can further guide the adjuvant treatment decision [68, 69]. For example, patients with a low OncotypeDX® recurrent score have a better prognosis, requiring only endocrine therapy, and biologically do not respond to chemotherapy and in fact would suffer toxicity without clinical benefit if given chemotherapy [70].

The clinical utility of ER/PR receptors as biomarkers does not stop there. For patients with higher stage hormone receptor positive breast cancer – large size, lobular histology, or lymph node involvement – the hormone receptor blocking agents have been used as neoadjuvant therapy [71, 72] The clinical outcome with this therapy still requires further evaluation [73–75]. These biomarkers also have a role in recurrent or metastatic ER/PR positive breast cancer patients (along with chemotherapy) as they predict response to endocrine therapy in a first, second, or third line setting. In advanced ER/PR positive breast cancer patients, endocrine therapy showed non-inferiority compared to chemotherapeutic agents [76, 77]. More importantly, endocrine therapeutic agents have activities even in the recurrent breast cancer patients who had been on adjuvant endocrine therapy prior to the recurrence [78].

There are various agents targeting the hormone receptor, and these drugs are used either alone or in combination with other therapies in advanced or metastatic breast cancer as standard of care. The details regarding the selection of the different agents have been well established via several milestones of research, however will not be discussed in this chapter [79, 80]. For more information about endocrine therapy in breast cancer, please refer to the following: St. Gallen recommendation, ASCO (American Society of Clinical Oncology), ESMO (European Society for Medical Oncology), NCCN (National Comprehensive Cancer Network) clinical practice guidelines for hormone positive breast cancer [81–85].

20.2.2 HER2/neu in Breast Cancer

HER2/neu (ErbB2) is a transmembrane glycoprotein receptor [86], which belongs to the EGFR family that includes – HER1 (ErbB1 = EGFR), HER2, HER3, and HER4. Each family member shares similar intracellular Tyrosine Kinase (TK) domains, but expresses distinct ligand binding extracellular domains. The HER2 receptor itself does not have the extracellular ligand-binding domain, and therefore its activation requires homo- or hetero- dimerization with HER1, HER3 for activation [87, 88]. The HER2 receptor was first cloned by three distinct groups of scientists including the group from Genentech in the mid 1980s [89, 90]. Soon afterwards, the location of the *HER2* gene loci was discovered on chromosome 17 [91], the same location as the proto-oncogene '*neu*' [90], which was later confirmed to be the same gene. HER2/neu overexpression has been recognized in several different cancers including breast, lung, head and neck, and GI, however it is most frequently so in breast cancer [92].

About 20–25 % of breast cancers have overexpression of HER2/neu [93, 94], and historically such overexpression was correlated with a poor clinical prognosis, regardless of ER/PR co-expression [94, 95]. These patients had almost a threefold increase in risk of death and distant metastasis, and conventional chemotherapy did not improve outcomes compared to those that did not have HER2 overexpression [95–97]. For a brief period of time, the HER2/neu receptor overexpression in breast cancer was only a prognostic marker, but more recently it has become of predictive value as well.

Assays to detect the HER2 receptor overexpression include gene-based assays, such as fluorescence in situ hybridization (FISH), Southern Blot, Polymerase Chain Reaction (PCR); and protein based assays, such as IHC and Western Blot [98]. The most widely accepted of these assays are IHC and FISH. In order to test for amplification of HER2, the FISH method measures the number of HER2 gene copies in comparison to a control, the centromere of chromosome 17. The discordance rate between IHC results and FISH results is as high as 20 %, and FISH testing is considered to be the most reliable test method [99, 100]. Many collaborative groups like ASCO (American Society of Clinical Oncology), College of American Pathology (CAP), the NCCN (National Cancer Comprehensive Network) HER2 Testing in Breast Cancer Task Force have been trying to standardize the proper testing and treatment selection guidelines based on the proper testing results [101, 102].

The discovery of trastuzumab changed the history of HER2/neu overexpressing in breast cancer from one of prognostic to one of predictive value. Several groups including Slamon et al. discovered a monoclonal mouse antibody that binds to p185, a form of the HER2 receptor [103]. In pre-clinical studies, HER2 receptor overexpression showed a very strong predictive correlation with the treatment of HER2 binding antibodies, and showed the regression of tumor growth. Trastuzumab, a humanized monoclonal antibody, was created from that parent drug in 1990 [104]. Within 3 years of the initial development of trastuzumab was tested in a phase III trial for metastatic HER2 receptor overexpressing breast cancer patients [105, 106]. Clinical trials showed significant improvement in the overall survival of metastatic HER2 overexpressing breast cancer patients when treated with trastuzumab, either as a single agent or in combination with chemotherapeutic agents. Given such striking improvement in outcome, trastuzumab was approved by the FDA in 1998.

Despite the role of the HER2 receptor as such a potent predictive marker of trastuzumab therapy, clinicians learned not all HER2 overexpressed breast cancers will respond to trastuzumab [107]. This lack of efficacy in a subgroup of HER2 positive breast cancers triggered the development of a biomarker in HER2 positive breast cancers based on the understanding of a resistance mechanism. There are several different resistance mechanisms postulated. One mechanism studied the overexpression of the HER2 heterodimerization partner, the HER3 receptor. Next, c-MET and IGF-1R have some role in resistance [108–110], as does the overexpression of the downstream pathway (PI3K-AKT-mTOR) of HER2. The overexpression or mutation of PTEN can bypass the blockage of the HER2 receptor [111]. Lastly, p95 – a truncated form of HER2/neu receptor that lacks the binding affinity to Trastuzumab was recognized as an important resistance mechanism [112]. So far, none of the fore-mentioned biomarkers succeed in helping the selection of treatment choice.

Of potential clinical benefit in the near future, however, is the extracellular domain (ECD) of the HER2 receptor, which is a truncated form of the intact receptor. Its advantage is that it can be measured in the serum [113, 114]. Given easier access to the serum sample compared to tissue biopsy to detect other biomarkers, the ECD has been extensively studied as a biomarker that can be followed in those with poor therapeutic response – as a predictive marker [114]. However, with the study of such biomarkers and pathways, HER2 targeted therapy entered into a new era with novel therapeutics that overcame the resistance to trastuzumab therapy [115, 116].

20.3 Conclusion

As the era of personalized/precision medicine and modern oncology advance in parallel, the development of biomarkers is essential. Ideal biomarkers are well validated and harbor important qualities. Good biomarker development is a key to successful clinical trials in early drug development. Biomarkers provide critical roles as diagnostic, prognostic, and predictive markers. These biomarkers have the potential to contribute greatly to improved clinical outcomes in cancer therapy, just as hormone (Estrogen/Progesterone) and HER2 receptors have in breast cancer. Limitations exists, however and future directions will need to involve novel techniques to detect functional subcategories of receptors, stratify receptors as predictive biomarkers based on different mutations, and visualize the distribution of normal receptors. Continued effort to develop receptors as comprehensive cancer biomarkers is core necessity in further development of modern oncology to be one step closer to a cure.

References

1. Strimbu K, Tavel JA (2010) What are biomarkers? Curr Opin HIV AIDS 5:463–466
2. Frank R, Hargreaves R (2003) Clinical biomarkers in drug discovery and development. Nat Rev Drug Discov 2:566–580
3. Atkinson A et al (2001) Biomarkers and surrogate endpoints: preferred definitions and conceptual framework. Clin Pharmacol Ther 69:89–95
4. Quintas-Cardama A, Cortes J (2006) Chronic myeloid leukemia: diagnosis and treatment. Mayo Clin Proc 81:973–988
5. Hegi ME et al (2005) MGMT gene silencing and benefit from temozolomide in glioblastoma. N Engl J Med 352:997–1003
6. Fasola G et al (1984) Serum LDH concentration in non-Hodgkin's lymphomas. Relationship to histologic type, tumor mass, and presentation features. Acta Haematol 72:231–238
7. Levis M, Small D (2003) FLT3: It does matter in leukemia. Leukemia 17:1738–1752
8. Italiano A (2011) Prognostic or predictive? It's time to get back to definitions! J Clin Oncol 29:4718
9. De Vita F et al (2010) Human epidermal growth factor receptor 2 (HER2) in gastric cancer: a new therapeutic target. Cancer Treat Rev 36(Suppl 3):S11–S15
10. Oldenhuis CN, Oosting SF, Gietema JA, de Vries EG (2008) Prognostic versus predictive value of biomarkers in oncology. Eur J Cancer 44:946–953
11. Sarker D, Workman P (2007) Pharmacodynamic biomarkers for molecular cancer therapeutics. Adv Cancer Res 96:213–268
12. Pan Y et al (2011) Evaluation of pharmacodynamic biomarkers in a Phase 1a trial of dulanermin (rhApo2L/TRAIL) in patients with advanced tumours. Br J Cancer 105:1830–1838

13. Mandrekar SJ, Sargent DJ (2010) Predictive biomarker validation in practice: lessons from real trials. Clin Trials 7:567–573
14. Floyd E, McShane TM (2004) Development and use of biomarkers in oncology drug development. Toxicol Pathol 32(Suppl 1):106–115
15. Beketic-Oreskovic L, Maric P, Ozretic P et al (2012) Assessing the clinical significance of tumor markers in common neoplasms. Front Biosci 4:2558–2578
16. Khleif SN, Doroshow JH, Hait WN (2010) AACR-FDA-NCI cancer biomarkers collaborative consensus report: advancing the use of biomarkers in cancer drug development. Clin Cancer Res 16:3299
17. Butler D (2008) Translational research: crossing the valley of death. Nat News 453:840–842
18. Sistare FD et al (2010) Towards consensus practices to qualify safety biomarkers for use in early drug development. Nat Biotechnol 28:446–454
19. Ferber G (2002) Biomarkers and proof of concept. Methods Find Exp Clin Pharmacol 24(Suppl C):35–40
20. Beckman RA, Clark J, Chen C (2011) Integrating predictive biomarkers and classifiers into oncology clinical development programmes. Nat Rev Drug Discov 10:735–748
21. Pagana KD, Pagana TJ (2014) Mosby's manual of diagnostic and laboratory tests. Elsevier, St. Louis
22. Brown R, Campagna L, Dunn J, Cagle P (1997) Immunohistochemical identification of tumor markers in metastatic adenocarcinoma: a diagnostic adjunct in the determination of primary site. Am J Clin Pathol 107:12–19
23. Voduc K et al (2010) Breast cancer subtypes and the risk of local and regional relapse. J Clin Oncol 28:1684–1691
24. Fox SB et al (1994) The epidermal growth factor receptor as a prognostic marker: results of 370 patients and review of 3009 patients. Breast Cancer Res Treat 29:41–49
25. Nicholson RI, Gee JMW, Harper ME (2001) EGFR and cancer prognosis. Eur J Cancer 37:9–15
26. Selvaggi G et al. (2004) Epidermal growth factor receptor overexpression correlates with a poor prognosis in completely resected non-small-cell lung cancer. Ann Oncol 15:28–32
27. Weigel MT, Dowsett M (2010) Current and emerging biomarkers in breast cancer: prognosis and prediction. Endocr Relat Cancer 17:245–262
28. Crowley E, Nicolantonio FD, Loupakis F, Bardelli A (2013) Liquid biopsy: monitoring cancer-genetics in the blood. Nat Rev Clin Oncol 10:472–484
29. Akca H et al (2013) Utility of serum DNA and pyrosequencing for the detection of EGFR mutations in non-small cell lung cancer. Cancer Genet 206:73–80
30. Kim H-R et al (2013) Detection of EGFR mutations in circulating free DNA by PNA-mediated PCR clamping. J Exp Clin Cancer Res 32:50
31. Fehm T et al (2007) Determination of HER2 status using both serum HER2 levels and circulating tumor cells in patients with recurrent breast cancer whose primary tumor was HER2 negative or of unknown HER2 status. Breast Cancer Res 9:R74
32. Loo L et al (2011) Highly sensitive detection of HER2 extracellular domain in the serum of breast cancer patients by piezoelectric microcantilevers. Anal Chem 83:3392–3397
33. Mortimer J et al (2012) Functional imaging of HER2-positive metastatic breast cancer using 64Cu DOTA-trastuzumab positron emission tomography (PET). Mortimer et al. 30(15):639 -- ASCO meeting abstracts. J Clin Oncol 30:639
34. Baum RP et al (2010) Molecular imaging of HER2-expressing malignant tumors in breast cancer patients using synthetic 111In- or 68Ga-labeled affibody molecules. J Nucl Med 51:892–897
35. Paik S et al (2006) Gene expression and benefit of chemotherapy in women with node-negative, estrogen receptor–positive breast cancer. J Clin Oncol 24 15:28–32
36. Stanford JL, Szklo M, Brinton LA (1986) Estrogen receptors and breast cancer. Epidemiol Rev 8:42–59
37. Althuis MD et al (2004) Etiology of hormone receptor–defined breast cancer: a systematic review of the literature Cancer Epidemiol Biomarkers Prev. 13:1558–1568
38. Miller K (2003) Estrogen and DNA damage: the silent source of breast cancer? J Natl Cancer Inst 95:100–102
39. Dunnwald LK, Rossing MA, Li CI (2007) Hormone receptor status, tumor characteristics, and prognosis: a prospective cohort of breast cancer patients. Breast Cancer Res 9:R6
40. Swain SM et al (2004) Estrogen receptor status of primary breast cancer is predictive of estrogen receptor status of contralateral breast cancer. J Natl Cancer Inst 96:516–523
41. Duffy MJ (2006) Estrogen receptors: role in breast cancer. Crit Rev Clin Lab Sci 43:325–347
42. Hayashi SI et al (2003) The expression and function of estrogen receptor alpha and beta in human breast cancer and its clinical application. Endocr Relat Cancer 10:193–202
43. Wang M et al (2009) Estrogen receptor beta mediates increased activation of PI3K/Akt signaling and improved myocardial function in female hearts following acute ischemia. Am J Physiol Regul Integr Comp Physiol 296:R972–R978
44. Park S, Song J, Joe CO, Shin I (2008) Akt stabilizes estrogen receptor alpha with the concomitant reduction in its transcriptional activity. Cell Signal 20:1368–1374
45. Vivanco I, Sawyers CL (2002) The phosphatidylinositol 3-Kinase – AKT pathway in human cancer. Nat Rev Cancer 2:489–501
46. Fuqua SAW et al (2003) Estrogen receptor β protein in human breast cancer: correlation with clinical tumor parameters. Cancer Res. 63:2434–2439
47. Mangelsdorf D et al (1995) The nuclear receptor superfamily: the second decade. Cell 83:835–839

48. Olivotto IA et al (2004) Time to stop progesterone receptor testing in breast cancer management. J Clin Oncol 22:1769–1770
49. Colozza M, Larsimont D, Piccart MJ (2005) Progesterone receptor testing: not the right time to be buried. J Clin Oncol 23:3867–3868; author reply 3869–3870
50. Fuqua SAW, Cui Y, Lee AV, Osborne CK, Horwitz KB (2005) Insights into the role of progesterone receptors in breast cancer. J Clin Oncol 23:931–932
51. Osborne CK, Yochmowitz MG, Knight WA 3rd, McGuire WL (1980) The value of estrogen and progesterone receptors in the treatment of breast cancer. Cancer 46:2884–2888
52. Mohsin SK et al (2004) Progesterone receptor by immunohistochemistry and clinical outcome in breast cancer: a validation study. Mod Pathol 17:1545–1554
53. Biswas DK, Cruz AP, Pardee AB (2000) Detection of the level of estrogen receptor and functional variants in human breast cancers by novel assays. Biotechniques 29(1056–1060):1062–1054
54. Claassen H et al (2001) Immunohistochemical detection of estrogen receptor alpha in articular chondrocytes from cows, pigs and humans: in situ and in vitro results. Ann Anat 183:223–227
55. Hanley KZ, Birdsong GG, Cohen C, Siddiqui MT (2009) Immunohistochemical detection of estrogen receptor, progesterone receptor, and human epidermal growth factor receptor 2 expression in breast carcinomas: comparison on cell block, needle-core, and tissue block preparations. Cancer 117:279–288
56. Reisenbichler ES et al (2013) Interobserver concordance in implementing the 2010 ASCO/CAP recommendations for reporting ER in breast carcinomas: a demonstration of the difficulties of consistently reporting low levels of ER expression by manual quantification. Am J Clin Pathol 140:487–494
57. Allred DC et al (2009) NCCN task force report: estrogen receptor and progesterone receptor testing in breast cancer by immunohistochemistry. J Natl Compr Canc Netw 7(Suppl 6):S1–S21; quiz S22–23
58. Hammond MEH et al (2010) American society of clinical oncology/college of American Pathologists Guideline recommendations for immunohistochemical testing of estrogen and progesterone receptors in breast cancer. J Clin Oncol 28:2784–2795
59. Houghton J et al (2003) Radiotherapy and tamoxifen in women with completely excised ductal carcinoma in situ of the breast in the UK, Australia, and New Zealand: randomised controlled trial. Lancet 362:95–102
60. Cummings SR et al (1999) The effect of raloxifene on risk of breast cancer in postmenopausal women: results from the more randomized trial. Multiple outcomes of raloxifene evaluation. JAMA 281:2189–2197
61. Vogel VG, Costantino JP, Wickerham DL, Cronin WM (2003) National surgical adjuvant breast and bowel project update: prevention trials and endocrine therapy of ductal carcinoma in situ. Clin Cancer Res 9:495s–501s
62. Perez EA et al (2006) Effect of letrozole versus placebo on bone mineral density in women with primary breast cancer completing 5 or more years of adjuvant tamoxifen: a companion study to NCIC CTG MA.17. J Clin Oncol 24:3629–3635
63. Dowsett M et al (2010) Meta-analysis of breast cancer outcomes in adjuvant trials of aromatase inhibitors versus tamoxifen. J Clin Oncol 28:509–518
64. van de Velde CJ et al (2011) Adjuvant tamoxifen and exemestane in early breast cancer (TEAM): a randomised phase 3 trial. Lancet 377:321–331
65. Ingle JN et al (2008) Intent-to-treat analysis of the placebo-controlled trial of letrozole for extended adjuvant therapy in early breast cancer: NCIC CTG MA.17. Ann Oncol 19:877–882
66. Goss PE et al (2008) Late extended adjuvant treatment with letrozole improves outcome in women with early-stage breast cancer who complete 5 years of tamoxifen. J Clin Oncol 26:1948–1955
67. Davies C et al (2013) Long-term effects of continuing adjuvant tamoxifen to 10 years versus stopping at 5 years after diagnosis of oestrogen receptor-positive breast cancer: ATLAS, a randomised trial. Lancet 381:805–816
68. Dowsett M et al (2013) Comparison of PAM50 risk of recurrence core with oncotype DX and IHC4 for predicting risk of distant recurrence after endocrine therapy. J Clin Oncol 31:29
69. Ellis MJ et al (2008) Outcome prediction for estrogen receptor–positive breast cancer based on postneoadjuvant endocrine therapy tumor characteristics. JNCI 100:1380–1388
70. Mamounas EP et al (2010) Association between the 21-gene recurrence score assay and risk of locoregional recurrence in node-negative, estrogen receptor–positive breast cancer: results from NSABP B-14 and NSABP B-20. J Clin Oncol 28:1677–1683
71. Goldhirsch A et al (2009) Thresholds for therapies: highlights of the St Gallen International Expert consensus on the primary therapy of early breast cancer 2009. Ann Oncol 20:1319–1329
72. Wolmark N, Wang J, Mamounas E, Bryant J, Fisher B (2001) Preoperative chemotherapy in patients with operable breast cancer: nine-year results from National Surgical Adjuvant Breast and Bowel Project B-18. J Natl Cancer Inst Monogr 30:96–102
73. Boughey JC et al (2009) Neoadjuvant chemotherapy in invasive lobular carcinoma may not improve rates of breast conservation. Ann Surg Oncol 16:1606–1611
74. Soucy G et al (2008) Surgical margins in breast-conservation operations for invasive carcinoma: does neoadjuvant chemotherapy have an impact? J Am Coll Surg 206:1116–1121
75. Mauri D, Pavlidis N, Ioannidis JP (2005) Neoadjuvant versus adjuvant systemic treatment in breast cancer: a meta-analysis. J Natl Cancer Inst 97:188–194

76. Fossati R et al (1998) Cytotoxic and hormonal treatment for metastatic breast cancer: a systematic review of published randomized trials involving 31,510 women. J Clin Oncol 16:3439–3460
77. Kaufmann M et al (1989) Goserelin, a depot gonadotrophin-releasing hormone agonist in the treatment of premenopausal patients with metastatic breast cancer. German Zoladex Trial Group. J Clin Oncol 7:1113–1119
78. Kurebayashi J et al (2000) Endocrine therapies for patients with recurrent breast cancer: predictive factors for responses to first- and second-line endocrine therapies. Oncology 59(Suppl 1):31–37
79. Yu B et al (2010) Changes in markers of ovarian reserve and endocrine function in young women with breast cancer undergoing adjuvant chemotherapy. Cancer 116:2099–2105
80. Boccardo F et al (2013) Switching to anastrozole versus continued tamoxifen treatment of early breast cancer: long term results of the Italian Tamoxifen Anastrozole trial. Eur J Cancer 49:1546–1554
81. Carlson RW, Hudis CA, Pritchard KI (2006) Adjuvant endocrine therapy in hormone receptor-positive postmenopausal breast cancer: evolution of NCCN, ASCO, and St Gallen recommendations. J Natl Compr Canc Netw 4:971–979
82. Burstein HJ et al (2010) American Society of Clinical Oncology clinical practice guideline: update on adjuvant endocrine therapy for women with hormone receptor-positive breast cancer. J Clin Oncol 28:3784–3796
83. Harbeck N, Thomssen C, Gnant M (2013) St. Gallen 2013: brief preliminary summary of the consensus discussion. Breast Care 8:102–109
84. Korman H, Lanni T Jr, Shah C et al (2013) Impact of a prostate multidisciplinary clinic program on patient treatment decisions and on adherence to NCCN guidelines: the William Beaumont Hospital experience. Am J Clin Oncol 36:121–125
85. Cardoso F, Kyriakides S, Penault-Llorca F (2013) Primary breast cancer: ESMO clinical practice guidelines for diagnosis, treatment and follow-up. Ann Oncol 24(Suppl 6):vi7–vi23
86. Yarden Y, Sliwkowski MX (2001) Untangling the ErbB signalling network. Nat Rev Mol Cell Biol 2:127–137
87. Kokai Y et al (1989) Synergistic interaction of p185c-neu and the EGF receptor leads to transformation of rodent fibroblasts. Cell 58:287–292
88. Wada T, Qian XL, Greene MI (1990) Intermolecular association of the p185neu protein and EGF receptor modulates EGF receptor function. Cell 61:1339–1347
89. Ullrich A et al (1984) Human epidermal growth factor receptor cDNA sequence and aberrant expression of the amplified gene in A431 epidermoid carcinoma cells. Nat Rev Mol Cell Biol 309:418–425
90. Coussens L et al (1985) Tyrosine kinase receptor with extensive homology to EGF receptor shares chromosomal location with neu oncogene. Science 230:1132–1139
91. Fukushige S et al (1986) Localization of a novel v-erbB-related gene, c-erbB-2, on human chromosome 17 and its amplification in a gastric cancer cell line. Mol Cell Biol 6:955–958
92. Van de Vijver M et al (1988) Neu-protein overexpression in breast cancer – NEJM 319:1239–1245
93. Lovekin C et al (1991) c-erbB-2 oncoprotein expression in primary and advanced breast cancer. Br J Cancer 63:439–443
94. Slamon DJ et al (1989) Studies of the HER-2/neu proto-oncogene in human breast and ovarian cancer. Science 244:707–712
95. Slamon DJ et al (1987) Human breast cancer: correlation of relapse and survival with amplification of the HER-2/neu oncogene. Science 235:177–182
96. Stal O et al (1995) c-erbB-2 expression and benefit from adjuvant chemotherapy and radiotherapy of breast cancer. Eur J Cancer 31a:2185–2190
97. Miles DW, Harris WH, Gillett CE, Smith P, Barnes DM (1999) Effect of c-erbB(2) and estrogen receptor status on survival of women with primary breast cancer treated with adjuvant cyclophosphamide/methotrexate/fluorouracil. Int J Cancer 84:354–359
98. Thor A (2001) HER2–a discussion of testing approaches in the USA. Ann Oncol 12(Suppl 1):S101–S107
99. Paik S et al (2002) Real-world performance of HER2 testing – national surgical adjuvant breast and bowel project experience. J Natl Cancer Inst 94:852–854
100. Perez EA et al (2006) HER2 testing by local, central, and reference laboratories in specimens from the north central cancer treatment group N9831 intergroup adjuvant trial. J Clin Oncol 24:3032–3038
101. Wolff AC et al (2007) American Society of Clinical Oncology/College of American Pathologists guideline recommendations for human epidermal growth factor receptor 2 testing in breast cancer. J Clin Oncol 25:118–145
102. http://www.nccn.org/JNCCN/PDF/her22006.pdf (2006)
103. Fendly BM et al (1990) Characterization of murine monoclonal antibodies reactive to either the human epidermal growth factor receptor or HER2/neu gene product. Cancer Res 50:1550–1558
104. Gajria D, Chandarlapaty S (2011) HER2-amplified breast cancer: mechanisms of trastuzumab resistance and novel targeted therapies. Expert Rev Anticancer Ther 11:263–275
105. Slamon DJ et al (2001) Use of chemotherapy plus a monoclonal antibody against HER2 for metastatic breast cancer that overexpresses HER2. N Engl J Med 344:783–792
106. Vogel C et al (2001) First-line, single-agent Herceptin(R) (trastuzumab) in metastatic breast cancer. A preliminary report. Eur J Cancer 37(Suppl 1):25–29
107. Lan KH, Lu CH, Yu D (2005) Mechanisms of trastuzumab resistance and their clinical implications. Ann N Y Acad Sci 1059:70–75
108. Lu Y, Zi X, Zhao Y, Mascarenhas D, Pollak M (2001) Insulin-like growth factor-I receptor signaling and

resistance to trastuzumab (Herceptin). J Natl Cancer Inst 93:1852–1857

109. Ritter CA et al (2004) Mechanisms of resistance development against trastuzumab (Herceptin) in an in vivo breast cancer model. Int J Clin Pharmacol Ther 42:642–643
110. Shattuck DL, Miller JK, Carraway KL 3rd, Sweeney C (2008) Met receptor contributes to trastuzumab resistance of Her2-overexpressing breast cancer cells. Cancer Res 68:1471–1477
111. Rexer BN, Arteaga CL (2012) Intrinsic and acquired resistance to HER2-targeted therapies in HER2 gene-amplified breast cancer: mechanisms and clinical implications. Crit Rev Oncog 17:1–16
112. Scaltriti M et al (2007) Expression of p95HER2, a truncated form of the HER2 receptor, and response to anti-HER2 therapies in breast cancer. JNCI 99:628–638
113. Leyland-Jones B, Smith BR (2011) Serum HER2 testing in patients with HER2-positive breast cancer: the death knell tolls. Lancet Oncol 12:286–295
114. Kruger JM et al (2013) Detection of truncated HER2 forms in formalin-fixed, paraffin-embedded breast cancer tissue captures heterogeneity and is not affected by HER2-targeted therapy. Am J Pathol 183:336–343
115. Verma S et al (2012) Trastuzumab emtansine for HER2-positive advanced breast cancer. N Engl J Med 367:1783–1791
116. Scheuer W et al (2009) Strongly enhanced antitumor activity of trastuzumab and pertuzumab combination treatment on HER2-positive human xenograft tumor models. Cancer Res 69:9330–9336

Part XI

Perspectives

The Role of CTCs as Tumor Biomarkers

21

Evi S. Lianidou, Athina Markou, and Areti Strati

Abstract

Detection of Circulating Tumor Cells (CTCs) in peripheral blood can serve as a "liquid biopsy" approach and as a source of valuable tumor markers. CTCs are rare, and thus their detection, enumeration and molecular characterization are very challenging. CTCs have the unique characteristic to be non-invasively isolated from blood and used to follow patients over time, since these cells can provide significant information for better understanding tumour biology and tumour cell dissemination. CTCs molecular characterization offers the unique potential to understand better the biology of metastasis and resistance to established therapies and their analysis presents nowadays a promising field for both advanced and early stage patients. In this chapter we focus on the latest findings concerning the clinical relevance of CTC detection and enumeration, and discuss their potential as tumor biomarkers in various types of solid cancers. We also highlight the importance of performing comparison studies between these different methodologies and external quality control systems for establishing CTCs as tumor biomarkers in the routine clinical setting.

Keywords

Breast cancer • Cancer stem cells • Circulating tumor cells (CTC) • Circulating tumour stem cells • CK-19 • Colorectal cancer • Epcam • Gastrointestinal Cancers • Hepatocellular carcinoma • Individualized treatment • Liquid biopsy • Lung cancer • Melanoma • Migrating cancer stem cells • Molecular characterization • Non-small-cell lung cancer (NSCLC) • Oncoproteomics • Overall survival (OS) • Pancreatic cancer • Peripheral blood • Predictive biomarkers • Prognostic biomarkers • Progression free survival (PFS) • Prostate cancer • Tumor biomarkers • Solid cancer

E.S. Lianidou (✉) • A. Markou • A. Strati
Analysis of Circulating Tumor Cells Lab, Lab of Analytical Chemistry, Department of Chemistry, University of Athens, 15771 Athens, Greece
e-mail: lianidou@chem.uoa.gr

R. Scatena (ed.), *Advances in Cancer Biomarkers*, Advances in Experimental Medicine and Biology 867, DOI 10.1007/978-94-017-7215-0_21

Abbreviation

AA	Abiraterone acetate
AR	Androgen receptor
BC	Breast cancer
CRPC	Castration-resistant prostate cancer
CA-15-3	Cancer antigen 15–3
CEA	Carcinoembryonic antigen
cfDNA	Cell free DNA
CTCs	Circulating Tumor Cells
CK-19	Cytokeratin-19
CK-7	Cytokeratin-7
DFS	Disease Free Survival
DTC	Disseminated tumor cells
EGFR	Epidermal growth factor receptor
EMT	Epithelial-Mesenchymal Transition
EQA	External quality assurance
CNA	Genome-wide copy-number aberration
HCC	Hepatocellular carcinoma
hTERT	Human telomerase reverse transcriptase
ISET	Isolation by size of epithelial tumour cells
LAPC	Locally advanced pancreatic carcinoma
LAHNC	Locally advanced head and neck cancer
LOH	Loss of heterozygosity
MBC	Metastatic breast cancer
mCRC	Metastatic colorectal cancer
NIH	National Institutes of Health
NSCLC	Non small cell lung cancer
OS	Overall Survival
PE	Pleural Effusion
PFS	Progression Free Survival
PSA	Prostate Specific Antigen
RT-PCR	Reverse transcriptase-polymerase chain reaction
SLN	Sentinel lymph node
SNP	Single-nucleotide polymorphism
SNUC	Sinonasal undifferentiated carcinoma
SCCHN	Squamous cell carcinoma of head and neck
TTF-1	Thyroid transcription factor 1
TGF-P	Transforming growth factor
TMPRSS2	Transmembrane protease serine 2

The major cause of cancer mortality is tumor metastasis and therefore there is a compelling need for the discovery and validation of novel biomarkers for cancer screening, diagnosis, prognosis and therapeutic monitoring [29]. The development of noninvasive methods to detect and monitor tumors continues to be a major challenge in oncology and the search for new and better non-invasive tumor biomarkers has become a holy grail of contemporary cancer research. As Dr Diamandis correctly has pointed out, "the journey of a cancer biomarker from the bench to the clinic is long, difficult and challenging and every step needs to be very carefully planned and executed in detail to succeed" [110].

The presence of tumor cells, circulating in blood of cancer patients was first reported by Thomas Ashworth in 1869 [5]. Nowadays, almost 150 years after this first report, the clinical and research potential of Circulating Tumor Cells (CTCs) is becoming widely recognized [118]. CTCs are indicators of residual disease and thus pose an increased risk of metastasis and poorer outcomes to those patients who are CTC-positive. The number of studies on CTCs published in peer reviewed journals is constantly rising during the last 15 years (Fig. 21.1).

CTCs represent cells that are shed in the circulation by primary or metastatic tumors and thus provide a "liquid biopsy" approach that enables frequent samplings of a patient's tumor and follow-up of patients during treatment. CTCs are in principle very different from all other established tumor biomarkers, since they represent a unique source of valuable information. By studying CTCs we can better understand tumour biology and tumour cell dissemination while their molecular characterization offers the unique potential to understand resistance to established therapies [79, 81].

CTC analysis is extremely challenging since CTCs are very rare, and the amount of available sample is very limited. Since CTC detection was shown to be of considerable utility in the clinical management of patients with solid cancers, a big variety of analytical systems for their isolation and detection have been developed [80, 108, 109, 163]. New areas of research are directed towards

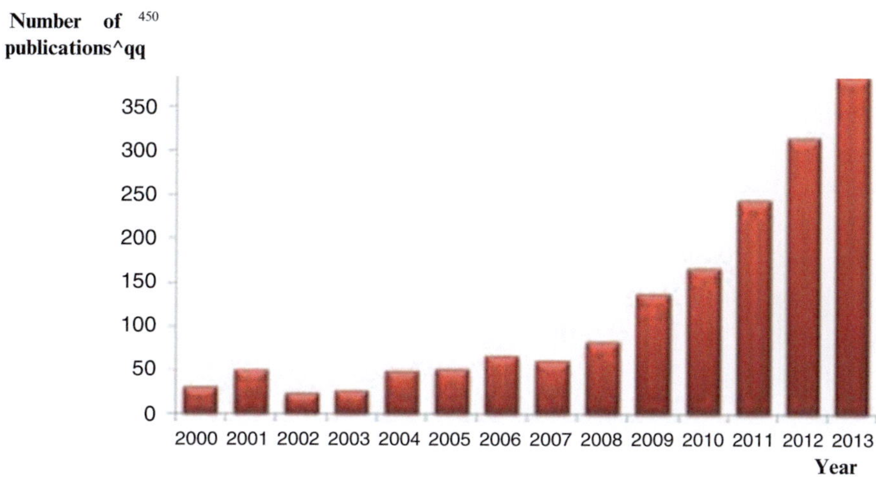

Fig. 21.1 Publications on CTCs during the last 13 years (http://www.ncbi.nlm.nih.gov/pubmed)

developing novel assays for CTC molecular characterization [3, 80, 120]. A high heterogeneity of CTC even among the same individuals has been observed by performing high dimensional single CTC profiling, and directly measuring gene expression in individual CTC without the common practice of pooling such cells [120]. Molecular studies on CTCs have often been limited by a low number of CTCs isolated from a high background of leukocytes. Improved enrichment techniques are now allowing molecular characterization of single CTCs, whereby molecular markers on single CTCs may provide a real-time assessment of tumor biomarker status from a blood test or "liquid biopsy", potentially eliminating the need for a more invasive tissue biopsy.

However, many questions still remain unanswered regarding the biology of CTC, the optimal method to enumerate and characterize them and the path to regulatory and general clinical acceptance of technology platforms currently under development [109].

In this chapter we focus on the latest findings concerning the clinical relevance of CTC detection and enumeration, and discuss their potential as tumor biomarkers in various types of solid cancers. We also discuss the different platforms available for CTC isolation, enumeration and molecular characterization, and highlight the importance of performing comparison studies between these different methodologies. Finally we discuss the importance of external quality control systems for establishing CTCs as tumor biomarkers in the routine clinical setting.

21.1 CTCs as Tumor Biomarkers

The clinical significance of CTC has been evaluated in many types of solid cancers, and the CTC enumeration test in metastatic breast, colorectal and prostate cancer has been cleared by the FDA almost a decade ago. There is a significant interest nowadays on examining CTCs as "surrogate" markers for potentially improved survival for regulatory purposes, and as prognostic or predictive biomarkers in a variety of solid cancers. In the official website of the National Institutes of Health (http://clinicaltrials.gov/ct2/home) our search (May 2014) based on the key word "Circulating Tumor Cells", revealed 587 ongoing clinical studies; when we searched for specific cancer types, a whole spectrum of studies evaluating the role of CTC as surrogate biomarkers was revealed (Fig. 21.2). These trials have different designs in various patient populations but are expected to be the pivotal trials for CTC implementation in the routine management of cancer patients [12, 13, 74]. The American Society of Clinical Oncology (ASCO) cited CTC and DTC

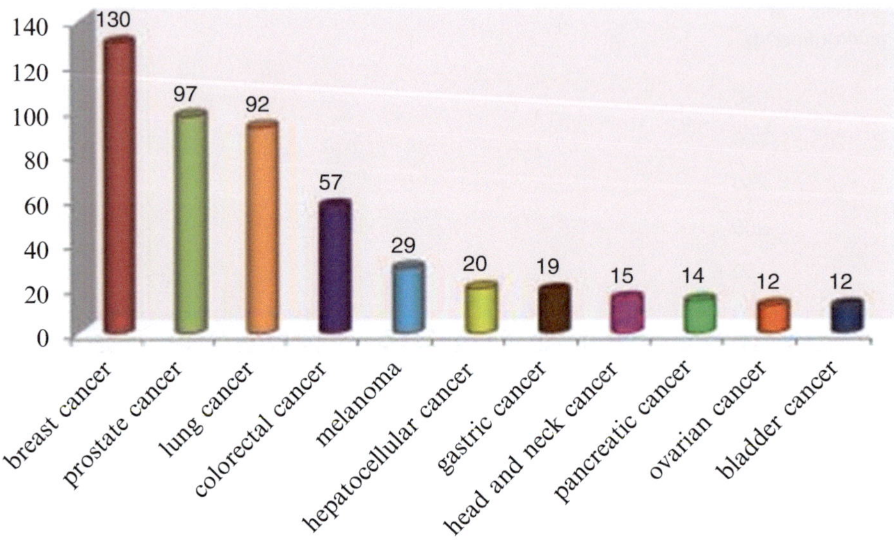

Fig. 21.2 Clinical studies that include CTCs analysis: in the official website of the National Institutes of Health (http://clinicaltrials.gov/ct2/home) our search on May 2014 on clinical studies, based on the key word "Circulating Tumor Cells", revealed 587 ongoing clinical studies

for the first time in its 2007 recommendations on tumor markers, however in the category of insufficient evidence to support routine use in clinical practice [51]. However, very recently, the American Joint Committee on Cancer has proposed a new category, M0(i+), for TNM staging in breast cancer (BC) defined as "no clinical or radiographic evidence of distant metastases, but deposits of molecularly or microscopically detected tumor cells (no larger than 0.2 mm) in blood, bone marrow, or other non-regional nodal tissue in a patient without symptoms or signs of metastases".

Below we are presenting the main studies performed so far on the clinical evaluation of CTCs as tumor biomarkers in various types of solid cancers.

21.1.1 Breast Cancer

In the official website of the NIH our search (May 2014) based on the key word "Circulating Tumor Cells AND breast cancer" revealed 130 studies (Fig. 21.2). The first comprehensive meta-analysis of published literature on the prognostic relevance of CTC in patients with early-stage and metastatic breast cancer clearly indicated that the detection of CTC is a reliable prognostic factor [164, 165].

21.1.1.1 Metastatic Breast Cancer

Cristofanilli and colleagues have shown by using the CellSearch System (Veridex, USA) that CTC represent an independent prognostic factor for Progression Free Survival (PFS) and Overall Survival (OS) in patients with metastatic breast cancer and that a cut-off of 5 CTC/7.5 ml of blood in these patients was highly predictive of clinical outcome [22]. This paper revolutionized the clinical applications of CTC in many types of cancer, since it led to the FDA clearance of the CellSearch assay that is standardized, semi-automated and not subjected to preanalytical errors. Since then, a plethora of clinical studies has verified the importance of CTC enumeration in metastatic breast cancer [41, 42, 98, 117, 155]. Liu et al. conducted a prospective study to demonstrate that CTC results correlate strongly with radiographic disease progression at the time of and in advance of imaging. They provided the first evidence of a strong correlation between CTC results and radiographic disease progression in patients receiving chemotherapy or endocrine therapy for MBC. These findings support the role of CTC enumeration as an adjunct to standard methods of monitoring disease status in MBC [85].

A very recent study assessed the clinical validity of CTC quantification for prognostication of patients with metastatic breast cancer by undertaking a pooled analysis of 1944 individual patient data. The authors contacted 51 European centers and asked them to provide reported and unreported anonymized data for individual patients with metastatic breast cancer starting a new line of therapy concerning PFS or OS, or both, and CTC quantification by the Cell Search method at baseline (before start of new treatment). The authors report that increased CTC counts 3–5 weeks after start of treatment, adjusted for CTC count at baseline, were associated with shortened PFS. Survival prediction was significantly improved by addition of baseline CTC count to the clinicopathological models The data collected confirmed the independent prognostic effect of CTC count on PFS and OS. CTC count also improves the prognostication of MBC when added to full clinic0pathological predictive models, whereas serum tumor markers do not. *CEA* and *CA 15–3* concentrations at baseline and during therapy did not add significant information to the best baseline model. [14].

In another recent prospective multicenter study a total of 254 MBC patients were enrolled at first diagnosis of metastatic disease or disease progression (before the start of a new treatment regimen). By using an EpCAM-independent enrichment approach, viable CTC releasing CK-19 as an epithelial cell marker were detected in the peripheral blood by the EPISPOT assay, and the FDA cleared CellSearch was used as the reference method. CTC detection using the EPISPOT assay has shown prognostic relevance of the presence of viable CTC. Interestingly, the combination of the EPISPOT and CellSearch assays was the strongest predictor of OS [127].

The presence of CTCs was found to be an effective measure of treatment efficacy and immune system function in MBC patients [18]. Green et al. report that that those patients with greater than 5 CTCs per 7.5 mL blood had significantly decreased responses by their immune cells when compared with those patients who had 5 CTCs or less. They also verified the already reported by many other groups correlation between disease progression and CTC-positive patients, indicating that those who have a positive test should be closely monitored by their clinician [46].

The detection and prognostic significance of CTCs in MBC in respect to the different immunehistochemical subtypes of breast cancer has been also recently evaluated. Peeters et al. report that the detection of EpCAM positive CTCs was not clearly associated with any of the immunehistochemical subtypes of breast cancer in patients with MBC before first-line treatment. Their data also suggest a lower prognostic significance of CTC evaluation in *HER2*-positive patients with MBC [112]. The French group, led by JY Pierga specifically evaluated the impact of CTC on brain metastasis outcome and has shown that there is a correlation between CNS metastasis response, outcome and early CTC clearance under targeted treatment of *HER2* positive MBC [115].

21.1.1.2 Early Breast Cancer

The prognostic value of CTC in axillary lymph node-negative breast cancer patients, based on a nested RT-PCR was already shown in 2002 [142]. By using a real time RT-qPCR assay for CK-19 mRNA [140, 141] CTC detection was shown to be an independent prognostic factor for reduced DFI and OS before [158], during [157] and after [156] chemotherapy in early breast cancer. Detection of CTC before adjuvant chemotherapy predicted for poor clinical outcome mainly in patients with ER-negative, triple-negative, and HER2-positive early-stage breast cancer [59]. When CTC were prospectively detected before and after neoadjuvant chemotherapy in a phase II trial it was found that detection of one or more CTC in 7.5 ml of blood before neoadjuvant chemotherapy can accurately predict OS [116]. A more recent study investigating the value of CTC detection during the first 5 years of follow-up in predicting late disease relapse, has shown that persistent detection of CTC was associated with an increased risk of late disease relapse and death in patients with operable breast cancer and indicates the presence of chemo-and hormonotherapy-resistant residual disease [133]. Lucci et al., prospectively collected data on CTC at the time of definitive surgery from chemonai've patients with stage 1–3 breast cancer. They enumerated CTC and assessed outcomes at a median follow-up of 35 months, and have shown that the presence of one or more CTC predicted for early recurrence and decreased overall survival in chemonai've patients with non-metastatic breast cancer [88].

These results were also recently confirmed by another study that was based on an RT-PCR molecular assay for CTC detection, the AdnaTest BreastCancer™ (AdnaGen AG, Germany). This assay is based on the detection of *EpCAM, HER2* and *MUC1* specific transcripts in enriched CTC-lysates. Mikulova et al. report that CTCs were detected in the peripheral blood of approximately 31 % of early stage breast cancer patients before therapy, while only 7 % of all patients remained CTCs positive after adjuvant therapy. There was no correlation between CTCs and tumor size, tumor grade, histological grade and receptor status [94].

21.1.1.3 CTC as Surrogate Markers for Treatment Response in Breast Cancer

Based on the current guidelines, in breast cancer, hormone therapy and anti-HER-2 therapies are prescribed according to the hormone (ER/PR expression) and *HER-2* status of the primary tumor. However, a growing body of evidence is showing that the hormone receptor and *HER-2* status in CTC can be different from that in the primary tumors and even change over time, especially during disease recurrence or progression in breast cancer patients [33, 34, 58, 122, 129, 139]. Based on that, re-evaluation of hormone receptor and HER-2 status by molecular characterization of CTC is a strategy with potential clinical application. An optimal individualized treatment could be selected by characterizing *ER* and *HER-2* status in CTC and comparing it to the primary tumor [124, 154].

Many research groups have already shown that HER2-positive CTCs can be detected in patients with HER2-negative primary tumors [34, 35, 58, 114, 122]. Ligthart et al. have recently developed an automated algorithm for evaluating HER-2 expression in CTC when using the CellSearch system. They report that HER-2 expression is very heterogeneous among CTC within each patient [82]. Georgoulias et.al were the first to investigate the effect of trastuzumab in HER2-negative patients that have CK(+)/HER2-positive CTC in a randomized phase II study. According to their results, administration of trastuzumab can eliminate chemotherapy-resistant CK19 mRNA-positive CTCs, reduce the risk of disease recurrence and prolong Disease Free Survival (DFS) [39].

However, to evaluate CTCs as a predictive biomarker and obtain clinically meaningful results large studies that are specifically designed around effective therapies are needed. This is very challenging, and difficult, because of the high cost and continuous changes in the molecular targeted therapies. Very recently the TREAT-CTC study (http://clinicaltrials.gov/ct2/results?term=TREAT-TC+study&Search=Search), is a randomized phase II trial for patients with HER2 negative primary BC who after completing (neo) adjuvant chemotherapy and surgery have detectable CTC in peripheral blood. The aim of the study is to see whether *HER2* directed therapy reduces relapses in women at high risk of recurrence, and for this reason women positive for CTC detection, as evaluated by using the CellSearch system, after neoadjuvant chemotherapy are randomly assigned to trastuzumab or a placebo. Moreover, the fact that breast cancer is a disease with clearly dinstict molecular subtypes[113] could be a reason why specific CTC counts or molecular phenotypes that are predictive for response to one therapy are not relevant for others.

Epithelial-Mesenchymal Transition (EMT) is an essential process in the metastatic cascade [10, 83]. CTC molecular characterization is highlighting the importance of EMT, a process which may be crucial for allowing tumors to invade into and grow at sites distant from the original site of tumor. The expression levels of EMT-inducing transcription factors have been determined in CTC in primary breast cancer patients [93].

Investigation of the apoptotic and proliferative status in CTC of breast cancer patients has shown that patients with metastatic and advanced disease had significantly lower numbers of apoptotic CTCs compared to patients with early breast cancer and that adjuvant chemotherapy reduced both the number of CTCs per patient and the number of proliferating CTCs [66]. Very recently Yu et al. have shown by serial monitoring of CTC in patients with breast cancer that these cells simultaneously expressed mesenchymal and epithelial markers, and that mesenchymal cells expressing known EMT regulators, including transforming growth factor (TGF)-P pathway components and the *FOXC1* transcription factor were associated with disease progression [162].

Similarly, the detection of CTCs expressing markers of stemness may also have important implications for treatment resistance. A major proportion of CTC of metastatic breast cancer patients show EMT and tumor stem cell characteristics [2] and CTC expressing *TWIST* and vimentin, were identified in patients with metastatic and early breast cancer patients [67]. The existence of a subpopulation of CTCs with putative stem cell progenitor phenotypes in patients with metastatic breast cancer has been shown by using triple-marker immunofluorescence microscopy [149]. Currently used detection methods for CTC are not efficient to identify this subtype of CTC which underwent EMT [68].

Moreover studies on the molecular characterization of CTCs have revealed that CTCs even within the same patient are heterogeneous. In non-metastatic breast cancer patients the expression of estrogen, progesterone and epidermal growth factor receptor (*EGFR*) by immunofluorescence experiments revealed heterogeneous expression of these hormonal receptors in samples from the same patients [100].

21.1.2 Prostate Cancer

In prostate cancer, CTC enumeration has been extensively studied and validated as a prognostic tool and has received FDA clearance for use in monitoring advanced disease. In the official website of the National Institutes of Health (http://clinicaltrials.gov/ct2/home) our search on May 2014 on clinical studies, based on the key word "Circulating Tumor Cells AND prostate cancer" revealed 97 studies. In patients with advanced prostate cancer, CTC enumeration by using the Veridex CellSearch™ system, at baseline and post-treatment, has been cleared by the FDA for quantifying the load of tumour cell dissemination. This test is prognostic of survival and is currently being implemented into routine clinical practice for estimating prognosis and monitoring treatment success [136]. The clinical utility of monitoring CTC changes with treatment, as an efficacy-response surrogate biomarker of survival, is currently being tested in large phase III trials, with the novel anti-androgen therapies abiraterone acetate and MDV3100. Molecular determinants can be identified and characterized in CTC as potential predictive biomarkers of tumor sensitivity to a therapeutic modality [23, 24].

The main CTC studies in advanced and localized prostate cancer, highlighting the important gains as well as the challenges posed by various approaches, and their implications for advancing prostate cancer management have been recently reviewed in detail [57].

21.1.2.1 Metastatic Prostate Cancer

Moreno et al. were the first to report in 2001 that CTC levels can be quantified in the circulation of patients with metastatic prostate cancer and that the change in the numbers of CTC correlates with disease progression with no diurnal variations [96]. Later, in 2007, Danila and colleagues reported that the number of CTC before therapy provides unique information relative to prognosis and that the shedding of cells into the circulation represents an intrinsic property of the tumor, distinct from the extent of the disease [25]. In 2008, data presented by de Bono and colleagues showed that CTC enumeration by using the CellSearch™ system has prognostic and predictive value in patients with metastatic castration- resistant prostate cancer (CRPC) and is an independent predictor of OS in CRPC, opening the way to the FDA clearance of this assay for the evaluation of CRPC [28]. CTC numbers, analyzed as a continuous variable, predict OS and provide independent prognostic information to time to disease progression and can be used to monitor disease status [105, 134].

Resel and colleagues analyzed the correlation between CTC levels and the Prostate Specific Antigen (PSA) level, Gleason score, and TNM stage in patients with metastatic hormone-sensitive prostate cancer and reported that CTC count in peripheral blood could provide a method for correctly staging prostate cancer and for assessing the prognosis of metastatic hormone-sensitive prostate cancer [128]. Combination of CTC and *PSA* velocity may offer insights into the prognosis and management of advanced PC [53, 131].

CTC enumeration was very recently prospectively validated in standard first-line docetaxel treatment for metastatic CRPC. S0421, a phase III trial of docetaxel plus prednisone with or without atrasentan, validated the prognostic utility of CTC enumeration for OS and disease response. Baseline CTC counts were prognostic, and rising CTCs at 3 weeks heralded significantly worse OS, potentially serving as an early metric to help redirect and optimize therapy in this clinical setting [43].

21.1.2.2 Early-Stage Prostate Cancer

Recently CTCs have been detected in early prostate cancer and may be a new surrogate candidate towards the decision whether to offer systemic or local treatment [31]. CTC tests may assist with clinical decision-making according to a pilot study that investigated whether CTC could be detected in early-stage prostate cancer patients receiving salvage radiotherapy using the CellSearch system. The results of this study demonstrated that CTC can be detected in early-stage prostate cancer and suggest the possibility that post-treatment reduction in CTC levels may be indicative of radiation therapy response [86]. Recent trials in patients with CRPC are incorporating the detection of CTC, imaging, and patient-reported outcome biomarkers in order to improve future drug development and patient management for patients [135].

21.1.2.3 CTCs as Surrogate Markers for Treatment Response in Prostate Cancer

Prostate cancer growth depends on androgen receptor (AR) signaling. Androgen ablation therapy induces expression of constitutively active androgen receptor splice variants that drive disease progression. Taxanes are a standard of care therapy in CRPC; A very recent study suggests that two clinically relevant AR splice variants, ARv567 and ARv7, differentially associate with microtubules and dynein motor protein, thereby resulting in differential taxane sensitivity in vitro and in vivo. They suggest that androgen receptor variants that accumulate in CRPC cells utilize distinct pathways of nuclear import that affect the antitumor efficacy of taxanes, suggesting a mechanistic rationale to customize treatments for patients with CRPC, which might improve outcomes [148].

Moreover, since persistence of ligand-mediated AR signaling has been documented in CRPC, abiraterone acetate (AA), an androgen biosynthesis inhibitor, was shown to prolong life in patients with CRPC already treated with chemotherapy. Miyamoto and colleagues have shown that measuring AR signaling within CTC may help to guide therapy in metastatic prostate cancer and highlight the use of CTC as liquid biopsy [95]. Leversha and colleagues have shown that FISH analysis of CTC can be a valuable, noninvasive surrogate for routine tumor profiling in patients with progressive castration-resistant metastatic prostate cancer [78]. Recent results by Darshan and colleagues suggest that monitoring AR subcellular localization in the CTC of CRPC patients might predict clinical responses to taxane chemotherapy [26]. Moreover, coding mutations in the AR gene that represent a possible mechanism underlying the development of CRPC have been identified in tissue samples from patients with advanced prostate cancer and have been also identified in CTC-enriched peripheral blood samples from CRPC patients [64].

Danila and colleagues studied the role of transmembrane protease, serine 2 (*TMPRSS2*)-v-ets erythroblastosis virus E26 oncogene homolog (ERG) fusion, an androgen-dependent growth factor, in CTC as a biomarker of sensitivity to AA [23, 24]. Hormone-driven expression of the ERG oncogene after fusion with *TMPRSS2* occurs in 30–70 % of therapy-naive prostate cancers. Molecular profiles of CTC with an analytically valid assay identified the presence of the prostate cancer-specific *TMPRSS2-ERG* fusion but did not predict for response to AA treatment [23, 24]. Attard and colleagues have used multicolor FISH to show that CRPC CTC, metastases, and prostate tissue invariably had the same ERG gene status as therapy-naive tumors and reported a significant association between ERG rearrangements in therapy-naive tumors, CRPC, and CTC and magnitude of PSA decline ($P = 0.007$) in CRPC patients treated with abiraterone acetate [6]. These findings demonstrate the role of CTC as surrogate marker that can be obtained in a routine practice setting [23, 24].

BRCA1 allelic imbalances were also detected among CTC in multifocal prostate cancer by using FISH analysis [9]. Especially, *BRCA1* losses might be one confounding factor initiating tumor dissemination and might provide an early indicator of shortened DFS [9]. The utility of CTC enumeration in hormone sensitive prostate cancer was recently shown by Goodman and colleagues, who enumerated CTC in 33 consecutive patients undergoing androgen deprivation therapy and reported that initial CTC values predict the duration and magnitude of response to hormonal therapy. CTC enumeration may identify patients at risk of progression to CRPC before initiation of androgen deprivation therapy [44].

Circulating endothelial cells, CTC and tissue factor levels alone and combined can predict early on OS in CRPC patients treated with docetaxel-based therapy [144]. Evaluation of the association between circulating objects positive for epithelial cell adhesion molecules and cytokeratin (EpCAM+CK+) that are not counted as CTC and survival in patients with prostate cancer has shown that each EpCAM+CK+CD45- circulating object showed a strong association with OS ($P < 0.001$) [21].

21.1.3 Lung Cancer

Lung cancer is the leading cause of cancer-related death worldwide. In the official website of the National Institutes of Health (http://clinicaltrials.gov/ct2/home) our search on May 2014 on clinical studies, based on the key word "Circulating Tumor Cells AND lung cancer" revealed 92 studies (Fig. 21.2). CTC detection in lung cancer in particular has proven difficult to perform, as CTCs in this type of cancer often present with non-epithelial characteristics. Moreover, as many detection methods rely on the use of epithelial markers to identify CTCs, the loss of these markers during EMT in certain metastatic cancers can render these methods ineffective.

21.1.3.1 Non-Small-Cell Lung Cancer (NSCLC)

Non-small-cell lung cancer (NSCLC) lacks validated biomarkers to predict treatment response. Zhu et.al evaluated the presence of EpCAM/MUC1 mRNA-positive CTCs in 74 non small cell lung cancer (NSCLC) patients and showed that DFS and OS was significantly reduced in patients with EpCAM/MUC1 mRNA-positive CTC preoperatively and postoperatively [166]. By using an EpCAM independent blood filtration system, the ISET (isolation by size of epithelial tumour cells) and immunofluorescence it was recently shown that hybrid CTCs with an epithelial/mesenchymal phenotype exist in patients with NSCLC and it is believed that their characterization should provide further insight on the significance of EMT in CTCs and on the mechanism of metastasis in patients with NSCLC [77]. Another single-center prospective study that investigated whether CTCs are detectable in patients with previously untreated, stage III or IV NSCLC and whether their detection could provide prognostic information and/or early indication of patient response to conventional therapy, came to the conclusion that CTCs are detectable in these patients and constitute a novel prognostic factor for this disease [76].

21.1.3.2 Small-Cell Lung Cancer (SCLC)

The clinical significance and molecular characteristics of CTCs and CTC clusters, termed circulating tumor microemboli (CTM), detected in patients with small-cell lung cancer (SCLC) undergoing standard treatment was evaluated. According to the results presented by Hou et al., both baseline CTC number and change in CTC number after one cycle of chemotherapy are independent prognostic factors for SCLC [56]

21.1.3.3 CTC as Surrogate Markers for Treatment Response in Lung Cancer

The group of Haber showed for the first time that lung cancer patients who's CTCs carried *EGFR* mutation known to cause drug resistance had faster disease progression than CTCs who lacked the mutation [89]. In late stage lung cancer patients *EGFR* mutations have been evaluated in single tumor cells enriched from blood using laser cell microdissection. In patients with advanced NSCLC mutational analysis with a 6-gene mutation panel *(EGFR, KRAS, BRAF, NRAS, AKT1,* and *PIK3CA)* were tested, where only one *EGFR* mutation (exon 19 deletion) was detected in CTC-derived DNA from the 38 patient samples analyzed [121].

The diagnostic test for ALK rearrangement in NSCLC for crizotinib treatment is currently done on tumor biopsies or fine-needle aspirations. Recently a group from the Institut de Cance'rologie Gustave Roussy attempted to avoid the need for a tissue sample to diagnose ALK-rearranged NSCLC by studying a novel ALK FISH method in CTCs. Pailler et al. recently detected ALK rearrangements in CTCs of patients with ALK-positive NSCLC by using a filtration technique and FISH, enabling both diagnostic testing and monitoring of crizotinib treatment. These results clearly suggest that CTCs harboring a unique ALK rearrangement and mesenchymal phenotype may arise from clonal selection of tumor cells that have acquired the potential to drive metastatic progression of ALK-positive NSCLC [106].

CellSearch™ technology was very recently adapted for the identification of tumor cells in Pleural effusions (PE) to assist in the diagnosis of malignant PEs. The pleural CellSearch™ assay may serve as a valuable addition to traditional cytology and provide useful information regarding the diagnosis of malignant effusions. Major advantages include that it is well standardized, relatively inexpensive, has a rapid turnaround, and is easily available [138].

21.1.4 Colorectal Cancer

In the official website of the National Institutes of Health (http://clinicaltrials.gov/ct2/home) our search on May 2014 on clinical studies, based on the key word "Circulating Tumor Cells AND colorectal cancer" revealed 57 studies (Fig. 21.2). The prognostic value of CTC and DTC in patients with resectable colorectal liver metastases or widespread metastatic colorectal cancer (mCRC) has been clearly shown in a meta-analysis study that was based on 12 studies [48].

A comprehensive literature search was used to identify studies reporting on the significance of CTCs in the postoperative blood of CRC patients. Based on this search, a systematic review examined the evidence for the use of CTCs as prognostic markers in CRP. In six out of nine studies examined the detection of postoperative CTCs was found to be an independent predictor of cancer recurrence [111].

21.1.4.1 Metastatic Colorectal Cancer

In a prospective multicenter study, CTC were enumerated in 430 patients with mCRC at baseline and after starting first-, second-, or third-line therapy by using the CellSearch system. According to this study, the number of CTC before and during treatment was an independent predictor of PFS and OS in patients with mCRC. Based on these results, the CellSearch assay was cleared by the FDA for mCRC [20]. It was further shown that CTC enumeration before and during treatment independently predicts PFS and OS in advanced colorectal cancer patients treated with chemotherapy plus targeted agents and provides additional information to CT imaging [153]. The clinical utility of CTC enumeration in improving the clinician's ability to accurately assess oxaliplatin-based chemotherapy treatment benefit and in expediting the identification of effective treatment regimens for individual patients was further shown [91].

Another study showed a strong correlation between CTC detection and radiographic disease progression in patients receiving chemotherapy for colorectal cancer [27]. Evaluation of the impact of immediate and differing surgical interventions on CTC and their compartmentalization or localization in different anatomic vascular sites has shown that surgical resection of metastases, but not radiofrequency ablation, immediately decreases CTC levels [65]. Another recent study has shown that the qualitative and quantitative detection of CTC is higher in the mesenteric venous blood compartments of patients with CRC [125].

Very recently, Barbazan et al. evaluated the clinical utility of six CTC markers (tissue specific and Epithelial to Mesenchymal Transition transcripts) both as prognostic and predictive tools in mCRC patients. CTC-markers identified therapy-refractory patients not detected by standard image techniques. Patients with increased CTC-markers along treatment, but classified as responders by computed tomography, showed significantly shorter survival times [8].

In another recent study, post-chemotherapeutic CTCs were detected in stage III colon cancer patients in order to identify those patients who were at high risk of relapse. By using human telomerase reverse transcriptase *(hTERT)*, *CK-19*, *CK-20,* and *CEA,* as the biomarkers to detect CTCs in 90 stage III colon cancer patients undergoing curative resection followed by mFOLFOX chemotherapy Lu et al. came to the conclusion that CTCs were independent predictors of post-chemotherapeutic relapse and that the persistent presence of post-chemotherapeutic CTCs in peripheral blood strongly correlated with reduced DFS and OS. The accuracy of detecting relapse in post-chemotherapeutic stage III colon cancer patients by analyzing the persistent presence of postchemotherapeutic CTCs was higher than that by postchemotherapeutic *CEA* levels chemotherapy [87].

21.1.4.2 Non-Metastatic Colorectal Cancer

The prognostic role of CTC in non-metastatic colorectal cancer is less clear than in mCRC. The low abundance of CTC in non-metastatic colorectal cancer requires very sensitive and specific detection methods. A recent review examined the possible clinical significance of CTC in non-metastatic colorectal cancer (TNM-stage I-III) with the primary focus on detection methods and prognosis. According to the findings reported, the presence of CTC in peripheral blood is a potential marker of poor disease-free survival in patients with non-metastatic colorectal cancer [150]. CTC detection might help in the selection of high-risk stage II colorectal cancer patient candidates for adjuvant chemotherapy, after enumerating CTC with the FDA-cleared CellSearch system [38].

Using *CEA, CK* and *CD133* as genetic markers, Iinuma et al. evaluated the clinical significance of CTCs as a prognostic factor for OS and DFS in the peripheral blood of patients with colorectal cancer who had undergone curative surgery. In the training sets, OS and DFS of patients who were positive for these markers were significantly worse than those of patients who were negative for these markers. At each staging analysis, OS and DFS of patients with Dukes' stage B or C cancer who were positive for *CEA/CK/CD133* were significantly worse than those of patients who were negative for these markers. In contrast, in patients with Dukes' stage A, no significant differences were seen between patients who were positive for these markers and those who were negative while in patients with Dukes' stage B and C cancer, *CEA/CK/CD133* demonstrated significant prognostic value. In validation sets, similar results were confirmed in patients with Dukes' stage B and C cancer. According to these data, in patients with Dukes' stage B and C CRC who require adjuvant chemotherapy, detection of *CEA/CK/CD133* mRNA in PB is a useful tool for determining which patients are at high risk for recurrence and poor prognosis [61]

21.1.4.3 CTC as Surrogate Markers for Treatment Response in Colorectal Cancer

The presence of *KRAS* and *BRAF* mutations reflect anti-EGFR therapy efficacy in metastatic colorectal cancer, and for this reason, primary tumors are analyzed for the presence of these specific mutations. However, discordances in respect to the mutation status of *KRAS* and *BRAF* in metastatic colorectal cancer patients between primary tumors, CTC and metastatic tumors have very important implications [97]. There is a lot of work being done towards this direction; using the CellSearch system, Gasch C et al. investigated EGFR expression, *EGFR* gene amplification and *KRAS, BRAF* and *PIK3CA* mutations in single CTC of patients with metastatic colorectal cancer [37]. When *KRAS* mutations were detected in single CTC isolated from metastatic colorectal cancer patients a mutational concordance between CTCs and primary tumor in 50 % of matched cases was reported [32]. *APC, KRAS,* and *PIK3CA* mutations that were found in CTCs were also present at subclonal levels in the primary tumors and metastases from the same patient [52]. *KRAS* mutation status was also examined in CTC of metastatic colorectal cancer patients [160].

Plastin3 is a novel marker for CTC undergoing EMT and is associated with colorectal cancer prognosis that was particularly strong in patients with Dukes B and Dukes C [161]. Patients with CTC positivity at baseline had a significant shorter median PFS compared with patients with no CTCs and a significant correlation was also founded between CTC detection during treatment and radiographic findings at the 6 month staging [27].

CTCs are promising markers for the evaluation and prediction of treatment responses in rectal cancer patients, superior to the conventional tumor marker *CEA*. When the clinical significance of CTCs in comparison to CEA was investigated in respect to prediction of treatment responses there was a close relationship between CTC levels and treatment outcomes but serum *CEA* did not have any correlation [145, 146].

21.1.5 Melanoma

In the official website of NIH our search on May 2014 based on the key words "Circulating Tumor Cells AND melanoma" revealed 29 studies (Fig. 21.2).

CTC have been detected in peripheral blood of patients with metastatic melanoma and are associated with advanced melanoma stage and poor patient outcome. When the expression of *MART-1, MAGE-A3,* and *PAX3* mRNA has been evaluated in CTC of stage IV melanoma patients by RT-qPCR 54 % of patients were positive and the presence of CTC was significantly associated with DFS and OS [54, 55]. Kiyohara E et al. have recently developed a multimarker quantitative real-time reverse transcriptase polymerase chain reaction (RT-qPCR) assay for detecting CTC directly from peripheral blood specimens without the need of separating CTC from leukocytes. This assay, that is based on four mRNA biomarkers *(MART-1/Melan-A, MAGE-A3,PAX3,* and *GalNAc-T)* has both high sensitivity and specificity for CTC in blood specimens, and its clinical significance for serial bleed assessment of CTC in clinical trials and for daily clinical usage has been evaluated [72]

Chiu CG et al. very recently provided the first detailed genome-wide copy-number aberration (CNA) and loss of heterozygosity (LOH)-based characterization of melanoma CTC and illustrated how CTC may be used as a novel approach for identification of systemic metastasis. They characterized 251 CNA in CTC and their comparative analysis demonstrated >90 % concordance in SNP profiles between paired CTC and tumor metastases. In particular, there were notable recurring CNA across patients. In exploratory studies, the presence of several top CTC-associated CNA was verified in distant metastasis (stage IV) suggesting that certain genomic changes are propagated from regional metastases to CTC and to distant systemic metastases [19]. Uveal melanoma is one of the most deadly diseases in ophthalmology for which markers able to predict the appearance of metastasis are needed. A recent study that investigated the role of CTC as a prognostic factor in this disease confirmed the role of CTC as a negative prognostic marker in uveal melanoma patients after a long follow-up period. Further characterization of CTC will help understanding metastasis mechanisms in uveal melanoma and even improve patient management [92].

21.1.5.1 Early Stage Melanoma

CTC analysis may be useful in discriminating melanoma patients who may benefit from aggressive adjuvant therapy or stratifying patients for adjuvant clinical trials. The outcomes of patients with melanoma who have sentinel lymph node (SLN) metastases can be highly variable, which has precluded establishment of consensus regarding treatment of the group. The detection of high-risk patients from this clinical setting may be helpful for determination of both prognosis and management. Hoshimoto S et al. evaluated the clinical utility of a multimarker RT-qPCR *(MART-1, MAGE-A3,* and *GalNAc-T)* assay for the detection of CTCs in 331 patients with melanoma diagnosed with SLN metastases that were clinically disease-free after complete lymphadenectomy in a phase III, international, multicenter clinical trial. Individual CTC biomarker detection ranged from 13.4 % to 17.5 % and there was no association of CTC status with known clinical or pathologic prognostic variables. However, the presence of two or more positive biomarkers was significantly associated with worse distant metastasis, DFS and reduced recurrence-free survival [54, 55]

Blood-based assays to detect melanoma progression by monitoring levels of CTC and cfDNA can be used to evaluate progress and therapy response in melanoma patients [147] while advances in the molecular analysis of CTC may provide insight into new avenues of approaching therapeutic options that would benefit personalized melanoma management [73]. Mutated BRAF was detected in 81 % of 21 assessed stage IV melanoma patients [71]. When single, isolated CTC from patients with melanoma have been subjected to *BRAF* and KIT mutational analysis, the *BRAF* sequences and KIT sequences identified in CTC were inconsistent with those identified in autologous melanoma tumours, showing clonal heterogeneity [132].

21.1.6 Hepatocellular Carcinoma

In the official NIH website our search (May 2014) on clinical studies, based on the key word "Circulating Tumor Cells AND hepatocellular cancer" revealed 20 studies (Fig. 21.2).

The clinical relevance of CTC in hepatocellular carcinoma (HCC) is lagging behind other major tumor types. Up to now there are just a few studies on CTCs and hepatocellular carcinoma but this list is continuously growing. Zhang et al. have recently reviewed existing and developing methodologies for CTC detection and describe the potential clinical impact of the identification and molecular characterization of CTC in HCC patients [164, 165]. Very recently, a remarkable variation of cells with epithelial, mesenchymal, liver-specific, and mixed characteristics and different size ranges were identifiable in the peripheral blood of HCC patients and the distribution of these cell subgroups varied significantly between different patient groups and was associated with therapeutic outcome [102]. By using the FDA cleared CellSearch™ system Schulze et al. investigated the prognostic relevance of EpCAM-positive CTCs in 59 patients with HCC and demonstrated a frequent presence of EpCAM-positive CTC in patients with intermediate or advanced HCC. The prognostic value of CTC detection in these cases for OS could have possible implications for future treatment stratification [137]. When the prognostic significance and the stem cell-like characteristics of EpCAM+ CTCs were identified prospectively in HCC patients undergoing curative resection, stem cell-like phenotypes were observed in EpCAM+ CTCs, and a preoperative CTC number of >2 cells/7.5 mL was found to predict for tumor recurrence in HCC patients after surgery, especially in patient subgroups with AFP levels of <400 ng/mL or low tumor recurrence risk [145, 146].

21.1.7 Pancreatic Cancer

The poor prognosis of pancreatic cancer patients is associated with the frequent and early dissemination of the disease, as well as late detection due to unspecific and late symptoms from the primary tumor. Pancreatic cancers frequently spread to the liver, lung and skeletal system, suggesting that pancreatic tumor cells must be able to intravasate and travel through the circulation to distant organs. Detection of CTC in peripheral blood may be a promising biomarker for the detection and prognosis of pancreatic cancer. In the official website of NIH our search on May 2014 based on the key word "Circulating Tumor Cells AND pancreatic cancer" revealed 14 studies (Fig. 21.2).

Tjensvoll et al., in a very recent review of previously reported studies on the clinical relevance of CTC detection in pancreatic cancer report that there is evidence that the presence of CTCs correlates with an unfavorable outcome [152]. Bidard et al. reported that CTC detection appears as a promising prognostic tool in locally advanced pancreatic carcinoma (LAPC) patients. In this study, CTC detection rates and prognostic value were evaluated in a prospective cohort of LAPC patients, using the CellSeach system. CTC positivity was associated with poor tumor differentiation and with shorter OS in multivariable analysis [12, 13]. However, as stated by Gall et al., with such low numbers of CTCs detected in LAPC patients, it is unclear whether CTCs can actually contribute toward tumor invasiveness and spread in such an aggressive cancer. Although this is a well- designed study, the small number of patients with detectable CTCs means that the statistical power is not great enough to make firm conclusions. Therefore, this expensive assay needs further investigation before being used a prognostic marker in patients with LAPC [36]

A very recent meta-analysis aimed to assess the prognostic value of CTC in patients with pancreatic cancer, including nine cohort studies with a total of 623 pancreatic cancer patients, 268 CTC-positive and 355 CTC-negative. This meta-analysis revealed that patients in the CTC-positive group were significantly associated with poor PFS. Furthermore, pancreatic cancer patients in the CTC-positive group also showed worse OS than those in the CTC-negative group [50]. Larger studies, as well as characterization of the CTC population, are required to achieve further insight into the clinical implications of CTC detection in pancreatic cancer patients.

21.1.8 Gastrointestinal Cancers

The clinical significance of CTC detection in gastrointestinal (GI) cancer remains controversial and the molecular biological characteristics of CTCs are poorly understood. In the official NIH website our search (May 2014) based on the key word "Circulating Tumor Cells AND Gastointestinal Cancers" revealed 19 studies (Fig. 21.2). In a recent study, a total of 87 patients with metastatic or recurrent GI cancer were prospectively enrolled. CTCs and their *HER2* status were assessed using the CellSearch System. The findings of this study suggest that it is critical to evaluate the *HER2* status of not only the primary tumour but also the CTCs because the metastasizing tumour cells are the primary target of systemic therapy [62].

21.1.9 Head and Neck

In the official website of NIH our search on May 2014 based on the key word "Circulating Tumor Cells AND head and neck cancer" revealed 15 studies (Fig. 21.2).

According to a prospective clinical follow-up study of patients with squamous cell carcinoma of head and neck (SCCHN) undergoing surgical intervention, patients with no detectable CTCs had a significantly higher probability of DFS [63]. The same group has shown recently, that in patients with SCCHN, the presence of CTCs correlates with worse disease-free survival [7]. This conclusion was based on results obtained after isolation of CTC by a purely negative enrichment methodology which does not depend on the expression of surface epithelial markers. According to another prospective multi-centric analysis that studied the possible role of CTC identification in locally advanced head and neck cancer (LAHNC), CTC were frequently identified in oro- and hypopharyngeal cancer and in sinonasal undifferentiated carcinoma, SNUC; A decrease in the CTC number or their absence throughout the treatment seems also to be related with non-progressive disease, after both complete or incomplete remission and with the proportion of patients alive and no evidence of disease [15, 159].

Current staging methods for squamous cell carcinomas (SCC) of the oral cavity (OSCC) need to be improved to predict the risk of individual patients. Grobe A et al. very recently assessed the prognostic significance of disseminated tumor cells (DTC) in bone marrow and CTC in peripheral blood from patients with OSCC. According to their findings both DTCs and CTCs are independent prognostic markers in patients with OSCC, predicting relapse with higher sensitivity at various disease stages than routine staging procedures [47].

21.1.10 Ovarian Cancer

In the official website of the NIH, our search (May 2014) based on the key word "Circulating Tumor Cells AND ovarian cancer" revealed 12 studies (Fig. 21.2).

Obermayr et al. identified a panel of six genes for the PCR-based detection of CTC in endometrial, cervical, and ovarian cancers and reported that by using this panel, they could detect 44 % of the cervical, 64 % of the endometrial and 19 % of the ovarian cancer patients [104]. The same group, in a more recent study identified novel markers for CTCs in patients with epithelial ovarian cancer, and evaluated their impact on clinical outcome. By using these markers they could detect CTC in 24.5 % of the baseline (before primary treatment) and 20.4 % of the follow-up samples (6 months after adjuvant chemotherapy) of which two thirds were identified by overexpression of the cyclophilin C gene (PPIC), and just a few by EpCAM overexpression. They report that the presence of CTCs at baseline correlated with the presence of ascites, sub-optimal debulking, and elevated CA-125 and HE-4 levels, whereas CTC during follow-up occurred more often in older and platinum resistant patients. PPIC positive CTCs during follow-up were significantly more often detected in the platinum resistant than in the platinum sensitive patient group, and indicated poor outcome independent from classical prognostic parameters [103].

By using the AdnaTest Breast Cancer commercially available test (Allere, USA) that is based on immunomagnetic enrichment and multiplex RT-PCR for selection and detection of CTCs Aktas et al., checked for CTC in the blood of 122 ovarian cancer patients at primary diagnosis and/or after platinum-based chemotherapy. They report that CTC positivity significantly correlated with shorter OS before surgery ($P=0.0054$) and after chemotherapy ($P=0.047$) [1]. Poveda et al. evaluated the correlation, between numbers of CTCs and PFS and OS, in a phase III study of pegylated liposomal doxorubicin (PLD) with trabectedin vs. PLD for relapsed ovarian cancer, by using the CellSearch system and reagents (Veridex). Results from this study indicated that elevated numbers of CTCs impart an unfavorable prognosis for ovarian cancer patients [119]. Recently, Liu et al. investigated whether CTCs, as detected and enumerated by the Veridex CellSearch™ system, could predict for clinical outcomes in women with newly diagnosed or recurrent epithelial ovarian cancer. According to their results, CTCs can be isolated from women with newly diagnosed or recurrent ovarian cancer, however, their numbers do not significantly correlate with clinical characteristics or patient outcomes [84].

21.1.11 Bladder Cancer

In the official website of NIH our search on May 2014 based on the key word "Circulating Tumor Cells AND bladder cancer" revealed 12 studies (Fig. 21.2). Nonmuscle-invasive bladder cancer is a tumor type characterized by early progression and a lack of prognostic markers and in this way it represents an optimal model to evaluate whether CTC assessment would be more beneficial in early stage cancer. Very recently, Raimondi C et al. reviewed whether CTCs may be used as a noninvasive, real-time tool for the stratification of early stage bladder cancer patients according to individual risk of progression [126].

Rink et al. prospectively detected and evaluated the biological significance of CTC in patients with bladder cancer, especially in those patients with non-metastatic, advanced bladder cancer using the CellSearch. Their findings suggest that the presence of CTC may be predictive for early systemic disease since CTCs were detected in 30 % of patients with non-metastatic disease [130]. Gradilone et al., have chosen to evaluate the prognostic significance of survivin-expressing CTC in patients with T1G3 bladder tumours since the prognosis of T1G3 bladder cancer is highly variable and unpredictable from clinical and pathological prognostic factors. They report that the presence of CTC was an independent prognostic factor for DFS in patients with T1G3 bladder cancer [45]. CTCs have also been shown to be present in the peripheral blood of patients with metastatic urothelial carcinoma. Guzzo et al. evaluated the ability of CTCs to predict extravesical disease in bladder cancer patients prior to radical cystectomy and came to the conclusion that CTC status is not likely to be a clinically useful parameter for directing therapeutic decisions in these patients [49].

21.1.12 Testicular Germ Cell Tumors

Germ cell tumors (GCTs) represent the most frequent malignancies among young men, but little is known about CTCs in these tumors. Nastaly et al., recently investigated the presence of CTCs in this tumor type, using two independent assays that target germ and epithelial cell-specific markers. For CTC detection, a combination of germ (anti-SALL4, anti-OCT3/4) and epithelial cell-specific (antikeratin, anti-EpCAM) antibodies was used because of the high heterogeneity of CTCs. Their results were correlated with disease stage, histology, and serum tumor markers. According to their findings, the inclusion of germ-cell specific markers improves CTCs detection in GCTs. CTCs occur frequently in patients with more aggressive disease, and there is a gradient of CTCs with decreasing numbers from the tumor-draining vein to the PB vessels [101].

21.1.13 Neuroendocrine Tumors

A recent single-center prospective study, aimed to determine the prognostic significance of CTCs in 176 patients with measurable metastatic neuroendocrine tumors (NETs). CTCs were measured using a semi-automated technique based on immune-magnetic separation of epithelial cell adhesion molecule-expressing cells. The presence of CTCs was associated with increased burden, increased tumor grade, and elevated serum chromogranin A (CgA). The presence of >one CTC was associated with worse PFS and OS; in multivariate analysis, CTCs remained significant when other prognostic markers, grade, tumor burden, and CgA were included. CTCs are a promising prognostic marker for patients with NETs and should be assessed in the context of clinical trials with defined tumor subtypes and therapy [69]

21.2 Quality Control Issues: Comparison of Different Methodologies

21.2.1 Analytical Methodologies for CTC Detection, Enumeration and Molecular Characterization

Since the detection of CTC has been shown to be of considerable utility in the clinical management of patients with solid cancers, a plethora of analytical systems for their isolation and detection have been developed and are still under development and their number is increasing at an exponential rate [80, 107–109, 163]. Since CTCs are very rare (1 CTC in 10^6–10^7 leukocytes) [151], in most cases they are specifically detected by using a combination of two steps: (a) isolation-enrichment and (b) detection. The only US Food and Drug Administration-cleared, commercially available CTC detection system is the CellSearch™ CTC test (Veridex, Raritan, NJ), which enriches CTCs by using particles that are coated with antibodies against EpCAM and is approved as a prognostic test in breast, colon, and prostate cancers.

The detailed presentation of these systems is beyond the scope of this review, especially since excellent reviews have been recently published on this topic (Pantel et al. 2012; Lianidou et al. 2011; [109, 163]; Alix-Panabieres et al. 2013).

21.2.2 Comparison Studies between Different CTC Assays

Advanced technologies developed for CTC isolation and detection are very promising for providing assays useful in oncological drug development, monitoring the course of disease in cancer patients, and in understanding the biology of cancer progression. However, the phenotypic heterogeneity of CTC and their low numbers in the bloodstream of patients, together with differences in pre-analytical sample processing, has led to the collection and accumulation of inconsistent data among independent studies [109]. Therefore, comparison of different methods for CTC enumeration and characterization by using the same samples is an important issue for the clinical use of CTC analysis as a liquid biopsy. However, as Powell et al. have recently shown, by performing a high dimensional single CTC profiling, CTC even within the ame patient are highly heterogeneous [120]. This heterogeneity of CTCs and their low numbers in the bloodstream of patients means that no standardized detection method currently exists. This, together with differences in pre-analytical sample processing, has led to the collection and accumulation of inconsistent data among independent studies.

We summarize here a number of recent studies that have focused on the comparison of different CTC methodologies, using the same clinical samples.

Andreopoulou et al. compared the CellSearch system and a molecular assay, the AdnaTest BreastCancer Select/Detect, to evaluate the extent that these assays differ in their ability to detect CTCs in the PB of MBC patients. The overall positive agreement between these two different methodologies was 73 % for CTC>2 and 69 % for CTC>5. These preliminary data suggest that theAdnaTest has equivalent sensitivity to that of the CellSearch system in detecting 2 or more CTCs. While there is concordance between these 2 methods, the AdnaTest complements the CellSearch system by improving the overall CTC detection rate and permitting the assessment of genomic markers in CTCs [4].

Khoja L et al. compared prospectively the utility of two platforms for CTC enumeration and characterisation in pancreatic cancer patients in a pilot exploratory study. Blood samples were obtained prospectively from 54 consenting patients and analysed by CellSearch and isolation by size of epithelial tumour cells (ISET). CellSearch exploits immunomagnetic capture of CTCs-expressing epithelial markers, whereas ISET is a marker independent, blood filtration device. CTC expression of epithelial and mesenchymal markers was assessed to explore any discrepancy in CTC number between the two platforms. According to their findings, ISET detects more CTCs than CellSearch and offers flexible CTC characterisation with potential to investigate CTC biology and develop biomarkers for pancreatic cancer patient management [70]

When three different CTC molecular assays were compared, using the same cDNAs throughout our study to avoid discrepancies due to pre-analytical errors all CTC assays gave similar results in about 70 % of cases. Better agreement was found in the metastatic setting, possibly explained by the higher tumor load in this group. Discordances could be attributed to the different gene transcripts used to evaluate CTC positivity. These results indicate the importance of CTC heterogeneity for their detection by different analytical methodologies [143].

The DETECT trial for metastatic breast cancer patients was designed to directly compare the prognostic impact of two commercially available CTC assays that are prominent representatives of immunocytochemical and RT-PCR based technologies. CTCs were assessed using both the AdnaTest Breast Cancer and the CellSearch system according to the manufacturers' instructions using 254 metastatic breast cancer patients. According to this study, when using the CellSearch system, there was a prognostic impact for OS even in the subgroups of patients with triple negative, HER2-positive and hormone receptor-positive/HER2-negative primary tumors while CTC-positivity assessed by the AdnaTest Breast had no association with PFS or OS. [98]

Gervasoni et al. compared the ability of three different methods to detect CTCs in the blood of colorectal cancer patients. Specifically, different aliquots of the same blood sample were screened for the presence of CTCs by a multimarker RT-PCR assay, the standardized CellSearch assay and dHPLC-based gene mutation analysis. In the population tested, none of the blood samples analysed appeared to be positive by all three methods. The samples which were positive for CTCs by the CellSearch assay did not overlap with those that were positive by dHPLC. Interestingly, however, all of these samples were positive when assessed by RT-PCR. Conversely, of the samples that resulted negative by RT-PCR analysis, none appeared to be positive by either of the other methods. These data, therefore, indicate that of the three methods tested, the multimarker RT-PCR assay provides maximal probability of CTC detection [40].

When CTCs were compared with classic serum tumor biomarkers (*CA 15–3, CEA* and lactate dehydrogenase) as prognostic markers in metastatic breast cancer, it was found that elevated CTCs before cycle 2 are an early predictive marker of poor PFS and OS, which could be used to monitor treatment benefit [117].

21.2.3 Quality Control Issues

Standardization of CTC detection and characterization methodologies is important for the incorporation of CTC into prospective clinical trials testing their clinical utility. Despite the attractiveness and potential convenience of using blood-based CTC assays to diagnose genomic alterations and follow response to therapy in solid cancers, these technologies face significant hurdles and have not been included as yet in the guidelines to supplement tissue-based diagnostics. The main issues with CTC assays are the lack of standardized methods to define and capture these cells and the technical challenges in capturing a few CTC among billions of non-cancerous circulating blood cells.

Critical issues concerning the standardized detection of CTC include: (a) the standardization of the pre-analytical phase such as sampling itself (eg sample volume, avoidance of epidermal epithelial cells co-sampling in case that epithelial markers such as CK-19 will be later used for CTC detection), sample shipping (stability of CTC under different conditions) and storage conditions (use of preservatives, or anticoagulants), (b) standardization of CTC isolation through use of spiking controls in peripheral blood, and (c) standardization of detection systems (d) inter-laboratory and intra laboratory comparison studies for the same samples. The development of international standards for CTC enumeration and characterization is also very important especially in imaging detection systems that are observer-dependent (Lianidou 2011; Parkinson 2012).

Kraan et al. evaluated the feasibility of performing an external quality assurance (EQA) of the entire CellSearch procedure from blood draw to interpretation of results in multiple laboratories. Blood samples from six cancer patients and controls were distributed to 14 independent laboratories to test between-laboratory, between-assay, and between-instrument variation. Additionally, between-operator variability was assessed through the interpretation of blinded images of all blood samples on a website. According to the results of this study, shipment and storage of samples had no influence on CTC values. Between-instrument and between-assay variation was low indicating high reproducibility. However, between-laboratory CV ranged from 45 to 64 %. Although inter-operator agreement on image interpretation (Fleiss' κ statistics) ranged from "substantial" to "almost perfect," image interpretation, particularly of samples containing high numbers of apoptotic cells, was the main contributor to between-laboratory variation. This multicenter study has shown the feasibility of an EQA program for CTC detection in patient samples, and the importance of continuation of such a program for the harmonization of CTC enumeration [75].

A very recent study evaluated the inter-reader agreement of the results obtained with the FDA-cleared CellSearch sytem for HER-2 in breast cancer, using exactly the same CTC images. For this reason, the same CellSearch images were sent to 22 readers from 15 academic laboratories and 8 readers from two Veridex laboratories. The inter-reader agreement for CTC definition was high, while reduced agreement was observed in M0 patients with low CTC counts. Continuous training and independent image review are required [60].

A recent manuscript summarized in a global aspect current thinking on the value and promise of evolving CTC technologies for cancer patient diagnosis, prognosis, and response to therapy, as well as accelerating oncologic drug development. According to Parkinson et al., moving forward requires the application of the classic steps in biomarker development-analytical and clinical validation and clinical qualification for specific contexts of use [109]. There is still a lot to be done for the automation, standardization, quality control and accreditation of analytical methodologies used for CTC isolation, detection and molecular characterization. When this goal is achieved, the next logical step will be to use CTC technologies to diagnose patients, select biomarker-based therapeutics, and monitor response to therapies using not only pathologic tissues but also CTCs.

21.3 Conclusions: Future Perpectives

The main advantage of CTC analysis is based on their unique potential to offer a minimally invasive "liquid biopsy" sample, easily obtainable at multiple time points during disease history which can provide valuable information on the very early assessment of treatment efficacy and can help towards establishing individualized treatment approaches that will improve efficacy with less cost and side effects for cancer patients [3, 80].

CTC downstream molecular characterization at the protein, DNA [16, 17] and RNA level, could now serve as a "liquid biopsy" approach and eventually offer additional information and even more a serious advantage over the conventional and well established tumor biopsy approach since peripheral blood samples can be frequently and sequentially obtained [3, 80].

Cell free DNA (cfDNA) circulating in plasma or serum of cancer patients has also been recently proposed as an alternative to CTCsliquid biopsy approach [11, 30, 90]. It has been recently shown that by using extremely powerful and highly sensitive detection techniques, the presence of specific mutations in plasma of cancer patients could give valuable information concerning response to specific molecular targeted therapies [99]. However, there is a substantial difference between these two approaches; CTCs are viable cells, circulating in blood, and understanding their biology in a holistic way, could give valuable information on the metastatic spread, elucidate their connection to cancer stem cells, and reveal active and possible targetable signalling networks, while cfDNA can give specific information as a circulating biomarker, for the presence or absence of specific alterations indicating therapy response.

Co-development of anticancer therapeutics with CTC-based diagnostics could enable clinical validation and qualification of CTC-based assays as companion diagnostics in the near future [123]. Further research on the molecular characterization of CTC will provide important information for the identification of therapeutic targets and understanding resistance to therapies. The molecular characterization of CTC is highly challenging especially in combination with next generation sequencing technologies that will enable the elucidation of molecular pathways in CTC and will probably lead to the design of novel molecular therapies targeting specifically CTC. Even if this is still far from being considered to be applied in a routine clinical setting, it holds a great promise for the future management of cancer patients.

References

1. Aktas B, Kasimir-Bauer S, Heubner M, Kimmig R, Wimberger P (2011) Molecular profiling and prognostic relevance of circulating tumor cells in the blood of ovarian cancer patients at primary diagnosis and after platinum-based chemotherapy. Int J Gynecol Cancer 21:822–830
2. Aktas B, Tewes M, Fehm T, Hauch S, Kimmig R, Kasimir-Bauer S (2009) Stem cell and epithelial-mesenchymal transition markers are frequently overexpressed in circulating tumor cells of metastatic breast cancer patients. Breast Cancer Res 11:R46

3. Alix-Panabieres C, Pantel K (2013) Circulating tumor cells: liquid biopsy of cancer. Clin Chem 59:110–118
4. Andreopoulou E, Yang LY, Rangel KM, Reuben JM, Hsu L, Krishnamurthy S, Valero V, Fritsche HA, Cristofanilli M (2012) Comparison of assay methods for detection of circulating tumor cells in metastatic breast cancer: AdnaGen AdnaTest BreastCancer select/detect™versus veridex cell search™ system. Int J Cancer 130(7):1590–1597. doi:10.1002/ijc.26111, Epub 2011 Nov 30
5. Ashworth TR (1869) A case of cancer in which cells similar to those in the tumours were seen in the blood after death. Med J Aust 14:146–147
6. Attard G, Swennenhuis JF, Olmos D, Reid AH, Vickers E, A'Hern R et al (2009) Characterization of ERG, AR and PTEN gene status in circulating tumor cells from patients with castration-resistant prostate cancer. Cancer Res 69:2912–2918
7. Balasubramanian P, Lang JC, Jatana KR, Miller B, Ozer E, Old M et al (2012) Multiparameter analysis, including EMT markers, on negatively enriched bloodsamples from patients with squamous cell carcinoma of the head and neck. PLoS One 7:e42048
8. Barbazan J, Muinelo-Romay L, Vieito M, Candamio S, Díaz-López A, Cano A, Gomez-Tato A, de Casares Cal MD, Abal M, Lopez-Lopez R (2014) A multimarker panel for circulating tumor cells detection predicts patient outcome and therapy response in metastatic colorectal cancer. Int J Cancer. doi:10.1002/ijc.28910 [Epub ahead of print]
9. Bednarz N, Eltze E, Semjonow A, Rink M, Andreas A, Mulder L et al (2010) BRCA1 loss preexisting in small subpopulations of prostate cancer is associated with advanced disease and metastatic spread to lymph nodes and peripheral blood. Clin Cancer Res 16:3340–3348
10. Bednarz-Knoll N, Alix-Panabieres C, Pantel K (2012) Plasticity of disseminating cancer cells in patients with epithelial malignancies. Cancer Metastasis Rev 31(3–4):673–687
11. Bettegowda C, Sausen M, Leary RJ, Kinde I, Wang Y, Agrawal N et al (2014) Detection of circulating tumor DNA in early- and late-stage human malignancies. Sci Transl Med 6(224):224ra24. doi:10.1126/scitranslmed.3007094
12. Bidard FC, Fehm T, Ignatiadis M, Smerage JB, Alix-Panabieres C, Janni W et al (2013) Clinical application of circulating tumor cells in breast cancer: overview of the current interventional trials. Cancer Metastasis Rev 32(1–2):179–188
13. Bidard FC, Huguet F, Louvet C, Mineur L, Bouche O, Chibaudel B et al (2013) Circulating tumor cells in locally advanced pancreatic adenocarcinoma: the ancillary CirCe 07 study to the LAP 07 trial. Ann Oncol 24:2057–2061
14. Bidard FC, Peeters DJ, Fehm T, Nole F, Gisbert-Criado R, Mavroudis D et al (2014) Clinical validity of circulating tumour cells in patients with metastatic breast cancer: a pooled analysis of individual patient data. Lancet Oncol 15(4):406–414. doi:10.1016/S1470-2045(14)70069-5, Epub 2014 Mar 11
15. Buglione M, Grisanti S, Almici C, Mangoni M, Polli C, Consoli F et al (2012) Circulating tumour cells in locally advanced head and neck cancer: preliminary report about their possible role in predicting response to nonsurgical treatment and survival. Eur J Cancer 48:3019–3026
16. Chimonidou M, Strati A, Malamos N, Georgoulias V, Lianidou ES (2013) SOX17 promoter methylation in circulating tumor cells and matched cell-free DNA isolated from plasma of patients with breast cancer. Clin Chem 59:270–279
17. Chimonidou M, Strati A, Tzitzira A, Sotiropoulou G, Malamos N, Georgoulias V et al (2011) DNA methylation of tumor suppressor and metastasis suppressor genes in circulating tumor cells. Clin Chem 57:1169–1177
18. Chinen LT, de Carvalho FM, Rocha BM, Aguiar CM, Abdallah EA, Campanha D, Mingues NB, de Oliveira TB, Maciel MS, Cervantes GM, Dettino AL, Soares FA, Paterlini-Brechot P, Fanelli MF (2013) Cytokeratin- based CTC counting unrelated to clinical follow up. J Thorac Dis 5(5):593–599. doi:10.3978/j.issn.2072-1439.2013.09.18
19. Chiu CG, Nakamura Y, Chong KK, Huang SK, Kawas NP, Triche T, Elashoff D, Kiyohara E, Irie RF, Morton DL, Hoon DS (2014) Genome-wide characterization of circulating tumor cells identifies novel prognostic genomic alterations in systemic melanoma metastasis. Clin Chem 60(6):873–885 [Epub ahead of print]
20. Cohen SJ, Punt CJ, Iannotti N, Saidman BH, Sabbath KD, Gabrail NY et al (2008) Relationship of circulating tumor cells to tumor response, progression-free survival, and overall survival in patients with metastatic colorectal cancer. J Clin Oncol 26:3213–3221
21. Coumans FA, Doggen CJ, Attard G, de Bono JS, Terstappen LW (2010) All circulating EpCAM+CK+CD45- objects predict overall survival in castration- resistant prostate cancer. Ann Oncol 21:1851–1857
22. Cristofanilli M, Budd GT, Ellis MJ, Stopeck A, Matera J, Miller MC et al (2004) Circulating tumor cells, disease progression, and survival in metastatic breast cancer. N Engl J Med 351:781–791
23. Danila DC, Anand A, Sung CC, Heller G, Leversha MA, Cao L et al (2011) TMPRSS2-ERG status in circulating tumor cells as a predictive biomarker of sensitivity in castration-resistant prostate cancer patients treated with abiraterone acetate. Eur Urol 60:897–904
24. Danila DC, Fleisher M, Scher HI (2011) Circulating tumor cells as biomarkers in prostate cancer. Clin Cancer Res 17:3903–3912
25. Danila DC, Heller G, Gignac GA, Gonzalez-Espinoza R, Anand A, Tanaka E et al (2007) Circulating tumor cell number and prognosis in progressive castration- resistant prostate cancer. Clin Cancer Res 13:7053–7058

26. Darshan MS, Loftus MS, Thadani-Mulero M, Levy BP, Escuin D, Zhou XK et al (2011) Taxane-induced blockade to nuclear accumulation of the androgen receptor predicts clinical responses in metastatic prostate cancer. Cancer Res 71:6019–6029
27. de Albuquerque A, Kubisch I, Stolzel U, Ernst D, Boese-Landgraf J, Breier G et al (2012) Prognostic and predictive value of circulating tumor cell analysis in colorectal cancer patients. J Transl Med 10:222
28. de Bono JS, Scher HI, Montgomery RB, Parker C, Miller MC, Tissing H et al (2008) Circulating tumor cells predict survival benefit from treatment in metastatic castration-resistant prostate cancer. Clin Cancer Res 14:6302–6309
29. Diamandis EP (2010) Cancer biomarkers: can we turn recent failures into success? J Natl Cancer Inst 102:1462–1467
30. Diaz LA Jr, Bardelli A (2014) Liquid biopsies: genotyping circulating tumor DNA. J Clin Oncol 32(6):579–586
31. Doyen J, Alix-Panabieres C, Hofman P, Parks SK, Chamorey E, Naman H et al (2012) Circulating tumor cells in prostate cancer: a potential surrogate marker of survival. Crit Rev Oncol Hematol 81:241–256
32. Fabbri F, Carloni S, Zoli W, Ulivi P, Gallerani G, Fici P et al (2013) Detection and recovery of circulating colon cancer cells using a dielectrophoresis-based device: KRAS mutation status in pure CTCs. Cancer Lett 335:225–231
33. Fehm T, Hoffmann O, Aktas B, Becker S, Solomayer EF, Wallwiener D et al (2009) Detection and characterization of circulating tumor cells in blood of primary breast cancer patients by RT-PCR and comparison to status of bone marrow disseminated cells. Breast Cancer Res 11:R59
34. Fehm T, Muller V, Aktas B, Janni W, Schneeweiss A, Stickeler E et al (2010) HER2 status of circulating tumor cells in patients with metastatic breast cancer: a prospective, multicenter trial. Breast Cancer Res Treat 124:403–412
35. Flores LM, Kindelberger DW, Ligon AH, Capelletti M, Fiorentino M, Loda M et al (2010) Improving the yield of circulating tumour cells facilitates molecular characterisation and recognition of discordant HER2 amplification in breast cancer. Br J Cancer 102:1495–1502
36. Gall TM, Frampton AE, Krell J, Jacob J, Stebbing J, Jiao LR (2013) Is the detection of circulating tumor cells in locally advanced pancreatic cancer a useful prognostic marker? Expert Rev Mol Diagn 13(8):793–796
37. Gasch C, Bauernhofer T, Pichler M, Langer-Freitag S, Reeh M, Seifert AM et al (2013) Heterogeneity of epidermal growth factor receptor status and mutations of KRAS/PIK3CA in circulating tumor cells of patients with colorectal cancer. Clin Chem 59:252–260
38. Gazzaniga P, Gianni W, Raimondi C, Gradilone A, Lo RG, Longo F et al (2013) Circulating tumor cells in high-risk nonmetastatic colorectal cancer. Tumour Biol 34(5):2507–2509
39. Georgoulias V, Bozionelou V, Agelaki S, Perraki M, Apostolaki S, Kallergi G et al (2012) Trastuzumab decreases the incidence of clinical relapses in patients with early breast cancer presenting chemotherapy-resistant CK-19mRNA- positive circulating tumor cells: results of a randomized phase II study. Ann Oncol 23:1744–1750
40. Gervasoni A, Sandri MT, Nascimbeni R, Zorzino L, Cassatella MC, Baglioni L, Panigara S, Gervasi M, Di Lorenzo D, Parolini O (2011) Comparison of three distinct methods for the detection of circulating tumor cells in colorectal cancer patients. Oncol Rep 25(6):1669–1703
41. Giordano A, Cristofanilli M (2012) CTCs in metastatic breast cancer. Recent Results Cancer Res 195:193–201
42. Giordano A, Egleston BL, Hajage D, Bland J, Hortobagyi GN, Reuben JM et al (2013) Establishment and validation of circulating tumor cell-based prognostic nomograms in first-line metastatic breast cancer patients. Clin Cancer Res 19:1596–1602
43. Goldkorn A, Ely B, Quinn DI, Tangen CM, Fink LM, Xu T, Twardowski P, Van Veldhuizen PJ, Agarwal N, Carducci MA, Monk JP 3rd, Datar RH, Garzotto M, Mack PC, Lara P Jr, Higano CS, Hussain M, Thompson IM Jr, Cote RJ, Vogelzang NJ (2014) Circulating tumor cell counts Are prognostic of overall survival in SWOG S0421: a phase III trial of docetaxel with or without atrasentan for metastatic castration-resistant prostate cancer. J Clin Oncol 32(11):1136–1142
44. Goodman OB Jr, Symanowski JT, Loudyi A, Fink LM, Ward DC, Vogelzang NJ (2011) Circulating tumor cells as a predictive biomarker in patients with hormone-sensitive prostate cancer. Clin Genitourin Cancer 9:31–38
45. Gradilone A, Petracca A, Nicolazzo C, Gianni W, Cortesi E, Naso G et al (2010) Prognostic significance of survivin-expressing circulating tumour cells in T1G3 bladder cancer. BJU Int 106:710–715
46. Green TL, Cruse JM, Lewis RE, Craft BS (2013) Circulating tumor cells (CTCs) from metastatic breast cancer patients linked to decreased immune function and response to treatment. Exp Mol Pathol 95(2):174–179. doi:10.1016/j.yexmp.2013.06.013, Epub 2013 Jul 4
47. Grobe A, Blessmann M, Hanken H, Friedrich RE, Schon G, Wikner J, Effenberger KE, Kluwe L, Heiland M, Pantel K, Riethdorf S (2014) Prognostic relevance of circulating tumor cells in blood and disseminated tumor cells in bone marrow of patients with squamous cell carcinoma of the oral cavity. Clin Cancer Res 20(2):425–433. doi:10.1158/1078-0432.CCR-13- 1101, Epub 2013 Nov 11
48. Groot KB, Rahbari NN, Buchler MW, Koch M, Weitz J (2013) Circulating tumor cells and prognosis of patients with resectable colorectal liver metasta-

ses or widespread metastatic colorectal cancer: a meta-analysis. Ann Surg Oncol 20:2156–2165
49. Guzzo TJ, McNeil BK, Bivalacqua TJ, Elliott DJ, Sokoll LJ, Schoenberg MP (2012) The presence of circulating tumor cells does not predict extravesical disease in bladder cancer patients prior to radical cystectomy. Urol Oncol 30:44–48
50. Han L, Chen W, Zhao Q (2014) Prognostic value of circulating tumor cells in patients with pancreatic cancer: a meta-analysis. Tumour Biol 35(3):2473–2480. doi:10.1007/s13277-013-1327-5, Epub 2013 Nov 12
51. Harris L, Fritsche H, Mennel R, Norton L, Ravdin P, Taube S et al (2007) American society of clinical oncology 2007 update of recommendations for the use of tumor markers in breast cancer. J Clin Oncol 25:5287–5312
52. Heitzer E, Auer M, Gasch C, Pichler M, Ulz P, Hoffmann EM et al (2013) Complex tumor genomes inferred from single circulating tumor cells by array-CGH and next-generation sequencing. Cancer Res 73:2965–2975
53. Helo P, Cronin AM, Danila DC, Wenske S, Gonzalez-Espinoza R, Anand A et al (2009) Circulating prostate tumor cells detected by reverse transcription-PCR in men with localized or castration-refractory prostate cancer: concordance with cell search assay and association with bone metastases and with survival. Clin Chem 55:765–773
54. Hoshimoto S, Faries MB, Morton DL, Shingai T, Kuo C, Wang HJ et al (2012) Assessment of prognostic circulating tumor cells in a phase III trial of adjuvant immunotherapy after complete resection of stage IV melanoma. Ann Surg 255:357–362
55. Hoshimoto S, Shingai T, Morton DL, Kuo C, Faries MB, Chong K, Elashoff D, Wang HJ, Elashoff RM, Hoon DS (2012) Association between circulating tumor cells and prognosis in patients with stage III melanoma with sentinel lymph node metastasis in a phase III international multicenter trial. J Clin Oncol 30(31):3819–3826
56. Hou JM, Krebs MG, Lancashire L, Sloane R, Backen A, Swain RK, Priest LJ, Greystoke A, Zhou C, Morris K, Ward T, Blackhall FH, Dive C (2012) Clinical significance and molecular characteristics of circulating tumor cells and circulating tumor microemboli in patients with small-cell lung cancer. J Clin Oncol 30(5):525–532
57. Hu B, Rochefort H, Goldkorn A (2013) Circulating tumor cells in prostate cancer. Cancers (Basel) 5(4):1676–1690
58. Ignatiadis M, Rothe F, Chaboteaux C, Durbecq V, Rouas G, Criscitiello C et al (2011) HER2-positive circulating tumor cells in breast cancer. PLoS One 6:e15624
59. Ignatiadis M, Xenidis N, Perraki M, Apostolaki S, Politaki E, Kafousi M et al (2007) Different prognostic value of cytokeratin-19 mRNA positive circulating tumor cells according to estrogen receptor and HER2 status in early-stage breast cancer. J Clin Oncol 25:5194–5202
60. Ignatiadis M, Riethdorf S, Bidard FC, Vaucher I, Khazour M, Rothe F, Metallo J, Rouas G, Payne RE, Coombes RC, Teufel I, Andergassen U, Apostolaki S, Politaki E, Mavroudis D, Bessi S, Pestrin M, Di Leo A, Campion M, Reinholz M, Perez E, Piccart M, Borgen E, Naume B, Jimenez J, Aura CM, Zorzino L, Cassatella MC, Sandri MT, Mostert B, Sleijfer S, Kraan J, Janni W, Fehm T, Rack B, Terstappen L, Repollet M, Pierga JY, Miller C, Sotiriou C, Michiels S, Pantel K (2014) International study on inter-reader variability for circulating tumor cells in breast cancer. Breast Cancer Res 16(2):R43 [Epub ahead of print]
61. Iinuma H, Watanabe T, Mimori K, Adachi M, Hayashi N, Tamura J et al (2011) Clinical significance of circulating tumor cells, including cancer stem-like cells, in peripheral blood for recurrence and prognosis in patients with Dukes' stage B and C colorectal cancer. J Clin Oncol 29:1547–1555
62. Iwatsuki M, Toyoshima K, Watanabe M, Hayashi N, Ishimoto T, Eto K, Iwagami S, Baba Y, Yoshida N, Hayashi A, Ohta Y, Baba H (2013) Frequency of HER2 expression of circulating tumour cells in patients with metastatic or recurrent gastrointestinal cancer. Br J Cancer 109(11):2829–2832
63. Jatana KR, Balasubramanian P, Lang JC, Yang L, Jatana CA, White E et al (2010) Significance of circulating tumor cells in patients with squamous cell carcinoma of the head and neck: initial results. Arch Otolaryngol Head Neck Surg 136:1274–1279
64. Jiang Y, Palma JF, Agus DB, Wang Y, Gross ME (2010) Detection of androgen receptor mutations in circulating tumor cells in castration-resistant prostate cancer. Clin Chem 56:1492–1495
65. Jiao LR, Apostolopoulos C, Jacob J, Szydlo R, Johnson N, Tsim N et al (2009) Unique localization of circulating tumor cells in patients with hepatic metastases. J Clin Oncol 27:6160–6165
66. Kallergi G, Konstantinidis G, Markomanolaki H, Papadaki MA, Mavroudis D, Stournaras C et al (2013) Apoptotic circulating tumor cells in early and metastatic breast cancer patients. Mol Cancer Ther 12:1886–1895
67. Kallergi G, Papadaki MA, Politaki E, Mavroudis D, Georgoulias V, Agelaki S (2011) Epithelial to mesenchymal transition markers expressed in circulating tumour cells of early and metastatic breast cancer patients. Breast Cancer Res 13:R59
68. Kasimir-Bauer S, Hoffmann O, Wallwiener D, Kimmig R, Fehm T (2012) Expression of stem cell and epithelial-mesenchymal transition markers in primary breast cancer patients with circulating tumor cells. Breast Cancer Res 14:R15
69. Khan MS, Kirkwood A, Tsigani T, Garcia-Hernandez J, Hartley JA, Caplin ME, Meyer T (2013) Circulating tumor cells as prognostic markers in neuroendocrine tumors. J Clin Oncol 31(3):365–372

70. Khoja L, Backen A, Sloane R, Menasce L, Ryder D, Krebs M, Board R, Clack G, Hughes A, Blackhall F, Valle JW, Dive C (2012) A pilot study to explore circulating tumour cells in pancreatic cancer as a novel biomarker. Br J Cancer 106(3):508–516
71. Kitago M, Koyanagi K, Nakamura T, Goto Y, Faries M, O'Day SJ et al (2009) mRNA expression and BRAF mutation in circulating melanoma cells isolated from peripheral blood with high molecular weight melanoma-associated antigen-specific monoclonal antibody beads. Clin Chem 55:757–764
72. Kiyohara E, Hata K, Lam S, Hoon DS (2014) Circulating tumor cells as prognostic biomarkers in cutaneous melanoma patients. Methods Mol Biol 1102:513–522
73. Klinac D, Gray ES, Millward M, Ziman M (2013) Advances in personalized targeted treatment of metastatic melanoma and non-invasive tumor monitoring. Front Oncol 3:54
74. Koyanagi K, O'Day SJ, Gonzalez R, Lewis K, Robinson WA, Amatruda TT, Wang HJ, Elashoff RM, Takeuchi H, Umetani N, Hoon DS (2005) Serial monitoring of circulating melanoma cells during neoadjuvant biochemotherapy for stage III melanoma: outcome prediction in a multicenter trial. J Clin Oncol 23(31):8057–8064
75. Kraan J, Sleijfer S, Strijbos MH, Ignatiadis M, Peeters D, Pierga JY, Farace F, Riethdorf S, Fehm T, Zorzino L, Tibbe AG, Maestro M, Gisbert-Criado R, Denton G, de Bono JS, Dive C, Foekens JA, Gratama JW (2011) External quality assurance of circulating tumor cell enumeration using the cell search(®) system: a feasibility study. Cytometry B Clin Cytom 80(2):112–118
76. Krebs MG, Sloane R, Priest L, Lancashire L, Hou JM, Greystoke A, Ward TH, Ferraldeschi R, Hughes A, Clack G, Ranson M, Dive C, Blackhall FH (2011) Evaluation and prognostic significance of circulating tumor cells in patients with non-small-cell lung cancer. J Clin Oncol 29(12):1556–1563
77. Lecharpentier A, Vielh P, Perez-Moreno P, Planchard D, Soria JC, Farace F (2011) Detection of circulating tumour cells with a hybrid (epithelial/mesenchymal) phenotype in patients with metastatic non-small cell lung cancer. Br J Cancer 105:1338–1341
78. Leversha MA, Han J, Asgari Z, Danila DC, Lin O, Gonzalez-Espinoza R et al (2009) Fluorescence in situ hybridization analysis of circulating tumor cells in metastatic prostate cancer. Clin Cancer Res 15:2091–2097
79. Lianidou ES, Markou A, Strati A (2012) Molecular characterization of circulating tumor cells in breast cancer: challenges and promises for individualized cancer treatment. Cancer Metastasis Rev 31:663–671
80. Lianidou ES, Markou A (2011) Circulating tumor cells in breast cancer: detection systems, molecular characterization, and future challenges. Clin Chem 57:1242–1255
81. Lianidou ES, Mavroudis D, Georgoulias V (2013) Clinical challenges in the molecular characterization of circulating tumour cells in breast cancer. Br J Cancer 108:2426–2432
82. Ligthart ST, Bidard FC, Decraene C, Bachelot T, Delaloge S, Brain E et al (2013) Unbiased quantitative assessment of Her-2 expression of circulating tumor cells in patients with metastatic and non-metastatic breast cancer. Ann Oncol 24:1231–1238
83. Lim J, Thiery JP (2012) Epithelial-mesenchymal transitions: insights from development. Development 139:3471–3486
84. Liu JF, Kindelberger D, Doyle C, Lowe A, Barry WT, Matulonis UA (2013) Predictive value of circulating tumor cells (CTCs) in newly-diagnosed and recurrent ovarian cancer patients. Gynecol Oncol 131:352–356
85. Liu MC, Shields PG, Warren RD, Cohen P, Wilkinson M, Ottaviano YL, Rao SB, Eng-Wong J, Seillier-Moiseiwitsch F, Noone AM, Isaacs C (2009) Circulating tumor cells: a useful predictor of treatment efficacy in metastatic breast cancer. J Clin Oncol 27(31):5153–5159
86. Lowes LE, Lock M, Rodrigues G, D'Souza D, Bauman G, Ahmad B et al (2012) Circulating tumour cells in prostate cancer patients receiving salvage radiotherapy. Clin Transl Oncol 14:150–156
87. Lu CY, Tsai H-L, Uen Y-H, Hu H-M, Chen C-W, Cheng T-L, Lin S-R, Wang J-Y (2013) Circulating tumor cells as a surrogate marker for determining clinical outcome to mFOLFOX chemotherapy in patients with stage III colon cancer. Br J Cancer 108(4):791–797
88. Lucci A, Hall CS, Lodhi AK, Bhattacharyya A, Anderson AE, Xiao L et al (2012) Circulating tumour cells in non-metastatic breast cancer: a prospective study. Lancet Oncol 13:688–695
89. Maheswaran S, Sequist LV, Nagrath S, Ulkus L, Brannigan B, Collura CV et al (2008) Detection of mutations in EGFR in circulating lung-cancer cells. N Engl J Med 359:366–377
90. Marzese DM, Hirose H, Hoon DS (2013) Diagnostic and prognostic value of circulating tumor-related DNA in cancer patients. Expert Rev Mol Diagn 13(8):827–844
91. Matsusaka S, Suenaga M, Mishima Y, Kuniyoshi R, Takagi K, Terui Y et al (2011) Circulating tumor cells as a surrogate marker for determining response to chemotherapy in Japanese patients with metastatic colorectal cancer. Cancer Sci 102:1188–1192
92. Mazzini C, Pinzani P, Salvianti F, Scatena C, Paglierani M, Ucci F, Pazzagli M, Massi D (2014) Circulating tumor cells detection and counting in uveal melanomas by a filtration-based method. Cancers (Basel) 6(1):323–332
93. Mego M, Mani SA, Lee BN, Li C, Evans KW, Cohen EN et al (2012) Expression of epithelial-mesenchymal transition-inducing transcription factors in primary breast cancer: the effect of neoadjuvant therapy. Int J Cancer 130:808–816
94. Mikulova V, Cabinakova M, Janatkova I, Mestek O, Zima T, Tesarova P (2014) Detection of circulating

tumor cells during follow-up of patients with early breast cancer: clinical utility for monitoring of therapy efficacy. Scand J Clin Lab Invest 74(2):132–142

95. Miyamoto DT, Lee RJ, Stott SL, Ting DT, Wittner BS, Ulman M et al (2012) Androgen receptor signaling in circulating tumor cells as a marker of hormonally responsive prostate cancer. Cancer Discov 2:995–1003
96. Moreno JG, O'Hara SM, Gross S, Doyle G, Fritsche H, Gomella LG et al (2001) Changes in circulating carcinoma cells in patients with metastatic prostate cancer correlate with disease status. Urology 58:386–392
97. Mostert B, Jiang Y, Sieuwerts AM, Wang H, Bolt-de VJ, Biermann K et al (2013) KRAS and BRAF mutation status in circulating colorectal tumor cells and their correlation with primary and metastatic tumor tissue. Int J Cancer 133:130–141
98. Muller V, Riethdorf S, Rack B, Janni W, Fasching PA, Solomayer E et al (2012) Prognostic impact of circulating tumor cells assessed with the cell search system and AdnaTest breast in metastatic breast cancer patients: the DETECT study. Breast Cancer Res 14:R118
99. Murtaza M, Dawson SJ, Tsui DW et al (2013) Non-invasive analysis of acquired resistance to cancer therapy by sequencing of plasma DNA. Nature 497:108–112
100. Nadal R, Fernandez A, Sanchez-Rovira P, Salido M, Rodriguez M, García-Puche JL et al (2012) Biomarkers characterization of circulating tumour cells in breast cancer patients. Breast Cancer Res 14:R71
101. Nastaly P, Ruf CG, Becker P, Bednarz-Knoll N, Stoupiec M, Kavsur R, Isbarn H, Matthies C, Wagner W, Hoppner D, Fisch M, Bokemeyer C, Ahyai S, Honecker F, Riethdorf S, Pantel K (2014) Circulating tumor cells in patients with testicular germ cell tumors. Clin Cancer Res 20(14):3830–3841. [Epub ahead of print]
102. Nel I, Baba HA, Ertle J, Weber F, Sitek B, Eisenacher M et al (2013) Individual profiling of circulating tumor cell composition and therapeutic outcome in patients with hepatocellular carcinoma. Trans Oncol 6:420–428
103. Obermayr E, Castillo-Tong DC, Pils D, Speiser P, Braicu I, Van Gorp T, Mahner S, Sehouli J, Vergote I, Zeillinger R (2013) Molecular characterization of circulating tumor cells in patients with ovarian cancer improves their prognostic significance – a study of the OVCAD consortium. Gynecol Oncol 128:15–21
104. Obermayr E, Sanchez-Cabo F, Tea MK, Singer CF, Krainer M, Fischer MB, Sehouli J, Reinthaller A, Horvat R, Heinze G, Tong D, Zeillinger R (2010) Assessment of a six gene panel for the molecular detection of circulating tumor cells in the blood of female cancer patients. BMC Cancer 10:666
105. Olmos D, Arkenau HT, Ang JE, Ledaki I, Attard G, Carden CP et al (2009) Circulating tumour cell (CTC) counts as intermediate end points in castration- resistant prostate cancer (CRPC): a single-centre experience. Ann Oncol 20:27–33
106. Pailler E, Adam J, Barthelemy A, Oulhen M, Auger N, Valent A, Borget I, Planchard D, Taylor M, Andre F, Soria JC, Vielh P, Besse B, Farace F (2013) Detection of circulating tumor cells harboring a unique ALK rearrangement in ALK-positive non-small-cell lung cancer. J Clin Oncol 31:2273–2281
107. Pantel K, Alix-Panabieres C, Riethdorf S (2009) Cancer micrometastases. Nat Rev Clin Oncol 6:339–351
108. Pantel K, Alix-Panabieres C (2012) Detection methods of circulating tumor cells. J Thorac Dis 4:446–447
109. Parkinson DR, Dracopoli N, Petty BG, Compton C, Cristofanilli M, Deisseroth A et al (2012) Considerations in the development of circulating tumor cell technology for clinical use. J Transl Med 10:138
110. Pavlou MP, Diamandis EP, Blasutig IM (2013) The long journey of cancer biomarkers from the bench to the clinic. Clin Chem 59(1):147–157. doi:10.1373/clinchem.2012.184614, Epub 2012 Sep 27. Review. PubMed
111. Peach G, Kim C, Zacharakis E, Purkayastha S, Ziprin P (2010) Prognostic significance of circulating tumour cells following surgical resection of colorectal cancers: a systematic review. Br J Cancer 102:1327–1334
112. Peeters DJ, van Dam PJ, Van den Eynden GG, Rutten A, Wuyts H, Pouillon L, Peeters M, Pauwels P, Van Laere SJ, van Dam PA, Vermeulen PB, Dirix LY (2014) Detection and prognostic significance ofcirculating tumour cells in patients with metastatic breast cancer according to immunohistochemical subtypes. Br J Cancer 110(2):375–383
113. Perou CM, Sørlie T, Eisen MB, van de Rijn M, Jeffrey SS, Rees CA, Pollack JR, Ross DT, Johnsen H, Akslen LA, Fluge O, Pergamenschikov A, Williams C, Zhu SX, Lønning PE, Børresen-Dale AL, Brown PO, Botstein D (2000) Molecular portraits of human breast tumours. Nature 406(6797):747–752
114. Pestrin M, Bessi S, Galardi F, Truglia M, Biggeri A, Biagioni C et al (2009) Correlation of HER2 status between primary tumors and corresponding circulating tumor cells in advanced breast cancer patients. Breast Cancer Res Treat 118:523–530
115. Pierga JY, Bidard FC, Cropet C, Tresca P, Dalenc F, Romieu G, Campone M, Mahier Ait-Oukhatar C, Le Rhun E, Gonçalves A, Leheurteur M, Domont J, Gutierrez M, Cure H, Ferrero JM, Labbe-Devilliers C, Bachelot T (2013) Circulating tumor cells and brain metastasis outcome in patients with HER2-positive breast cancer: the LANDSCAPE trial. Ann Oncol 24(12):2999–3004

116. Pierga JY, Bidard FC, Mathiot C, Brain E, Delaloge S, Giachetti S et al (2008) Circulating tumor cell detection predicts early metastatic relapse after neoadjuvant chemotherapy in large operable and locally advanced breast cancer in a phase II randomized trial. Clin Cancer Res 14:7004–7010
117. Pierga JY, Hajage D, Bachelot T, Delaloge S, Brain E, Campone M et al (2012) High independent prognostic and predictive value of circulating tumor cells compared with serum tumor markers in a large prospective trial in first-line chemotherapy for metastatic breast cancer patients. Ann Oncol 23:618–624
118. Plaks V, Koopman CD, Werb Z (2013) Cancer. Circulating tumor cells. Science 341(6151):1186–1188
119. Poveda A, Kaye SB, McCormack R, Wang S, Parekh T et al (2011) Circulating tumor cells predict progression free survival and overall survival in patients with relapsed/recurrent advanced ovarian cancer. Gynecol Oncol 122:567–572
120. Powell AA, Talasaz AH, Zhang H, Coram MA, Reddy A, Deng G et al (2012) Single cell profiling of circulating tumor cells: transcriptional heterogeneity and diversity from breast cancer cell lines. PLoS One 7(5):e33788
121. Punnoose EA, Atwal S, Liu W, Raja R, Fine BM, Hughes BG et al (2012) Evaluation of circulating tumor cells and circulating tumor DNA in non-small cell lung cancer: association with clinical endpoints in a phase II clinical trial of pertuzumab and erlotinib. Clin Cancer Res 18:2391–2401
122. Punnoose EA, Atwal SK, Spoerke JM, Savage H, Pandita A, Yeh RF et al (2010) Molecular biomarker analyses using circulating tumor cells. PLoS One 5:e12517
123. Punnoose EA, Lackner MR (2012) Challenges and opportunities in the use of CTCs for companion diagnostic development. Recent Results Cancer Res 195:241–253
124. Rack B, Juckstock J, Gunthner-Biller M, Andergassen U, Neugebauer J, Hepp P et al (2012) Trastuzumab clears HER2/neu-positive isolated tumor cells from bone marrow in primary breast cancer patients. Arch Gynecol Obstet 285:485–492
125. Rahbari NN, Bork U, Kircher A, Nimitz T, Scholch S, Kahlert C et al (2012) Compartmental differences of circulating tumor cells in colorectal cancer. Ann Surg Oncol 19:2195–2202
126. Raimondi C, Gradilone A, Gazzaniga P (2014) Circulating tumor cells in early bladder cancer: insight into micrometastatic disease. Expert Rev Mol Diagn 14(4):407–409. doi:10.1586/14737159.2014.908119, Epub 2014 Apr 10
127. Ramirez JM, Fehm T, Orsini M, Cayrefourcq L, Maudelonde T, Pantel K, Alix-Panabieres C (2014) Prognostic relevance of viable circulating tumor cells detected by EPISPOT in metastatic breast cancer patients. Clin Chem 60(1):214–221
128. Resel FL, San Jose ML, Galante Romo I, Moreno SJ, Olivier GC (2012) Prognostic significance of circulating tumor cell count in patients with metastatic hormone-sensitive prostate cancer. Urology 80:1328–1332
129. Riethdorf S, Fritsche H, Muller V, Rau T, Schindlbeck C, Rack B et al (2007) Detection of circulating tumor cells in peripheral blood of patients with metastatic breast cancer: a validation study of the cell search system. Clin Cancer Res 13:920–928
130. Rink M, Chun FK, Minner S, Friedrich M, Mauermann O, Heinzer H et al (2011) Detection of circulating tumour cells in peripheral blood of patients with advanced non-metastatic bladder cancer. BJU Int 107:1668–1675
131. Saad F, Pantel K (2012) The current role of circulating tumor cells in the diagnosis and management of bone metastases in advanced prostate cancer. Future Oncol 8:321–331
132. Sastre J, Vidaurreta M, Gómez A, Rivera F, Massutí B, López MR et al (2013) Spanish Cooperative Group for the Treatment of Digestive Tumors. Prognostic value of the combination of circulating tumor cells plus KRAS in patients with metastatic colorectal cancer treated with chemotherapy plus bevacizumab. Clin Colorectal Cancer 12:280–286
133. Saloustros E, Perraki M, Apostolaki S, Kallergi G, Xyrafas A, Kalbakis K et al (2011) Cytokeratin-19 mRNA-positive circulating tumor cells during follow-up of patients with operable breast cancer: prognostic relevance for late relapse. Breast Cancer Res 13:R60
134. Scher HI, Jia X, de Bono JS, Fleisher M, Pienta KJ, Raghavan D et al (2009) Circulating tumour cells as prognostic markers in progressive, castration- resistant prostate cancer: a reanalysis of IMMC38 trial data. Lancet Oncol 10:233–239
135. Scher HI, Morris MJ, Larson S, Heller G (2013) Validation and clinical utility of prostate cancer biomarkers. Nat Rev Clin Oncol 10:225–234
136. Schilling D, Todenhofer T, Hennenlotter J, Schwentner C, Fehm T, Stenzl A (2012) Isolated, disseminated and circulating tumour cells in prostate cancer. Nat Rev Urol 9(8):448–463
137. Schulze K, Gasch C, Staufer K, Nashan B, Lohse AW, Pantel K et al (2013) Presence of EpCAM-positive circulating tumor cells as biomarker for systemic disease strongly correlates to survival in patients with hepatocellular carcinoma. Int J Cancer 133:2165–2171
138. Schwed Lustgarten DE, Thompson J, Yu G, Vachani A, Vaidya B, Rao C, Connelly M, Udine M, Tan KS, Heitjan DF, Albelda S (2013) Use of circulating tumor cell technology (CELLSEARCH) for the diagnosis of malignant pleural effusions. Ann Am Thorac Soc 10(6):582–589
139. Sieuwerts AM, Mostert B, Bolt-de Vries J, Peeters D, de Jongh FE, Stouthard JM et al (2011) mRNA and microRNA expression profiles in circulating tumor cells and primary tumors of metastatic breast cancer patients. Clin Cancer Res 17:3600–3618

140. Stathopoulou A, Gizi A, Perraki M, Apostolaki S, Malamos N, Mavroudis D et al (2003) Real-time quantification of CK-19 mRNA-positive cells in peripheral blood of breast cancer patients using the lightcycler system. Clin Cancer Res 9:5145–5151
141. Stathopoulou A, Ntoulia M, Perraki M, Apostolaki S, Mavroudis D, Malamos N et al (2006) A highly specific real-time RT-PCR method for the quantitative determination of CK-19 mRNA positive cells in peripheral blood of patients with operable breast cancer. Int J Cancer 119:1654–1659
142. Stathopoulou A, Vlachonikolis I, Mavroudis D, Perraki M, Kouroussis C, Apostolaki S et al (2002) Molecular detection of cytokeratin-19-positive cells in the peripheral blood of patients with operable breast cancer: evaluation of their prognostic significance. J Clin Oncol 20:3404–3412
143. Strati A, Kasimir-Bauer S, Markou A, Parisi C, Lianidou ES (2013) Comparison of three molecular assays for the detection and molecular characterization of circulating tumor cells in breast cancer. Breast Cancer Res 15(2):R20
144. Strijbos MH, Gratama JW, Schmitz PI, Rao C, Onstenk W, Doyle GV et al (2010) Circulating endothelial cells, circulating tumour cells, tissue factor, endothelin-1 and overall survival in prostate cancer patients treated with docetaxel. Eur J Cancer 46:2027–2035
145. Sun W, Huang T, Li G, Shen W, Zhu J, Jin Q, Zhao J, Jia C, Zhang Z (2013) The advantage of circulating tumor cells over serum carcinoembryonic antigen for predicting treatment responses in rectal cancer. Future Oncol 9(10):1489–1500
146. Sun YF, Xu Y, Yang XR, Guo W, Zhang X, Qiu SJ et al (2013) Circulating stem cell-like epithelial cell adhesion molecule-positive tumor cells indicate poor prognosis of hepatocellular carcinoma after curative resection. Hepatology 57:1458–1468
147. Tanaka R, Koyanagi K, Narita N, Kuo C, Hoon DS (2011) Prognostic molecular biomarkers for cutaneous malignant melanoma. J Surg Oncol 104:438–446
148. Thadani-Mulero M, Portella L, Sun S, Sung M, Matov A, Vessella RL, Corey E, Nanus DM, Plymate SR, Giannakakou P (2014) Androgen receptor splice variants determine taxane sensitivity in prostate cancer. Cancer Res 74(8):2270–2282
149. Theodoropoulos PA, Polioudaki H, Agelaki S, Kallergi G, Saridaki Z, Mavroudis D et al (2010) Circulating tumor cells with a putative stem cell phenotype in peripheral blood of patients with breast cancer. Cancer Lett 288:99–106
150. Thorsteinsson M, Jess P (2011) The clinical significance of circulating tumor cells in non-metastatic colorectal cancer–a review. Eur J Surg Oncol 37:459–465
151. Tibbe AG, Miller MC, Terstappen LW (2007) Statistical considerations for enumeration of circulating tumor cells. Cytometry A 71:154–162
152. Tjensvoll K, Nordgard O, Smaaland R (2014) Circulating tumor cells in pancreatic cancer patients: methods of detection and clinical implications. Int J Cancer 134:1–8
153. Tol J, Koopman M, Miller MC, Tibbe A, Cats A, Creemers GJ et al (2010) Circulating tumour cells early predict progression-free and overall survival in advanced colorectal cancer patients treated with chemotherapy and targeted agents. Ann Oncol 21:1006–1012
154. Turner N, Pestrin M, Galardi F, De Luca F, Malorni L, Di Leo A (2014) Can biomarker assessment on circulating tumor cells help direct therapy in metastatic breast cancer? Cancers (Basel) 6(2):684–707
155. Wallwiener M, Hartkopf AD, Baccelli I, Riethdorf S, Schott S, Pantel K et al (2013) The prognostic impact of circulating tumor cells in subtypes of metastatic breast cancer. Breast Cancer Res Treat 137:503–510
156. Xenidis N, Ignatiadis M, Apostolaki S, Perraki M, Kalbakis K, Agelaki S et al (2009) Cytokeratin-19 mRNA-positive circulating tumor cells after adjuvant chemotherapy in patients with early breast cancer. J Clin Oncol 27:2177–2184
157. Xenidis N, Markos V, Apostolaki S, Perraki M, Pallis A, Sfakiotaki G et al (2007) Clinical relevance of circulating CK-19 mRNA-positive cells detected during the adjuvant tamoxifen treatment in patients with early breast cancer. Ann Oncol 18:1623–1631
158. Xenidis N, Perraki M, Kafousi M, Apostolaki S, Bolonaki I, Stathopoulou A et al (2006) Predictive and prognostic value of peripheral blood cytokeratin-19 mRNA-positive cells detected by real-time polymerase chain reaction in nodenegative breast cancer patients. J Clin Oncol 24:3756–3762
159. Yang L, Lang JC, Balasubramanian P, Jatana KR, Schuller D, Agrawal A, Zborowski M, Chalmers JJ (2009) Optimization of an enrichment process for circulating tumor cells from the blood of head and neck cancer patients through depletion of normal cells. Biotechnol Bioeng 102(2):521–534
160. Yen LC, Yeh YS, Chen CW, Wang HM, Tsai HL, Lu CY et al (2009) Detection of KRAS oncogene in peripheral blood as a predictor of the response to cetuximab plus chemotherapy in patients with metastatic colorectal cancer. Clin Cancer Res 15:4508–4513
161. Yokobori T, Iinuma H, Shimamura T, Imoto S, Sugimachi K, Ishii H et al (2013) Plastin3 is a novel marker for circulating tumor cells undergoing the epithelial-mesenchymal transition and is associated with colorectal cancer prognosis. Cancer Res 73:2059–2069

162. Yu M, Bardia A, Wittner BS, Stott SL, Smas ME, Ting DT et al (2013) Circulating breast tumor cells exhibit dynamic changes in epithelial and mesenchymal composition. Science 339:580–584
163. Yu M, Stott S, Toner M, Maheswaran S, Haber DA (2011) Circulating tumor cells: approaches to isolation and characterization. J Cell Biol 192:373–382
164. Zhang L, Riethdorf S, Wu G, Wang T, Yang K, Peng G et al (2012) Meta-analysis of the prognostic value of circulating tumor cells in breast cancer. Clin Cancer Res 18:5701–5710
165. Zhang Y, Li J, Cao L, Xu W, Yin Z (2012) Circulating tumor cells in hepatocellular carcinoma: detection techniques, clinical implications, and future perspectives. Semin Oncol 39(4):449–460
166. Zhu WF, Li J, Yu LC, Wu Y, Tang XP, Hu YM, Chen YC (2014) Prognostic value of EpCAM/MUC1 mRNA-positive cells in non-small cell lung cancer patients. Tumour Biol 35(2):1211–1219

Index

A

Adjuvant chemotherapy, 149–151, 165, 239, 254, 264, 294–296, 303–305, 307, 312, 345–347, 351, 355
Alpha-fetoprotein (AFP), 180, 185
Alpha-fetoprotein-L3 (AFP-L3), 180–182, 184–190
  clinical performance, 187–188
Alpha-fetoprotein isoforms, 185
A-methylacyl-coenzyme racemase (AMACR), 286
Amine precursor uptake and decarboxylation (APUD) tumors, 129, 132, 319
Analysis of body fluids, 48–50
Androgen deprivation therapy (ADT), 320, 349

B

Bax, 298, 299, 302–303
BC200, 271
Bcl-2, 265, 298, 299, 302–303
Biomarkers, 10–12, 15–19, 30, 53–55, 62, 71, 179, 235–236, 252–254
  determination, 49, 53–55
  failures, 19, 20
Bladder cancer, 61, 165–166
Brain cancer, 62
Breast cancer, 62, 64, 198
  follow-up, 206, 211

C

CA15.3, 198–209, 211–216
CA 19-9
  biochemical structure, 247–257
  measurement, 249–252
CA 125, 12, 30, 32–34, 233–240
  clinical use, 229–241
  measurement, 33, 236
  nadir, 237
CA549, 198–201, 212
  epigenetics, 69–70
  glucose metabolism, 116–117
  prognosis, 64, 236–237, 352
  stem cells, 6, 180, 359
Cancer control studies, 15, 19
Carcinoids, 135, 138, 319
Catestatin, 318, 319
CD40, 302, 306
Cerebrospinal fluid (CSF), 11, 48, 49, 68, 129, 130, 132, 139
Cervical cancer, 29, 60, 62, 64, 68, 167
Chemotherapy, 13, 14, 36, 119, 135, 149–151, 163–165, 167, 206, 211, 212, 214, 215, 217, 236, 237, 239, 252, 254, 257, 293–298, 300, 301, 303–307, 309–311, 331, 332, 345, 346, 348, 350, 351, 355
Chip-based microfluidic assay, 186–187
Chromacin, 318
Chromatin, 14, 60, 64, 65, 67, 71, 268
Chromofungin, 318
Chronic hepatitis, 180
Circulating free DNA, 330
Circulating miRNAs, 67, 267–268
Circulating tumor cells (CTC), 4, 21, 216–219, 286–288, 330, 341–359
  detection, 21, 217, 356
Cirrhosis, 30, 31, 66, 180, 181, 183, 188, 189, 234, 250
Cisplatin, 294–301, 303–310
CK-19, 345, 351, 358
Clinical assay development, 16–18
Clinical interferences, 249–251
Clinical outcome, 209
Clinical performance, 188
Clinical response, 13, 17, 215, 303, 304, 309, 348
Clinical uses, 6, 10–15, 17, 71, 103, 104, 162–168, 170, 186, 238, 240, 241, 257, 357
Colorectal cancer, 34–35, 64–65
Core fragment of hCGβ, 166
C-reactive protein (CRP), 306
Criteria for disease screening, 28
CTCs. *See* Circulating tumor cells (CTC)
CYFRA21.1, 200–202, 207, 214
Cytokeratins, structure, 198–200, 202, 206, 218

D

Data normalization, 53
Des-gamma-carboxy prothrombin (DCP), 185
Diagnosis, 15, 28, 61–71
Diagnostic tool, 41–55, 267, 268, 281, 282
  in prostate cancer, 95

R. Scatena (ed.), *Advances in Cancer Biomarkers*, Advances in Experimental Medicine and Biology 867, DOI 10.1007/978-94-017-7215-0

Disseminated tumor cells (DTCs), 217–219, 355
detection, 217–219
DUPAN-2, 255

E
Early detection, 255, 263
Early malignancy, 29, 36
Emmprin, 298–302
EMT. *See* Epitelial-mesenchymal-transition (EMT)
Endometrial cancer, 62
ENO1, 128
ENO2, 128
ENO3, 128
Epidermal growth factor receptor (EGFR) mutations, 330, 350
Epigenetic Inhibitors, 70–71
Epigenetics, 60
Epigenomic biomarkers, 67–69
Epitelial-mesenchymal-transition (EMT), 6, 218, 269, 270, 346, 347, 349, 352
Estrogen receptor, 148, 150, 264–266, 330, 331
Excision repair cross-complementing 1 (ERCC1, 297–299, 302, 304–305)

F
Faecal occult blood testing (FOBT), 29, 30, 34, 35
Feces analysis, 49–50
5a-reductase inhibitor, 285
Follow-up pancreatic cancer, 253, 254, 257
Free PSA (fPSA), 5, 96, 100

G
Gas chromatography, 45
Gastric cancer, 30, 60, 62, 65, 70, 149, 166, 252, 292
Gastrointestinal cancers, 166, 200, 250, 254, 354
GE25, 318
Gene therapy, 287
Genomic instability, 13, 60, 64, 66
Germ cell tumors, 164, 356
Gestational trophoblastic disease, 15, 163
Gestational trophoblastic neoplasia (GTN), 35–36
Gleason score, 67, 98, 101, 103, 281, 284, 348
Glioma, 64, 119, 149
Golgi membrane protein 1 (GOLM1), 286

H
hCGβcf, 166, 167
Head and neck cancers, 62, 65–66, 168, 354–355
HE4. *See* Human epididymis protein 4 (HE4)
Hepatocellular cancer (HCC)
biomarkers, 182, 188, 190
risk factors, 183–187
HER2/neu, 308, 328–330, 332–333
Her2neu/ERBB2, 266
High-performance liquid chromatography (HPLC), 44
Histone, 62, 65, 66, 70
Hook effect, 321
Hormonal therapy, 266, 349
Hormone receptor status, 265
Human chorionic gonadotrophin (hCG)
α-subunit, 161
antibodies specificity, 169–170
β-subunit, 161, 162
biochemical structure, 160–161
biological functions, 161–162
in clinical practice, 162–163
determination, 163, 164, 169
in other non-trophoblastic cancer, 165–168
Human epidermal growth factor receptor 2 (HER-2), 298, 301, 302, 305–307, 346, 358
Human epididymis protein 4 (HE4), 12, 238–239, 241

K
Ki-67, 118, 294, 298–300, 302, 303
Kidney cancer, 48, 49, 62, 66
K-ras, 83, 255

L
Lactate dehydrogenase (LDH), 116
activity in clinical practice, 120–121
biochemistry, 116
in hematological diseases, 120–121
isoenzymes, 117, 118
in lung cancer, 121–122
in melanoma, 121
Lactate dehydrogenase-A (LDH-A), 118
let-7 miRNA, 266
Leukemia and lymphoma, 61–64
Level of evidence, 85, 148, 183
Linearity, 17, 85, 131
Liquid biopsy, 21, 22, 342, 343, 348, 357, 359
Liquid chromatography, 44
Liver cancer, 62, 66
Liver fibrosis, 183
Long non coding RNA, 22, 270–271
Lung cancer, 62, 133, 349

M
Macrophage inhibitory cytokine (MIC-1), 255
Mass spectrometry, 17, 44–47, 50, 52, 131, 239, 297
MCA
Mucin-like carcinoma associated antigen (MCA)
Medullary thyroid carcinomas (MTC), 319, 320
Melanoma, 67, 82, 116, 121, 138, 139, 352, 353
MDR1. *See* Multidrug resistance gene 1 (MDR1)
Membrane-associated mucins (MAMs), 230–232
Metabolite extraction, 47
Metabolites, 43, 45
Metabolomics, 42–43, 47–53
data analysis tools, 52
datasets, 50, 53, 54
technologies, 42, 53
workflow, 47

Metallothionein (MT), 307
Metastasis, 184, 268–270
Methodological interferences, 251
Methylation, 61, 62, 65–68
MicroRNA, 4, 21, 22, 60, 264
MiR-9, 257, 266, 270
MiR-10b, 265, 268
MiR-16, 63, 67, 256, 265, 268
MiR-21, 256, 265, 268, 269
MiR-29, 63, 67, 268
MiR-31, 270
MiR-145, 265, 268
MiR-195, 63, 67, 268
MiR-200 family, 269
MiR-335, 270
MiR-451, 268
MiRNAS and breast cancer, 264–265
Molecular characterization, 20, 342, 343, 346, 347, 353, 359
Molecular forms of PSA, 96–98, 100
MUC16, 231, 233
  biochemical structure, 231
Mucin-like carcinoma associated antigen (MCA), 198–201, 206, 208
Mucins, 198–200, 230–233, 248, 255
  biological functions, 231–233
  and cytokeratins, 197–219
  structure, 230–231
Multiparametric MRI (mpMRI), 107–108
Multidrug resistance gene 1 (MDR1), 63, 297–299, 302, 304–305

N

Neuroblastomas, 319
Neuroendocrine tumors (NETs), 319, 356
Neuron-specific enolase (NSE)
  assays in body fluids, 129–132
  biochemical properties, 126–127
  as biomarker, 125–139
  in brain damage, 137–138
  clinical indications, 132–133, 139
  in gastroenteropancreatic neuroendocrine tumours, 136
  in lung cancer, 133
  mapping and gene function, 127–129
  in melanoma, 138
  in neuroblastoma, 136–137
  in neuroendocrine tumours, 135–136
  in seminoma, 138
Non-small-cell lung cancer (NSCLC), 349
Novel therapeutics, 333
Nuclear magnetic resonance (NMR) spectroscopy, 44–46
Nuclear receptors, 330

O

Oncology personalized medicine, 89
OVA1 algorithm, 239–241
Ovarian cancer, 32–34, 66–67, 235, 236
Ovarian cancer monitoring, 236–237

P

p53, 117, 255, 302, 303, 306, 308–311
PAI-1, 146–152
Pancreastatin, 318
Pancreatic cancer, 44, 61, 63, 67, 150, 151, 238–239, 248, 250–257, 353–354, 357
Parastatin, 318
PCA3, 103, 104, 278–287
  nomogram, 103
Percent free PSA, 100, 281
Performance characteristics, 104, 182, 187–189, 236
Peripheral blood, 358
Pharmacodynamic markers, 13
Phase 1 clinical studies, 85
Phase 2 clinical studies, 84
Phase 3 clinical studies, 83–89
Pheochromocytomas, 319
Plasma analysis, 48
Preclinical exploratory studies, 15–16, 183
Predictive biomarker, 12, 82, 89
Premalignant lesions, 13, 29
Primary metabolites, 43
Progesterone receptors, 12, 150, 265, 266, 330–332
prognostic biomarkers, 12, 48, 189
Prognostic markers, 11, 12
Progression free survival (PFS), 344
ProPSA, 100–101
Prospective screening studies, 18–19
Prostate biopsy, 95, 101, 106, 108, 279, 281, 283
Prostate cancer, 11, 12, 30–33, 63, 67, 94, 95, 98–101, 103–105, 107–108, 150, 166, 235, 278–287, 347–349
Prostate cancer antigen 3 score, 285
Prostate health index, 100–101
Prostate specific antigen (PSA), 5, 12, 30–32, 95–108, 278, 280–286, 348, 349
  Biology, 96
  cut-off value, 106
  derived parameters, 101–103
  assays, 98
  density, 101
  doubling time, 101
  kinetics, 101–103
  physiology, 96
  velocity, 101

Q

Quality control issues, 358–359

R

REG-4, 255
Reproducibility, 17, 35, 42, 48, 85, 131, 181, 187, 239, 329, 358
Retrospective longitudinal repository studies, 15, 18
Risk assessment, 13
Risk of Ovarian Malignancy Algorithm (ROMA), 239–241

S

Saliva analysis, 49
Screening, 12, 14–15, 28–36, 102, 105–106, 235–236, 252–253, 283
  advantages, 28–29
  for cancer, 29–30
  limitation, 28–29
  tests, 34
Secondary metabolites, 43
Secreted mucins, 230
Sensitivity, 99, 134, 181–182, 188, 203, 205–207, 218–219, 234, 251–252
Serpinin, 318
Serum analysis, 48
sialylated Lewis a antigen, 248
Skin cancer, 63
Smac/DIABLO, 298, 302, 307
SPINK1, 286
Statistical analysis
Stratification, 87, 108
Surveillance, 179–183, 189
Survivin, 298–302

T

Testicular germ cell tumors, 164, 165, 356
Tissue NSE expression, 129
Tissue polypeptide antigen (TPA), 199–203, 206–209, 211, 212, 214–216, 298, 301–304
Tissue polypeptide-specific antigen (TPS), 134, 199–202, 207, 209, 212, 214–216
TLX3 gene, 309
Transmembrane-serine protease gene (TMPRSS2), 104, 285–287, 349
  ERG gene fusion, 103, 104
Transcription factor TFAP2α, 306
Translational medicine, 83
Transmembrane-serine protease, 285
Tumor biomarkers, 6, 13, 122, 341–359
Type 1 biomarkers, 328
Type 2 biomarkers, 328

U

uPA/PAI-1
  as biomarkers, 149–151
  in breast cancer, 148–151
uPAR, 146–152
Urine analysis, 49, 279–281
Urokinase-type plasminogen activator (uPA), 146–152
  activity and lymph node involvement, 148
  PAI-1 expression, 148, 149

V

Validation, 15–19
Vasostatin I, 318
Vasostatin II, 318

W

Warburg effect, 7, 42, 116, 117
WE14, 318

MIX
Papier aus verantwortungsvollen Quellen
Paper from responsible sources
FSC® C105338

FSC
www.fsc.org

If you have any concerns about our products,
you can contact us on
ProductSafety@springernature.com

In case Publisher is established outside the EU,
the EU authorized representative is:
Springer Nature Customer Service Center GmbH
Europaplatz 3, 69115 Heidelberg, Germany

Printed by Libri Plureos GmbH
in Hamburg, Germany